Oxford Specialty Training:
Training in Obstetrics &
Gynaecology

DATE DUE

0 2 JUN 2017		
2 7 SEP 2017		
		PRINTED IN U.S.A.

Oxford Specialty Training: Training in Obstetrics & Gynaecology

Edited by

Ippokratis Sarris

Specialist Registrar in Obstetrics & Gynaecology
London Deanery
London

Susan Bewley

Consultant in Obstetrics & Maternal Fetal Medicine
Guy's & St Thomas' NHS Foundation Trust
and
Honorary Senior Lecturer
Kings College London
London

Sangeeta Agnihotri

Consultant Gynaecologist & Obstetrician (Maternal Medicine)
Whipps Cross University Hospital Trust
London

Foreword by

Sabaratnam Arulkumaran

Professor and Head of Obstetrics and Gynaecology
St George's University of London
St Georges Hospital
London

Series Editor

Matthew D Gardiner

Research Fellow in Plastic and Reconstructive Surgery
Kennedy Institute of Rheumatology
Imperial College London

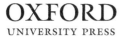

OXFORD
UNIVERSITY PRESS

OXFORD
UNIVERSITY PRESS

Great Clarendon Street, Oxford OX2 6DP

Oxford University Press is a department of the University of Oxford.
It furthers the University's objective of excellence in research, scholarship,
and education by publishing worldwide in

Oxford New York

Auckland Cape Town Dar es Salaam Hong Kong Karachi
Kuala Lumpur Madrid Melbourne Mexico City Nairobi
New Delhi Shanghai Taipei Toronto

With offices in

Argentina Austria Brazil Chile Czech Republic France Greece
Guatemala Hungary Italy Japan Poland Portugal Singapore
South Korea Switzerland Thailand Turkey Ukraine Vietnam

Oxford is a registered trade mark of Oxford University Press
in the UK and in certain other countries

Published in the United States
by Oxford University Press Inc., New York

British Library Cataloguing in Publication Data

Data available

Library of Congress Cataloging in Publication Data

Data available

Typeset by Cepha Imaging Private Ltd, Bangalore, India
Printed in Great Britain
on acid-free paper by
Ashford Colour Press Ltd.

ISBN 978-0-19-921847-9

7 9 10 8

Foreword

There is a need for a concise book for those at a junior level of Obstetrics & Gynaecology which will give them the basic physiology, training in pathology, how women present with conditions, and how one should diagnose and manage them. Training in Obstetrics & Gynaecology gives precisely this information. It covers a wide spectrum of gynaecology and obstetrics in a very succinct manner. The line diagrams, tables, flowcharts, and colour photographs make it easy to understand the condition and its management. The book itself is styled in such a manner that a junior doctor could recognize a condition or equipment when seen for the first time.

The text boxes which indicate the technical skills needed for one to manage the condition are extremely useful. The chapters have clear recommendations to further reading, often RCOG or NICE guidelines. These are quite relevant for any practising clinician as they are evidence-based. Not only is it a useful book for trainees but it will be useful for those who are in advanced training as well as practising clinicians. It is very easy to read and gives the essential knowledge in each topic. I enjoyed reading this book. It gave me a quick revision of obstetrics & gynaecology. It will be useful for medical students because the clear illustrations will help them to understand the subject well.

Not many books deal with topics such as consent, chaperones, and dealing with complaints. This is most welcome because these are taught less in medical schools or postgraduate courses but are essential for junior doctors. The section on risk management is useful as every hospital has risk management procedures, and the junior doctor should understand the detailed process. The book includes ethics and legal issues in obstetrics & gynaecology. One section deals with what to do when things go wrong, when doctors can be exposed if they are not knowledgeable about what to do next. A very good book, not only for juniors in training, but useful for medical students and for those in advanced years of training.

Sabaratnam Arulkumaran
Professor and Head of Obstetrics & Gynaecology
St. George's University of London
St Georges Hospital
London

Oxford Specialty Training Series

The recent upheaval in training and education has left junior doctors much to contend with, including a new career structure, online curricula, and workplace-based assessments. The need for resources that reflect these changes is great. Other books have become outmoded and although the Internet offers access to boundless medical material, little is tailored to the needs of specialty trainees. Fear not, change is coming; the *Oxford Specialty Training Series* has arrived.

The series encompasses core specialty books as well as basic science and revision texts that directly follow their respective Royal College curriculum. *Training in Obstetrics and Gynaecology* exemplifies their compact, but comprehensive style. It has self-contained double-page spreads with a clear layout incorporating high quality illustrations. These features make information easy to access and digest. In addition, the editorial team and contributing authors are drawn from both trainees and senior clinicians to ensure the content is both relevant and of a high standard.

The *Oxford Specialty Training Series* should see you through the first few years of specialty training whether on the ward, in the clinic, or revising for specialty exams. I believe that that regardless of your specialty, *Oxford Specialty Training* gives you the best possible chance of success in your chosen career.

Matthew D. Gardiner

Series Editor

Basic Sciences in Obstetrics and Gynaecology covers core anatomy and physiology relevant to both the practice of obstetrics and gynaecology and the MRCOG.

Visit our website for details of forthcoming self-assessment titles www.oup.com/uk/medicine/ost/

Preface

'Everyone who is born holds dual citizenship, in the kingdom of the well and in the kingdom of the sick'
Susan Sontag, writer (1933–2004)

'Is it a girl or a boy?'—the first and most defining of questions in our lives, asked in those moments of wonder that we, as obstetricians and gynaecologists, are privileged to share. Still, for too many women in the world, biology truly is destiny and can be tragic. International agencies now frame avoidable maternal death as one of the basic human rights. Many of women's gains in modern society rest on control and containment of their obstetric and gynaecological health.

We can be justly proud that so many doctors in O&G have helped and continue to help women; whether by developing contraception, delivering babies, saving mother's lives in childbirth, providing safe termination or sterilization, ameliorating pelvic pain or menstrual loss, enhancing fertility, restoring continence or removing cancers. Even when we cannot make things better, we have a vital caring role when women are hurting or harmed, whether by miscarriage, stillbirth, rape, violence, infertility, infidelity, metastasis or complications of their diseases, or even the treatments.

Our specialty is particularly endowed with a wide ranging scientific basis, plenty of evidence-based medical, surgical, and psychological interventions, a host of sensitive issues relating to identity, and strewn with legal and ethical pitfalls for the unwary. We are enriched by wise and experienced teachers, challenging colleagues, multidisciplinary teammates, and an occasional sense of humour to endure the long nights and hard times.

This book distils current knowledge. The principles of good medical practice do not change though the content and delivery of training do. The restructured curriculum (found at www.rcog.org.uk) clearly states the key topics for each subject and level of training. It outlines clinical, technical, and generic skills that will be needed to progress through O&G training. With the curriculum at its core, this book will provide you with a foundation for the knowledge, skills, and attitudes that will guide your (career-long) learning.

The editorial team consists of a trainee, a new and an established consultant working in different settings. We have tapped into a heady mixture of both the best experts in the UK (including non-O&G) and the fresh, upcoming generation of specialists. Every chapter has been written by a team of training and established practitioners but always with the trainees' needs, curriculum, and goals in mind.

All the editors and contributors love the specialty and we hope to pass on some of that enthusiasm through the pages. Any special insights or wisdom you gain from the book will have come from patients we've attended or teachers who inspired us. Maybe paying attention to the 'tips' will even help you avoid making the mistakes we made.

Whatever motivates you to learn, we hope you enjoy the book and welcome any feedback on how it might be improved in the future.

How to use this book

'There is no short cut, nor 'royal road' to the attainment of medical knowledge'
John Abernethey, surgeon (1764–1831)

There is a simple layout with a double page spread for each key topic and plenty of cross-referencing. Core clinical and technical skills, as well as landmark research papers, have been placed in separate boxes which are clearly labelled. Where definitive evidence-based guidance exists, this is clearly marked (e.g. grade A recommendation, etc.).

We begin with a chapter on the key non-clinical skills and legal and ethical framework you need to be a good doctor. The clinical sections start with the transitions that make women, well… women! This covers women's development and the beginning and end of reproductive life. The book is then divided, roughly chronologically, by chapters on the patient journey that women may take during their reproductive and gynaecological lifetime. These examine sexual health, fertility, early pregnancy, later complications, and the unique diseases of women.

Acknowledgements

We thank Fiona Goodgame at Oxford University Press (OUP) for commissioning us and for all the work, support, and encouragement that so many people (our 'midwives') put into the production and birth whilst we struggled, particularly in the final transition stage! In particular, we should like to thank Matt Gardiner, Tom King, and Tracey Mills, the artists, production and marketing teams, and especially the many anonymous reviewers whose valuable feedback helped raise the quality of the final manuscript.

We are eternally grateful to the contributors particularly for all their hard work. Other doctors who made smaller but vital contributions in terms of advice, literature review, drafting or manuscript commenting were Colin Duncan, Sue Milne, David Gillanders, Meekai To, Ramesh Kuppusamy, Alistair Milne, Ailsa Gebbie and Inez von Rège. Although too many to name, we thank all the secretaries, supporters, and corridor-consultation colleagues who also helped. Whatever faults remain are ours.

The project would not have been possible without the support of our families and friends to whom we owe an enormous debt of gratitude (and time!) … until the next edition.

Ippokratis Sarris

Susan Bewley

Geeta Agnihotri

Contents

Detailed contents

Contributors

Imelda Balchin
Academic Clinical Fellow
UCL Institute for Women's Health
London

Gregory Benchetrit
Senior House Officer in Obstetrics & Gynaecology
London Deanery
London

Maggie Blott
Consultant in Obstetrics & Maternal Medicine
University College London Hospitals NHS Trust
London

Eamonn Breslin
Specialist Registrar in Obstetrics & Gynaecology
North Central London Deanery
London

Peter Brocklehurst
Director, National Perinatal Epidemiology Unit &
Professor of Perinatal Epidemiology, University of Oxford
Oxford

Sarah Creighton
Consultant Gynaecologist
University College London Hospitals NHS Trust
London

Hilary Critchley
Professor of Reproductive Medicine & Consultant Obstetrician and
Gynaecologist
University of Edinburgh and Royal Infirmary
Edinburgh

Melanie Davies
Consultant Obstetrician & Gynaecologist
University College London Hospitals NHS Trust
London

Tim Draycott
Consultant Obstetrician & Gynaecologist
Southmead Hospital
Bristol

Greta Forster
Lead Clinician, Haven Whitechapel & Consultant in
Genitourinary Medicine
Barts & the London NHS Trust
London

Robert Freeman
Consultant Gynaecologist & Obstetrician & Honorary Reader
Peninsula College of Medicine and Dentistry
Derriford Hospital
Plymouth

Gabriella Gray
Specialist Registrar in Obstetrics & Gynaecology
Guy's and St Thomas' NHS Foundation Trust
London

Shelley Haynes
Specialist Registrar in Obstetrics & Gynaecology
London Deanery
London

Kathryn Hillaby
Subspecialty Trainee
Pan-Birmingham Gynaecological Cancer Centre
Birmingham

Tony Hollingworth
Consultant Obstetrician & Gynaecologist
Whipps Cross University Hospital Trust
London

Andrew Horne
Clinical Lecturer in Obstetrics & Gynaecology
University of Edinburgh and Royal Infirmary of Edinburgh

Tracey Johnston
Consultant in Fetal Maternal Medicine
Birmingham Women's Hospital
Birmingham

Jacqueline Maybin
Clinical Research Fellow in Obstetrics & Gynaecology
University of Edinburgh and Royal Infirmary of Edinburgh

Rona McCandlish
Epidemiologist, Maternal Health
National Perinatal Epidemiology Unit, University of Oxford
Oxford

Lina Michala
Clinical Fellow in Paediatric & Adolescent Gynaecology
UCL Institute for Women's Health
London

Tim Mould
Consultant Gynaecological Oncologist
UCLH Gynaecological Cancer Centre
UCL Institute for Women's Health
London

Helen Nicks
Specialist Registrar in Obstetrics & Gynaecology
London Deanery
London

Millicent Nwandison
Specialist Registrar in Obstetrics & Gynaecology
London Deanery
London

Stephen Robson
Professor of Fetal Medicine
Newcastle University
Newcastle

Rehan Salim
Subspeciality Trainee in Reproductive Medicine
UCHL, London Deanery
London

Dimitrios Siassakos
Specialist Registrar in Obstetrics & Gynaecology, South West
Deanery, Severn Institute & Clinical
Fellow in Medical Education, Bristol North Academy, University of
Bristol
Bristol

Ruben Trochez-Martinez
Specialist Registrar in Obstetrics & Gynaecology
and Honorary University Fellow
South West Peninsula Deanery and Peninsula
College of Medicine and Pentistry
Exeter

Symbols and abbreviations

AAA	Arterio-arterial anastomoses		CEA	Carcinoembryonic antigen
ABC	Airway, breathing, circulation		CEMACH	Confidential Enquiry into Maternal and Child Health
ABG	Arterial blood gas		CEMD	Confidential Enquiry into Maternal Death
ACE	Angiotensin-converting enzyme		CESDI	Confidential Enquiry into Stillbirth and Deaths in Infancy
ACTH	Adrenocorticotrophic hormone			
ADE	Anti-epileptic drug		CHD	Congenital heart disease
ADP	Adenosine diphosphate		CI	Confidence interval
AFE	Amniotic fluid embolism		CIN	Cervical intraepithelial neoplasia
AFI	Amniotic fluid index		cm	Centimetres
AFL	Acute fatty liver of pregnancy		CM	Cardiomyopathy
AFP	Alpha fetoprotein		CMV	Cytomegalovirus
AFV	Amniotic fluid volume		CNS	Central nervous system
A & E	Accident & emergency department		CNST	Clinical Negligence Scheme for Trusts
AIDS	Acquired immunodeficiency disorder		CO	Cardiac output
AIS	Adenocarcinoma in situ (cervix)		COCP	Combined oral contraceptive pill
ALS	Advanced life support		CO_2	Carbon dioxide
ALSO	Advanced Life Support in Obstetrics		COS	Controlled ovarian stimulation
ALO	Actinomyces-like organisms		CPD	Cephalopelvic disproportion
ALP	Alkaline phosphatase		CRP	C-reactive protein
ALT	Alanine aminotransferase		CS	Caesarean section
AMH	Anti-Müllerian hormone		CT	Computerized tomography
APGAR	Apgar score		CTG	Cardiotocograph
APH	Antepartum haemorrhage		CTPA	CT pulmonary angiogram
APTT	Activated partial thromboplastin time		CVA	Cerebrovascular accident
ARDS	Acute respiratory distress syndrome		CVP	Central venous pressure
ARM	Artificial rupture of membranes		CVS	Chorionic villus sampling
ART	Assisted reproduction technology		CXR	Chest X-ray
ASB	Asymptomatic bacteriuria		DC	Dichorionic
ASRM	American Society of Reproductive Medicine		DCDA	Dichorionic diamniotic
AST	Aspartate aminotransferase		DES	Diethylstilboestrol
ATFP	Arcus tendineous fascia pelvis		DHT	Dehydroepiandrosterone
AUS	Artificial urinary sphincters		DIC	Disseminated intravascular coagulopathy
AV	Aortic valve		DNA	Deoxyribonucleic acid
AVM	Arteriovenous malformation		DO	Detrusor overactivity
BD	bis die (two times a day)		DSD	Disorder of sex development
BP	Blood pressure		DUB	Dysfunctional uterine bleeding
BFLUTS	Bristol female lower urinary tract symptoms		DV	Domestic violence
BHIVA	British HIV Association		DVT	Deep vein thrombosis
BMD	Bone mineral density		DZ	Dizygotic
BMI	Body mass index		EBV	Epstein–Barr virus
BPM	Beats per minute		EC	Emergency contraception
BSO	Bilateral salpingo-oophorectomy		ECG	Electrocardiogram
BV	Bacterial vaginosis		Echo	Echocardiogram
BV	Blood volume		ECV	External cephalic version
CAH	Congenital adrenal hyperplasia		EDD	Expected date of delivery
CAIS	Complete androgen insensitivity syndrome		EFM	Electronic fetal monitoring
CCF	Congestive cardiac failure			

EFW	Estimated fetal weight
ELISA	Enzyme-linked immunoassay
EMG	Electromyography
ESM	Ejection systolic murmur
EUA	Examination under anaesthesia
FBC	Full blood count
FBS	Fetal blood sampling
FDPs	Fibrin degradation products
Fe	Iron
FEV_1	Forced expiratory volume in 1 second
FFN	Fetal fibronectin
FFP	Fresh frozen plasma
FGM	Female genital mutilation
FGR	Fetal growth restriction
FH	Fetal heart
FHR	Fetal heart rate
FISH	Fluorescent *in situ* hybridization
FM	Fetal movements
FSE	Fetal scalp electrode
FSH	Follicle-stimulating hormone
FT4	Free T4 (thyroxine)
FTA	Fluorescent treponemal antibody test
FTP	Failure to progress
FVS	Fetal varicella syndrome
GA	General anaesthetic
GBS	Group B streptococcus
GFR	Glomerular filtration rate
GGT	Gamma glutamyl transferase
GMC	General Medical Council
GnRH	Gonadotrophin-releasing hormone
GP	General practitioner (family doctor)
G&S	Group and save
GU	Genitourinary
GUM	Genitourinary medicine
h	hour
HAART	Highly active antiretroviral therapy
HAV	Hepatitis A virus
Hb	Haemoglobin
HbA1C	Glycosylated haemoglobin
HBV	Hepatitis B virus
HCG	Beta human chorionic gonadotrophin
HCT	Haematocrit
HCV	Hepatitis C virus
HDN	Haemolytic disease of the newborn
HDU	High dependency unit
HDV	Hepatitis D virus
HELLP	Haemolysis, Elevated liver enzymes, Low platelets
HF	Heart failure
Hg	Mercury
HIV	Human immunodeficiency virus
HMB	Heavy menstrual bleeding
HPA	Health Protection Agency

HPV	Human papilloma virus
HR	Heart rate
HRT	Hormone replacement therapy
HSG	Hysterosalpingogram
HVS	High vaginal swab
HyCoSy	Hysterosalpingo-contrast sonography
IA	Intermittent auscultation
ICS	International Continence Society
ICIQ	International consultation on incontinence questionnaire
ICIQ-SF	International consultation on incontinence questionnaire short form
ICIQ-VS	International consultation on incontinence vaginal symptoms questionnaire
IHD	Ischaemic heart disease
IM	Intramuscular
IMB	Intermenstrual bleeding
INR	International normalized ratio
IOL	Induction of labour
IPPV	Intermittent positive-pressure ventilation
I-QOL	Incontinence quality of life
ISC	Intermittent self-catheterization
ISD	Intrinsic sphincter deficiency
ISI	Incontinence severity index
ITU	Intensive therapy (care) unit
iu	International units
IUCD	Intrauterine contraceptive device
IUD	Intrauterine death
IUI	Intrauterine insemination
IUP	intrauterine pregnancy
IUS	Intrauterine contraceptive system
IV	Intravenous
IVC	Inferior vena cava
IVF	*In vitro* fertilization
IVH	Intraventricular haemorrhage
IVIG	Intravenous immunoglobulin
IVS	Posterior intravaginal slingoplasty
IVU	Intavenous urography
JVP	Jugular venous pressure
K	Potassium
kg	Kilogram
KHQ	King's health questionnaire
l	Litre
LA	Local anaesthetic
LA	Left atrium
LAH	Left atrial hypertrophy
LDA	Low-dose aspirin
LDH	Lactate dehydrogenase
LFT	Liver function test
LH	Luteinizing hormone
LLETZ	Large loop excision of the transformation zone
LMP	Last menstrual period
LMWH	Low molecular weight heparin

LNG	Levonorgestrel
LNG-IUS	Levonorgestrel intrauterine contraceptive system (Mirena)
LOA	Left occipitoanterior
LOP	Left occipitoposterior
LOT	Left occipitotransverse
LSCS	Lower segment caesarean section
LV	Left ventricle
LVEF	Left ventricle ejection fraction
MAP	Mean arterial pressure
MC	Monochorionic
MCDA	Monochorionic diamniotic
MCHC	Mean corpuscular haemoglobin concentration
MCMA	Monochorionic monoamniotic
MCV	Mean corpuscular volume
MDT	Multidisciplinary team
mg	Milligrams
$MgSO_4$	Magnesium sulphate
MI	Myocardial infarction
min	Minute(s)
ml	Millilitres
mm	Millimetres
mmHg	Millimetres of mercury
MOET	Managing Obstetric Emergencies and Trauma
MPA	Medroxyprogesterone acetate
MRI	Magnetic resonance imaging
MRKH	Mayer–Rokitansky–Kuster–Hauser syndrome
MSU	Midstream urine (specimen)
MSV	Mauriceau–Smellie–Veit manoeuvre
MUI	Mixed urinary incontinence
MVP	Maximum vertical pool
MZ	Monozygotic
Na	Sodium
NAATs	Nucleic acid amplification tests
NB	*nota bene* (take note)
NBM	Nil by mouth
NEC	Necrotizing enterocolitis
NET	Norethisterone acetate
NHS	National Health Service
NICE	National Institute of Clinical Excellence
NNT	Number needed to treat
NNU	Neonatal unit
NSAIDS	Non-steroidal anti-inflammatory drugs
NSCSA	National sentinel caesarean section audit
NT	Nuchal translucency
NYHA	New York Heart Association
O_2	Oxygen
OA	Occipitoanterior
OAB	Overactive bladder syndrome
OC	Obstetric cholestasis
OD	*omni die* (once a day)
O/E	On examination
O&G	Obstetrics & gynaecology

OGTT	Oral glucose tolerance test
17-OHP	17-hydroxyprogesterone
OHSS	Ovarian hyperstimulation syndrome
OP	Occipitoposterior
OT	Occipitotransverse
P_{abd}	Abdominal pressure
$PaCO_2$	Partial pressure of CO_2 in arterial blood
PAIS	Partial androgen insensitivity syndrome
PaO_2	Partial pressure of O_2 in arterial blood
PAP	Pulmonary artery pressure
PCA	Patient-controlled anaesthesia
PCB	Postcoital bleeding
PCO	Polycystic ovary
PCOS	Polycystic ovarian syndrome
PCR	Polymerase chain reaction
PCR	Protein:creatinine ratio
P_{det}	Detrusor pressure
PE	Pulmonary embolism
PEP	Pruritic eruption of pregnancy
PEP	Postexposure prophylaxis
PFMT	Pelvic floor muscle training
PG	Prostaglandin
PH	Pulmonary hypertension
PID	Pelvic inflammatory disease
PIH	Pregnancy-induced hypertension
Plts	Platelets
PMB	Postmenopausal bleeding
PMS	Premenstrual syndrome
PO	*Per os* (by mouth)
POF	Premature ovarian failure
POP	Progesterone-only pill
POP	Pelvic organ prolapse
POP-Q	Pelvic organ prolapse quantification system
PPH	Postpartum haemorrhage
PPROM	Preterm prelabour rupture of membranes
PPV	Positive predictive value
PR	*Per rectum* (by rectum)
PR	Pulmonary regurgitation
PROM	Prelabour rupture of membranes
PRN	*pro re nata* (as required)
PSM	Pansystolic murmur
PSTT	Placental site trophoblastic tumour
PT	Prothrombin time
PTB	Preterm birth
PTL	Preterm labour
PV	*Per vaginum* (by vagina)
P_{ves}	Bladder pressure
PVL	Periventricular leukomalacia
PVR	Pulmonary vascular resistance
PVR	Past void residual
QDS	*Quater die sumendum* (four times a day)
QoL	Quality of life
Q_{ura}	Urine flow

RA	Right atrium
RBBB	Right bundle branch block
RCA	Royal College of Anaesthetists
RCM	Royal College of Midwives
RCOG	Royal College of Obstetricians and Gynaecologists
RCPCH	Royal College of Paediatrics and Child Health
RCT	Randomized controlled trial
RDS	Respiratory distress syndrome
Rh	Rhesus
RhD	Rhesus D
RHF	Right heart failure
RHP	Right heart pressure
RIBA	Recombinant immune blot assay
RNA	Ribonucleic acid
ROA	Right occipitoanterior
ROM	Rupture of membranes
ROP	Right occipitoposterior
ROT	Right occipitotranverse
RPR	Rapid plasmin reagin
RR	Relative risk
RV	Right ventricle
RVH	Right ventricular hypertrophy
s	Second(s)
SARC	Sexual assault referral centre
SC	Subcutaneous
SCJ	Squamocolumnar junction
SD	Standard deviation
SFH	Symphyseal–fundal height
SGA	Small-for-gestational age
SHBG	Sex hormone-binding globulin
SIDS	Sudden infant death syndrome
SIRS	Systemic inflammatory response syndrome
SLE	Systemic lupus erythematosus
SPD	Symphysis pubis dysfunction
SROM	Spontaneous rupture of membranes
SSF	Sacrospinous fixation
SSRI	Selective serotonin reuptake inhibitor
STI	Sexually transmitted infections
STV	Short-term variability
SUI	Stress urinary incontinence
SUIQQ	Stress and urge incontinence and quality of life questionnaire
SVR	Systemic vascular resistance
SVT	Supraventricular tachycardia
T4	Thyroxine
TAH	Total abdominal total hysterectomy
TAH & BSO	Total abdominal hysterectomy and bilateral salpingo-oophorectomy
TB	Tuberculosis
TBG	Thyroid-binding globulin

TDS	*ter die sumendun* (three times a day)
TED	Thromboembolic disease
TEDS	Thromboembolic deterrent stockings
TENS	Transcutaneous electrical nerve stimulation
TFT	Thyroid function test
TOP	Termination of pregnancy
TOT	Transobturator tape
TPHA	*Treponema pallidum* haemagglutination test
TSH	Thyroid-stimulating hormone
TT	Thrombin time
TTP-HUS	Thrombotic thrombocytopenic purpura-haemolytic uraemic syndrome
TTTS	Twin-to-twin transfusion syndrome
TV	*Trichomonas vaginalis*
TVS	Transvaginal scan
TVT	Tension-free vaginal tape
TZ	Transformation zone
UAE	Uterine artery embolization
UDCA	Ursodeoxycholic acid
U&E	Urea and electrolytes
UH	Unfractionated heparin
UI	Urinary incontinence
UISS	Urinary incontinence severity score
UKOSS	UK Obstetric Surveillance System
URTI	Upper respiratory tract infection
US	Ultrasound
USI	Urodynamic stress urinary incontinence
USS	Ultrasound scan
UTI	Urinary tract infection
UUI	Urge urinary incontinence
URP	Urethral retro-resistance pressure
UV	Ultraviolet light
VAIN	Vaginal intraepithelial neoplasia
VB	Vaginal birth
VBAC	Vaginal birth after caesarean section
VC	Vena cava
VCU	Video cystourethrography
VDRL	Venereal disease reference laboratory
VE	Vaginal examination
VEGF	Vascular endothelial growth factor
VIN	Vulval intraepithelial neoplasia
V_{infus}	Volume of fluid infused in the bladder
V/Q	Ventilation/perfusion scan
VTE	Venous thromboembolism
VVA	Veno-venous anastomoses
VVS	Vulval vestibulitis syndrome
vWF	Von Willebrand factor
VZV	Varicella zoster virus
VZIG	Varicella zoster immunoglobulin
WCC	White cell count
WHO	World Health Organization

Symbols

⊕   Risk factors and contraindications

◎   Technical and clinical skills

◎   Classification and differential diagnoses

➲   Landmark research

Levels of evidence

Ia	Obtained from meta-analysis of randomized controlled trials
Ib	Obtained from at least one randomized controlled trial
IIa	Obtained from at least one well-designed, controlled, non-randomized study
IIb	Obtained from at least one well-designed, quasi-experimental study
III	Obtained from well-designed, non-experimental descriptive studies
IV	Obtained from expert committee reports or opinions and/or clinical experience of respected authorities

Grades of recommendations

A	At least one randomized controlled trial (Evidence levels Ia, Ib)
B	Availability of well controlled clinical studies, but no randomized clinical trials (Evidence levels IIa, IIb, III)
C	Evidence obtained from expert committee reports or opinions and/or clinical experiences of respected authorities. An absence of directly applicable good quality clinical studies (Evidence level IV)

Adapted from the Royal College of Obstetricians and Gynaecologists Guidelines: Clinical Governance Advice

Chapter 1

Non-clinical professional skills

Contents

Covered elsewhere

- Breaking bad news (see Section 15.1)

1

1.1 Communication with patients and confidentiality

Introduction

Knowledge and surgical skill are paramount to ensuring good clinical practice. However, effectiveness as a doctor is equally dependent on non-technical skills that underpin relationships with patients and colleagues, good standing in the profession, and the ability to cope when things go wrong. Acquisition of these other skills is necessary for all doctors, but many are particularly relevant to O&G owing to the intimate nature of the caseload.

This chapter draws on the GMC document *Good Medical Practice* (2006), discusses underpinning principles, and provides information on how to ensure that you deliver the best possible care to your patients. *Good Medical Practice* demands clinical competence and maintenance of clinical skills from practising doctors. Doctors are required to put the safety and interests of their patients at the heart of their practice. Equal importance is placed on good communication and probity. Guidance relevant to O&G is emphasized.

Communication with patients

The trust that patients place in doctors is a unique privilege. Communication is central to the patient–doctor relationship and is:

- Essential to elicit a precise and complete history
- The basis for making the right diagnosis, which in turn is
- Necessary for prescribing the right treatment and hence ensuring compliance
- Closely dependent on trust
- Especially important in O&G

Our patients' problems are often deeply personal and not easy to talk about, especially in certain cultures. Intimate, sometimes uncomfortable, investigations and procedures are necessary. Few people meet a perfect stranger and tell intimate problems and fears within a few minutes!

Despite scientific and technical advances, doctoring remains a 'people profession'. There is great satisfaction from relieved, happy, and grateful patients with successful outcomes following treatment. Whether by instinct or personality, some doctors are natural communicators. Others develop it by hard work. Good communication is best viewed as a skill to be developed alongside clinical skills. It is learnt by observation, supervision, and practice. Watch senior colleagues known to be good communicators listening and talking to patients. Ask and analyse what to do about your own skills. When the phrase 'poor historian' is used, does it mean the patient or does it really refer to the history-taker? Replace blame with relishing a challenge. Take time at the end of a consultation to consider what did or did not go well. It is hard to be a good doctor, and impossible to be perfect. Professionalism demands we strive to be better tomorrow than yesterday.

Examine where your strengths and weaknesses lie and improve accordingly. Eighty per cent of communication is through body language. It is a performance and takes rehearsal after rehearsal and feedback to get right. Good communication should not increase consultation time; it will make more effective use of it. Good communication requires good listening, concentrating on what the patient says and her demeanour. Remember to support the information you give with written material.

Assessment of communication skills is an important part of postgraduate training. Remember that feedback (good and bad) is necessary to develop. Criticism in this area is hard to accept and may leave trainees dismayed; they may feel misrepresented despite receiving similar comments from several team members. The way we are perceived often differs from the way we imagine ourselves. In order to improve, negative feedback must be assimilated and used constructively.

The seven key communication skills expected

- *The greeting* (it is important to introduce yourself and acknowledge the continuity of your relationship if you have met the patient before)
- *Beginning the interview* (mention the purpose and time available)
- *Eliciting a full account of the patient's problem* (ask clear questions and find out any concerns)
- *Receiving communication* (check what the patient means)
- *Offering a full account of the patient's problems* (have you got them all and have you got them right?)
- *Checking that the patient understood the advice* (ask her to repeat the information)
- *Ending the interview* (sum up and check if the patient wishes to add anything more)

Good habits to get into

- Pay attention to detail, let the patient speak
- Resist the urge to interrupt or control the conversation
- Do not fake attention (or confidence). Illness gives patients acuity—they will find you out and be mistrustful
- Try to avoid interruptions (leave bleeps at the reception if possible)
- Watch for non-verbal communication (patient looking at her partner before answering, eye contact)
- Don't shy away from difficult questions. Ask them directly and plainly, so the patient knows you can handle the answer. This is best done once rapport is established, after you have gained the patient's trust, even though this may mean coming back to the subject later
- Never find fault with the patient (if she presented late, she knows that and may be upset enough)
- Do not take notes (you will appear distracted even if you can listen and write simultaneously)
- Try to replace the concept of a 'difficult patient' with one of 'a patient with difficult problems'

The above principles apply to all specialities.

Obstetrics and gynaecology differs from other specialties

- It is a combination of a medical and surgical specialty with a high psychosocial component
- The caseloads are extremely diverse (which makes our profession exciting). One moment you may deal with a young woman with exceptionally heavy periods and the next you rush a mother to theatre for an emergency CS to save the life of her baby
- The majority of women are fit and well. This changes the dynamics of the relationship and adds a different meaning to patient choice
- There is a second 'patient' in pregnancy. The wellbeing of the baby is extremely important irrespective of the ethical debate regarding moral status (see Section 1.12)
- There is a family unit, primarily in obstetrics, but also in gynaecology, and outcomes have complex effects on the whole family. Partners and relatives have an interest in being involved. The first duty is always to the patient
- There is a strong cultural component to how women, sexuality, menstruation, childbirth and death are regarded. The UK has a complex cultural mix. While it is not possible to be expert on all beliefs and customs, it is important to be aware that they exist and to be sensitive to them

Confidentiality

The obligation of confidentiality is set in civil law and is a GMC requisite for good practice.

Why is it important?

- The promise of confidentiality is central to the doctor–patient relationship. Breaking the promise betrays trust
- Confidential information is privileged, i.e. it would not have been disclosed were there not a prior promise
- The diagnostic and therapeutic process is hindered if patients keep information hidden
- It is in the public interest to maintain confidentiality, as breaking this will diminish the faith of society in the medical profession

A breach of patient confidentiality will result in disclosure of confidential information. Most breaches occur by accident but are no less damaging to the patient and yourself.

Be careful

- Do not leave notes open on the reception desk or the trolley while you go into a room or answer a bleep (see Figure 1.1)
- Ensure your phone conversations cannot be overheard
- Do not discuss patients in public areas (e.g. lifts)

Disclosure

Confidential information may sometimes be needed. In such cases, conflicting interests must be balanced. This is usually done by public consultation or the courts.

Should you find yourself in a dilemma, seek advice from a senior consultant and your defence organization. You must usually warn your patient if you intend to disclose, and give her a chance to do so herself.

HIV-positive women

The UK Department of Health initiated a policy consultation on the confidentiality of HIV and sexual health records because:

- Since 2003 nine people were imprisoned for reckless transmission of HIV
- An underlying principle in the care of people with HIV is the need for a secure and confidential environment in which sensitive issues can be fully discussed
- GMC guidance to doctors on *Serious Communicable Diseases* states: 'you may disclose information to a known sexual contact where you have reason to believe that the patient has not informed that person and cannot be persuaded to do so. In such circumstances you should tell the patient before you make the disclosure'
- Also, 'confidential medical information may be disclosed to other health workers if failure to disclose would put them at serious risk of infection'

In HIV pregnancy the situation differs somewhat because:

- By law the duty of care is to the woman not her partner
- The unborn child has no legal rights
- Women come for care and support and advice on reducing the transmission to the baby
- It is crucial that confidentiality be guaranteed
- Confidentiality helps compliance with medication and fetal surveillance because the woman feels safe
- Women are often dependent on their partners

In practical terms

- The decision to whom and how the diagnosis is disclosed must be made following discussion with the woman, taking care to respect her wishes
- Gaining trust and cooperation is a process, not an event, and there is rarely an urgency to disclose
- Generally genitourinary medicine (GUM) services are more familiar with encouraging disclosure and this should be dealt with by an experienced multidisciplinary team (MDT) and not a junior doctor or midwife
- The HIV diagnosis need not be written in the handheld notes without agreement. Alternatives include codes for health professionals, e.g. 'on antiviral therapy', 'viral illness', 'avoid invasive procedures in labour', and 'see confidential birth plan (sealed envelope)'
- The diagnosis is not automatically disclosed to the GP
- The woman should be strongly encouraged to inform her GP to facilitate follow-up of both mother and baby

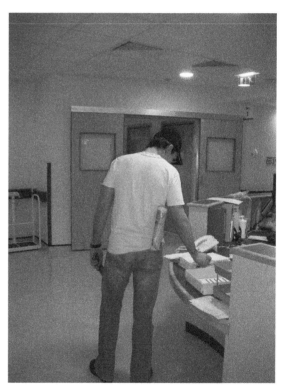

Fig. 1.1 Who can see or overhear? Most breaches of confidentiality are inadvertent. Always ensure that you do not leave notes around.

Further reading

www.bhiva.org for guidelines about management of HIV-positive pregnant women.

www.gmc-uk.org for guidance about confidentiality, disclosures, serious communicable disorders.

1.2 Consent and chaperones

Consent

- Ensures a relationship of confidence and trust between patient and doctor
- Is a legal requirement (English consent law)
- Is only valid if the patient is adequately informed and competent. It must be given voluntarily
- Must be obtained when examining, treating or caring for a competent patient
- Requires competence

To be competent, an individual must be able to understand, in simple language, the nature of the treatment, the associated risks, benefits, and alternatives, including the consequences of not receiving the treatment, and be able to retain the information long enough to make a decision.

Forms of consent

- Implied or verbal for simple examination
- Express verbal consent for intimate examination must be sought and documented in notes (a chaperone should be present irrespective of the doctor's gender)
- There is no legal requirement for written consent (except in mental health and fertility), but the RCOG advises it for all interventions under anaesthesia
- In the case of loss of the consent form, it is easier to defend a claim with a fully informed discussion documented in the notes than with an inadequate form

Who should take consent

- It is the responsibility of the medical professional carrying out the intervention to make sure that valid, informed consent has been obtained
- Consent may be sought on behalf of a colleague if the person consenting is able to carry out the procedure or has been trained to obtain consent

Information given during consent

- Full explanation in simple terms of the condition, its prognosis, likely consequences of no treatment, alternatives, and any diagnostic uncertainties
- Name and details of the procedure, including subsidiary procedures (e.g. catheter, pain relief, thromboprophylaxis), anaesthesia, recovery, hospital stay, impact on daily life and removal, storage, and examination of tissue
- Intended benefits and how the intervention will help
- Serious risks: in O&G these include thromboembolism, return to theatre, inadvertent trauma to the bowel, bladder, ureter, and death
- Frequent risks such as infection, bleeding, bruising, scarring, and adhesions
- Measures taken to minimize and prevent the occurrence of complications
- Other procedures that may become necessary: blood transfusion, biopsy of a mass, oophorectomy, hysterectomy at myomectomy or after CS, proceeding to laparotomy during laparoscopy, and additional surgery to repair any accidental damage
- Anaesthesia and its risks: although the anaesthetist will discuss these with the patient on the day of the intervention, information should be given before
- If the patient is non-English-speaking, all above information must be conveyed via an interpreter, ideally a professional and not a family member or child. This can be supported with visual aids, patient leaflets or video tapes

- Consent should be a two-stage process. The first stage in clinic is provision of information, allowing time for deliberation. Consent is finalized at the second stage, on the day of the procedure, after any additional questions

Unexpected findings at operation

- The scope of the consent should not be exceeded without further discussion with the woman even if this means a second operation
- A potentially viable pregnancy should not be terminated without consent unless this is to save the mother's life
- In an emergency, when consent cannot be obtained, only procedures immediately necessary to save life or avoid significant deterioration of health should be undertaken

Women in labour

- As much information as possible should be given during the antenatal period
- If consent is to be obtained in labour (for vaginal examinations, epidural anaesthesia, operative delivery), this should be done between contractions
- Consent to irreversible procedures, including sterilization, should be deferred, unless fully discussed with a senior clinician during the antenatal period
- Normally, written consent should be obtained for emergency CS. When this is not possible, verbal consent should be witnessed and documented in the notes
- If a competent woman refuses an intervention (including blood transfusion or CS with full understanding of the consequences for herself or the fetus), her wishes have to prevail

Chaperones

- Vaginal examination (VE) is intrusive and intimate
- Before doing a VE, consider whether it is necessary
- Most problems and litigation arise from unnecessary examinations, rather than unchaperoned ones
- If the examination will not alter your management, you may want to refrain
- A chaperone should be available for the gynaecological examination irrespective of the doctor's gender
- The purpose of chaperoning is to reassure, support and assist the woman, assist with any procedures, safeguard against unnecessary discomfort during examination, and incidentally protect the doctor if there are subsequent allegations of misconduct
- Ideally, the chaperone should be a professional, unrelated to the patient, or the parent in case of a minor
- If a chaperone is not available, this should be explained and an alternative appointment offered if required
- If the patient is non-English speaking, an interpreter/patient advocate is needed
- The presence and identity of the chaperone should be recorded in the notes. If declined by the patient, this must be clearly documented too

Further reading

www.gmc-uk.org Seeking patients' consent: the ethical considerations. Maintaining boundaries. Intimate examinations.

www.rcog.org.uk Gynaecological examinations: guidelines for specialist practice.

What is a team?

All aspects of the specialty require team working and are vital to ensure good care. Working well within a multidisciplinary team (MDT) is a quintessential part of being an obstetrician/gynaecologist. Obstetricians, midwives, anaesthetists, paediatricians, haematologists, and a wide variety of other specialists need to work together. In an acute emergency, the obstetrician will lead the team. It helps to understand how teams form and work.

Four stages in the development of a team

- **Forming**: early testing. Members are polite but guarded; they find out about each other's skills and agenda, e.g. first weekend on-call in a new unit
- **Storming**: controlled conflict when roles and goals are agreed, e.g. the same 'difficult' doctor or midwife is on duty. You need to work together
- **Norming**: the team starts to get organized, the roles are established, and issues that affect performance are addressed, e.g. accepting that normal women do not need to be formally reviewed by a doctor
- **Performing**: mature phase. The team works in an effective, flexible, and supportive way, e.g. everyone works together in shoulder dystocia

Effective team members learn to work with people with a variety of skill mix and experience, and will make quick and accurate judgements about their ability. They will learn to listen to opinions that differ from their own and will question some decisions in the interest of patient safety. Personal pride and ego have no place on labour ward.

Strategies to help communication and prevent conflict

- Be respectful and professional
- Listen intently to the other person
- Do not interrupt or second-guess
- Try to understand the other person's viewpoint
- Check by paraphrasing and ask 'is that what you mean?'
- Acknowledge the other person's feelings. This does not necessarily mean agreement, but builds trust and promotes problem-solving
- Be cooperative, assume good faith, make joint decisions
- Look for shared concerns and common ground
- State your feelings and worries
- Avoid accusations and be consistent
- Be open to evaluation and criticism
- Learn to say: 'I was wrong'
- Give yourself time. Do not take it personally
- Remember that conflict resolution is a gradual process
- Start with immediate issues that can be resolved, then take the next step and address the next issue

Handover

Nowhere is teamwork more critical than on labour ward. In the current shift system, teams form and dissolve every 8–12 h, yet with skill the team can be effective and satisfying.

The shift starts and finishes with handover, the key to continuity of care. Ward rounds should be conducted every 6 h, but the ward needs continuous and meticulous assessment and time-keeping.

The good obstetrician is proactive, not reactive, and works alongside midwives to think ahead. Many difficult situations can be foreseen.

The aim is to convey to the oncoming team the information accumulated about the women and the pending problems requiring attention.

It allows the oncoming team to prioritize the cases.

Handover time should be protected, emergencies allowing.

This is a good opportunity for juniors to present cases and develop management skills, so delay non-urgent jobs.

Do:
- Update the board immediately before handover
- Remember to look up results of tests
- Have all members of both teams present at handover
- Handover in a room (area) away from public ears
- Handover extra information gathered during your shift (patients lose trust if they need to repeat themselves)
- Handover antenatal and postnatal cases needing attention
- Ask questions—if management deviated from usual there may be a good reason
- Write down what is said
- Thank your colleagues as you take over
- Be gracious if there are jobs left over—you are fresh

Do not:
- Interrupt the speaker; wait until they have finished
- Go on about very exciting events that took place but have no bearing on the current state—however much you need to share or show off
- Criticize the management—it is neither the time nor the place

The ward round

After handover, there should be a ward round. Go through the board and prioritize:

- High-risk women ('no maternal deaths on my watch')
- Then identify fetal risk ('no stillbirths on my watch')
- Aim to see all patients so you are clear about workload
- Remember low-risk inductions tucked away
- Manage your time efficiently
- Sometimes helpful to discharge low-risk or post-natal women first to help midwifery staffing
- Keep an eye on the clock to be sure you see all high-risk women quickly

If several cases demand immediate attention, delegate tasks.

Delegating

Several patients may need attention at the same time, and tasks must be shared between team members.

Some pointers:
- Know and use your MDT members' skills, e.g. ask a senior midwife advice on social factors or to check a CTG
- Instruct clearly: 'Can you see this woman?' is vague; 'Please check the pulse, BP and blood loss. Establish IV access and take bloods for FBC and G&S' is clear
- Ask for feedback: 'please return in X min to tell me about...'
- At times you will need to ask your seniors for help. Do not hesitate to ask as patient safety is paramount

Other colleagues

The obstetric anaesthetist

- The obstetric anaesthetist is an invaluable member of the team and experienced at assessing women who have collapsed, fitted or have serious medical problems or strict fluid balance regimens

- You must always inform the anaesthetist about seriously ill patients or those who may need to go to theatre
- The urgency of delivery in a CS must be clearly communicated to the anaesthetist. 'Section for fetal distress' is vague. 'Section for cord prolapse. Knife-to-skin by 10.15' is clear and allows the anaesthetist to make the safety judgement about spinal or general anaesthetic. You must be ready and scrubbed, but not exert undue pressure whilst the anaesthetic is being administered
- Try not to 'delegate' cannulation or other chores to the anaesthetist; although they are happy to help with difficult or urgent IV access, ask politely

Communicating with senior colleagues

This is usually the on-call consultant. They inevitably vary in availability and approachability. Remember that patient care is your first priority. If you feel you need help, or even when you are simply uncertain or unhappy, you must ask for it. It is OK to ask for help for difficult clinical, management, communication or even political problems.

- Check who is on call
- See the patient
- Never rely solely on what you were told
- Start the investigations and primary measures necessary
- Have all the facts (and notes) at hand
- Give the consultant a few pointers regarding the patient as they may already be aware of the case
- Be clear about the need for the consultant to come in
- Treat night and day the same—if you'd ask in the day for help with this problem, then ring at night
- Do not leave messages with patient details; say 'please call/bleep ASAP'

Criticism

In day-to-day work, problems arise and bad outcomes, mistakes or errors of judgement occur. From time to time there will be criticism: from within, from patients or colleagues.

- Learn to deal with criticism and the emotions that go with bad outcomes (guilt, denial, and blame)
- Be open—if people have made the effort to talk to you, assume it is because they care
- Take time out and think things through
- If it is a communication failure with a patient or colleague, apologize and talk to them to clarify the issue
- If your management has deviated from normal, look up the guideline or the evidence

- Write a reflective note for yourself and your learning
- It is human to err and wise seniors recognize this
- We cannot go backwards or undo the past
- The aim is not to make the same mistake again
- Distinguish critique (analysis), constructive criticism (how to learn and do better) and destructive criticism (point-scoring)
- Learn the art of respectful feedback: 'private criticism and public praise'
- Avoid the dark arts of put-downs, sarcasm, and undermining
- Report abuses of power

'Not so constructive' criticism

- Do not put up with unclear 'concerns' coming via an intermediary. Find the person who has initiated the criticism and discuss it directly
- You are allowed to acknowledge that you are upset, but maintain a calm, polite, and collected stance
- If you feel the criticism is unfair, check with your educational supervisor or a senior colleague
- Severe, repeated or persistent criticism may amount to bullying and harassment. Take advice from the people above, your trade union or defence organization
- Do not be overwhelmed by the negative. See it as the opportunity to improve

Do not complain about or criticize colleagues or other departments in public. 'The place is going downhill' does not inspire the trust of patients or relatives who are seeking help. There are more professional routes by which to express concerns (see Section 1.6).

Further reading

Griffiths M. Communicating with colleagues. *BMJ Careers* 2005; **331**:110.

Srivastava D. Communicating with the on-call consultant. *BMJ Careers* 2006; **332**:189–90.

www.kingsfund.org,uk Safe births: everybody's business 2008. Most recent enquiry into teams and systematic approach required to maintain safety.

www.popan.org.uk Prevention of professional abuse network (or WITNESS), a UK charity concerned with breaches of trust in professional relationships. They work with organizations to improve public protection and support people whose trust has been broken. WITNESS runs a helpline, support, and advocacy services, provides professional boundaries training, and undertakes research and policy work.

Finding reading material

Some people visit libraries regularly to browse. Others buy books or subscribe to paper journals. The key is to open the packets as they arrive and read some or all of the contents.

Alternatively, to keep up to date continuously with the literature you may choose to have email alerts of contents tables or, for a small price, subscribe to a service which selects and summarizes new papers in O&G. You can then read the summaries (and at least be aware that a paper has just been published) or ask the library for a full text if you want to explore it in depth.

Another way to find papers is to perform a literature search to answer a specific clinical question to inform or change your practice (e.g. for treating a specific patient or contributing to a guideline). Cochrane Reviews, Medline, and RCOG guidelines are good starting points.

Critical appraisal

The following questions need to be considered

- *What is the study about?* The clinical question should be immediately evident and important
- *Was the study original?* Most clinical studies are not. The practical question to ask is 'what does this study add to our knowledge?' This study may be more rigorous in its methodology, bigger or have longer follow-up, or the addition of the data may significantly add to a meta-analysis of previous studies
- *Methodology.* This refers to the type of study performed (recruitment of subjects, inclusion and exclusion criteria, what intervention was studied, how the outcome was measured and whether systematic bias was avoided or minimized)
- *Was the assessment blind?* That is, did the assessor of the outcome know which group the subject belonged to?
- *Were statistical questions correctly dealt with?* Were the conclusions adequate based on the results?

Types of study

- *Randomized control studies*: these are the preferred design for any intervention. As systematic bias is eliminated, the differences found should be attributable to the intervention. It is not always possible (or ethical) to conduct such studies. They also have some disadvantages: monetary and time cost, which may lead to sponsorship from drug industry and influence of the research agenda; patient groups who do not understand or agree with the research will be excluded; failures in randomization or blinding of the assessors
- *Non-randomized controlled trials* will carry bias in selection of subjects and assessors
- *Cohort studies*: in this type of study, two (or more) groups of people are selected on the basis of the differences in exposure to a particular agent and followed up to see how many in each group develop a certain disease. The validity of the study depends on the way the cohorts were chosen. Few studies succeed in choosing perfectly comparable cohorts
- *Case–control studies*: patients with a particular condition are identified and 'matched' to controls without the condition. Data is collected and comparisons made. Both cohort and case–control studies are concerned with aetiology rather than treatment. Again, the critical step is the selection of cases and controls. As long as the characteristics of the selected groups are made available, it is up to the reader to use common sense to decide whether the baseline differences invalidate or weaken the conclusions
- *Cross-sectional surveys*: where a number of subjects are assessed to answer a clinical question

- *Case reports:* can raise awareness of important clinical phenomena

The hierarchy of evidence

1. Systematic reviews and meta-analyses
2. Randomized controlled studies with definitive results
3. Randomized controlled studies with non-definitive results
4. Cohort studies
5. Case–control studies
6. Cross-sectional surveys
7. Case reports

Statistical analysis

Statistical validity of a paper does not start with the analysis of the results and even less with the 'magical' P value, but with the design of the study.

Most of us struggle with the understanding of the calculations and leave these to computer programmes.

A few questions are, however, important (if not picked up by the peer review process before publication).

- Are the groups compared *comparable*? The study should include a table of the baseline characteristics of the groups studied. This should show that either there are no significant differences or the right adjustments have been made
- Is the sample size adequate to power the study? The *power calculation* (chance of detecting a difference) should be undertaken before the study and will be a function of the magnitude of the clinical difference to be measured. If you want to measure a small difference and have a high chance of proving that the effect is due to the intervention, a large number of subjects will be required
- What kind of data were measured? The statistical data are either parametric (they represent distinct numbers from a normal distribution) or non-parametric (look at a rank order without considering the exact differences between ranks)
- Were the data normally distributed? Normal distribution refers to the symmetrical bell shape distribution of most biological phenomena. Non-normal or skewed data can be transformed mathematically (e.g. logarithmically) to give a normal distribution. This is a valid 'manipulation' necessary before applying statistical tests designed for normally distributed data
- Were the correct tests chosen for the data?
- Were the results correctly interpreted?

A few definitions

- **Correlation:** when two or more characteristics are measured on the same people, we want to know whether one is associated with another. Correlation means linear association. It can be positive, negative or non-existent. Positive correlation is when the variables tend to increase together. For two variables this is usually represented in a scatter diagram. If the scatter points lie around an imaginary line, a correlation exists. The magnitude of the correlation is defined by the distance at which the points scatter from the line (not the slope or angle). A coefficient of correlation (the r value) can be calculated and this will have a value and a sign (positive or negative)
- **Regression** refers to a mathematical equation that allows one variable (target) to be predicted from another (the independent variable) if a linear association between variables exists
- **Causation** is not equivalent to either of the above. For causation to be likely there should be a specific, strong, consistent association, biologically and epidemiologically plausible, supported by experimental research (preferably in humans) and dose- and time-dependent effects

- **Probability (or P value):** although considered the cornerstone of statistical significance by many, this simply tells us what are the chances that the observed effect could arise by chance. If the study were repeated 100 times, for a P value of 0.05, a different conclusion would be supported on 5 occasions. The smaller the P value, the less chance that the effect arose by chance. These are, however, cut-off values. Confidence intervals are a better expression of probability
- **Confidence intervals:** a 95% confidence interval tells us that there is a 95% chance that the differences between the observed effects are within two certain limits. The closer the two values, the more exact the study. The higher the value, the more likely that the effect is proven. If the interval crosses zero, the trial may be classified as a negative trial
- **Statistical significance does not equate to clinical significance:** as clinicians, although we must know the numbers, we must also see beyond them. Sometimes we see trends which may not reach statistical significance. On the other hand, tiny but statistically significant differences from huge trials may not be useful in clinical practice
- **Absolute and relative risks are different for individual patients:** common sense must inform us. In clinical practice the numbers translate into real morbidity and mortality rates. Doubling the chance of getting heads when tossing a coin is no longer a gamble. Doubling of a very tiny number, or risk, is still a very tiny number
- **Number needed to treat (or harm):** this is a measure indicating how many patients would require a form of treatment to reduce the expected number of cases of a certain endpoint by one (e.g. the number of CS to prevent one death from vaginal breech delivery). It is defined as the inverse of the absolute risk reduction. It must always specify the comparator, the therapeutic outcome, and the duration of treatment that is necessary to achieve the outcome

Further reading

Greenhalgh et al. How to read a paper. *BMJ* 1997; **315:** weekly from 19 July-20 September. An excellent series of articles.

www.ncbi.nlm.nih.gov National Center for Biotechnology Information with medical literature databases.

www.jameslindlibrary.org A website about the history of fair tests in healthcare.

Definition

Clinical governance underpins care in the NHS; by ensuring high quality responsive systems, the NHS can provide good clinical care. Quality assurance, a way of assessing good practice, is crucial to ensure that the right things get done, while the wrong things cease to happen. From the professional's point of view, care must be effective, efficient, and achievable within the available resources. From the patients' point of view (as individuals and groups), care must be relevant to the need and convenience of the patient and her family, and must be socially acceptable and equitable.

Quality assurance cannot be left to happen in a fragmented manner or on an ad hoc basis. Individual organizations within the NHS must continually look to improve the quality of services and raise standards of care. The NHS must also be accountable to its users for the service it provides.

The framework (a collection of methods and systems) by which this is achieved, reported, and monitored is called clinical governance.

Clinical governance is about:
- Delivering the right care
- In a safe environment
- Using your resources effectively
- Improving clinical skills
- Evaluating and re-evaluating our practice

A clear understanding of clinical governance is important to clinical practice and to becoming a good and safe doctor.

This section concentrates on those aspects which are important for the early years of training: evidence-based medicine, clinical audit, risk management, training, and appraisal.

Evidence-based medicine

This phrase was coined by the McMaster Medical School in Canada in the 1980s.

Definition

Many definitions exist but the one most commonly cited is 'the conscientious, explicit and judicious use of current best evidence in making decisions about the care of individual patients'. In simple terms, this means integrating best external evidence with individual clinical expertise.

- Best evidence: relevant good quality clinical research, especially patient-centred
- Individual clinical expertise: both proficiency and judgement acquired through experience in taking histories, recognizing signs, and making a diagnosis. It includes the thoughtful identification and compassionate use of the patient's beliefs, rights, and preferences in making clinical decisions
- Proficiency and judgement have to coexist. Without clinical experience, the knowledge of evidence may be inapplicable and therefore unsuitable for the particular patient. Without use of best evidence, the experience may be biased, become rapidly out of date and to the detriment of the patient

Evidence-based medicine requires four steps:
- Formulation of a clear clinical question from the patient's problem
- Search of the literature for the relevant clinical articles
- Evaluation (critical appraisal) of the evidence for validity and usefulness
- Implementation of useful findings in clinical practice

Is your practice evidence-based?

Evaluating one's own performance should be the final step in the process described.

You should ask whether you have:
- Identified and prioritized the clinical, psychological, and social problems of your patient from her perspective
- Performed a sufficiently competent and complete examination to establish the likelihood of competing diagnoses
- Considered additional factors
- Where necessary, sought relevant evidence from systematic reviews, guidelines, and clinical trials
- Assessed and taken into account the completeness, strength of the evidence, and its relevance to your patient
- Presented the pros and cons to the patient in a manner she can understand, and incorporated the patient's conditions in the recommendations

The challenge(s)

- Patients rarely have only one clear problem. This is particularly true for chronic conditions (e.g. uterovaginal prolapse), or for complex medical problems in difficult social settings
- Clinical experience is more of an 'art' which cannot be dissected into a set of objective and measurable components
- The greatest challenge will always be to provide 'the right intervention at the right time in the right place to the right patient'

It is impossible to answer such complex questions with the simple methodology of clinical audit. It has been proposed that the question 'is your practice evidence-based?' would be better reformulated as 'how evidence-based is your practice?'

Clinical audit

Definition

Audit is an important component of clinical governance. It is defined as 'the systematic and critical analysis of quality of medical care, including diagnosis, treatment, use of resources and effects on quality of life for the patient'.

- Audit improves patient care. In essence, it asks 'are we doing the right things in the right way?'
- It is a contractual requirement for all doctors in the NHS and one must prove an active involvement for career progress
- It should be open and non-confrontational and, when effective, will lead to implementation of change and improvement

The audit process

Audit is a cyclical process. The components of the cycle are:
- Observing clinical practice (to set the audit theme)
- Setting standards of care, guidelines, and protocols using existing research or evidence
- Monitoring clinical practice against these standards
- Comparing practice to standards and implementing change
- Supporting changes and improvements to patient care as a result
- Re-audit, to see what difference the implemented changes have made to outcomes (closing the loop)

This should be a continual process.

Special audits can, and indeed should, also look at:
- The 'patient journey', i.e. following patients from the time of referral to the time of discharge (e.g. a couple referred by the GP for infertility through clinics, investigation, counselling, and IVF)

- Multidisciplinary care (this may identify flaws in referral, communication between specialties)
- Patient satisfaction

NHS trusts attach great value to such audits and to the doctors who carry them out well

Audit in practice (how to do it)

Design
- What is the purpose of the audit?
- Identify the standards and outcome measures (national and local guidelines, literature search)
- Pilot the audit (i.e. look at a small number of notes and see whether the audit is feasible: are the data available, collectable?)
- Register with the audit office of the institution
- Design a proforma—this is a sheet of paper or computer spreadsheet which contains all the questions you want answered
- Set a deadline

Collect the data
- If your audit is retrospective, you will need the medical notes or information stored on the computer. This is an area where you can and should get help from medical records, the audit office, or IT support.
- If the audit is prospective, make sure you have disseminated the proforma and made your colleagues aware it exists (e.g. ask the clinic clerk to attach it to every set of notes, or intercalate it with the consent forms if you are auditing emergency CS)

Results
- Analyse the data collected
- Draw the conclusions—does the practice measure up to the standards?
- Make recommendations
- Present your audit at a departmental meeting (the audit office can be a great asset in analysing the data, help with statistics and graphs for the presentation). Make sure your presentation is well prepared as this is a time to show your ability

Tips for involvement
- Aim for one quality audit a year, rather than a poor one every 6 months
- In your first year, try to join a senior, or a team of senior trainees who are running an interesting audit. This way, in return for your work, you will learn how it is done well and may even get published. It is also a great opportunity to show a senior (who may be your future consultant) that you are committed and hardworking and to establish contacts

- Do an audit by yourself in the second year. By now you should have an area of interest and have learned the methodology (how to design a proforma, etc.)
- In your third year and onwards, you should be able to conduct an audit enlisting help from your junior colleagues. This will help them and is a simple but valuable opportunity for you to learn to delegate, motivate, and supervise
- A good alternative is to carry out one of the regular departmental audits. This is a programme of rolling audits, many of them in the second or third cycle, some of them required by the Clinical Negligence Scheme for Trusts (CNST)
- Finally, make sure you keep a copy of the audits you conduct. At appraisals and interviews you may be asked to talk about your involvement and how your audit has changed practice in the department. Be honest. Good audits and good answers to these questions will set you apart at the interview

Further reading

Gibbons A, Dhariwal D. Audit for doctors: how to do it. *BMJ* 2003; **327**:51–2.

Greenhalgh T. Is my practice evidence-based? *BMJ* 1996; **313**:957–8.

Sackett DL et al. Evidence based medicine: what it is and what it isn't. *BMJ* 1996; **312**:71–2.

⊙ Box.1.1 The seven pillars of clinical governance

- **Clinical effectiveness**, in which clinicians use an evidence-based approach, benchmark their practice against others, and make use of recent evidence and guidelines
- **Clinical audit**, which aims to evaluate how current practice conforms to the guidelines and what the effect of the practice is on the outcomes
- **Patient and public involvement:** services and care are aimed at patients. Their experience and involvement is essential to improvement, and patient satisfaction is an important measure of outcome
- **Risk management systems** monitor adverse events and aim to prevent them by undertaking risk assessment and learning from adverse events
- **Staff management**, including appropriate organizational culture for the appraisal and development of staff and the handling of poor performance
- **Training**, including continuous professional development
- **Resource management** (funds, equipment, buildings): information (and information systems) to support delivery of healthcare

1.6 Risk management

Definition

The culture and processes that aim to recognize, prevent, and manage adverse effects.

- Healthcare, especially maternity, is susceptible to risk
- There is a recognized need to reduce harm and this should be done in a systematic and consistent way
- In the UK, recent impetus for this approach was provided by the report *An Organization with a Memory*, which emphasized the need to learn from clinical error
- It is aimed at improving patient safety and quality of care
- Risk can result from clinical or non-clinical (administrative, buildings, equipment, transport) errors
- It conforms with the principle of 'first, do no harm…'
- Risk identification—what could go wrong?
- Risk analysis—what would be the impact?
- Risk treatment—what could we do and what would it cost?

Common misconceptions

- *Risk management is primarily about avoiding or mitigating legal claims and financial burdens.* No, but it is true that improving the quality of care should reduce claims
- *Risk management is only about reporting bad incidents.* No, identification of potential adverse effects and their prevention is as important. Sometimes it is easier to learn when there is no bad outcome, just a 'near miss'
- *It is done by, and is important to, managers.* Yes, but it is equally important to clinicians, as enhancing health and reducing risk are our prerogative. This is an area where active clinicians have a decisive say
- *Filling in a risk management form is criticizing someone.* No, in a true 'no-blame' culture, the full facts are established before judgements are made. Human error occurs within a context. Reflective practitioners will want to strengthen safety systems, the training and learning

Risk assessment, failure mode, and effects analysis

Prospective risk identification is an interesting concept borrowed from aviation, which can be applied to healthcare as it is a rigorous risk assessment tool.

- Examine the process in detail and outline each step
- Identify ways in which it could go wrong (failure modes)
- Establish the consequences (effects)
- Identify the possible contributory factors
- Rate each of these in terms of frequency, likelihood, and severity of the consequences
- Identify the existing controls (factors acting to prevent, detect, monitor, mitigate risk)
- Use the ratings to prioritize risk, decide which ones are acceptable and which need treatment
- Devise an action plan

Root cause analysis

Retrospective risk identification (also called the London Protocol) has the following steps:

- Identify the incident and decide to investigate; select members of the team to investigate
- Gather data (clinical records, theatre logs, statements, protocols)
- Determine chronology
- Identify the care delivery problems (e.g. failure to act, incorrect decision, communication)
- Identify the contributory factors (e.g. inadequate training, lack of supervision, unsafe equipment)

- Devise an action plan

Whether we try to 'model' risk prospectively or look back through the events of a reported incident, the concept and steps are similar. Some of the steps are common.

Which incidents to report?

All maternity and gynaecology services have an extensive list of suggested triggers for incident reporting. A special form is available. It is a good habit to familiarize yourself and use it. Put simply, any outcome which deviates from expected should raise the possibility of triggering incident reporting. Online reporting systems such as Datix exist. It is also important to report and learn from 'near-misses'.

Further information is gathered from:

- Complaints and claims
- Staff consultation, clinical audit
- Confidential Enquiries
- RCOG guidelines
- National Patient Safety Agency alerts
- Healthcare Commission

Risk analysis and treatment

Risk analysis assigns a risk score based on the severity of the incident and likelihood of recurrence. The appropriate response will then be devised and will receive priority based on the score. Junior trainees have less involvement in these latter processes, but need to be familiar with two aspects.

No blame

The aim of investigation is not to apportion blame for the incident but to reduce the risk of recurrence.

Investigators are people with extensive experience of clinical work, and should be familiar with the role of human error.

Learning from adverse incidents

There is little point in reporting and investigating incidents if the results are not disseminated accordingly.

Adverse incidents rarely happen because doctors, nurses or midwives are bad.

Often, seemingly small errors added to failures in communication set off a cascade of events leading to catastrophic results.

Feedback to staff is therefore important, and should be done in regular departmental risk meetings.

It is important for all doctors to keep a copy of any serious untoward clinical incident they are involved in and to have a copy of the final report.

Personal reflection is an important way of learning from these incidents.

Organizational requirements

Risk is best managed within a framework (clinical governance) and integrated with audit, training, and complaints handling.

A safety culture is the most important, with strong leadership, teamwork, and communication both within the team and with the patients. This has been addressed in the document *Towards safer childbirth*, which describes organizational standards of quality and safety in maternity and gynaecology.

Each department should have a written risk management strategy and a designated lead. The team should include a lead (senior) clinician, a trainee doctor, a nurse/midwife, a neonatologist, and the unit manager. The team should be responsible for linking the risk management in the unit with hospital or nationwide strategies.

Risk management can be applied at all levels:

- Senior management will be concerned with general strategies (such as provision of care in rapid access clinics, wards, theatres, histology to ensure adequate access to services in case of suspected gynaecological cancer)
- A team of managers and clinicians may trace the patient's journey through various systems, e.g. from the GP referral, via rapid access clinic, to hospital (surgery, adjuvant therapy) and back to GP care with adequate follow-up
- Individual clinicians will look at the risks involved with the operations, e.g. planning procedures jointly with bowel surgeons
- All staff, from porters and secretaries to consultants and professors, should be able to point out faults and flaws in systems, unhelpful or dangerous behaviours, errors and bad outcomes, and have their constructive ideas for improvements heeded

There are two further aspects of national relevance of which all obstetrician–gynaecologists must be aware:

- Clinical Negligence Scheme for Trusts (CNST)—a system of set standards to prevent and reduce clinical risk and litigation in all acute care
- The Confidential Enquiry into Maternal Deaths (CEMD), a national 'audit' investigating the causes with a view to collective learning from the most serious outcomes

Clinical Negligence Scheme for Trusts

Administered by the NHS Litigation Authority, CNST provides an indemnity to members and their employees in respect to clinical negligence events that occurred after April 1995. It is funded by contributions paid by member trusts and provides means for the NHS trusts to fund the cost of medical negligence litigation. The aim is to minimize the overall cost to the NHS and thus maximize the resources available for patient care by defending unjustified actions robustly and settling justified actions efficiently.

CNST has set safety standards for each area of care. There are standards specific to maternity (see below). Each trust will pay a set amount of monetary contributions into the Scheme. However, a discount is available based on attainment of the standards:

- Compliance at level 1   10%
- Compliance at level 2   20%
- Compliance at level 3   30%

An assessment is made by a body of assessors every 2 years for level 1 and every 3 years for levels 2 and 3.

The CNST Maternity Standards fall into eight areas:

- Standard 1: *organization*—meaning clearly defined local arrangements and accountability for implementing clinical risk management. This will include the existence of a written maternity services risk management strategy, a nominated lead professional for clinical risk management, clear lines of communication and accountability, a lead consultant, and midwifery manager for labour ward
- Standard 2: *learning from experience*—i.e. the maternity services proactively use internal and external information to improve clinical care. In practical terms, this relates to the reporting of adverse incidents and near misses, review of summarized incident reports, applications of recommendation from national Confidential Enquiries, and evidence of lessons learned from incidents, i.e. implemented changes
- Standard 3: *communication*—refers to the expectations that women are informed by competent professionals of all aspects

and options concerning their treatment and care, and there are clearly documented systems for management and communication between professional staff. This includes the existence of a clearly identified lead professional for each woman, an agreed mechanism of referral to a consultant, personal handover on labour ward, monitoring of decision-to-delivery interval for emergency CS, and early referral system for fetal anomalies
- Standard 4: *clinical care*—refers to the existence of clear guidelines. These have to be evidence-based, referenced, multidisciplinary care pathways for the key conditions (and include fetal monitoring, high dependency, general anaesthetic, stillbirth) and a systematic approach to audit
- Standard 5: *management systems*—to ensure the competence and training of all staff. This includes attendance at induction training, CTG training, 'skills and drills' for major obstetric emergencies, resuscitation
- Standard 6: *a comprehensive system of record-keeping and auditing record-keeping*—this will include secure storage of CTGs, legible, signed, chronological record-keeping and evidence of improvement of the record-keeping by audit at least every 12 months
- Standard 7: *a clinical risk management system is in place and operational*—this has to start with risk assessment and continue with evidence of progression and achievement of action points
- Standard 8: *staffing levels*—it is necessary to have clear arrangements for the statutory supervision of midwives, dedicated obstetric anaesthetic services in all consultant units, sufficient medical leadership and experience to provide a reasonable standard of care

The role of the trainee
Make sure you:
- Report incidents promptly
- Take part in clinical risk meetings
- Know the guidelines
- Participate in clinical audit
- Have a high standard of record-keeping
- Are up to date with 'skills and drills' training
- Produce statements promptly

CNST understands that the role of the clinician is crucial when investigating a negligence claim. The panel of solicitors need to know what would happen at a trial to work out the chances of success.

They need to know:
- The facts (what you did)
- The reasoning behind the decisions you made
- What the notes say

Most claims are settled out of court, but when investigated, the most important aspects of your care will be scrutinized. The two most important aspects are contemporaneous record-keeping and compliance with guidelines.

Further reading
www.dh.gov.uk An organization with a memory. June 2000.

www.kingsfund.org,uk Safe births: everybody's business 2008. Most recent enquiry into teams and systematic approach required to maintain safety.

www.rcog.org.uk Improving patient safety: risk management for maternity and gynaecology.

Analysis of serious untoward clinical incidents enables clinicians to determine whether these occurred despite good clinical care or whether there was an element of substandard care. Investigation and in-depth analysis identifies at what level and why systems fail, and comparison of similar incidents identifies common themes from which national recommendations can be made to reduce similar events occurring in the future. Clinical audit is an essential part of everyday practice. Collection of outcomes and comparison of these outcomes against predetermined standards facilitates good clinical care.

The Confidential Enquries into Maternal Deaths (CEMD) and Stillbirths and Deaths in Infancy (CESDI) are essential reading for every obstetrician and gynaecologist. The Confidential Enquiry into Maternal and Child Health (CEMACH) is the national body that now facilitates this process.

Background

In 1952, the system of local reporting of maternal deaths was replaced by a superior national system, the CEMD, with anonymity encouraging full analysis and reflection on what could be improved. A report generated from information provided by this enhanced system is published every 3 years and allows for dissemination of the findings and recommendations with the aim of reducing or containing maternal mortality by improving practice. The Enquiry examines all maternal deaths and identifies common themes. A working knowledge of this document is a crucial part of working as an obstetrician or gynaecologist. The reports are thought to have had an important role in reducing maternal deaths in the UK. This is the longest running professional self-evaluation in the world.

CEMACH is commissioned by NICE, but is an independent body with its own board, comprising obstetricians, gynaecologists, midwives, anaesthetists, pathologists, psychiatrists, and paediatricians. *Why Mothers Die* (2004) has been renamed *Saving Women's Lives* (2007).

Methodology

The Enquiry is an observational and self-reflective study. It is not a classical audit, has no disease denominators, and little statistical power. However, it represents the 'tip of the iceberg' of bad outcomes and contains many relevant, valuable lessons for practice.

Definitions

- **Maternal death**: death of a woman while pregnant, or within 42 days from its end, from causes related to or aggravated by pregnancy
- **Direct maternal death:** death resulting from obstetric complications
- **Indirect maternal death:** death resulting from previous disease, or disease developed in pregnancy, but not caused by direct obstetric causes
- **Late maternal death**: death resulting from any of the above causes from 42 days to 1 year after the end of pregnancy
- **Coincidental maternal death:** resulting from unrelated causes in pregnancy and puerperium
- **Pregnancy-related deaths** are deaths resulting from any cause while pregnant or within 42 days from the end of pregnancy

The objectives of the report include:

- Assessment of the main causes of maternal death
- Identification of any avoidable factors
- Production of a report to disseminate the findings
- Recommendations to improve clinical care
- Suggestions for future areas for research and audit

The Enquiry has an important *local* role in supporting clinical governance. Trusts must:

- Ensure that maternal deaths are subject to local review and critical incident reporting
- Develop or regularly update multidisciplinary guidelines for the management of complications during pregnancy
- Review and modify, where necessary, the existing provision of maternity care
- Promote local audit and clinical governance

At *national* level the Enquiry

- Helps inform government policy
- Informs guideline development by the relevant colleges (RCOG, RCM, RCA, RCPCH)
- Sets minimum standards of care
- Informs the postgraduate training syllabus

The report is highly regarded *internationally* for its thoroughness. Most countries only use death certificate data and live births as the denominator to obtain an official maternal mortality rate. Doing this in the UK would halve the true rate.

Each major cause of death has a dedicated chapter with:

- Summary of key recommendations
- A historical review of the cause in previous reports and changes made since
- A summary of the cases for the triennium, with in-depth analysis of the causes, risk and contributory factors, and standards of care
- Vignettes or stories that illuminate the reader
- Learning points
- Guidelines relevant to the field with specific recommendations and assessment tools

Confidential Enquiry findings 2003–2005

There were 295 deaths and 2 114 004 maternities.

The combined overall mortality rate (see Figure 1.2) was 14 deaths/ 100 000 maternities (13.1 and 11.4 for the two previous triennia).

The rise may be caused by a variety of factors such as increasing age and obesity, better reporting, increasing numbers of new migrants, chance, or an increase in the number of women receiving substandard care.

Mortality rates and main causes of death

- The maternal mortality rate for both indirect and direct deaths increased, although this increase was not statistically significant
- The overall rate of indirect deaths is higher than that of direct deaths although the gap is decreasing
- The most common cause of direct deaths continues to be thromboembolism, followed by amniotic fluid embolism which has risen inexplicably
- There were non-significant increases in mortality rates from thromboembolism, pre-eclampsia/eclampsia and genital tract sepsis, and apparent slight declines in rates of death from haemorrhage and direct uterine trauma
- Cardiac disease was the most common cause of indirect deaths, as well as maternal deaths overall, overtaking psychiatric (which rose owing to improved ascertainment)
- At least 360 existing children and 160 live newborns lost their mother to a direct or indirect maternal death. Of these, a third were already in care

Risk factors for maternal deaths 2003–2005

- **Social disadvantage:** one-third of all women who died were either single and unemployed or in a relationship where both partners were unemployed. Women with partners who were unemployed, many of whom had features of social exclusion, were up to seven times more likely to die
- **Poor communities:** women living in the most deprived areas were five times more likely to die than women from the most affluent areas
- **Late booking and poor attendance:** 17% of women who died from direct or indirect causes booked after 22 weeks or missed >4 appointments
- **Minority ethnic groups:** black African women, including asylum seekers and newly arrived refugees, have a six times greater mortality than white women. Black Caribbean and Middle Eastern women also had a lesser but significantly higher rate than white women
- **Obesity:** more than half of all women who died were obese, and 15% were morbidly obese
- **Domestic violence:** 14% of the women who died self-declared that they were subject to violence in the home
- **Child protection:** 10% lived in families known to child protection services
- **Substance abuse:** 11% of the women had problems with substance misuse (of whom 60% were registered addicts)
- **Substandard care** was identified in 64% and 40% of direct and indirect deaths, respectively. A number of healthcare professionals failed to identify and manage common medical conditions or potential emergencies outside their immediate area of expertise. Resuscitation skills were also considered poor in some cases
- **Lack of cross-disciplinary or cross-agency working or communication:** this included poor or non-existent team working, poor interpersonal skills, inappropriate or too short consultations by phone, the lack of sharing of relevant information between health professionals, including between GPs and the maternity team. The lack of sharing of significant information regarding a risk of self-harm and child safety between health and social services was particularly noted.

Recommendations for local maternity services 2003–2005

- Maternity services should be approachable and flexible
- Asylum seekers and refugees are particularly vulnerable
- Women should be educated on the importance of seeking antenatal care early
- Professional interpreters should be used for women who do not speak English (not family members)
- Coordinated multidisciplinary and multi-agency care should be available for women with complex problems, bearing in mind that one midwife should stay closely in contact to support the woman
- Women at risk of developing clinical problems should not be delivered in isolated units
- Dedicated obstetric anaesthesia should be available in all consultant obstetric units

Top 10 recommendations 2003–2005

Many lessons from previous reports were repeated (see above), but specific auditable recommendations were made.

1) *Pre-conception counselling*, both opportunistic and planned, should be provided for women with pre-existing serious medical or mental health conditions which may be aggravated by pregnancy. This includes obesity and especially prior to fertility treatment

2) Services should be *accessible* and welcoming. The booking visit and hand-held record should be completed by 12 weeks

3) Women should be seen *within 2 weeks* if >12 weeks

4) *Migrants* from poor countries who have not had a full medical examination in the UK should have one, including cardiovascular examination. Ask sensitively about female genital mutilation (FGM)

5) Women with systolic BP >160 mmHg require *antihypertensive treatment*. Consider initiating treatment at lower BP if rapid deterioration or severe hypertension anticipated

6) *Caesarean:* although CS is sometimes safer, mothers must be advised that CS is not a risk-free procedure and can cause problems in current and future pregnancies. Women with previous CS must have placental localization to exclude placenta praevia. If present, try to identify accreta and the development of safe management strategies

7) To optimize clinical skills, providers must ensure that all *clinical staff learn from any critical events* and serious untoward incidents and document this

8) Clinical staff must undertake regular, written, documented and audited *training*

9) Routine use of a national *obstetric early warning* chart will help in the timely recognition, treatment, and referral of women who have, or are developing, a critical illness (in O&G, emergency, and critical care settings)

10) Guidelines for the management of obesity, sepsis, and early pregnancy pain and bleeding

Further reading

The full report is available at www.cemach.org or as hard copy from the RCOG bookshop.

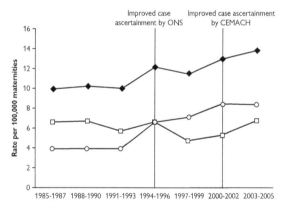

Fig. 1.2 Maternal mortality rates per 100 000 maternities and the dates of improved systems for case ascertainment, United Kingdom 1985–2005. ONS, Office for National Statistics. (Reproduced from Gwyneth Lewis, Summary and overall findings, p. 5, 2007, with the permission of the Confidential Enquiry into Maternal and Child Health.)

Introduction

One of the most challenging aspects of a doctor's work is dealing with loss and breaking bad news. Although some themes are similar for breaking bad news, e.g. in palliative care and in oncology (see Section 15.1), this topic has been written focusing around fetal loss. Maternal death and death of non-pregnant women in the gynaecology setting is fortunately a very rare event and it will be dealt with by the most senior doctors. Junior doctors in their first years of training will be involved with bereaved parents. Routine postgraduate training in bereavement work is often poor. Patients and staff alike do not want additional people present at these very difficult consultations. However, to gain the necessary training it is important to be present. Junior doctors should accompany the consultant, listen to the discussion, observe, and learn. Remember to get senior help and support. There should never be an expectation that trainees manage these complex situations alone.

Expectations are such that most parents anticipate falling pregnant easily, are unaware of the risks of early loss, and expect the safe delivery of a healthy baby. The unanticipated death of an eagerly awaited infant *in utero* or around the time of birth is very traumatic. The care parents receive will influence how they are able to both cope with and come to terms with the experience.

A few general principles refer to understanding grief and how to conduct yourself around parents who have experienced recent loss. Royal College guidelines ask that doctors treat fetal loss at any gestation in the same way. Although medical issues may differ, it should be treated with the same compassion at any gestation. Care given to the woman and her family has a major impact on her recovery.

The mother (or both parents) experiences a range of powerful feelings and is entitled to expect her carers to be able to cope with these emotions. The natural progression of grief and mourning involves four stages:

- **Denial:** sense of shock and disbelief, patients often question the reality and wish time could be reversed
- **Pain and distress**: they may be confused by medical information and anticipatory information (what may follow) at this time. They may be hurt, angry, trying to find someone to blame, guilty, or fearful that losing the baby may be equated to having done something bad
- **Realization:** this is the beginning of realization of loss, and may be associated with depression and apathy, tearfulness, and exhaustion
- **Acceptance:** readiness to accept loss and move on to new activities, including contemplation of further pregnancy

Early pregnancy loss
(see Section 5.6)

Often, women will see the most junior doctor on arrival. The trainee needs to respond on two levels: medical and emotional. If the bleeding is heavy and/or the pain severe, one may feel rushed to resolve the physical problem. There are also the time constraints in A&E where one may have several similar cases waiting.

- There is a need for explanation both of the diagnosis and the interventions that may be needed
- Be clear without being blunt (even in an emergency). There are many aspects in the way a doctor communicates. Body language (sit down next to woman, do not appear to be in a hurry), tone of voice, an introductory phrase ('I'm afraid it's bad news', 'I am very sorry...' rather than 'we need to take you to theatre')
- Do not minimize the loss ('There is no baby really' or 'It was just a blood clot' are not helpful comments)

- Offer emotional help even if only in the form of a leaflet or support group's website

Stillbirth
(see Section 8.30)

The events during the 'crucial hours' preceding and following the death of the baby have been identified as most significant for the emotional outcome for women. This puts the responsibility for women's mental wellbeing with the obstetric team.

It is not high-technology expert attention, but gentle, considerate care that is expected. Most units have midwives who specialize, or have a special interest, in bereavement and fetal loss. They have great experience and training and most likely time to dedicate. Midwives will provide the parents with mementos, will involve other professionals and religious representatives. As in all other aspects of labour care, midwives and doctors bring complementary skills.

When seeing recently bereaved parents

- Allow parents time before you see them. Let them settle in the room, recover from shock or anaesthetic and formulate questions in their minds (take guidance from the midwife as to when to review them)
- Be prepared—read the notes in advance and know the facts
- Change into clean scrubs or preferably normal clothes (blood on clothes or shoes after a traumatic delivery is frightening and not appropriate)
- Leave your bleep outside
- Ask the midwife caring for the mother to accompany you. When you first walk into the room she will introduce you, which will make it easier for the parents to accept your presence
- Sit down next to the mother (don't stand above her), offer your condolences, say something simple such as 'I am very sorry for your loss'
- Try to make eye contact or, if it feels appropriate, gently touch her shoulder or hold her hand
- Be comfortable with tears and long silences
- Offer a simple account, in small increments, with openness to answer further questions at any time
- Do not be afraid to give a bleep number or secretary's extension. Patients will rarely contact you but will appreciate availability

Regarding labour and delivery

- Allow the woman as much choice as possible in method of induction and delivery (some limitations on the medications used refer to live fetuses and may be exceeded in the case of the fetal demise)
- Make sure you respond promptly to any concern regarding medical problems (bleeding, pyrexia)
- Ensure that adequate pain relief is available and working efficiently (involve the anaesthetist early)
- Be considerate in handling the baby if you are delivering (instrumental delivery may be necessary and shoulder dystocia may be encountered)

Medical care

Perinatal death can be associated with significant maternal morbidity. The mother may have undergone a major operation or be in a critical condition. Both maternal health and emotional support are important considerations.

The partner will often be very frightened and anxious. This may be expressed as aggression. Never respond with aggressive comments. Remember he too has just lost his baby and his partner is ill. Take time to support and reassure him, keep him abreast of developments and try to ensure he has someone with him.

Cultural and religious issues

- Make use of support services. Most hospitals will have patients' advocates, volunteers, chaplains, and other religious representatives. Take care not to make assumptions. It is better to ask parents to determine their preferences.

Termination of pregnancy

(see Section 5.9)

Termination requires a special mention as a bereavement. This is a complex issue. The legal right for women to choose not to continue with pregnancy was hard won. There is a wide range of firmly held beliefs amongst women and professionals alike whether abortion is morally right or wrong. Doctors choosing gynaecology and obstetrics have to think about it continually. Women do not make decisions to terminate a pregnancy lightly and are entitled to grieve. There needs to be an understanding of the difficult circumstances in which women find themselves. The decision includes several dimensions: reason for being pregnant, making the decision, the pressure of time, the procedure, and the aftermath with (usually) lack of follow-up care. Doctors and nurses may conscientiously object to being directly involved in the termination. They have a right to be supported by their colleagues in this, but still have a duty of care to women (see Section 1.12).

How to cope on a personal level

Look again at the four stages of grief described above, as these refer to the doctor as well when things go wrong, and the hoped-for good outcomes are lost.

While your experience does not in any way compare to that of the patient, you may experience a similar succession of emotions and a sense of loss. Support is mostly informal and not always readily available.

- **Talk to your immediate colleagues:** this is not easy. If you heard of a colleague who was involved in a stillbirth, pick up the phone, seek out your colleague, and offer them to talk through the events. You can offer to hold the bleep for a short time to allow them a break. Ask, 'Are you ok?'
- **Seek help from your seniors:** it would be expected of your consultant to offer a debrief and support, but this may not be always the case. Find someone with whom you feel comfortable. As you progress through your career you may have identified a consultant with whom you worked in the past who has now become a mentor or a senior colleague
- **Seek confidential counselling:** your GP, occupational health or hospital counsellors may be available and very helpful
- **Take time off:** you may feel you need a break. Do not regard this as a sign of weakness: on the contrary, you have a duty to yourself and your patients. If you feel overwhelmed, it is in everybody's best interest that you take rest. A complete break from work is only helpful if it is short. If you require extended time, a 'phased return' (when you return for certain duties, or indirectly supervised at first) may be more appropriate.

1.9 Domestic violence

Definition

Threatening behaviour, violence or abuse (psychological, physical, sexual, financial, or emotional) between adults who are or have been intimate partners or family members, regardless of gender or sexuality.

Domestic violence (DV) includes forced marriage, female genital mutilation, and 'honour crimes'.

A highlighted issue

DV has moved in 30 years from an unspoken topic to a recognized serious crime that government, statutory bodies, and voluntary organizations tackle together.

The first safe house for women and children opened in 1971. In 2003–2004, Women's Aid estimate 18 600 women and 23 000 children were accommodated and supported by 400 refuges in the UK.

Demographics

DV is an important issue because:

- It affects one in four women at some point in their lives
- 88% of victims are female
- DV can affect men and same-sex relationships
- It can be perpetrated by extended family members
- It is an increasing problem for teenagers
- It often starts or worsens in pregnancy
- DV accounts for 16% of all violent crime (over one in four actual and one in eight grievous bodily harm reports)
- DV has more repeat victims than any other crime
- Victims are assaulted 35 times before involving the police
- DV can escalate to murder and be a factor in suicide
- Annually, DV costs the UK economy £23 billion
- Over 100 women and 30 men are killed per year
- In the 2003–2005 Confidential Enquiry (CEMACH) 19 women were murdered by their partner during pregnancy or shortly after delivery
- Of ~500 000 DV-related calls to the police, ~7000 result in a prosecution
- One hundred and ten thousand DV incidents were reported to the Metropolitan Police in 2005
- Worldwide, DV is the largest cause of morbidity in women aged 19–44, more than war, cancer or road traffic accidents
- DV is a factor in the lives of many of our patients and colleagues
- DV affects the presentation and management of patients, so awareness may improve clinical care
- Witnessing and advice may be the start of social change

Patterns

DV can occur at any stage of a relationship. It is rarely a one-off, with a pattern of abusive and controlling behaviour where the abuser seeks power over the victim. In one study, the first incident of DV occurred after 1 year in 51%, between 3 months and 1 year in 30%, between 1 and 3 months for 13%, and less than 1 month for 6%.

In a group of pregnant women attending primary care in East London, 15% reported DV during their pregnancy. In 40% of them the violence had started during their pregnancy.

Indicators of possible DV in pregnancy

- Late booking
- Poor or non-attendance at antenatal clinics
- Repeat attendance at antenatal clinics, GP's surgery or A&E departments for minor injuries or 'vague/non-existent' complaints
- Repeat presentation with depression, anxiety, self-harm, and psychosomatic symptoms
- Minimalization of signs of violence on the body
- Recurrent sexually transmitted infections
- Unexplained admissions
- Non-compliance with treatment regimes
- Early self-discharge from hospital against advice
- Constant presence of the partner, who may answer questions on behalf of the woman and refuse to leave, but equally may be very charming
- The woman appears evasive or reluctant to speak or disagree in front of her partner

Effects of domestic violence

Effects on victim

DV has a wide variety of manifestations and presentations, ranging from non-specific symptoms and signs, e.g. insomnia and anxiety, to more specific presentations due to acts of violence against women, e.g. injury to the breasts. Depression, drug and alcohol misuse, and other mental health problems are also associated with, and may be exacerbated by, DV.

Effects on children

Children who have experienced, witnessed or lived with DV are at risk. They are more likely to suffer poverty, homelessness, and detrimental effects on short-term welfare and long-term life chances. Children witness about 75% of abusive incidents where there is DV. Young children may become anxious, complain of abdominal pain or start bed-wetting. They may find it difficult to sleep. Older boys tend to express distress outwardly and can become aggressive and disobedient. They may themselves use violence to try to solve problems. Girls are more likely to internalize their distress, becoming withdrawn. They may complain of vague symptoms, and are more likely to self-harm or develop eating disorders.

Routine enquiry and disclosure

Asking the question

Asking about DV uncovers hidden issues, changes the perceived acceptability of violence in a relationship, makes it easier for the woman to disclose, changes the health professional's knowledge and attitude towards DV, and reduces social stigma. Routine questioning has a high level of acceptability.

- Only 50% will tell voluntarily, most likely to the police
- Women may present with injuries to A&E or their GP. Female victims of DV are three times more likely to access emergency medical services
- Victims may have suspicious bruises/scars on examination
- Enquiries about relationships and DV should be more routine as part of the social history
- All pregnant women should be asked about DV at the booking visit (see Section 6.3) and see a midwife on their own, without their partner, at least once
- If you suspect DV, talk to the woman in a supportive environment without her partner
- Ask if anyone is hurting her, offer support and follow up, and remember to document the consultation (but not in hand-held notes)
- After disclosure a woman may take no immediate action, but validation and empathy may be the first step in the path to change. If requested, facilitate referral to DV services, the police or social services
- Gain consent to share the information with her GP. Remember the impact on children and consider child protection issues

- Women who disclose DV should be regarded as 'high risk' and cared for by multidisciplinary teams
- Safety of the woman and any children must be paramount at all times

Why don't women just leave?

- It is not a simple thing to do
- She may still care for her partner and hope for change
- She may blame herself and feel ashamed
- Low self-esteem results from constant undermining, name-calling, and abuse
- She is often deliberately isolated from her family, friends, and support
- She may be scared of the future; financial security, housing, or believe it is better for the children
- She may be unsure of her options for help
- She will be in more danger, as the greatest risk of homicide is at, or after, the point of separation
- Of women who leave their partners, 76% report post-separation violence

Good practice to support women

- Waiting rooms with messages or posters about DV encourage women to feel safe to tell their stories
- Detailed information about local DV services, Women's Aid or Refuge can be kept in areas entered only by women (e.g. toilets)
- DV specialists can help with refuge accommodation, childcare, advice about solicitors, etc.
- Talk to the woman alone
- Never ask about relationships or abuse in front of the partner, friends, family or even small children
- Use an interpreter (e.g. phone) for non–English-speakers
- Refugees are especially vulnerable as they may have no secure residency, money or entitlement to public funds even to enter safe refuges
- Ask direct questions: 'are there any stresses at home?', 'is anyone frightening you?', 'were you hit or hurt?', 'who by?' This will show the woman that you are able to handle disclosure
- Be gentle, sympathetic, listen, and do not judge
- Do not feel that you need to give good advice or solve her problem—it is complex. You can facilitate by putting her in contact with the support agencies
- If a woman discloses DV, assess her safety. Is she safe to go home? Has the partner threatened her or worse?
- Ask particularly about the use of weapons, sexual assault, and threats to kill as these are associated with severe violence and death
- Offer a phone in a private room where she will not be disturbed or heard. Let her ring the support agency and allow her to make plans. Pop back to offer support, but do not influence her decision
- Keep a clear concise account
- If there is fighting on the ward, call security. Diffuse the situation if you can but stay safe
- Do not intervene. Do not tackle the partner, even if the woman asks you, as he may become aggressive. Instead, refer to the agencies mentioned below
- The process of change has to come from the woman
- We have a duty of care to the woman, to act in her interest, and advise her but we cannot act for her
- Refer child protection concerns to relevant agencies
- Intervention is only part of the solution

A woman needs to believe that she will be taken seriously for disclosure to take place. She needs to know that she has options and practical resources available, e.g. housing, legal support, etc. A woman may make several attempts to leave an abusive relationship before finally doing so. If a woman feels that she will be excluded from ongoing support if she does not leave, she is unlikely to seek help from that person/organization again. It is very important to be supportive and non-judgemental. There are additional barriers for women from ethnic minorities, including language and family expectations.

Prevention

Government National Report action points:
- Information sharing guidance for professionals
- An NHS Domestic Violence Coordinator
- National awareness campaigns
- Educating young people at school
- Domestic Violence, Crime and Victims Act 2004
- Police guidelines on investigating DV. Arrest and prosecution no longer rely on a victim's statement
- Training for magistrates and policies on DV within the CPS
- Perpetrator programmes within the Probation Service and, since 2004, a phone line for perpetrators who seek help
- Specialist DV courts since 2004—currently seven running
- National phone line for the lesbian, gay, bisexual, and transgender communities

Useful contacts
- English National DV Helpline 0808 2000 247
- Northern Ireland Women's Aid 24-hr DV Helpline 028 9033 1818
- Scottish Domestic Abuse Helpline 0800 027 1234
- Wales Domestic Abuse Helpline 0808 80 10 800
- Male Advice and Enquiry Line 0845 064 6800
- The Dyn Wales/Dyn Cymru Helpline 0808 801 0321
- The Samaritans 08457 909090
- Parentline 0808 800 2222

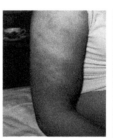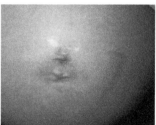

Fig. 1.3 Injuries from an assault by the partner that led to stillbirth.

Further reading

Bewley S, Friend J, Mezey G (eds.) Violence Against Women. RCOG Press, 1997.

www.dh.gov.uk DH 4126161. Responding to domestic violence. A handbook for health professionals. December 2005

www.homeoffice.gov.uk (guidance for practitioners).

www.victimsupport.org.uk

www.refuge.org.uk and www.womensaid.org.uk can be viewed by women in confidence and are not traceable on computers.

www.cemach.org Why mothers die 2000–2002 and Saving mothers lives 2003–2005.

Clinical errors

Errors will continue to occur in medical practice, in spite of techno-logical advances and risk management mechanisms. When they occur they are investigated and systems put in place to try to mini-mize the possibility of the same mistake recurring. Many patients think that their doctors are infallible as, of course, there is no other way they could trust them with their lives.

When things have gone wrong there is first a sickening realization which is agonizing. The doctor may feel singled out, replay the events over and over, and have agonies of self-doubt or, alternatively, deny any responsibility.

It has been written very fittingly: 'although patients are the first victim of medical mistakes, doctors are wounded by the same errors; they are the second victims...'

The three main emotions

For both doctors and patients (see Figure 1.4), these are:

- **Guilt** (What did I do wrong? It's all my fault. I shouldn't have done x, y, z)
- **Denial** (it's not so serious, the patient is exaggerating)
- **Blame** (it was all someone else's fault, no-one handed over, it was the night staff)

After the realization that a mistake has been made there is emo-tional turmoil, which can bring down a doctor and end his or her career. Obstetrics is a particularly exposed specialty from this point of view.

The more reflective and sensitive doctors are most affected, whilst uncaring and unbothered doctors fail to learn or improve with time. The unconditional support of family, peers, and senior colleagues is paramount in surviving this period.

Support

For the junior doctor, the first port of call is the educational super-visor. Unfortunately, the allocation of the 'educational supervisor' is arbitrary and so is the relationship some have with their trainees. We have all identified consultants whom we respect and see as role models. If we are lucky, we will 'click' with them, demonstrate our commitment to the profession and to the shared principles, and profit from their support throughout our careers. They are mentors.

Do not hesitate to ask for help from them. Undoubtedly, they have been through exactly what you are going through, and will be able to do two things: support and advise you and, with great feeling, reassure you that obstacles and set-backs can be overcome.

Sometimes all a doctor needs at a dark point in their career is to hear from someone they really admire, 'I've been there too', 'you are a good doctor, we are all forged and tested through the fire', 'everyone makes mistakes and the patient can't forgive you', or 'you have to forgive yourself and just not make the same mistake again'.

There is little organized support to help trainees cope in these difficult situations. There are counsellors in each hospital, who are trained to provide confidential support to all staff.

Three basic principles are very important:

- The right way to deal with a colleague's mistake is in private, without reproach but with support ('public praise, private criticism')
- As doctors we have the trust of our patients and with this comes the duty to tell them about the mistakes made

- As educators we have the duty to look for the near-misses even when there is no bad outcome, to try and learn from them, and to prevent future error

It has been suggested that facing up to a mistake is a process involving confession, restitution, and absolution. Confession is terrifying but necessary, especially if the error has caused harm. It is also a doctor's ethical obligation to be honest and report the mistake. Dreading punishment and patient anger are normal feelings.

Practical actions

- Be honest
- Talk to a senior doctor (this could be the consultant on call, or the patient's consultant)

If the patient or family is not aware of the mistake, the importance of disclosure should be discussed. You, or preferably a more objec-tive senior, will need to talk to the patient, or at worst to the family. It is best to do this with senior involvement as junior doctors often overestimate or underestimate their part in a bad outcome.

The talk will have to include:

- An explanation in simple terms
- A description of the consequences and measures taken to remedy
- An expressed personal regret
- An apology
- Preparedness to answer questions
- Preparedness to empathize with and receive emotional reactions

You may need to talk to parents of a baby who died or who was delivered in poor condition owing to unrecognized fetal distress.

How does anyone correctly judge or say 'I regret that I misjudged or missed signs on the heart tracing that your baby might be distressed. If we had noticed, we may have delivered the baby earlier. I am dev-astated to be responsible and can only tell you how sorry I am'? Upset patients are not helped by excessive frankness, defensiveness or 'Don't blame me, I didn't do anything wrong, it was someone else's fault'. Maybe simply asking 'can I answer any questions?' would be the most helpful approach.

In these rare and extremely difficult situations you must talk to and get advice from the senior clinician involved before talking so directly to the parents. Judgements about responsibility cannot be made objectively by those involved at the time or in the heat of the event, particularly without the full facts.

Writing a statement

After an untoward clinical incident the clinicians involved will be asked to provide a statement. This is a document describing your involvement in the clinical management of the event.

You should:

- Obtain the medical records (not write from memory)
- Provide a factual description of your involvement
- Describe exactly what happened, in chronological order and who was present
- Sign and date each page
- Return your statement within the deadline

You should not:

- Report on what you heard second-hand
- Speculate on what may have been the outcome if the manage-ment had been different
- Describe what you may have been thinking at a certain time or speculated later

Dealing with complaints

Complaints about care are increasing owing to:

- Patient expectation; this may be particularly true for pregnancy as childbirth is seen as a safe and happy event by the woman and her partner
- Unavoidable inefficiencies; wards do not run smoothly and the NHS is affected by staffing problems
- Communication failures
- The popular press, who concentrate on publicizing failures of care rather than more mundane daily successes

Complaints fall into two main areas:

- Against members of staff (commonly doctors) or the hospital, by dissatisfied patients or relatives
- About the whole team, medical outcomes, administrative services or the hospital as a whole. These are often initiated by patients or patients' organizations

The majority of complaints start informally. Patients express their dissatisfaction with staff at the time of their visit or admission. This is by far the best time to address them.

A complaint is not a medicolegal claim (yet). It is important that it is handled well. Do not underestimate your role as a junior doctor in handling complaints. Remember we all become involved at some point in our careers. Patients and relatives are usually understanding and forgiving as long as they feel the truth is not being concealed.

- Find out what happened
- Offer an explanation promptly
- Deal with the situation sympathetically
- Offer a carefully phrased apology. This is not an admission of liability
- Do not say 'I'm sorry you feel like that'; say 'I'm sorry for the wait, for what happened...' or 'It was not our intention to upset you'

- Minor criticism should be dealt with by conciliation, not confrontation
- Involve the senior or appropriate manager at the earliest opportunity

If things go wrong, you may find yourself in the frontline when the complainant is angry.

Some points to remember:

- Try to be honest
- Allow plenty of personal space. Don't stand too close or over them, as this could be perceived as threatening
- Acknowledge feelings. Once they know you understand that they are angry, there is no need for them to prove their anger
- Indicate that you are listening—partly by waiting to hear everything, partly by reflecting the language and concerns expressed
- Consider taking notes or providing follow-up
- Avoid questioning or interrupting an angry person
- Remember that you may be physically threatened, position yourself nearer the door so that you can leave quickly if need be
- Use simple techniques, such as repetition ('the broken record') to express yourself calmly and persistently
- You can take some wind out of the angry complainant's sails by acknowledging the truth in what they are saying 'I can see that', 'that would be disappointing/distressing'
- Ask 'Is there anything that you would like me to do?'

Further reading

Wu AW. Medical error: the second victim. The doctor who makes the mistake needs help too. *BMJ* 2000; **320**:726–7.

Wu AW. Doctors are obliged to be honest with their patients. *BMJ* 2001; **322**:1238–9.

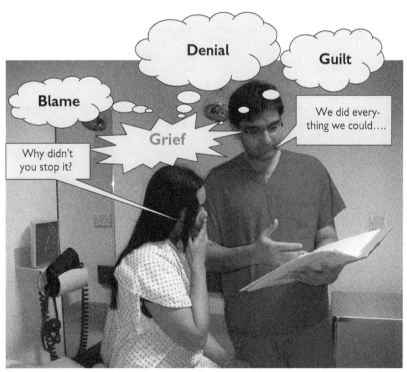

Fig. 1.4 The main emotions for both patient and doctor when things go wrong.

The law in the four countries of UK is different to that in other European countries. There is no single code relevant to our profession. Abortion and assisted conception are regulated by Acts of Parliament and within the criminal law. On the other hand, law in medical negligence, like much of the English law, is made by judges—the common law. Parliament delegates the regulation of the practice and the disciplining of doctors to the General Medical Council.

Medical negligence

The Bolam test

- In medical litigation the main question is whether or not a doctor has provided the standard of reasonable care required by the law
- The standard was established by the courts based on the Bolam test (named after a patient in 1954)
- The ruling said: 'a doctor is not guilty of negligence if he has acted in accordance with the practice accepted as proper by a responsible body of medical men (sic) skilled in that particular art...'
- It follows that if a medical practice is endorsed by a responsible body of peers, the Bolam test is satisfied and the doctor has met the criteria set by the law

Endorsement

- The principle has been upheld repeatedly to test a wide range of medical issues, including diagnosis, treatment, information disclosure, and ethics
- In addition, a House of Lords ruling in 1985 established that medical negligence cannot be found by preferring the opinion of one body of professionals to that of another. This is an acknowledgement of the differences of opinion and practice within the medical profession

Criticism

- The main criticism is that the test does not try 'what ought to be done' but 'what is done'. An action, even if taken by most people, could still be negligent
- It is heavily reliant on medical testimony
- Critics argue that the standard should be established independently
- The Bolam test is considered the only test available for medical knowledge and expertise in diagnosis and treatment, but
- In issues involving ethics, or information disclosure and the fundamental rights of individuals, it may be more appropriate that the courts decide the accepted standard and that doctor is envisaged as a professional but not the 'moral arbiter'

The Bolitho principle

- Named after Bolitho, a 2-year-old who suffered brain damage after a cardiac arrest. The decision of the paediatric registrar not to attend to the patient was based on the judgement that medical intervention would not have changed the outcome. This decision was supported by an impressive body of professionals
- However, the judge ruled that for the court to accept the opinion of the body of professionals, such opinion has to have a logical basis—thus the courts reserve the right to say that, even if all doctors do something, that still does not mean it is acceptable
- In practical terms, the first stage of the judgment would be to assess whether the decision had responsible peer support, based on an approach that was structured, reasoned, and defensible (in keeping with Bolam). The second stage is to assess the validity of the course of action and that of rejecting the competing ones
- The emergence of independent guidance and standards of good practice would enable the courts to utilize the Bolitho principle more proactively, moving from a 'defensible' to a 'justifiable' standard

Fraser competence

In 1985, Mrs Gillick, the mother of a 15-year-old girl, challenged the decision of a doctor to provide contraception to her daughter without informing her. The ruling in this case brought about the rules for assessing competence in children (named after the ruling judge, Lord Fraser):

- Any child below the age of 16 can give consent when they reach the necessary maturity and the intelligence to understand fully the intervention and the consequences of the decision
- If a child is deemed 'Fraser-competent' after receiving appropriate information, the consent is valid
- Intelligence and ability to understand will vary greatly with both the child and intervention, so competence must be carefully ascertained
- Doctors should always encourage children to inform their parents

Abortion Act

History

- Abortion has been a criminal offence since 1861, when Parliament passed the Offences Against The Person Act
- In 1929 the Infant Life Preservation Act amended the law, stating it would no longer be a felony if abortion was carried out in good faith and for the sole purpose of saving the mother
- The Bourne case was heard in 1938, named after the doctor who performed an abortion on a girl who was pregnant as a result of gang rape. It was the first case in which abortion was deemed acceptable to preserve a woman's mental health
- After this, women had abortions for urgent medical reasons. Wealthier women could afford to see a psychiatrist, but poor ones still resorted to illegal methods; 40 women died each year because of their complications

The Abortion Act 1967

The Act was introduced after intense political campaigning. It placed the responsibility for abortion not with the woman, but with doctors. The framework remains that abortion is a crime except when it is legal; for it to be legal, two doctors must be of the opinion made in good faith that:

- one of the clauses (see below) has been fulfilled
- it is performed on licensed premises
- it is notified

The law recognizes the following five situations in which the termination of a pregnancy is permitted:

A. The continuance of the pregnancy would involve risk to the life of the pregnant woman greater than if the pregnancy were terminated

B. The termination is necessary to prevent grave permanent injury to the physical and mental health of the pregnant woman

C. The pregnancy has not exceeded its 24th week and that the continuance of the pregnancy would involve risk, greater than if the pregnancy were terminated, of injury to the physical and mental health of the pregnant woman

D. The pregnancy has not exceeded its 24th week and the continuation of the pregnancy would involve risk, greater than if the pregnancy were terminated, of injury to the physical or mental health of any existing child(ren) of the family of the pregnant woman

E. There is substantial risk that if the child were born it would suffer from such physical or mental abnormalities as to be seriously handicapped

The law is open to interpretation, and medical practice changes gradually with time. Occasionally the law is challenged or clarified in the Courts, and it can be changed by Parliament. Presently doctors are asked to weigh risk. Two doctors will have to be in agreement that one of the clauses is satisfied. While termination for social reasons or maternal request is still theoretically illegal, clause C has effectively made such terminations widely possible and within the law.

The Human Fertilization and Embryology Act 1990

This Act is broadly based on the recommendations of the Warnock Committee (created by Parliament to make recommendations for regulation of reproductive techniques). It provides a complex code of law controlling all procedures related to human embryos. It is an Act that established the Human Fertilization and Embryology Authority, which has powers to license and control any unit or person carrying out:

- The creation and keeping of an embryo
- The storage of gametes
- The placing of sperm or eggs in a woman
- Research on embryos

The HFE Act amended the Abortion Act of 1967. Before 1990 abortion could not be performed legally after the gestational age of viability. In 1990 this was limited to 24 weeks' gestation. However, the amended Abortion Act allows termination without time limit where:

- The termination is necessary to save the life or protect the health of the woman from grave permanent injury, or
- There is substantial risk that the child will be seriously handicapped

The words substantial and seriously have not yet been defined by the Courts.

Further reading

http://www.rcog.org.uk The care of women requesting abortion, 2004.

A consideration of the law and ethics in relation to late termination for fetal abnormality. RCOG Press, 1998.

http://www.hfea.gov Code of Practice

www.veradrake.com Award winning film directed by Mike Leigh, 2004.

Working in O&G means being involved with maternal and fetal morbidity and death, abortion, infertility, cancer, sexuality, and other complex, difficult issues.

We deal with the most intimate aspects of women's lives and must take the attendant responsibility seriously.

Ethical dilemmas are an everyday occurrence and include:

- Keeping confidences (of young girls, the unfaithful, or women with STIs or HIV)
- Whether to undertake certain procedures (abortion, maternal request for CS)
- How to advise patients when they face tough decisions (such as IVF or terminations for fetal abnormality)
- Whether any form of paternalism is appropriate

Many young doctors are poorly prepared for the ethical dilemmas. No doubt they have a strong sense of right and wrong and (hopefully) all are good and moral people. The challenge is both to work out what they as individuals believe and to assist our patients make the right choices for themselves, based on their values and beliefs, even if not fully shared or comprehensible. Recognizing that the views of the doctor and the patient may be very strongly influenced by personal, cultural, and religious factors, the doctor also needs to be able to remain professional and supportive of the patient even if beliefs differ. When asked 'what do you think about…?' it is a balanced, objective, and professional argument which is required.

There are a number of different frameworks and tools to use by which to analyse ethics; some look at duties, others rights, and others outcomes. One version claims that 'four principles' cover all ethical questions: autonomy, beneficence (doing good), non-maleficence (avoiding harm), and justice. Another version suggests that encouraging virtues will be adequate (i.e. compassionate, caring, prompt, skilled, empathic, honest, and non-judgemental doctors). Probably the best thing is to keep alert and attentive to the ethical dimensions of everyday work.

How to get out of ethical trouble

The best way to get out of ethical trouble is not to get into it. It is important to recognize 'the queasy feeling' when you feel something is not quite right, that there is some uncomfortable pressure to do something unusual or outside one's reasonable expertise. The only clue might be the startled look on the receptionist, medical student or nurse's face. It might be a sinking, gnawing pain in the pit of your stomach before doing a procedure or ringing a rude colleague. Or it might be the desperate desire to please a pleading patient or aggressive relative. Watch out!

- Take stock, defer a final decision, and agree to meet again to review the question (whether that's in 5 minutes, an hour, tomorrow or in a clinic in a week's time)
- It is best to acknowledge that the problem is complex and one needs further advice from a senior colleague
- Clinical knowledge is paramount, as ethical questions revolve around medical problems; this is the reason why medical professionals are called upon to make decisions with ethical dimensions—some things turn on the medical facts of large or small risks or benefits, and doctors are entrusted to act ethically with their patients' interests in the forefront of their mind
- Do not be pressured into acting beyond your level of competence, but refer to colleagues when this is in the best interest of the patient
- Document your concerns closely and contemporaneously
- If stuck, get second opinions (from seniors, medical experts, legal or ethics committee)

Abortion

The central ethical question in abortion is the moral worth of the fetus and the question 'when does life begin?'

The moral arguments are simple only in the following extremes:

- Abortion is always morally wrong because life starts at conception and no human being has the right to take life. The counterargument might be that at no time before birth (or maybe viability) is the fetus an independent human being, therefore it does not require the absolute respect for life that the mother (our patient) does
- Abortion is never morally wrong because no woman should be forced to use her body against her will. The counterargument is that a woman has a duty to her vulnerable fetus (particularly if she could have had an abortion and did not) who will grow into a child and has interests that need protecting regardless of her preferences or the needs of her body

In a pluralist society, such as the UK, with law that both protects fetuses and permits abortion (with increasing stricture with rising gestation), the moral approach can be seen as lying between these two extremes with a gradualist approach to fetal moral worth.

Real life very seldom offers extreme or simple situations. Quite often in our profession, both mother and doctor place a great value on the fetus, but they still might accept late abortion for rape, maternal cardiac conditions, severe pre-eclampsia or fetal abnormality. How in our system of moral values do doctors and patients deal with the abortion? Both 'fundamentalist' positions have merit depending on one's beliefs. The challenge for an obstetrician or gynaecologist is not to use the consulting room to promulgate one view or another, nor to convince one or other side (these things can be done 'out of hours' just as other citizens), but to live within the law in a democratic society where the only recognized medical conscientious objection is to abortion.

It is important for the gynaecologist to determine how he or she feels about the issues and deal fairly and honestly with the patient who asks for advice about abortion. Gynaecologists are allowed to follow their own beliefs and not be forced to engage in abortion (a practice that they may consider morally wrong), but they should remember that at all times they have a duty to arrange cover for the process with a colleague and are obliged to care for the woman should any complications arise.

Further reading

Bewley S. Ethics in maternal–fetal medicine. In: Rodeck C, Whittle M (eds). Fetal Medicine, 2nd edn. Churchill Livingstone, 2009.

www.rcog.org.uk (for ethical guidance, hot topics).

www.bma.org.uk

Chapter 2

Reproductive transitions:
development, adolescence, and menopause

Contents

Covered elsewhere

- Physiology of the menstrual cycle (see Section 12.1)
- Basic anatomy of the female pelvis and perineum (see Section 12.2)

2.1 Embryology of the genital tract

The genital tract develops in close association with the urinary system. Lateral to the mesonephric ducts (also known as Wolffian ducts) lie the paramesonephric or Mullerian ducts that lead to the formation of the female internal genitalia.

The chromosomal sex of an embryo is determined at conception with the fertilization of the ovum by an X or Y chromosome-containing sperm. Nevertheless, the morphological differentiation into male or female begins around week 7 when the undifferentiated gonad becomes a testis or an ovary.

Gonads

The gonad starts forming in week 5 of embryonic life, as a thickening in the medial side of each mesonephros. Primordial germ cells migrate from the yolk sac to the gonadal ridge by week 6.

In the chromosomally female embryo (XX), the gonad develops into an ovary, which becomes identifiable by week 10. The fetal ovary produces no hormones.

In a chromosomally male embryo, a part of the Y chromosome, known as the *sry* gene, is responsible for the differentiation of the gonad into a testis. By week 8, the testes produce two hormones:

- Testosterone, the male sex hormone that drives the formation of male genitalia, and
- Anti-Mullerian hormone (AMH) that suppresses the development of Mullerian ducts

Internal genitalia

In the absence of testosterone and AMH, the development of female internal genitalia occurs. The cranial parts of the Mullerian ducts become the Fallopian tubes. Their caudal ends fuse medially (under the level of the mesonephros) to become the uterovaginal primordium and eventually forms the uterus and upper vagina. The Wolffian ducts regress (see Figure 2.1).

External genitalia

The external genitalia develop from the genital tubercle, the labioscrotal swellings, and the urogenital folds. These are undifferentiated in both sexes until week 9. The default development of the undifferentiated external genitalia is towards the female phenotype. In the absence of a hormonal stimulus, the genital tubercle becomes the clitoris, the labioscrotal swellings form the labia majora, and the urogenital folds form the vestibule and the lower part of the vagina.

In the male embryo the external genitalia virilize under the stimulation of dihydrotestosterone (DHT), which is a potent derivative of testosterone. The genital tubercle becomes the penis and the labioscrotal swellings fuse to form the scrotum. The urogenital folds fuse along the ventral surface of the penis and include the urethra, so that the urethral opening is positioned at the tip of the penis (see Figure 2.2).

The fetus is identifiable as female or male by week 10 of its life. This corresponds with the 12th week of gestation.

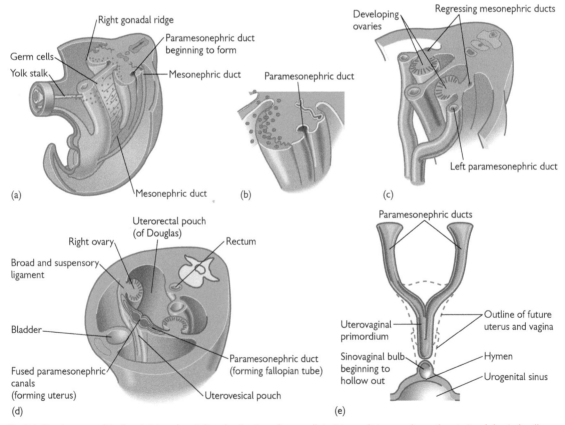

Fig. 2.1 Development of the female internal genitalia. a, b migration of germ cells to intermediate mesoderm of posterior abdominal wall, where the indifferent gonad is formed; c, d development of ovary and paramesonephric duct; e development of vagina. Reproduced from the *Oxford Textbook of Functional Anatomy*, Vol. 2 by Patricia MacKinnon and John Morris (© Oxford University Press 2005).

INDIFFERENT STAGE

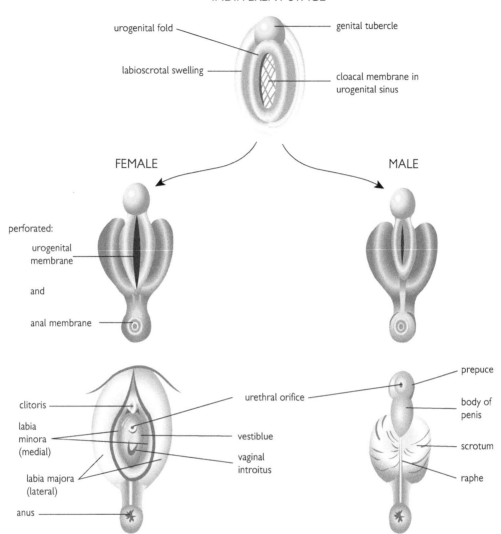

urogenital fold

genital tubercle

labioscrotal swelling

cloacal membrane in
urogenital sinus

FEMALE

MALE

perforated:

urogenital
membrane

and

anal membrane

clitoris

labia
minora
(medial)

labia majora
(lateral)

anus

urethral orifice

vestiblue

vaginal
introitus

prepuce

body of
penis

scrotum

raphe

Fig. 2.2 Development of the perineum (external genitalia). Reproduced from the *Oxford Textbook of Functional Anatomy*, Vol. 2 by Patricia MacKinnon and John Morris (© Oxford University Press 2005).

2.2 Ambiguous genitalia at birth

Definition
The genitalia are considered ambiguous when they have an atypical appearance and it is impossible to determine the sex of the baby by inspecting them.

Incidence
Estimated at 1:4000.

Pathophysiology
The terminology of these conditions is currently under review in an attempt to agree a system which is both medically accurate and acceptable to patients. The current accepted terminology is disorders of sex development (DSD).

The cause of ambiguous genitalia is either virilization of a karyotypically XX infant (46XX DSD) or under-masculinization of an XY infant (46XY DSD).

The following conditions can cause ambiguous genitalia in an infant with a normal female karyotype (46XX):
- Congenital adrenal hyperplasia (CAH)
- Exposure in utero to increased maternal androgens (exogenous or endogenous)
- Placental aromatase deficiency

Causes of ambiguous genitalia in an infant with a normal male karyotype (46XY) are:
- Partial gonadal dysgenesis
- Complete androgen insensitivity syndrome (CAIS)
- Partial androgen insensitivity syndrome (PAIS)
- Defect in testosterone biosynthesis
- 5-alpha-reductase deficiency

In some cases, testicular and ovarian tissue is found simultaneously, either in the same or in opposite gonads.

The karyotype is most commonly 46XX, but XX/XY mosaicism is found in 20%. The condition is known as ovotesticular DSD (previously true hermaphroditism).

Clinical evaluation

History
- Drugs taken by the mother during pregnancy, e.g. progestogens cause virilization and cyproterone acetate (found in Dianette®) causes undermasculinization
- Virilization in the mother during pregnancy, e.g. poorly controlled maternal CAH. Placental aromatase deficiency leads to increased fetal adrenal androgens which in turn cross the placenta, virilizing both the mother and the fetus
- Family history, e.g. CAH (autosomal recessive), PAIS (X-linked) or consanguinity

Examination
The following should be assessed systematically.
- Size of the phallus or clitoris (<1 cm) and presence of erectile tissue assessed by palpation
- Position of the urethral meatus on the phallus or perineum (level of hypospadias)
- Presence of a vaginal orifice
- Colour and rugosity of the genital folds

Hyperpigmentation suggests CAH because of excessive production of melanocyte-stimulating hormone. Rugosity suggests androgen exposure.
- Fusion of genital folds
- Presence of a palpable gonad within the genital folds or the inguinal region

The degree of ambiguity can be classified into five Prader stages (see Table 2.1).

Table 2.1 Prader stages	
Stage	Degree of sexual ambiguity
1	Isolated clitoromegaly
2	Narrow vestibule with separate urethral and vaginal opening
3	Single urogenital sinus/labia majora partially fused
4	Micropenis
5	Isolated crypto-orchidism

Investigations
- Fluorescent in situ hybridization (FISH) to detect Y chromosome sequences. Results can be available within 6–8 h
- Karyotyping
- Serum 17-hydroxyprogesterone levels (17-OHP) (are high in CAH)
- Urea and electrolytes (abnormal in salt-losing CAH)
- Synacthen test (stimulation with synthetic ACTH and measurement of plasma 17-OHP concentration)
- Basal and gonadotrophin-releasing hormone (GnRH)-stimulated follicle-stimulating hormone (FSH) and luteinizing hormone (LH) levels
- Basal and beta human chorionic gonadotrophin (HCG)-stimulated androgen levels (uniform high androgen levels in PAIS, disproportionate rise of testosterone precursors versus low levels of testosterone in inborn errors of testosterone metabolism)
- AMH (low in dysgenetic gonads)
- Ultrasonography of the pelvis to assess the presence of a uterus and ovaries
- Examination under anaesthetic (EUA) with vaginoscopy and cystoscopy. This is used to assess the morphology of the urogenital sinus (see Figure 2.3). The presence or absence of a vagina and its level of communication to the urethra and the urethral sphincter is ascertained
- Culture of genital skin to evaluate the number of androgen receptors and their affinity to androgens

Management

Treatment of salt-wasting crisis
Almost half of the newborns with ambiguous genitalia suffer with CAH and are at risk of life-threatening salt-losing crises.

Hypoglycaemia and electrolyte imbalances should be assessed and treated urgently. Lifelong steroid treatment will be required.

Gender assignment
At birth, parents should be told that there is a difficulty in deciding the gender of the baby.

Speculations on the gender and prognosis should be avoided until a full clinical evaluation has taken place.

Once a diagnosis is available, the doctors and family should decide on the sex of rearing.

The decision is usually guided by the anatomy of the infant and the future reproductive and sexual potential.

Gonadectomy
In susceptible cases, the gonads should be removed in childhood to prevent virilization. Not all cases of 46XY DSD will be virilized. However, gonadectomy is necessary in cases that have been assigned

to a female sex of rearing and where there is a potential for the child to respond to increased circulating androgens in puberty. This is likely in partial gonadal dysgenesis, PAIS, and defects in testosterone biosynthesis. Dysgenetic gonads have a 30% risk of developing malignancy and therefore gonadectomy is recommended as soon as the diagnosis is made. In CAIS the testes are normal and the malignancy risk low (approximately 3%). In this situation the gonads can be left *in situ* until after puberty. This allows spontaneous puberty and also means the children themselves can be involved in any surgical decisions.

Feminizing genital surgery

The two main aspects of feminizing surgery are the reduction of clitoral size and the opening of the vaginal canal. The latter allows passage of menstrual blood flow (if a uterus is present) and enables penetrative sexual intercourse.

The timing of such operations is a matter of debate. There is increasing evidence that genital surgery should be delayed as much as possible. Surgery performed on the vagina in infancy usually requires revision at adolescence. Surgery on the clitoris can have a detrimental effect on later sexual sensitivity and sexual function. By deferring surgery until adolescence the patient can be involved in the decision-making. However, western society does not accommodate a middle gender and delaying the operation can cause significant psychological distress to the child's parents and carers who may prefer to 'fix' the discordant appearance as soon as possible despite possible long-term risks to sexual function.

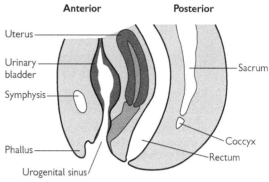

Fig. 2.3 Diagram of urogenital sinus, depicting the common opening of the urethra and vagina on the perineum.

Congenital adrenal hyperplasia (CAH)

Incidence
- Estimated incidence in the UK: 1:10 000 births

Genetics
- Enzyme deficiency in the corticosteroid production pathway
- In 90% of cases the deficient enzyme is 21-hydroxylase, followed in frequency by 11β-hydroxylase

Pathophysiology
Production of cortisol is decreased. ACTH is increased as a result of negative feedback and this leads to hyperplasia of the adrenal gland. Increased levels of 17-hydroxyprogesterone (17-OHP) are shunted towards the production of androgens.

Diagnosis
- Raised serum levels of 17-OHP
- In equivocal cases the levels of cortisol and 17-OHP are measured 30 and 60 minutes after the administration of synthetic ACTH (synacthen test)

Presentation and management
If both cortisol and corticosterone are deficient, the child is at risk of a salt-losing crisis and needs immediate treatment with hydrocortisone.

In a female infant there can be varying degrees of virilization, with clitoral enlargement, scrotal appearance of the labia majora, and a single urogenital sinus (see Figure 2.4).

The vagina can join the posterior wall of the urethra at varying levels, leading to a low or a high defect. The vagina will have to be reconstructed surgically to allow sexual intercourse. A flap vaginoplasty is performed when the defect is low. In cases of a high defect, the operation is more complex and may require a combined perineal and abdominal approach. Vaginal surgery is usually combined with clitoral reduction in a feminizing genitoplasty.

There is current controversy about the appropriate need for, and timing of, surgical intervention.

In cases of late onset CAH, virilization may only occur in puberty. The presentation of these cases can be similar to polycystic ovarian syndrome.

Partial and complete androgen insensitivity

Incidence
- 1:40–60 000 births
- CAIS > PAIS

Genetics
- X-linked inheritance in two-thirds of cases

Pathophysiology
There is normal testicular production of androgens but abnormal androgen receptors. Virilization of external genitalia is incomplete or absent because it is dependent on androgen receptor activity.

As the testes produce AMH, Mullerian structures regress.

The Fallopian tubes, uterus, and upper two-thirds of the vagina are absent.

Presentation
In CAIS the genitalia will have a normal female appearance and the commonest presentation is primary amenorrhoea. In PAIS there can be varying degrees of virilization, ranging from defects in spermatogenesis and isolated hypospadias to ambiguous genitalia.

The gonads are usually undescended. They may be located in the inguinal canal and first presentation can be that of a phenotypically female infant with bilateral inguinal hernias.

During puberty some degree of virilization occurs in PAIS but not in CAIS. In CAIS, pubic and axillary hair are absent.

Diagnosis
- 46XY karyotype
- Normal rise of testosterone after HCG stimulation test in the presence of ambiguous genitalia or normal female external genitalia

Management
Once the correct diagnosis of CAIS is established the main initial management is psychological. Disclosure of the XY karyotype to the patient is essential as well as the information that she will never menstruate or carry a pregnancy. In addition, gonadectomy should be considered (see Section 2.2). If performed, then replacement oestrogen therapy will be necessary. The vagina is usually shortened and will need expansion to allow penetrative sexual intercourse. This is usually achieved with vaginal dilatation. However, surgery is sometimes necessary.

If a PAIS patient is reared as female, then gonadectomy should be performed prior to adolescence to avoid virilization. Other issues, such as psychological support, full disclosure, and vaginal dilatation, are as for CAIS.

5α-reductase deficiency

Incidence
- Unknown (much rarer than CAIS and PAIS)
- Geographical variation reported
- Increases with consanguinity

Pathophysiology
There are at least five types. They all lack the enzyme that converts testosterone to dihydrotestosterone (DHT). DHT is a potent androgen that is required for fetal genital virilization.

Presentation
- Female or ambiguous genitalia at birth
- Virilization during puberty

Diagnosis
- Normal basal and HCG-stimulated testosterone, decreased DHT
- Measurement of 5α-reductase activity in genital skin fibroblasts

Management
- If the child is reared as female, gonadectomy should be performed before adolescence to avoid virilization
- In those reared as males, surgery may be required to treat hypospadias
- Psychosexual support
- Genetic counselling

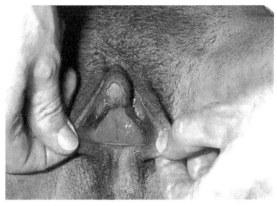

Fig. 2.4 Ambiguous genitalia. Late presentation of CAH. Clitoromegaly and single opening of vagina and urethra, Prader stage 3.

Further reading

Androgen Insensitivity Support Group website www.aissg.org

Congenital Adrenal Hyperplasia Support Group website www.cah.org.uk

2.4 Congenital uterine and vaginal anomalies

Incidence

It is estimated that between 0.5 and 6% of women may have a uterine anomaly. This varies, depending on the population studied and the diagnostic method used.

Pathophysiology

Uterine anomalies are the result of abnormal development of the Mullerian ducts during embryogenesis.

Classification

The classification most widely used is the revised American Society of Reproductive Medicine (ASRM) classification (see Box 2.1 and Figure 2.5).

Clinical evaluation

History

- Primary amenorrhoea with or without cyclical abdominal pain, because of obstructed menstruation (imperforate hymen, transverse vaginal septum, vaginal or cervical agenesis, uterine agenesis)
- Dysmenorrhoea (non-communicating obstructed horn)
- Dyspareunia (transverse or longitudinal vaginal septum)
- Subfertility
- Recurrent miscarriages
- Obstetric complications (preterm delivery, abnormal lie)

In the majority of cases there are no symptoms or associated history.

Examination

- Shortened vagina
- Absent or double cervix on vaginal examination
- Palpable pelvic mass in case of an obstructed uterine horn or obstructed vagina

Investigations

- Ultrasonography (two- or three-dimensional)
- Hysterosalpingogram (HSG)/saline infusion sonohysterography
- MRI
- Laparoscopy
- Hysteroscopy

Management

Depends on the anomaly and the symptoms caused.

Imperforate hymen or low transverse vaginal septum (see Section 2.8)

Surgical resection of the hymen or septum is curative. Care must be taken to excise the whole septum or re-stenosis can occur.

Cervical agenesis

Symptoms are caused by menstrual blood accumulating within the uterus. The young girl presents with primary amenorrhoea and cyclical pain that gradually worsens. This is further aggravated by endometriosis caused by retrograde menstruation.

Traditional treatment was hysterectomy, but there is increasing experience in performing anastomosis of the uterus to the vagina which preserves fertility. The operation can also be performed laparoscopically.

Non-communicating rudimentary uterine horn with functioning endometrium

In these cases, menstrual blood accumulates within the uterine horn, causing dysmenorrhoea. Often, the diagnosis is delayed as the girl has cyclical menses. Treatment is excision of the horn, which can be an open or laparoscopic procedure. GnRH analogues are used preoperatively to alleviate symptoms by suppressing menstruation and also to thin the endometrium, thus facilitating the operation.

Septate or subseptate uterus

If a uterine septum is thought to be contributing to pregnancy loss it can be resected hysteroscopically. Simultaneous laparoscopy is advised to decrease the risk of perforation and to assess the exact anomaly of the uterus.

Bicornuate uterus (see Figure 2.6)

In the past, bicornuate uterus was treated using a Strassmans' operation to unite the two cavities. However, this procedure is now largely abandoned as there is no evidence that it improves fertility. The obstructed uterine horn is best removed laparoscopically.

Although there is a link between a uterine septum, or bicornuate uterus, and pregnancy complications, it is not clear at present whether surgical treatment is of benefit. Theoretically, removing a uterine septum allows a pregnancy to implant into a healthy part of the uterine cavity. Nevertheless, the scar tissue itself may lead to miscarriage and abnormal placentation. Randomized controlled trials are required to draw appropriate conclusions. Until then, treatment should be individualized (see also Section 5.6).

Women with a uterine anomaly, particularly cases of unilateral hypoplasia or agenesis (type II anomaly), should undergo imaging of their renal tract. Up to 50% have associated renal malformations such as unilateral renal agenesis, renal duplications or ectopy.

Mayer–Rokitansky–Kuster–Hauser syndrome (MRKH)

Definition

Absent or rudimentary uterus or bilateral rudimentary horns on either side of the pelvic wall (see Figure 2.7).

Incidence

- 1:4–6000

Pathophysiology

- Multifactorial

Presentation

- Normal development of secondary sexual characteristics (indicating normal ovarian function)
- Primary amenorrhoea
- Short vagina
- Associated with renal and skeletal anomalies

Management

- Psychological support to help come to terms with the diagnosis and the inability to bear children
- Interventions to enlarge the vagina and enable normal sexual life
- Fertility is possible via surrogacy

Vaginal agenesis or hypoplasia

Aetiology

Vaginal agenesis may occur due to MRKH or androgen insensitivity.

Treatment

Treatment is required to enable vaginal penetrative intercourse and is best delayed until puberty when the patient can be involved with the decisions and can comply with the proposed dilatation regime.

Conservative

Initial treatment should be by dilatation therapy. This entails the insertion of plastic moulds of increasing size within the vaginal dimple and applying mechanical pressure. The results are satisfactory in the majority of patients, although good motivation and compliance are required.

Surgical

A variety of techniques are available using different graft tissue.

Williams vaginoplasty

A U-shaped incision is made on the perineum and the edges are sutured to create a horizontal pouch on the perineum. This procedure is no longer performed as it creates an unsatisfactory shallow exterior vagina.

McIndoe–Reed procedure

A cavity is dissected between the urethra and rectum and lined with a split-thickness skin graft mounted on a mould. The skin is usually obtained from the buttocks. The mould is left *in situ* for 7–10 days initially. Thereafter, the woman is instructed to insert regular vaginal dilators. Once sexually active she will need to use lubrication. Vaginal stenosis is common and the skin graft donor site can leave ugly and unacceptable scarring.

Bowel vaginoplasty

A segment of sigmoid is mobilized at laparotomy, maintaining its vascular supply, and is passed through a cavity created between the urethra and rectum. The caudal end of the intestinal graft is then sutured to the introitus and the distal part is closed to create a blind pouch.

Davydov procedure

A vaginal passage is created and then lined by pelvic peritoneum which is sutured at the introitus and closed distally to form a pouch. The mobilization of the peritoneum can be done laparoscopically.

Laparoscopic Vecchietti procedure

An acrylic olive is placed in the vaginal dimple. The olive has sutures which are passed laparoscopically through the vesicorectal space to the abdominal wall. The sutures are then mounted on a tension device and the olive is gradually pulled. The neovagina is formed over several days.

There are no randomized controlled studies to compare outcomes of different vaginoplasties.

Whatever the surgical technique, the woman will need to use dilators when she is not in a sexual relationship to avoid stenosis of the neovagina.

Squamous cell carcinoma and adenocarcinoma can develop in the neovagina created by McIndoe or bowel vaginoplasty. Therefore women that undergo these procedures will need annual follow-up.

> **Box 2.1 ASRM classification**
>
> - Type I: segmental hypoplasia or agenesis, involving the vagina, cervix, uterus or tubes
> - Type II: unilateral hypoplasia or agenesis
> - Type III and IV: failure of fusion of Mullerian ducts
> - Type V: non-resorption of midline septum
> - Type VI: arcuate uterus
> - Type VII: anomalies relating to *in utero* diethylstilboestrol (DES) exposure

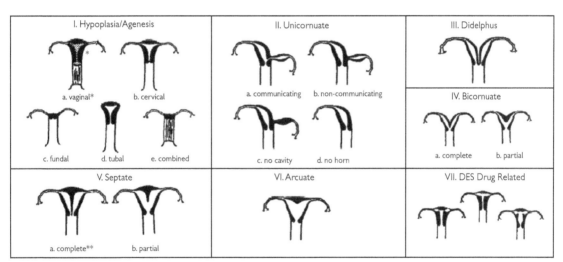

* Uterus may be normal or take a variety of abnormal forms.

** May have two distinct cervices

Fig. 2.5 ASRM classification of uterine anomalies. Reprinted from *Fertility Sterility* 49(6):944–55, American Fertility Society. ©1988, with permission from the American Society for Reproductive Medicine.

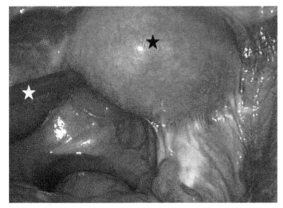
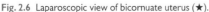

Fig. 2.6 Laparoscopic view of bicornuate uterus (★).

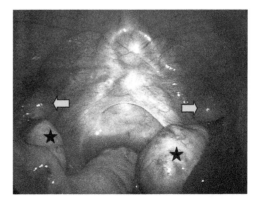

Fig. 2.7 MRKH syndrome. Rudimentary uterine buds (⇨) seen adjacent to the ovaries (★).

2.5 Vulval disorders in prepubertal girls

Vulvovaginitis

Definition
Vulvovaginitis is inflammation of the vulva and vagina with associated discharge.

Incidence
The exact incidence is unknown. However, it is the commonest gynaecological problem in young girls.

Pathophysiology
Prepubertal girls do not have a physiological discharge, in contrast to adult women.

Infectious agents
The most commonly isolated organisms are group A haemolytic streptococcus and *Haemophilus influenzae*.

Threadworms can cause vulvovaginitis and the usual symptom is nocturnal perianal itching.

Candida is rare in prepubertal girls, but it may be isolated in diabetics, after a recent course of antibiotics, or if still wearing nappies.

Chlamydia trachomatis, *Neisseria gonorrhoea*, and *Trichomonas vaginalis* are sexually transmitted and suggest sexual abuse. *Gardnerella vaginalis* can be sexually transmitted but can also be present in the absence of sexual abuse.

Foreign bodies
Rare and are usually toilet paper or small toys.

Dermatological conditions
Contact dermatitis, eczema, lichen sclerosis.

Non-specific aetiology
In the majority of girls no specific agent is identified, and the symptoms are caused by local irritants such as bubble baths or tight underwear.

Risk factors
Reasons the prepubertal girl is prone to vulvovaginitis:
- Thin vaginal mucosa
- Alkaline pH
- Absence of vulval fat pads
- Absence of pubic hair
- Close proximity of vagina to anus
- Poor hygiene

Clinical evaluation
History
- Vaginal discharge (>90%)
- Pruritus
- Soreness
- Dysuria
- Bleeding (rare symptom and should prompt further examination)

Examination
- Inflammation and redness
- Vaginal discharge
- Excoriations

Investigations
- Swabs should be taken for microscopy and culture
- Examination under anaesthesia is required in cases where symptoms are severe or refractory to treatment

Management
- Antibiotics are given if a pathogen is isolated
- Consider treating empirically for threadworms
- General advice on good hygiene of the area (e.g. front-to-back cleaning after using the toilet)
- Avoidance of irritants, such as bubble bath and harsh soaps
- Loose cotton underwear should be preferred to tight synthetic underwear
- Careful evaluation for sexual abuse, especially in cases where a sexually transmitted organism is isolated

The family can usually be reassured that the symptoms will disappear with puberty and that there will be no long-term sequelae from the condition.

Labial adhesions

Definition
Adhesions between the labia minora.

Incidence
The condition occurs in an estimated 1–3% of prepubertal girls. Labial adhesions are never present at birth and the peak incidence is between the first and second year of life.

Pathophysiology
The exact cause is unknown, but it is probably related to a combination of low oestrogen levels and local inflammation. Vulval irritation and scratching denude the thin skin covering the labia which then agglutinates.

Risk factors
- Nappy (diaper) dermatitis
- Poor hygiene

Clinical evaluation
History
Minor adhesions are usually asymptomatic.

With more severe cases, urine accumulates behind the fused labia, leading to urinary symptoms such as:
- Post-micturition dribble
- Dysuria
- Recurrent urinary infections
- Urinary retention

Examination
The labia are fused from the level of the posterior fourchette towards the urethra.

A thin avascular membrane is visible in the midline where the tissues have fused.

Investigations
No investigations are required to make the diagnosis.

Management
If the child is asymptomatic, treatment is not required. The adhesions will resolve spontaneously with puberty.

The following may be necessary:

Local oestrogen cream application
A small amount of oestrogen cream is applied to the labia in the midline daily for a maximum of 6 weeks. Parents need to be aware that a small amount of oestrogen is absorbed and can lead to systemic side effects such as vaginal spotting, breast swelling, and tenderness.

Surgical separation
In severe cases or those refractory to oestrogen treatment, the labia can be separated surgically under local or general anaesthetic.

Oestrogen cream should be used postoperatively to prevent recurrence.

Recurrence is very common following both hormonal and surgical treatment. Complete resolution may not occur until the onset of puberty.

Lichen sclerosus
(see also Section 13.9)

Lichen sclerosus is usually associated with postmenopausal age. Nevertheless, it can also present in childhood with partial or complete resolution at puberty.

Definition
Hypotrophic dystrophy of the vulva.

Incidence
Estimated as 1:900.

Risk factors
- Autoimmune disorder
- Infections
- Local trauma

Clinical evaluation
History
- Vulval soreness
- Pruritus

Examination
- Flat ivory-coloured plaques in the perianal and vulval area
- Atrophy of the skin
- Skin fragility can lead to bleeding and the appearance of 'blood blisters'. These appearances can lead to suspicion of genital trauma and sexual abuse so it is important to be clear about the diagnosis
- Extragenital lesions can be identified in 10% of cases, usually on the upper trunk, breasts, neck, and face

Investigations
Skin biopsy is rarely required in childhood, and the diagnosis can be made on the typical skin appearance.

Management
- Topical corticosteroids. Usually a potent corticosteroid is required until remission of symptoms, followed by maintenance with a less potent agent and less frequent application
- Local emollients

Unlike adult lichen sclerosus, there is no confirmed risk of progression to squamous cell carcinoma of the vulva.

Symptoms commonly resolve at puberty. It is not known whether this group of children is at greater risk of postmenopausal lichen sclerosus.

Box 2.2 Normal vaginal flora in prepubertal girls

- Has not been well studied in prepubertal girls
- It is therefore sometimes difficult to define which organisms are pathological if isolated in the secretions of symptomatic girls
- Mixed anaerobes, diphtheroids, and Staphylococcus epidermidis are probably normal commensals
- Lactobacilli are more likely to be present in older children approaching puberty

Puberty

Definitions
Puberty is the period between childhood and adulthood when reproductive and sexual development and maturation occurs.

Anatomical and physiological changes that occur:

- Breast development (thelarche)
- Pubic hair growth (adrenarche)
- Axillary hair growth
- Growth spurt
- Onset of menstruation (menarche)

Demographic details
The average age of menarche occurs at 12.3 years in African girls and 12.8 years in western Caucasian girls.

Physiology
During childhood the hypothalamo–pituitary–ovarian axis remains quiescent, and the levels of GnRH and FSH and LH are almost undetectable.

Puberty is initiated by intrinsic and extrinsic factors. Its onset is influenced by heredity, race, ethnicity, gender, body weight, fat mass composition, nutrition, and exercise levels.

Leptin, a metabolic hormone produced by adipose tissue in response to fat deposition, also plays a permissive role in the development of puberty.

The degree of breast and pubic hair development is described in five Tanner stages. Tanner 1 is the prepubertal stage and Tanner 5 is the mature, adult development (see Figure 2.8).

Between the ages of 7 and 9 years the GnRH secretory system becomes activated. GnRH is secreted in pulsations of higher amplitude and frequency. GnRH stimulates the production of LH and FSH by the pituitary, and these promote follicular growth and steroidogenesis in the ovary. GnRH, LH, and FSH are initially only produced nocturnally and lead to a moderate rise in circulating oestrogen levels. This leads to breast budding, which is usually the first sign of puberty. Thelarche precedes menarche (the onset of menstruation) by an average of 2–3 years as it is only after the GnRH pulsations extend to daytime that ovulation and the menstrual cycle can be established.

The appearance of pubic hair in girls is dependent primarily on adrenal androgen production. The rise in the secretion of androgens by the adrenal gland (adrenarche) occurs independently to the pituitary–ovarian maturation. Adrenarche usually follows thelarche by a few months, although the opposite can also occur, particularly in African girls.

During puberty, and parallel to the adrenal and gonadal maturation, growth hormone production also rises. This leads to a pubertal growth spurt. Figure 2.9 shows the age range for pubic hair and breast development, height spurt, and menarche.

Precocious puberty

Definition
Precocious puberty is defined as onset of pubertal development before the age of 8 (girls) or 9 years (boys).

Female to male ratio = 5:1.

Pathophysiology
Precocious puberty is classified as the following:

Central, gonadotrophin-dependent or true precocious puberty

- 80% of cases
- This may be caused by brain tumours or central nervous system malformations
- In the majority of cases, though (approximately 75%), a cause is not found and the precocious onset of puberty is idiopathic

Peripheral precocious puberty or pseudopuberty

- 20% of cases
- Pseudopuberty is always pathological and is caused by:
  - Hormone-producing ovarian tumours
  - Exogenous administration of oestrogen
  - McCune Albright syndrome

The latter is caused by a mutation of the G protein gene. This leads to its continuous activation despite the absence of a hormonal stimulation. The classic triad of the syndrome is polyostotic fibrous dysplasia, café-au-lait skin lesions, and gonadotrophin-independent precocious puberty.

Clinical evaluation

Investigations

- **Serum gonadotrophin levels** (LH and FSH): these are suppressed with peripheral causes of precocious puberty and elevated with central ones
- **Brain imaging** in cases of central puberty: to detect a lesion (e.g. a tumour or hamartoma)
- **Pelvic and abdominal imaging** to detect ovarian or adrenal tumours

Management
Usually this is the remit of the paediatric endocrinologist.

Treatment is required to slow growth velocity and avoid early skeletal maturation. Furthermore, early development of secondary sexual characteristics can be distressing to a young girl.

If produced by a lesion, surgical resection can be attempted.

Pubertal development may be suppressed with GnRH analogues. GnRH analogues are longer acting than endogenous GnRH and, when given continuously, lead to downregulation of pituitary GnRH receptors and suppression of gonadotrophin production (LH and FSH).

Further reading

Parent AS, Teilmann G, Juul A, Skakkebaek NE, Toppari J, Bourguignon JP. The timing of normal puberty and the age limits of sexual precocity: variations around the world, secular trends and changes after migration. *JP Endocrine Reviews* 2003; **24(5):**668–93.

Ress M. Menarche when and why? *Lancet* 1993; **342:**1375–6.

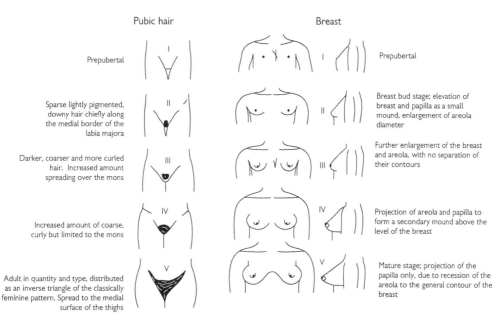

Fig. 2.8 Marshall and Tanner stages of breast and pubic hair development. Adapted from McVeigh E, Homburg R, and Guillebaud J. *The Oxford Handbook of Reproductive Medicine and Family Planning*, Oxford University Press, 2008. Original data from Marshall WA and Tanner JM. *Archives of Disease in Childhood* 1969; 44:291–303.

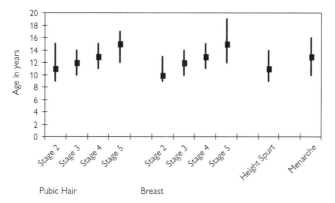

Fig. 2.9 Age for breast and pubic hair Tanner stages, compared with age for menarche and height spurt. (Means ± 2 SD). Redrawn from Marshall WA and Tanner JM. *Archives of Disease in Childhood* 1969; 44: 291–303, with permission from the BMJ Publishing Group.

> ### ➔ Box 2.3 Secular trends in age at menarche
>
> Age at onset of menarche has decreased considerably over the past century, from 17 years to less than 13 currently. The average decrease has been by 3–4 months per decade. This trend was consistent until the 1960s in the western world, probably indicating improving nutritional and socioeconomic conditions.
>
> Over the past few decades the trend has either arrested or reversed.
>
> In the developing world, the secular trend towards reduction of age at menarche is still obvious, and is sometimes more pronounced than that previously seen in the developed world.

2.7 Delayed puberty

Definition
Delayed puberty is the absence of all secondary sexual characteristics by the age of 14 years.

Pathophysiology
Delayed puberty is caused either by a central defect or the result of non-functioning gonads. These are classified as:

- Hypogonadotrophic hypogonadism
- Hypergonadotrophic hypogonadism

Hypogonadotrophic hypogonadism
No pituitary or hypothalamic stimulation of the gonad, and low FSH.

- Constitutional delay, often following a familial pattern
- Chronic illness, such as diabetes, chronic renal failure or cystic fibrosis. Optimizing the underlying condition usually allows for puberty to progress
- Anorexia nervosa
- Excessive exercise
- Kallman's syndrome (see below)
- Hydrocephalus or central nervous system tumours
- Pituitary adenomas (usually prolactinomas)
- Panhypopituitarism

Hypergonadotrophic hypogonadism
Non-functioning gonad with high FSH.

- Abnormal gonadal development
- Turner syndrome (see below)
- Swyer syndrome (see below)
- Premature ovarian failure
- Following chemotherapy or radiotherapy
- Galactosaemia
- Autoimmune
- Infections

Management
Induction of puberty is usually achieved by administering small doses of ethinyl oestradiol, i.e. 2 µg, one-tenth of the content of the combined oral contraceptive pill (COCP), initially at night time. The dose is increased at 6-monthly intervals until breakthrough vaginal bleeding occurs. At that point the girl should be started on a standard combined oestrogen and progestogen preparation.

Introducing high doses of oestrogen to a prepubertal girl is not advisable, as it may cause irreversible abnormal breast development.

In cases of hypogonadotrophic hypogonadism, puberty can be induced by pulsatile gonadotrophins administered via a subcutaneous pump.

Long-term hormone replacement is required, either in the form of the COCP or hormone replacement therapy (HRT).

Kallman's syndrome

Incidence
- Female:male ratio = 7:1
- Female   1:7500
- Male   1:50 000

Genetics
X-linked disorder owing to a mutation to the *Kal-1* gene.

Pathophysiology
Dysgenesis of the olfactory bulbs and abnormal development of GnRH neurons, which also originate from the nasal region during embryogenesis.

Clinical features
- Delayed puberty
- Anosmia or hyposmia

- Commonly there are associated midline structural defects and mental restriction

Turner syndrome

Incidence
- 1:2500 female live births

Genetics
- 45XO

Clinical features
Prenatally:
- Cystic hygroma, non-immune hydrops fetalis, and fetal growth restriction

Postnatally:
- Short stature; adult height is 20 cm below the female average
- Gonadal failure, occurring in most cases before the onset of puberty, although in one-third of patients it occurs after menarche
- Widely spaced nipples (shield chest)
- Short and webbed neck, low hairline
- Lymphoedema
- Associated cardiac and renal anomalies (coarctation of the aorta, horseshoe kidney)
- Endocrine problems (hypothyroidism, insulin resistance)
- Individuals with Turner syndrome have a female gender identity

Diagnosis
Karyotype. At least 20 cells should be examined because of the likelihood of mosaicism.

Management
- Administration of growth hormone to improve adult height
- Induction of puberty
- Long-term hormone replacement
- Childbearing possible with ovum donation

Swyer syndrome

Incidence
- Unknown, but rare

Genetics
- 46XY
- Mutation in *Sry* gene in 10%
- Unknown cause in remaining

Clinical features
- Gonadal dysgenesis, failure of testes to develop in embryonic life. No testosterone or anti-Mullerian hormone (AMH) is produced
- External genitalia are female
- Uterus and Fallopian tubes are present
- Absence of pubertal development
- Tall stature
- 30% risk of developing a gonadal malignancy (dysgerminoma) which can occur at any age

Diagnosis
Karyotype, assessment for mutation in *Sry* gene.

Management
- Induction of puberty
- Gonadectomy as risk of malignancy
- Long-term hormone replacement
- Childbearing is possible with ovum donation

2.8 Menstrual dysfunction in adolescence

Primary amenorrhoea

Definition
- Absence of menstruation
- Investigated at age 14 years if there are no secondary sexual characteristics or age 16 in a girl with normal secondary sexual characteristics

Incidence
Primary amenorrhoea occurs in 3–4%.

Pathophysiology—classification
- Anatomical
- Ovarian
- Pituitary
- Hypothalamic
- Amenorrhoea secondary to systemic disorders

Clinical evaluation

History
- Chronic systemic illness such as diabetes, cystic fibrosis, renal failure
- History of delayed puberty or menarche in mother or siblings
- Anosmia (suggestive of Kallman's syndrome)
- Excessive exercise or competitive sports
- Anorexia nervosa
- Childhood cancer requiring chemotherapy or radiotherapy
- Cyclical pelvic pain

Examination
- Stature
- Body mass index (BMI)
- Breast development
- Presence of pubic and axillary hair
- Inguinal masses
- Hirsutism and evidence of virilization

Investigations
- FSH and LH levels
- Oestradiol level
- Peripheral blood karyotype
- Pelvic ultrasound and MRI

Approach
The presence or absence of secondary sexual characteristics along with gonadotrophin levels help make an initial assessment of the possible causes of amenorrhoea. Normal breast development usually indicates that there is normal ovarian function, or that there has been at some point.

Gonadotrophins are low when there is a dysfunction of the hypothalamus or pituitary, whereas they rise in the case of a failing gonad.

Normal levels of gonadotrophins suggest that the ovarian–pituitary–hypothalamic axis is functioning normally. In these cases, an anatomical defect causes the amenorrhoea.

A girl with primary amenorrhoea falls into one of four categories.

1. Absent breast development and low FSH
Delayed puberty and amenorrhoea are caused by a central defect. It may also be constitutional, especially where there is a history of delayed menarche in the mother or other siblings. (See Section 2.7)

2. Absent breast development and high FSH
The defect lies in the gonad which has no hormonal or reproductive potential.

A karyotype is required to differentiate:
- Turner syndrome (45XO)—see Section 2.7
- Premature ovarian failure (46XX)
- Swyer syndrome (46XY)—see Section 2.7

These girls have a uterus, which can sometimes be missed on initial assessment because of its small prepubertal size.

3. Normal breast development and high FSH
In this category puberty is arrested. Performing a karyotype and imaging of the pelvis will help differentiate the following two conditions:
- Premature ovarian failure (46XX, uterus present)
- Complete androgen insensitivity (CAIS) (46XY, absent uterus—see Section 2.3)

Patients with CAIS are also identified by the absence of adult type pubic and axillary hair which are androgen-dependent. The vagina is short.

4. Normal breast development and normal FSH
The hypothalamic–pituitary–ovarian axis is normal and the amenorrhoea is caused by an anatomical defect.

Imaging of the pelvis is required to assess the presence of the uterus and to classify the girl in to either of two categories:
- Absent uterus (Mayer–Rokitansky–Kuster–Hauser syndrome, see Section 2.4)
- Obstructive anomaly leading to obstructed menstruation (imperforate hymen, vaginal septum, vaginal agenesis, cervical agenesis)

Management
The management of amenorrhoea depends on the cause.
- Hormone replacement may be required for induction of puberty and to protect from osteoporosis in the long term
- Interventions may be required to expand the vagina to allow sexual intercourse (e.g. in CAIS and MRKH)
- There may be longstanding sexual and fertility implications in all but those due to constitutional delay and imperforate hymen. Psychological support will be necessary to help the adolescent and her family come to terms with the diagnosis
- Fertility can be achieved by assisted conception in the form of ovum donation or surrogacy

Imperforate hymen

Incidence
- 1:4000

Aetiology
Failure of the hymenal septum to perforate in fetal life.

Clinical evaluation

History
- Primary amenorrhoea and cyclical pelvic pain
- Urinary retention secondary to urethral compression from the distended vagina

Examination

At birth
- Hydrocolpos: this is diagnosed either antenatally on ultrasound or at birth as the vagina fills with mucus and becomes palpable abdominally or leads to urinary retention

In adolescence

- Normal secondary sexual characteristics
- Palpable pelvic mass
- Bulging bluish membrane on parting the labia (see Figure 2.10)

Investigations

- Pelvic ultrasound scan
- No further investigation is required except in the cases where a transverse vaginal septum is suspected. In these cases an MRI will localize the level of the obstruction and help plan the operation

Management

Cruciate incision to the hymen (see Figures 2.11 and 2.12).

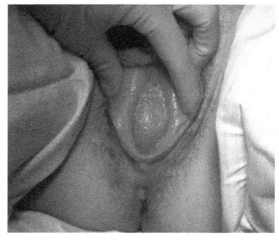

Fig. 2.10 Imperforate hymen.

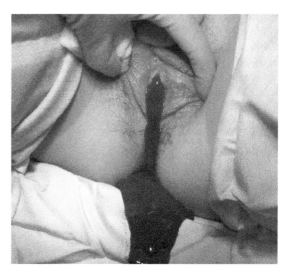

Fig. 2.11 Imperforate hymen after incision with old blood draining.

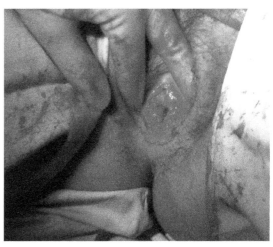

Fig. 2.12 Hymen post-procedure.

2.9 Dysfunctional uterine bleeding and dysmenorrhoea in adolescence

Dysfunctional uterine bleeding (DUB)
(see also Sections 12.3 and 12.4)

Definition
DUB is heavy and irregular menstrual bleeding that occurs secondary to anovulation.

Heavy menstrual bleeding is defined as a menstrual loss of more than 80 ml per cycle.

Aetiology
In the months following menarche the ovary has not yet reached its full maturity, and cycles are usually anovulatory. The endometrium is stimulated from unopposed oestrogen, and becomes thick and unstable. It breaks down, causing bleeding that is both heavy and irregular. Endometrial pathology is rare in this age group.

In certain cases, a bleeding diathesis may first present with menorrhagia.

Incidence
85% of cycles are anovulatory in the first year after menarche.

Clinical evaluation
History
- Irregular and long cycles (>35 days)
- Prolonged bleeding
- Flooding
- Missing school or sporting activities during menses
- Tiredness

Examination
- Signs of anaemia (pallor, tachycardia)

Investigations
- Full blood count
- Thyroid function tests
- Coagulation studies
- Pelvic ultrasound

Management
During menstruation
Antifibrinolytic agents (tranexamic acid) and prostaglandin synthetase inhibitors (mefenamic acid).

Cyclical progestogen
Supplementation with a cyclical progestogen for 6 months to 1 year. This can be done in either of two forms:
- Combined oral contraceptive pill (COCP)
- Cyclical administration of a progestogen for at least 21 days in each cycle

Although norethisterone acetate is a potent progestogen and is very effective in treating DUB, it is also moderately androgenic. Therefore the less potent (and less androgenic) medroxyprogesterone acetate is usually the drug of choice.

Management of acute excessive vaginal bleeding
- Hospital admission
- Resuscitation
- Blood transfusion
- Oral high-dose progestogens (i.e. norethisterone acetate 10 mg TDS), followed by a lower maintenance dose once the bleeding has reduced
- If the progestogens fail to control the bleeding, then IV conjugated oestrogen can be tried (0.625 mg Premarin IV) or
- Recombinant factor VIIa

Dysmenorrhoea
(see also Sections 13.1 and 13.2)

Definition
Pain during menstruation is a common symptom in adolescence. It is usually associated with ovulatory cycles. The pain typically starts a few months to a year after menarche.

Incidence
There are no accurate figures, but it is estimated that up to 60% of adolescents complain of dysmenorrhoea.

Classification
- Primary dysmenorrhoea (present from menarche and is idiopathic)
- Secondary dysmenorrhoea

Pathophysiology
In primary dysmenorrhoea, pain is the result of uterine contractions that occur during menstruation as a response to local release of prostaglandins. Occasionally, the contractions result as a response to heavy menstrual flow.

Secondary dysmenorrhoea can be caused by endometriosis or obstructed menstruation.

Clinical evaluation
History
Pain starting prior to, or at the onset of, menstruation and subsiding by the third day of menstruation.

Investigations
Ultrasound imaging may be required in severe cases to rule out Mullerian obstruction.

Management
Medical treatment
- Mefenamic acid 500 mg TDS PO
- COCP OD PO

Surgical treatment
Where medical treatment has failed, it is reasonable to proceed to further investigation with a diagnostic laparoscopy to rule out endometriosis.

2.10 Menopause

Definitions

Menopause: defined by the World Health Organization (WHO) as the permanent cessation of menstruation resulting from a loss of ovarian follicular activity, after 1 year of amenorrhoea.

It signifies a woman's last menstrual period and therefore the end of her reproductive life.

Premenopause: the time interval leading up to menopause. It is characterized by anovulatory cycles.

Climacteric: the time interval between the reproductive and the non-reproductive life. It encompasses the menopause.

Premature menopause or premature ovarian failure: menopause occurring before a woman is 40 years of age.

Demographic details

The average age for a woman to undergo menopause in the UK is 50.5 years. It occurs earlier in smokers by up to 1 year compared to non-smokers. Unlike menarche, whose average age has decreased over the past decades (see Section 2.6), the age of menopause has remained unchanged.

Premature ovarian failure occurs in approximately 1% of women. The incidence is higher in women with autoimmune disease, Down's, and Turner's syndromes.

Physiology

Unlike sperm production in men, women are born with all of the gametes they will ever produce.

During the fetal period the total number of oocytes is 6–8 million. By birth the number has reduced to 1.5–2 million, and by puberty only 300 000–600 000 are available for ovulation. This number continues to decrease gradually until the late thirties. Beyond this time the number of oocytes dramatically falls until there are no more suitable follicles for reproduction and the menopause ensues. Simultaneously, there is a fall in the ability of the ovary to produce oestrogens (especially oestradiol) and progestogens. This leads to an increase in the level and pulsatile release of FSH from the pituitary in an effort to stimulate the ovary to produce oestrogens. In essence, end-organ failure occurs.

Menopause can also be induced iatrogenically. This occurs as a result of surgery (bilateral oophorectomy), medical therapy (gonadotrophin-releasing hormone (GnRH) analogues), chemotherapy, and radiotherapy. Only surgical menopause is always permanent.

Symptoms are caused by a relatively oestrogen-deficient state and the increase in the pulsatile release of FSH. They are most prevalent in the first 12 months. After this period, the above hormone changes revert back to normal where forms of non-ovary-produced oestrogen predominate.

Diagnosis

In an amenorrhoeic woman over 50 years of age, an FSH level of >30 iu/dl is indicative of menopause. In women <50 years, two FSH levels of >30 iu/dL taken a few weeks apart should be used to diagnose menopause. In this age group it is not unusual for a single raised FSH to be caused by the normal FSH/LH surge (see Section 12.1).

Clinical evaluation

History

Vasomotor instability

- Hot flushes
- Night sweats

These (especially hot flushes) are caused by the increase in the pulsatile release of FSH. Eventually, levels revert to normal and the vasomotor instability subsides.

Genital symptoms

- Dyspareunia
- Vulval itching
- Prolapse

These are due to vaginal atrophy and dryness.

Urological symptoms (50% of women)

- Urinary frequency
- Dysuria
- Recurrent UTIs
- Urinary incontinence (occasionally)

Psychological

All of which may be the result of disturbed sleep.

- Fatigue
- Depression
- Mood instability
- Decreased libido
- Insomnia
- Short-term memory loss

The nature, severity, and duration of symptoms vary widely between women.

Examination

Findings are variable and depend on when the woman is seen in relation to the onset of menopause. The vulva, vagina, and cervix are commonly atrophic (see Figure 2.13).

Investigations

LH and FSH blood serum levels. Premenopausal values are 3–10 iu/dl on days 3–5 of the cycle.

Management

Approximately 10% of women seek medical help.

The main aim is symptom relief. Treatments are varied and many are untested. These include pharmacological agents, alternative therapies, psychological support, and lifestyle alterations. The diversity of existing methods is a sign that no one good treatment option exists when dealing with this unavoidable stage in a woman's life.

Hormone replacement therapy (HRT)

This includes combined HRT (an oestrogen with a progestogen) and oestrogen-only HRT (see Section 2.11).

Topical vaginal oestrogens

These can aid in relieving genital symptoms caused by atrophy, e.g. dyspareunia (**A**). Systemic absorption is minimal, thus they can be used in women with an intact uterus. See also vaginal atrophy in Section 13.9.

Venlafaxine

Venlafaxine is a serotonin and noradrenaline reuptake inhibitor. It has been shown to have a beneficial effect on vasomotor symptoms. However, many women find that the associated nausea outweighs the benefits.

Clonidine

Clonidine is an α-agonist. Once the mainstay of treatment, it has now been shown to have a limited effect on vasomotor symptoms.

Selective oestrogen reuptake modulators (SERMs)

See Section 2.11.

Tibolone

Tibolone is a synthetic steroid which has weak oestrogenic, progestogenic, and androgenic action. It has a beneficial effect on hot flushes (**A**) and vaginal atrophy (**B**). Long-term effects, e.g. breast cancer, are unknown.

Exercise
Evidence shows that regular aerobic exercise such as swimming and walking can relieve menopausal symptoms.

Diet
Diets high in antioxidants and low in caffeine and alcohol have a positive effect on vasomotor symptoms.

Phytoestrogens
These are naturally occurring oestrogen-like compounds. They have been proven to reduce hot flushes greatly. Large amounts are present in soya.

Red clover (Trifolium pratense)
Five randomized controlled trials (RCTs) concerning its use have shown improvement in the vasomotor symptoms of menopause.

St John's Wort (Hypericum perforatum)
This reduces the psychological symptoms of menopause. It is thought that this is because of its SSRI-like (selective serotonin reuptake inhibitor) effect. It has not been proven to relieve the vasomotor symptoms.

Acupuncture
A small RCT showed a significant reduction in vasomotor symptoms in women who use acupuncture for treatment of menopausal symptoms. However, subsequent studies have not confirmed these findings.

Other herbal remedies
Other herbal remedies include Ginkgo biloba, ginseng, dong quai, black cohash, and evening primrose oil.

With the exception of HRT and SERMs, no other treatments have been shown to prevent osteoporosis. It should be noted that there are recognized drug interactions with the herbal remedies, and little is known of the ideal minimal dosage or long-term effects.

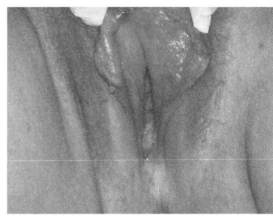

Fig. 2.13 Atrophic vulva. Note the pallor and dryness.

2.11 Hormone replacement therapy

Definition
HRT is the exogenous administration of female sex hormones to replace those that the body no longer produces.

Physiology
The purpose of HRT is primarily to replace oestrogens. This decreases the pulsatile release of FSH (by negative feedback), leading to reduction of the vasomotor symptoms. In addition, oestrogen replacement directly reverses vaginal atrophy.

Unopposed oestrogens cause endometrial hyperplasia which increases the risk of endometrial carcinoma. Progestogen prevents the development of endometrial hyperplasia. Therefore any woman with an intact uterus should be prescribed combined HRT, containing both an oestrogen and a progestogen.

Combined HRT can be given either as a continuous regimen (oestrogen and progesterone daily) or a sequential one (oestrogen daily with progestogen 10–14 days per month). The latter causes monthly withdrawal bleeding.

Controversies surrounding HRT
Recently there has been much controversy regarding HRT. It was previously prescribed for both symptom relief and for osteoporosis prevention. HRT was prescribed for up to 10 years in some cases. However, recent research has linked the use of HRT with an increased risk of breast cancer and venous thromboembolism.

Osteoporosis and HRT
Osteoporosis is a disease characterized by low bone mass and deterioration of bone tissue. The WHO (World Health Organization) defines osteoporosis as a bone density of more than 2.5 standard deviations below the average adult mean. It is assessed by dual energy X-ray absorption (DEXA), usually of the lower spine or head of femur. Postmenopausal women with osteoporosis are recommended to take 1500 mg of calcium and 400–800 iu of vitamin D daily.

New drugs such as bisphosphonates, which inhibit osteoclasts, are replacing HRT as first line prevention of osteoporosis. SERMs (selective oestrogen reuptake modulators) were previously thought to have no effect on the endometrium. However, a recent large scale study suggests otherwise. Caution should therefore be used in prescribing these to postmenopausal women.

Duration of treatment
Between 40 and 50% of women discontinue treatment within 1 year of starting and 65–70% within 2 years.

Counselling women prior to prescribing HRT
- Fully inform of intended benefits as well as risks of taking HRT (see Box 2.4)
- Indications are: hot flushes, night sweats, and vaginal dryness (A)
- It prevents osteoporosis and fractures but it is not a first line treatment for these
- It prevents colorectal cancer with a risk reduction of one-third. However, this is unquantified in the high-risk groups and it is unknown what happens once HRT is stopped. Thus, prevention of colorectal cancer is not a recommendation
- Should not be used for the prevention of myocardial infarction or Alzheimer's disease
- It increases the risk of breast cancer
- It increases the risk of venous thromboembolism (VTE). The risk increases 2-fold with the highest risk in first year. However, absolute risk is small (background is 1.7 per 1000 women over 50 years not on HRT per year). In a woman with a personal history of VTE, HRT should be avoided. SERMs carry the same risk. (RCOG Green Top Guideline No. 19)
- It increases the risk of endometrial cancer if oestrogen-only HRT is used with an intact uterus
- It increases the risk of (mainly ischaemic) cerebrovascular accidents
- It increases the risk of coronary heart disease
- It increases the risk of dementia (women >65 years old) and gallbladder disease
- Use for shortest time possible (<5 years). Long-term use should be assessed on an individual basis annually
- In premature menopause, use until the average age of menopause
- Contraindicated in breast cancer
- Use with a progestogen if the woman has an intact uterus
- If postmenopausal for over a year, then continuous regimens can be used. Prior to this, sequential regimens should be used to prevent irregular bleeding (ovarian oestrogen production is still fluctuating)
- HRT is not a contraceptive. Even though fertility is reduced after the age of 40 years, perimenopausal women taking HRT should also use appropriate contraception

HRT comes in a variety of forms. Tablets, patches, gels, and implants are all widely used. The most appropriate form depends on the patient.

> **Box 2.4 Summary of risks and benefits of combined HRT**
>
> For every 10 000 women taking combined HRT per year
> - 8 more will develop breast cancer
> - 6 more will have a heart attack
> - 7 more will have a stroke
> - 18 more will develop a thromboembolism
> - 1.5 more will develop ovarian cancer
> - 5 fewer will have a hip fracture
> - 6 fewer will develop colorectal cancer
>
> Source: Women's Health Initiative study

Further reading
www.consensus.nih.gov State of the Science Conference on Management of Menopause-Related Symptoms 2005.

www.rcog.org Menopause and hormone replacement—study group statement. Chapter 29. Consensus views arising from the 47th study group: menopause and hormone replacement 2004.

www.rcog.org.uk RCOG Green Top Guideline 19. Hormone replacement therapy and venous thromboembolism 2004.

www.the-bms.org The British Menopause society.

→ Box 2.5 Landmark research

The million women study (www.millionwomenstudy.org)

Study design

A multicentre, population-based prospective cohort study of women aged 50 years and over invited to routine breast cancer screening in the UK. It examined general reproductive health and specifically the effect of HRT on breast and endometrial cancers compared to never-users.

Outcomes

These are a selected few; for further outcomes see www.million womenstudy.org.

Breast cancer

Although the connection of breast cancer and HRT was previously known, this was the first trial to quantify the risk.

- The background incidence of breast cancer in postmenopausal women is 32 cases per 1000 women
- There were 5 extra cases per 1000 women after 10 years of oestrogen-only HRT usage
- There were 19 extra cases per 1000 women after 10 years of combined oestrogen/progesterone HRT usage
- Neither the method of administration nor the pattern (cyclical versus continuous) influences the risk

Endometrial cancer

- The background incidence of endometrial cancer is 5 cases per 1000 postmenopausal women aged between 50 and 65 years
- There were 2 fewer cases per 1000 women on continuous combined oestrogen/progestogen HRT between the ages 50 and 65 years
- There were 4 extra cases per 1000 postmenopausal women on oestrogen-only HRT between the ages 50 and 65 years

Criticism of the study

- Poorly designed trial. Previous oestradiol use was not accounted for. Even women who had recently stopped oestradiol were included in the never-used oestradiol group
- The risk of endometrial cancer persists for many years after the cessation of HRT, which is not the case for breast cancer
- The background incidence of breast cancer was reported to be lower in both the perimenopausal and postmenopausal groups compared to the premenopausal group, even though the incidence of breast cancer increases with increasing age

→ Box 2.6 Landmark research

Women's Health Initative (WHI) study (www.whi.org)

Study design

A multicentre, prospective cohort study looking at the general health in postmenopausal women in the USA. Through RCTs it assessed the effect of HRT, diet modification, calcium, and vitamin D supplements on heart disease, fractures, breast, and colorectal cancer. The duration of the study is approximately 6 years.

Outcomes

These are a selected few; for further outcomes see www.whi.org.

Breast cancer

Combined oestrogen and progestogen given to women with an intact uterus.

- 245 of the 8506 women on combined HRT, and 185 of the 8102 women on placebo, developed breast cancer, resulting in a 28% increase in risk of breast cancer with combined HRT

Oestrogen-only, given to women who had a hysterectomy.

- The rate of breast cancer in this group was 28 of 10 000 per year versus 34 of 10 000 per year in the placebo group. The difference is not statistically significant

Venous thromboembolism (VTE)

Combined oestrogen and progestogen

- Over the period of the study, 167 women given combined HRT (3.5 per 1000 person years) and 76 given placebo (1.7 per 1000 person years) developed VTE, or, 18 in 10 000 additional women developed VTE per year when using combined HRT

Oestrogen-only

- 111 women given oestrogen-only (30 of 10 000 per year) and 86 women given placebo (22 of 10 000 per year) developed a VTE. The risk was highest during the first 2 years from commencement of HRT

Cerebrovascular accident

Strokes are increased regardless of years since menopause and when HRT is commenced.

Coronary heart disease

Risk is not increased if HRT is started <10 years after the menopause, but there is an increased risk if commenced later.

As this is a prospective trial, results are constantly being released and updated.

Criticism of the study

- The average age of the participants was 62.5 years old. This is significantly higher than the average age of 50.5 years at which a woman goes through the menopause
- The participants were not appropriately screened and therefore there were women with significant co-morbidities such as hypertension and previous malignancy

2.12 Postmenopausal bleeding

Definition
Postmenopausal bleeding (PMB) is defined as vaginal bleeding in a woman 12 months or more after her last menstrual cycle.

Incidence
- A common complaint, accounting for 5% of gynaecology outpatients clinic visits annually
- Average age for referral is 60–69 years
- It is important to exclude endometrial hyperplasia and cancer. It is estimated that a GP will see one case of endometrial cancer every 6–8 years, although the incidence is rising
- Abnormal perimenopausal bleeding, including postcoital or intermenstrual loss, needs to be investigated
- The majority (90%) of cases of PMB are due to benign conditions

Clinical evaluation
History
- Full obstetric and gynaecology history, including LMP, menarche, and smear history
- Past medical history, including clotting disorder and previous malignancy
- Family history of gynaecological malignancies
- Drug history, including anticoagulants or aspirin, use of HRT and Tamoxifen

Examination
- Abdominal examination for the presence of masses
- Bimanual vaginal examination for adnexal masses
- Speculum examination looking for cervical lesions, trauma or evidence of vaginal atrophy

Investigations
- FBC
- Coagulation screen (if appropriate)
- Transvaginal ultrasound scan (TVS)
- Endometrial biopsy, e.g. Pipelle™ biopsy
- Hysteroscopy (outpatient or day case procedure) ± endometrial biopsy

Management
An endometrial thickness measurement of 5 mm or less is associated with endometrial atrophy. Irrespective of HRT use, 96% of women with endometrial cancer, and 92% of women with endometrial disease (hyperplasia, polyps, and submucous fibroids), will have an abnormal endometrial thickness (>5 mm).

The high sensitivity of TVS makes it an effective non-invasive test for triaging women with vaginal bleeding who do not require endometrial biopsy.

Conversely, its relatively poor specificity means that an abnormal endometrial thickness measurement needs to be followed up by a second stage test in the form of either an outpatient endometrial biopsy with a Pipelle™ (see also Section 12.3) or with a hysteroscopy (see also section 12.7 and 15.5).

Endometrium >5 mm or recurrent episodes of bleeding
(see Figures 2.14 and 2.15)
Hysteroscopy and endometrial biopsy are indicated.

If submucous fibroids and endometrial polyps are found, they should be resected as a day case procedure (see also Section 12.7).

Anaemia should be treated with oral iron supplements. Those who are symptomatic (and Hb <7 g/dl) should be considered for a blood transfusion.

In suspected endometrial cancer, refer to the gynaecological oncologist when the histology is available; see Figure 2.16 (also see Section 15.5).

Endometrium <5 mm (see Figure 2.16)
No need for further investigation.

Unless bleeding persists, the majority of patients with no abnormality on TVS will have an atrophic genital tract on speculum examination consistent with atrophic vaginitis. This may be treated with a short course of topical oestrogen—unless contraindicated (e.g. previous irritation, previous breast cancer). The role topical oestrogens play in the development of endometrial cancer is uncertain, hence yearly review is recommended. If there has been no further PMB, treatment may be stopped. Vaginal moisturizers can be used in some cases (e.g. Replens® which has a high pH and keeps the vagina moisturized for 2–3 days).

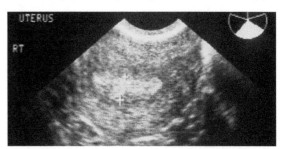

Fig. 2.15 Thick endometrium measuring 6.6 mm. Hysteroscopy revealed a normal uterine cavity and no evidence of malignancy on biopsy.

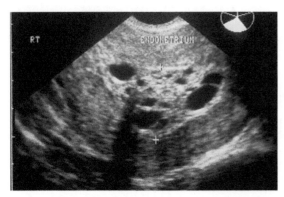

Fig. 2.14 Thick, cystic endometrium measuring 26 mm. Pipelle™ biopsy in clinic revealed endometrial cancer.

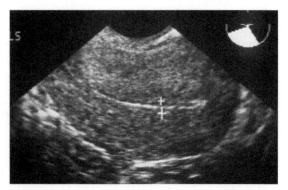

Fig. 2.16 Thin endometrium measuring 3.2 mm. Atrophic vaginitis was treated with topical oestrogen. There were no subsequent episodes of PMB.

Chapter 3

Sexual health

Contents

Covered elsewhere

49

3.1 Vaginal discharge—general approach

This is a common presenting complaint. It may be physiological or pathological.

Pathophysiology

The normal flora of the vagina changes under the influence of oestrogen. The presence of oestrogen leads to a glycogen-rich environment, which favours acid-tolerant organisms and lactobacilli. Glycogen is broken down to lactic acid, causing the pH of the vagina to be <4.5. Other bacteria commonly present include:

- Anaerobic cocci
- Diphtheroids
- Coagulase-negative staphylococci
- α-haemolytic streptococci

Some colonizing organisms are potential pathogens:

- β-haemolytic streptococci, e.g. *Strep. agalactiae*
- *Actinomyces* spp.

The vagina has a delicate environment and anything that can upset the balance may lead to the lactobacilli being lost, e.g. douching, the use of strongly perfumed soaps, etc. Other flora can then increase which may lead to bacterial vaginosis.

Women who have symptoms of vaginal discharge are often worried about sexually transmitted infections (STIs). However, vaginal discharge is poorly predictive of an STI.

Demographics

All women of reproductive age will have normal physiological discharge and this will vary throughout their cycle. A careful history of changes throughout the month may discover the discharge is physiological (see Section 4.7).

75% of women will have discharge secondary to vulvovaginal candidiasis at some point during their reproductive life.

Aetiology

The causes of vaginal discharge are:

Physiological

The quality and quantity may alter in cycles, over time, and with hormonal influences, e.g. menarche, the combined oral contraceptive pill, pregnancy and menopause

Infective

- Candida albicans
- Bacterial vaginosis

STIs:

- Trichomonas vaginalis
- Chlamydia trachomatis
- β-haemolytic streptococcus
- Neisseria gonorrhoeae
- Cervical herpes (primary infection)
- Cervical warts
- Syphilitic chancre
- Toxic shock syndrome
- Mycoplasmas

Non-infective

- Cervical ectropion
- Cervical polyps
- Neoplasm
- Retained products of conception
- Retained tampon or foreign body in vagina
- Oestrogen deficiency
- Trauma

- Allergy
- Fistulae

Clinical assessment

History

Full gynaecological, cervical smear, obstetric, and medical history.

Important points about the discharge:

- Colour
- Consistency
- Amount
- Odour (enquire if it changes after sex)
- Onset
- Duration
- Similar symptoms before
- Change with cycle
- Exacerbating factors
- Any recent change in contraception, e.g. COCP, POP, coil
- Associated symptoms, e.g. itching, dyspareunia, dysuria, fever, intermenstrual or postmenopausal bleeding (IMB or PCB)
- Current medications, e.g. antibiotics, immunosuppressives
- Diabetes

A full sexual history should be taken sensitively and in confidence, warning the woman that she can expect some personal questions. Always invite people who are attending with the woman to leave.

Points in the history which may indicate an STI are:

- Multiple partners in the last 6 months (usual length of contact tracing)
- Recent partner change
- Unprotected sexual intercourse with a new partner or a number of partners
- Recurrent symptoms
- Symptoms in the partner
- Other symptoms such as abdominal pain, menstrual problems, postcoital bleeding (PCB), rash, dyspareunia, arthralgia

Useful tip

Explore the woman's concerns and expectations. She is less likely to re-present with physiological discharge if listened to.

Examination

- External inspection of the genitalia for colour, odour, and erythema
- Speculum examination: structures (lateral walls, cervix), discharge (amount, consistency, colour, area affected, e.g. anterior or posterior fornix). Remember to exclude foreign bodies, and triple swabs should be taken at the same time (see below)
- Bimanual examination, if indicated, to assess cervical excitation, adnexal tenderness, and uterine tenderness. If present consider pelvic inflammatory disease (PID)
- Abdominal palpation

Investigations

Referral to a genitourinary medicine (GUM) clinic is ideal for thorough investigation of those thought to be at risk of STIs.

- Swabs should be sent for microscopy, culture, and sensitivity. Chlamydia swabs can be sent for nucleic acid amplification technique tests (see Figure 3.1)

High vaginal swab (HVS) to test for bacterial vaginosis (BV), candidiasis, and *Trichomonas vaginalis*.

This should be taken from the lateral walls and posterior fornix. It may be transported in charcoal medium immediately to the laboratory. If not, store at 4°C for up to 48 h. The swab is then used for microscopy, Gram stain slide to look for candida and BV. Wet microscopy can be prepared by dipping the HVS into saline which can identify candidal pseudohyphae and *Trichomonas*. The HVS is then plated on medium for culture.

Endocervical swab to test for chlamydia.

Endocervical charcoal swab to test for gonorrhoea.

As gonorrhoea infects the columnar cells, an endocervical swab should ideally be taken for microscopy, culture, and sensitivities.

- Microscopy, if in a GU clinic, of dry and wet slides can be done at the time of examination
- pH of the vagina if no bleeding at the time
- Cervical smear, if indicated
- Urine dipstick and MSU
- If the patient does not want to be examined, vulvovaginal swabs can be self-taken or a first void urine sent for chlamydia testing
- Serological tests for syphilis if any ulceration is seen
- Swabs for herpes simplex if ulcers are seen
- HIV test

Management

This depends on the cause and is discussed individually in Sections 3.2 and 3.3.

It is important to treat based on a diagnosis from tests rather than on the clinical appearance of the discharge.

Persistent discharge with negative cervical cytology and STI screen results can be difficult to manage. It is worth considering:

- Spermicides and lubricants which worsen the symptoms. If so, change method of contraception
- If there is a cervical ectropion (with normal cervical cytology), intravaginal acetic acid and, occasionally, cryocautery may be used for symptom relief
- Menopausal atrophy increases the likelihood of infective vaginitis, so topical use of oestrogen creams may improve the condition of the epithelium and reduce susceptibility

- Underlying gynaecological disease, e.g. endometrial polyps and malignancy
- Psychosexual causes

Useful Tips

Swabs for STIs can be taken during menstruation. Bacterial vaginosis, *Trichomonas vaginalis*, and candidiasis are difficult to exclude while menstruating, and the pH of the vagina cannot be assessed. However, gonorrhoea and chlamydia tests are reliable. The patient may prefer not to be examined while menstruating. Follow-up should be offered.

If not in a GUM clinic it is important to explain what you are testing for and how the results are obtained. How will the patient receive treatment and how will partner notification take place if the results show an STI? As there is a social stigma around STIs, the GUM clinic setting with trained health advisors is ideal.

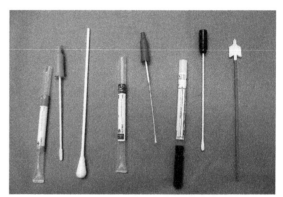

Fig. 3.1 Examples of commonly used swabs. From left → right: pink swab used for endocervical sampling for chlamydia testing with swab to clean cervical mucus prior to sampling; blue swab used for urethral chlamydia test in men; charcoal swab used for taking HVS and endocervical sample for gonorrhoea; cervical brush for smear sampling.

3.2 Vaginal discharge—bacterial vaginosis and thrush

Bacterial vaginosis (BV)

Demographics
BV is the commonest cause of abnormal discharge in women of childbearing age. The prevalence ranges from 5 to 50% depending on the population. In the UK, the condition can be found in 12% of pregnant women attending antenatal clinic and in 30% of women undergoing termination. It is commoner in sexually active women, black women, smokers, and those with an IUCD.

Pathophysiology
BV is not an STI but is caused by an overgrowth of predominantly anaerobic organisms, e.g. *Gardnerella vaginalis*, *Prevotella* species, and *Mycoplasma hominis* in the vagina. These replace the lactobacilli and alter the pH of the vagina, increasing it to as high as 7.0. It can resolve spontaneously.

Presentation
Symptoms and signs
- Offensive fishy smelling discharge, often worse after intercourse
- Not usually associated with vulval itching or irritation
- Thin white or grey discharge in the vagina which may be offensive smelling

Diagnosis
There are different criteria for diagnosis.
- Amsel criteria: at least three of the following four
  - characteristic discharge
  - clue cells on wet slide microscopy
  - pH >4.5
  - fishy odour on adding alkali to slide
- Hay and Ison criteria look at the vaginal smear microscopy; from normal with lactobacilli, ranging through to grade 3, which is BV with few or absent lactobacilli. This spectrum of normal to BV means some women who have symptoms will have intermediate grade flora on microscopy. If they are symptomatic they should be treated

Management
- Advise against douching and using feminine hygiene products, strong soaps or shower gels, etc.
- Reassure patients regarding the normal flora in the vagina and how delicate the area is. Support to change behaviours is required
- If symptomatic or undergoing a surgical procedure, the woman should be treated with one of the following:
  - metronidazole 400–500 mg BD PO 7 days
  - metronidazole 2 g stat PO
  - intravaginal metronidazole gel OD for 5 days
  - intravaginal clindamycin cream 2% OD for 7 days
  - clindamycin 300 mg BD PO for 7 days
- The cure rates are 70–80%
- Patients should be warned not to use alcohol while taking metronidazole and for 48 h afterwards
- Clindamycin cream can weaken condoms, so another contraceptive method should be used
- For recurrent BV treatment options, include metronidazole at the beginning and end of each period and Aci-Jel at menstruation, but it can be difficult to control
- There is no evidence to support treating partners

Complications
- Having BV may be predictive of subsequent PID associated with gonorrhoea or chlamydia
- Associated with post-termination endometritis
- Vaginal cuff cellulitis after vaginal hysterectomy
- Recurrence is common

In pregnancy
BV is associated with, but not causative of, late miscarriage, pre-term birth, preterm premature rupture of membranes, and postpartum endometritis. Symptomatic women should be treated with metronidazole. There is no evidence to support routine antenatal swabs and treatment in asymptomatic women to prevent pre-term birth.

Candida albicans (thrush)

Demographics
Over 75% of women will suffer with vulvovaginal candidiasis at some point, some recurrently. It can be exacerbated by antibiotic treatment and synthetic underwear, and is commoner in diabetic patients.

Pathophysiology
Candida is a yeast that can be found as a commensal organism. It may or may not be sexually transmitted. It may overgrow or it may colonize the vagina by spread from the perineum and perianal area, causing an infection. This happens especially if the normal flora of the vagina is affected by antibiotics. Vulvovaginal candidiasis is caused by *Candida albicans* in 80–92% of cases, but other species can cause it, e.g. *Candida glabrata*.

Presentation
Symptoms and signs
- Vulval itching
- Soreness
- Vaginal discharge, which may be curdy and thick
- Superficial dyspareunia
- External dysuria (from local irritation to skin)
- Erythema
- Fissuring
- Satellite lesions, small white plaques
- Oedema of vulva

Investigations
- pH of vagina 4.0–4.5
- Microscopy from anterior fornix or lateral wall may show spores or pseudohyphae (see Figure 3.2)
- Culture on Sabouraud's medium via high vaginal swab (HVS)

Management
- Avoid local irritants, e.g. perfumed products
- Cotton underwear advised
- Treat a positive swab result, if symptomatic. Around 10–20% of women who may harbour Candida are asymptomatic
- All topical and oral azole therapies are 80–95% effective
- Pessaries should be used at night and the patient should be warned to expect increased discharge
- The effect of most pessaries on latex barrier methods of contraception is not known but may be damaging. Inform patients to abstain or use alternative contraception

Complications
- Recurrence, defined as four or more symptomatic episodes yearly, occurs in <5% of women with candidiasis. It is associated with diabetes, immunodeficiency, corticosteroid use, and antibiotic therapy. Treatment can be maintenance, e.g. fluconazole 100 mg

weekly for 6 months or clotrimazole pessary 500 mg weekly for 6 months

In pregnancy
- Asymptomatic colonization is common (30–40%)
- Symptomatic candidiasis is commoner throughout
- Treatment with topical azoles is recommended
- Longer courses may be necessary
- Oral treatment is contraindicated

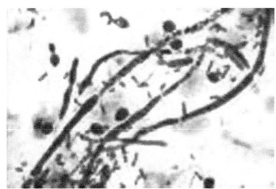

Fig. 3.2 Gram smear of *Candida* spores and pseudohyphae. Reproduced with permission from *The Oxford Handbook of Genitourinary Medicine, HIV, and AIDS*, edited by R Pattman et al. ©Oxford University Press, 2005.

Further reading

McDonald H et al. Antibiotics for treating BV in pregnancy. *Cochrane Database of Systematic Reviews* 2005; **1:** Art no CD000262.

Young GL, Jewell D. Topical treatment for vaginal candidiasis in pregnancy. *Cochrane Database of Systematic Reviews* 2000; **2:**CD225.

www.bashh.org.uk British association for sexual health and HIV.

www.hpa.org.uk Health Protection Agency for latest prevalence figures for infections.

3.3 Vaginal discharge—gonorrhoea, trichomonas, and chlamydia

Gonorrhoea

Demographics
There were estimated to be 62 million cases of gonorrhoea globally in 1995. There were 18,700 new cases diagnosed in the UK in 2007 (Health Protection Agency figures).

Pathophysiology
Neisseria gonorrhoea is a sexually transmitted Gram-negative diplococcus which infects the mucous membranes of the urethra, endocervix, rectum, pharynx, and conjunctiva. It is also known to infect vaginal epithelium in prepubescent girls. It infects the columnar epithelium in these sites. It can also infect Bartholin's glands. The incubation period is 3 days.

Presentation
Symptoms and signs
- ~50% asymptomatic
- Mucopurulent vaginal discharge (commonest symptom, in up to 50%)
- Lower abdominal pain may be present (up to 25%)
- Dysuria (12%) but not frequency
- IMB ± PCB
- Easily induced endocervical bleeding on examination
- Pelvic or low abdominal tenderness (<5%)
- No abnormal findings on examination

Investigations
Microscopy and culture are the commonly used diagnostic methods. Microscopy can directly visualize Gram-negative diplococci and facilitate early treatment. Nucleic acid amplification tests (NAATs) can be used but are not routine in most hospitals.

Endocervical swabs are the gold standard. Self-taken vulvovaginal swabs and urine can be used to test using a NAAT.

Management
- Full sexual health screen
- Partner notification covering the preceding 3 months (dependent on the sexual history)
- Avoid sex until clear and partner has been treated
- Treat uncomplicated infection with a stat dose of ceftriaxone 250 mg IM or cefixime 400 mg PO or spectinomycin 2 g IM
- Gonorrhoea may be resistant to penicillin and ciprofloxacin; most resistant infections are acquired in the UK
- Data for 2004 show 11% resistance to penicillin, 45% to tetracyclines, and 14% to ciprofloxacin
- Local treatment regimens should be consulted
- Up to 40% of women also have chlamydia, so concurrent treatment for chlamydia is recommended
- Follow-up should be offered to confirm resolution of symptoms, to enquire about compliance and adverse reactions, and to complete partner notification
- A test of cure should be at least 3 days after treatment if culture or 2 weeks after treatment if using NAATs

Complications
- PID (<10%)
- Haematogenous spread to infect skin and joints leading to arthralgia, arthritis, and tenosynovitis
- Disseminated gonococcal infection is rare (<1%)

In pregnancy
It is important to treat as it can cause infection in the neonate and endometritis in the mother. The above antibiotic regimens can be used, as can amoxicillin plus probenecid—no one regimen has been shown to be more effective than another.

In the neonate
The infections caused are:
- Gonococcal ophthalmia neonatorum (notifiable)—usually appears within 21 days of delivery
- Disseminated gonococcal infection causing sepsis and arthritis. Usually presents 7–28 days after delivery
- Scalp abscess has been described following use of a fetal scalp electrode (FSE)
- Vaginitis, proctitis, and urethritis have been described
- Partner notification—the parents should be screened
- Notifiable disease

Trichomonas

Demographics
Trichomonas vaginalis (TV) is less common than chlamydia and gonorrhoea, with 6000 new cases diagnosed in 2007 in the UK.

Pathophysiology
TV is an STI. The protozoan parasite may be found in the vagina, urethra, and Bartholin's glands. The incubation period is 4 to 28 days.

Presentation
Symptoms and signs
- Asymptomatic (10–50%)
- Vaginal discharge in up to 70%. (Tip: the classical frothy yellow discharge only occurs in 10–30% of these)
- Vaginal itching
- Dysuria and low abdominal pain
- Offensive odour
- Vulvitis and vaginitis
- 2% have the classical 'strawberry cervix'
- Between 5 and 15% will have no examination abnormalities

Investigations
- Direct observation of wet smear slide from posterior fornix
- Culture will be positive in 95%
- Trichomonads can be seen on cervical smears
- More recent polymerase chain reaction (PCR)-based diagnostic tests have sensitivities and specificities approaching 100%

Management
- Avoid sex until both partners treated
- Full sexual health screen
- Metronidazole 2 g stat PO or 400–500 mg BD PO for 7 days is the recommended regimen, with a cure rate of 95%
- Spontaneous cure rate without treatment is 20%
- It is important to advise patients on metronidazole to avoid alcohol for 48 h after treatment because of the possibility of disulfiram-like reaction with vomiting

- For resistant infections, seek advice from genitourinary medicine (GUM). Successful treatments include high dose metronidazole IV and nonoxinol pessaries

Complications
- Enhanced HIV transmission
- Problems in pregnancy

In pregnancy
- TV is associated with pre-term delivery and low birth weight
- Metronidazole is relatively contraindicated in the first trimester, although there is no data showing increased teratogenicity. The benefit of systemic treatment is likely to outweigh the risk.

In the neonate
Neonates may develop a vulvovaginitis as a result of passing through the vagina of an infected mother (5%). Infection beyond the first year of life suggests sexual contact and this should be investigated.

Chlamydia

Demographics
Chlamydia is the commonest curable STI. In the UK in 2007 approximately 122,000 new cases were diagnosed (Health Protection Agency figures). Between 5 and 10% of women <24 years in the UK are currently thought to be infected. It is frequently asymptomatic, and ongoing transmission in the community is therefore sustained.

Pathophysiology
Infection is through penetrative sexual intercourse. The *Chlamydia trachomatis* bacterium is an obligate intracellular organism. It attaches to, and is internalized in, endocytic vesicles. It can infect the cervix, urethra, rectum, Bartholin's glands, pharynx, and eye. Infections may persist or resolve spontaneously. The incubation period ranges from 1 day to 6 weeks.

Presentation
Symptoms and signs
- Asymptomatic in 70%
- PCB or IMB
- Lower abdominal and pelvic pain
- Purulent vaginal discharge
- Mucopurulent cervicitis, contact bleeding on swab or smear
- Dysuria

Investigations
Nucleic acid amplification tests (NAATs) are the gold standard (95% sensitivity). They are more sensitive and specific than enzyme immunoassays.

If unconfirmed result, treat and retest.

Ideally:
- Endocervical swab—rotate the swab 360° in the os
- Vulvovaginal self-taken swab (sensitivity of 90%)
- Urine samples can be taken, using first catch specimen (sensitivities vary from 65 to 100%)

Useful tip
NAATs remain positive in treated individuals up to 5 weeks after treatment. This may represent the presence of nucleic acid from non-viable organisms rather than active infection.

Management
- First line treatment is a stat dose of azithromycin 1 g PO or 7 days of doxycycline 100 mg BD PO
- Alternatively, erythromycin 500 mg BD PO for 14 days/ofloxacin 200 mg BD PO or 400 mg OD PO for 7 days
- Partner notification for previous 6 months or, if no change of partner in past 6 months, most recent partner
- Abstain from sex until 7 days after both partners treated

- Full sexual health screen ideal
- No indication for removal of IUCD unless severe PID
- Test of cure is only recommended in pregnant or breastfeeding women; after azithromycin or doxycycline treatment >95% will be negative on retesting

Complications
- PID in 10–40% of those untreated
- Tubal infertility
- Ectopic pregnancy
- Chronic pelvic pain
- Fitz-Hugh-Curtis syndrome (Figure 3.3 and Section 3.9)
- Reactive arthritis

In pregnancy
- No good evidence that chlamydia is associated with early pregnancy loss
- There is an association with ectopic pregnancy
- An association exists with premature rupture of membranes and low birth weight. Treatment improves the outcome
- If positive, treat with erythromycin 500 mg QDS PO 7 days first line or amoxicillin 500 mg TDS PO 7 days. Azithromycin 1 g PO stat is unlicenced hence use with caution
- After treatment, the woman must have a test of cure, i.e. a retest 6 weeks after treatment

In the neonate
- Transmission to the neonate at birth can cause neonatal conjunctivitis ± pneumonia
- Studies have shown that up to 50% of babies develop an eye infection and 10–20% a pneumonia after normal vaginal delivery in a woman with cervical infection
- Symptomless vaginal and rectal infection is found in ~15% of these neonates and can persist for up to 1 year or longer
- Chlamydia found in older children raises the suspicion of sexual contact. It is a notifiable disease

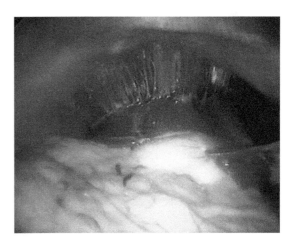

Fig. 3.3 Laparoscopic view of perihepatic adhesions seen in Fitz-Hugh-Curtis syndrome.

Further reading

Brocklehurst P. Antibiotics for gonorrhoea in pregnancy. *Cochrane Database of Systematic Reviews* 2002; **2**: CD000098.

Brocklehurst P. Interventions for treating genital *Chlamydia trachomatis* infection in pregnancy. *Cochrane Database of Systematic Reviews* 2006; **4**: CD000054.

3.4 Vulval ulceration

This is a common presenting complaint of concern to patients which may have a huge impact on their sexual function.

Aetiology

Infective

- Herpes simplex
- Syphilis (primary and secondary)
- *Neisseria gonorrhoeae*
- *Trichomonas vaginalis* vaginitis
- Severe candidiasis (immunocompromised)
- Herpes zoster affecting the lumbar or spinal roots
- *Chlamydia trachomatis* and lymphogranuloma venereum (common in tropical countries)
- Tuberculosis
- Cytomegalovirus
- Chancroid (commoner in developing world, caused by *Haemophilus ducreyii*)
- Donovanosis of granuloma inguinale (caused by *Klebsiella granulomatis*, commoner in developing world)
- *Schistosoma haematobium*

Non-infective

- Eczema or dermatitis
- Lichen planus (see Section 13.10)
- Lichen sclerosus (see Section 13.9)
- Stevens–Johnson syndrome
- Vulval squamous cell carcinoma (see Section 15.11)
- Vulval intraepithelial neoplasia (see Section 15.11)
- Trauma
- Crohn's disease
- Aphthous ulcers
- Behcet's disease
- Pemphigus vulgaris
- Pemphigoid
- Strachan's syndrome (orogenital ulceration, sensory neuropathy, amblyopia of unknown aetiology)
- Drugs, e.g. foscarnet (used to treat CMV infection in immunocompromised patients)
- Idiopathic

The commonest causes in the UK are herpes, severe candidiasis, and trauma. Most other causes are very rare.

The incidence of syphilis in the UK is increasing.

Clinical assessment

History

- Onset
- Duration
- Single lesion or multiple
- Site
- Previous similar episodes
- Exudate
- Itching
- Pain or no pain
- Symptoms in partner
- Eye symptoms
- Any ulceration anywhere else
- Recent foreign travel and sexual contacts abroad
- Urinary symptoms
- Lymphadenopathy noticed

A full sexual history should be taken in privacy. Warn the woman that she can expect to be asked some personal questions which are routine. Always invite people who are attending with the woman to leave. A woman may wish a relative to be there during the history but this might interfere with confidentiality.

Points in the history which may indicate an STI is likely are:

- Multiple partners in the last 6 months (usual length of contact tracing)
- Partner change recently
- Unprotected sexual intercourse with a new or a number of partners
- Recurrent symptoms
- Symptoms in the partner
- Recent travel history

Other symptoms—enquire about abdominal pain, menstrual problems such as intermenstrual and postcoital bleeding, rash, dyspareunia, arthralgia.

A full gynaecological, cervical smear, obstetric, medical, and family history should be taken.

Examination

- External inspection of the genitalia
- Speculum examination—inspect the lateral walls and the cervix for ulceration. If it is too painful to insert a speculum, treat and bring back for follow-up at a later date
- Look for foreign bodies
- Eye and mouth examination
- Palpate for lymphadenopathy
- Bimanual examination to assess cervical excitation, adnexal tenderness, and uterine tenderness. Think of PID
- Abdominal palpation
- Inspect the perianal area

Investigations

For thorough investigation of those thought to be at high risk of STIs, referral to a GU clinic is ideal.

- Swab from ulcers to test for Herpes simplex type 1 or 2. This can be very painful and patients may not tolerate it
- Dark ground microscopy of serum from ulcer to look for *Treponema pallidum*

Management

Management depends on the cause and is discussed individually in the relevant sections.

Tips

- Genital ulceration is likely to be due to herpes
- However, syphilis serology should always be taken at presentation and repeated at follow-up >6 weeks later
- It is important to explain what you are testing for and how to obtain the results
- Positive results require treatment, including advice about the importance of compliance and future prevention
- Partner notification should be carried out, ideally in the setting of a GUM clinic with trained health advisors
- There is a social stigma around STIs, and counselling is important.

3.5 Herpes simplex virus (HSV)

Demographics
- 10% of the population has had genital herpes
- In total, 26, 000 new cases were diagnosed in the UK in 2007 (Health Protection Agency figures)
- 1:4 of those infected is asymptomatic
- 1:2 has mild symptoms and 1:4 present with moderate to severe symptoms

HSV type 1—commonly causes orolabial herpes ('cold sores'). After childhood, if there has been no exposure to HSV-1, it is equally likely to affect genital or oral areas. Genital infection with type 1 or 2 may be indistinguishable. Prior infection with HSV-1 modifies the first infection by HSV-2.

HSV type 2—commonly affects the genitals; 7% of the UK population are seropositive.

Pathophysiology
The incubation period is 1–2 weeks. Some people are symptomatic at the time of primary infection, while others develop symptoms at a later date. This means infections can be unknowingly passed onto partners and therefore appear in monogamous relationships.

HSV is a chronic, lifelong condition. After infection the virus becomes latent in the local sensory ganglion. Periodically it can be reactivated. If it causes symptoms it will affect the same area.

Recurrence rates decline over time but the pattern is variable between individuals. There can be trigger factors, e.g. stress, menstruation, UV light.

HSV-2 recurs more frequently, average four times/year, and there is more viral shedding. Active lesions indicate viral shedding and high infectivity, but there is evidence of asymptomatic shedding. It is transmitted through skin contact, and from mouth to the genital area with oral sex.

Presentation
Symptoms and signs
Primary
- Fever and myalgia
- Dysuria (may result in urinary retention)
- Vaginal discharge
- Painful ulceration, usually multiple blisters and ulcers of vulva, cervix, anal area (see Figure 3.5)
- Inguinal lymphadenopathy

Secondary
- Asymptomatic
- Single or multiple painful ulcers, usually less painful than primary infection and affecting the same area
- Prodromal symptoms, e.g. tingling in the area in 50% of those with recurrences

Systemic symptoms are commoner in primary infection.

Clinical assessment
Investigations
- Virus detection by swabbing the base of the lesion. The swab must be taken to the laboratory immediately and kept at 4°C. To increase the chance of a positive result in HSV the ulcers need to be swabbed as early as possible. Culture, PCR or antigen detection can be used
- Serology—one sample at the time of infection should be negative and a follow-up sample up to 3 months later should be positive. However, type 1 or 2 cannot be easily ascertained. Patients may have been exposed to Herpes simplex in the past,

making both tests positive. Therefore serology is not widely used and not recommended
- Exclude other causes of ulceration
- Always take syphilis serology at presentation and after 6 weeks at follow-up

Management
Primary occurrence
- Saline bathing, advice to pass urine in the bath, drying with a cool hairdryer may help relieve symptoms, topical anaesthetic agents should be used with caution to avoid potential sensitization
- First episodes are often more severe. If the patient presents within 5 days or has developing lesions she should be treated with oral antiviral agents. Aciclovir, valaciclovir and famciclovir reduce the severity and duration of symptoms
- Recommended regimens are:
  - Aciclovir 200 mg 5 times/day for 5 days
  - Famciclovir 250 mg TDS for 5 days
  - Valaciclovir 500 mg BD for 5 days
- If vomiting or unable to swallow, consider IV treatment
- If in urinary retention, catheterization is indicated. Suprapubic catheterization is preferred to reduce pain and prevent ascending infection
- Condoms are not 100% protective as they may not cover the entire area affected
- Transmission is commoner from men to women
- Full sexual health screen
- Partner notification
- Counselling is important about the natural history, transmission, asymptomatic shedding, and protection for partners
- Herpes serology can be used in discordant partners to clarify risk, e.g. when wanting to conceive

Secondary
- The COCP can be tricycled to avoid menstruation which may trigger recurrences
- Avoid tampon use while symptomatic
- Episodic treatment can be used with prodromal symptoms
- Suppressive continuous low-dose treatment, e.g. aciclovir 400 mg BD may be indicated, for a maximum of 1 year

Complications
- Aseptic meningitis
- Autonomic neuropathy—urinary retention

See Section 8.25 for pregnancy and neonatal management of HSV.

Further reading
RCOG. Genital herpes in pregnancy—management. Green top guideline no. 30, 2007. www.rcog.org.uk

www.herpes.org.uk (patient support/ information).

www.herpesalliance.org.uk (patient support/information).

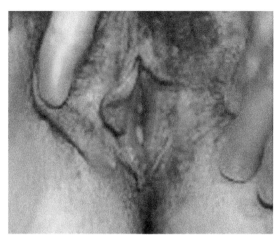

Fig. 3.4 Vulval herpes infection. Reproduced with permission from
The Oxford Handbook of Genitourinary Medicine, HIV, and AIDS, edited
by R Pattman et al. ©Oxford University Press, 2005.

3.6 Syphilis

Demographics

The introduction of penicillin had a dramatic effect in reducing the incidence of syphilis in the late 20th century, but the number of new cases increased 10-fold in England and Wales between 1996–2002. In 2007, nearly 3000 new cases of primary and secondary syphilis were diagnosed. The WHO estimates 12 million new cases annually in developing countries.

Pathophysiology

The bacterium *Treponema pallidum* can be spread by sexual contact, close contact with lesions or by vertical transmission. The incubation period is 9–90 days.

Primary syphilis is ulceration at the site of inoculation (usually the genitals, perianal area or mouth). The initial lesion is a solitary purple papule from infiltration of the dermis with lymphocytes and plasma cells. Inflammatory changes lead to necrosis. An ulcer forms, containing treponemes, and is highly infectious. This stage may be asymptomatic or undetected by the woman (on her cervix).

Secondary syphilis develops after 1–6 months and is a systemic illness but there can also be skin involvement.

Early latent syphilis is asymptomatic and is of <2 years' duration.

Late latent syphilis is asymptomatic and is of >2 years' duration.

Gummatous syphilis refers to necrotic nodules or plaques which develop 3–12 years after primary infection.

Neurosyphilis occurs 10–20 years after primary infection.

Meningovascular syphilis can appear early and as part of secondary syphilis or late, after 2–20 years.

Cardiovascular syphilis, including aortic regurgitation, angina and aneurysms, occurs 10–40 years after infection.

Presentation

Symptoms and signs

Primary
- Solitary painless ulcer (see Figure 3.6)
- Inguinal lymphadenopathy—rubbery and non-tender
- Patients may not notice the lesion

Secondary
- Generalized lesions affecting skin and mucous membranes
- Symmetrical and non-itchy lesions which can be macular, papular, and, rarely, pustular
- The pustular lesions are grey and are described as snail track ulcers on mucosal surfaces
- The signs of secondary syphilis can be widespread but may also only affect the genital area
- Malaise, fever, anorexia
- Generalized lymphadenopathy
- Hepatitis
- Iritis
- Meningitis
- Optic neuritis

Clinical assessment

Investigations
- Dark ground microscopy from the ulcer in primary syphilis or lesion in secondary syphilis to look for Treponema pallidum. Ideally, 3 separate specimens from 3 different days should be examined. Patients should avoid antiseptic or soaps containing antibacterial agents on the affected area. If necessary, they can bathe with salt water
- Serological tests are either non-specific (non-treponemal) or specific (treponemal)

Non-specific tests
VDRL (venereal disease reference laboratory) and RPR (rapid plasmin reagin)
- Useful for monitoring treatment and diagnosing reinfection
- Detect antibody (reagin) in the serum and this is usually positive 3–5 weeks after contraction of the infection
- ↓ titres occur with treatment response but can decay naturally
- ↑ titres occur with treatment failure and reinfection
- False positives occur in pregnancy, old age, acute infection with mumps, measles, herpes, after immunization against yellow fever and typhoid, and in autoimmune disease. Acute causes for false positive results will be negative on re-testing after 6 months. Chronic causes, e.g. old age, will remain positive over 6 months
- Positive in yaws, Bejel and pinta

Specific tests
T. pallidum EIA (enzyme immunoassay test), FTA (absorbed fluorescent treponemal antibody test), and TPHA (*T. pallidum* haemagglutination test)
- Useful to confirm diagnosis, especially at first diagnosis
- EIA tends to be used for screening
- FTA is not used regularly
- Remain positive throughout life even after treatment
- FTA and EIA are usually the first to become positive, between 3 and 4 weeks after infection

Management
- Refer to specialist GUM clinic
- Undertake a full sexual health screen
- Partner notification, screening children
- Primary and secondary syphilis: benzathine penicillin as a single injection or 10 days of procaine penicillin
- If penicillin allergy, doxycycline can be used
- The Jarisch–Herxheimer reaction is common in treatment of primary and secondary syphilis. Flu-like symptoms and a fever may develop after the first injection, usually after 3–12 h, and skin lesions can become more widespread. Reassurance, NSAIDs, and paracetamol can be used and treatment should be continued

Complications
- Development of neurosyphilis
- Development of meningovascular syphilis
- Development of cardiovascular syphilis

Adequate treatment of primary, secondary, and latent syphilis should prevent progression of the disease.

In pregnancy (see also Section 6.7)
- Penicillin is effective in the treatment of syphilis in pregnancy and prevention of congenital syphilis, but the optimal regimen is not clear
- It may be indicated to admit the pregnant woman until after the second penicillin injection to monitor for Jarisch–Herxheimer reaction

In the neonate
Fetal syphilis can be detected *in utero* in mothers who have positive serological tests in pregnancy. Ultrasound may show hydrops fetalis, polyhydramnios, placental thickening, skin thickening, serous cavity effusions, hepatomegaly, and splenomegaly. After birth, manifestations can be divided into early (under 2 years) and late. The many manifestations can last into later life.

Serological follow-up is indicated, as passive maternal transfer may occur until seronegative.

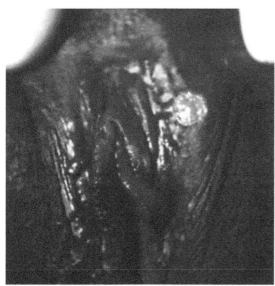

Fig. 3.5 Primary syphilitic chancre. Image reproduced courtesy of the CDC.

Further reading

Walker GJA. Antibiotics for syphilis diagnosed during pregnancy. *Cochrane Database of Systematic Reviews* 2007; **3:** Art. No. CD001143.

Mcmilan A, Young H, Ogilvie M, Scott G. *Clinical Practice in Sexually Transmissible Infections.* London Saunders, 2002.

3.7 Genital warts

Demographics

Genital warts, condyloma acuminata, are common.

There were about 30, 000 new cases in the UK in 2007.

Pathophysiology

Genital warts are caused by human papillomaviruses (HPV), a group of DNA viruses from the papovavirus family. There are hundreds of subtypes:

- Types 6 and 11 are the commonest cause of benign genital disease
- Types 16, 18, 31, 33, and 35 can also be the cause

They are usually transmitted by sexual contact, but transmission can be by autoinoculation (transfer from another area of affected skin on the same individual), e.g. hand to genital.

They are commonly found at the introitus and vulval area, but can be on the cervix, perianal area, anus, and rectum.

The incubation period is variable, ranging from 2 weeks to 18 months.

Clinical assessment

History

- Usually painless lumps (see Figure 3.7)
- Can be solitary or multiple
- Often noticed once a partner is symptomatic
- Full sexual history

Examination

- Full screen as increased risk of other STIs
- Cervical lesions are not usually visible to the naked eye but can be seen on colposcopy
- Cervical smears as routine
- HPV testing is not offered routinely. It is useful for determining risk of, and for the early detection and treatment of, HPV infection-related changes which can lead to CIN

Investigation

Diagnosis is based on clinical features.

Differential diagnosis

- Molluscum contagiosum
- Sebaceous cysts
- Tumours
- Condylomata lata of secondary syphilis

Management

There are many options for treating warts.

- Do nothing and wait for the immune system to recognize the infection
- Condom use reduces transmission but does not provide complete protection (as skin-to-skin contact)
- Podophyllotoxin, a cytotoxic agent, 10–15% strength is applied to the affected area twice/week. After application it should be washed off about 4 h later as it is irritating and may cause burns to healthy skin. It can also have side effects of peripheral neuropathy, coma and hypokalaemia if large quantities are administered. Patients can self-administer 0.5% podophyllin to the affected area twice a day for 3 days and repeat once a week for up to 4 weeks
- Glacial trichloroacetic acid 80–90% can be used weekly if podophyllin has been ineffective, in a specialist clinic. The surrounding skin is protected with petroleum jelly
- Cryotherapy or electrocautery
- Imiquimod is an immune response modifier that induces a cytokine response. It can be applied to the lesions three times a week and is washed off 10 h after. The treatment can be used for up to 16 weeks
- Fluorouracil, a DNA antimetabolite, as a 5% cream. Use is limited as it can cause neovascularization and vulval burn
- Interferons have been used but are expensive and show no better response
- Patience may be required on behalf of both patient and doctor, as some warts are very difficult to treat
- Treat a small group at a time if large numbers

Complications

- Association with cervical neoplasia (types 16, 18, 31, 33, 35, 39, 45, 51, 52, 56, and 58). Routine 3-yearly screening should be carried out (see Section 15.2)
- Warts often increase in pregnancy
- Recurrence is common

In pregnancy, breast feeding and the neonate

- Vertical transmission is rare. They can cause laryngeal papillomas in neonates. The incubation period is about 3 months, but they can develop from 2 weeks up to 12 years later. It is not clear if these are acquired transplacentally, intrapartum or postpartum. Genital warts are not an indication for CS unless sufficiently large to cause obstruction
- Podophyllin should not be used in pregnancy as it may be teratogenic
- Fluorouracil and imiquimod should be avoided
- The best treatments during pregnancy and postnatally are cryotherapy and electrocautery
- Reassure that warts are likely to decrease postnatallyt

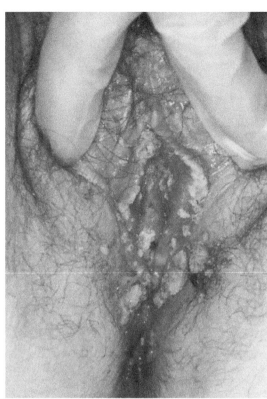

Fig. 3.6 Vulval warts. Image reproduced courtesy of the CDC/Joe Millar.

3.8 Molluscum contagiosum, pubic lice, and scabies

Molluscum contagiosum

Demographics

Molluscum contagiosum is common. It can be seen in outbreaks at schools, between siblings, at swimming pools, etc. There were 17,000 cases diagnosed in the UK in 2007.

Pathophysiology

- The condition is caused by a pox virus
- It is spread by close bodily contact, towels or clothing, and sexual contact
- There is an incubation period of 2–12 weeks

Clinical assessment

History
- Usually multiple lesions
- Small 2–5-mm pearly white papules with a dimple in the centre (umbilicated), but can be smooth
- Lesions affecting the face are more likely if immunocompromised, e.g. in HIV-positive patients

Examination
Diagnosis is made by clinical assessment (see Figure 3.8).

Investigations
- Virus cannot be cultured successfully
- Material expressed shows viral inclusions on Giemsa staining or on electron microscopy
- Always carry out a full STI screen
- HIV test (opportunistic) in all, but especially if facial lesions

Differential diagnosis
As for warts (see Section 3.7).

Management

- Leave as they are self-limiting and usually resolve over a period of several months
- Cryotherapy or electrocautery
- Phenol applied with the end of a sharpened orange stick to the central 'dimple' of the lesions
- The aim is to cause tissue destruction and viral demise as well as alerting the host defences to recognize the infection
- There is no need for contact tracing unless another STI is diagnosed
- Repeat treatments are often needed

Complications

- No complications but cosmetically distressing
- In immunocompromised patients the lesions can become large, and secondary infection can be a problem

In pregnancy and breastfeeding
Leave alone or treat with cryotherapy or electrocautery

Pediculosis pubis

Aetiology

- The crab louse *Phthirus pubis* is transmitted by close body contact
- The incubation is 5 days to several weeks
- Adult lice infest strong hairs of the pubic area, body hair, eyelashes, and eyebrows
- It is a different species from head and body louse infestation
- The adult is 1–2 mm long
- It sucks blood and the hypersensitivity from the bite causes itching
- The female lays eggs at the base of the hairs, termed 'nits'.

Clinical assessment

History
- Asymptomatic
- Itching due to hypersensitivity

Examination
- Adult lice visible
- Nits visible attached to hair
- Blue macules may be visible at feeding sites

Investigation
Diagnosis is clinical. Examination under a light microscope can be useful in determining exact morphology.

Management

- Avoid close body contact until patient and partner treated
- Full STI screen indicated
- Lotions are more effective than shampoos and should be applied to all body hair, including beards and moustaches. A second application may be advisable after 3–7 days
- Malathion 0.5%—apply and leave for at least 12 h
- Permethrin 1%—apply and wash out 10 min later
- Phenothrin 0.2%—apply and wash off 2 h later
- Carbaryl 1%—apply and wash off 12 h later
- Lice can be removed individually or with petroleum jelly
- Avoid shaving as this may exacerbate itching

Follow-up
- Reinfection is a complication if partner not treated
- Patients should be re-examined after 1 week
- Reassure that dead nits may remain adherent to hairs and that re-treatment is not required

In pregnancy and breastfeeding
Permethrin is safe to use in both situations.

Scabies

Pathophysiology

Infestation by the mite *Sarcoptes scabiei*. The clinical features are caused by the female burrowing in the stratum corneum of the skin, laying eggs, and defaecating. A hypersensitivity to the intestinal enzymes causes itching. This can take up to 4–6 weeks to develop and is often worse at night. The female is about 0.3 mm long and can be seen as a black dot to the naked eye. Transmission is by close bodily contact, not necessarily sexual.

Clinical assessment

History
- Itching worse at night
- In a first infection this can take 4–6 weeks to develop, but in reinfection can be within a few hours

Examination
- Silver lines 5–15 mm long where mites have burrowed, e.g. clefts of fingers, wrists, elbows, and genitals. They often have a scaling appearance
- Papules or nodules as a result of itching which may not be near the burrows

Investigations
- Clinical diagnosis
- Scrapings from burrows may be examined under a light microscope to reveal mites

Management

- Avoid body contact until patient and partner treated
- Offer a full STI screen
- Contact tracing arbitrary for the last 2 months
- Permethrin 5% or malathion 0.5% should be applied to the whole body and left for 12 h
- Reassure that even after successful treatment the itch may persist for several weeks
- Antihistamines may help itching
- Wash contaminated clothes, towels, and bedding at 50°C
- Mites separated from the host die after 72 h

Useful tip: in HIV-positive patients, crusted lesions may contain Norwegian scabies and pose a risk of transmission.

Follow-up

No follow-up is needed. New burrows need new treatment.

In pregnancy and breastfeeding

Permethrin is safe to use.

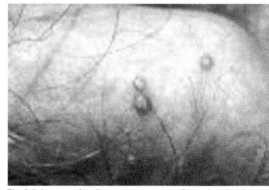

Fig. 3.7 Lesions of molluscum contagiosum. Reproduced with permission from *The Oxford Handbook of Genitourinary Medicine, HIV, and AIDS*, edited by R Pattman et al. ©Oxford University Press, 2005.

3.9 Pelvic inflammatory disease

Definition
Pelvic inflammatory disease (PID) is the result of infection ascending from the endocervix, causing endometritis, salpingitis, parametritis, oophoritis, tubo-ovarian abscess, and/or pelvic peritonitis.

Demographics
PID is a disease of sexually active women. Statistics vary with populations examined; the incidence is higher in urban rather than rural areas. Peak incidence is 20 per 1000 (20–24-year-olds).

Aetiology
Gonorrhoea and chlamydia are the main causative agents. *Garderella*, *Mycoplasma* and anaerobes have also been implicated. Gonorrhoea accounts for 14% of PID in Britain. There is up to a 40% risk of chlamydia with gonococcal infections.

Pathophysiology
Infection ascends from the endocervix and vagina into the uterus, tubes, and surrounding structures. Inflammation causes adhesion formation and damage to tubal epithelium.

An intrauterine contraceptive device (IUCD) increases the risk of developing PID in the first few weeks after insertion.

The use of the COCP had been regarded as protective against symptomatic PID. However, retrospective case-control and prospective studies have shown an increased incidence of asymptomatic chlamydia cervical infection and this may mask endometritis.

Clinical assessment
Women may present acutely or chronically to their GP, GUM clinic, emergency department or gynaecology outpatients for investigation of pain or subfertility.

History
- Lower abdominal pain
- Deep dyspareunia
- Abnormal vaginal bleeding
- Abnormal vaginal or cervical discharge
- History of STIs in the past

Useful Tip
HIV-positive women may have more severe symptoms.

Examination
Clinical findings may include all, any or none, of:
- Pyrexia of >38°C
- Lower abdominal tenderness, usually bilateral
- Adnexal tenderness on bimanual vaginal examination
- Cervical excitation on vaginal examination

Useful tip
Cervical excitation is the equivalent of rebound tenderness in the abdomen, i.e. a sign of peritonism. To elicit it, put a finger either side of the cervix and push it gently to one side and then the other. If this causes pain there is cervical excitation. This manoeuvre causes pulling on the ipsilateral broad ligament and thus can also localize the 'peritonism' to the left or right.

Investigations
PID can be symptomatic or asymptomatic. Clinical diagnosis is less sensitive and specific than laparoscopic (positive predictive value 65–90%).

- Take triple swabs—high vaginal (trichomonas vaginalis, candida, bacterial vaginosis) and endocervical swabs (gonorrhoea, chlamydia). Positive swabs support the diagnosis, negative ones do not exclude it. The endocervical gonorrhoea swab should be sent for culture or a nucleic acid amplification test (NAAT). The endocervical chlamydia swab should also be processed using a NAAT, e.g. PCR. A urethral swab for chlamydia and gonorrhoea or a first catch urine may also improve diagnostic yield
- Microscopy, if available, for gonorrhoea
- No endocervical or vaginal pus cells on microscopy has a negative predictive value of 95%
- ↑CRP, ↑ESR and ↑WCC support the diagnosis
- Blood cultures if there is a pyrexia of >38°C
- Laparoscopy can support the diagnosis but may not identify mild tubal inflammation or endometritis. It can be valuable in excluding other diagnoses. Although considered the gold standard, laparoscopy will not diagnose 15–30% of PID (see Figure 3.9)
- Ultrasound can be useful, especially with Doppler as it can identify inflamed, dilated tubes, and tubo-ovarian masses
- MRI can assist diagnosis but the evidence is limited
- There is insufficient evidence for the use of endometrial biopsy as a routine diagnostic test

Differential diagnosis
- Ectopic pregnancy must be excluded using a urine pregnancy test or serum HCG
- Acute appendicitis
- Bleeding or torsion of an ovarian cyst
- Endometriosis
- UTI

Useful tip
Nausea and vomiting are present in most patients with appendicitis, but in only 50% of those with PID. Cervical excitation is present in 25% of women with appendicitis.

Management
Delay in diagnosis and treatment, even of a few days, increases the risk of sequelae, which include infertility, ectopic pregnancy, and chronic pelvic pain.

Medical
- Analgesia
- Rest if severe disease
- Consider admission if surgical emergency cannot be excluded, severe symptoms, pregnant, oral therapy cannot be tolerated, or patient is not responding to oral treatment
- Mild to moderate disease—outpatient oral antibiotic treatment with follow-up (see Box 3.1)
- Moderate to severe disease—admit for IV antibiotics. Change to oral therapy 24 h after clinical improvement (see Box 3.2)
- Broad-spectrum antibiotics are required to cover gonorrhoea, chlamydia, and anaerobic infection
- Randomized controlled trial evidence regarding removal of IUCD is limited. An IUCD may be left in situ in women with mild PID but should be removed in severe disease
- Remember to assess the risk of pregnancy as emergency contraception may be needed

Useful Tips
- If using gentamicin, remember to take levels in order to avoid toxicity and monitor renal function
- Ofloxacin should be avoided in women <18 years where bone development still occurs (owing to calcium chelation)
- Remember to warn women on the COCP to use other forms of contraception
- In patients with drug allergies, use an alternative regimen
- HIV-positive patients should have the same regimen

- If intolerable side effects occur, e.g. gastrointestinal symptoms, metronidazole can be stopped in mild to moderate PID
- Avoid ofloxacin in patients with gonococcal PID as there is increased quinolone resistance in the UK

Surgical

Laparoscopy or laparotomy may be considered if:
- No response to therapy
- Clinically severe disease
- Presence of a tubo-ovarian abscess

It can help early resolution by dividing adhesions and/or draining pelvic abscesses.

US-guided aspiration of pelvic fluid collections is less invasive and may be equally effective.

In both situations, swabs should be sent for microscopy, culture, and sensitivities.

Complications

- Fitz-Hugh-Curtis syndrome, defined as right upper quadrant abdominal pain and perihepatitis, occurs in 10–15% of women with PID. Laparoscopic division of hepatic adhesions can be performed, but there is no evidence that this is better than antibiotics alone (see Figure 3.2)
- Chronic pelvic pain, including deep dyspareunia and sexual dysfunction
- Increased risk of ectopic pregnancy
- Subfertility owing to tubal damage

Approach

Understandably, there are likely to be questions about cause, especially if presenting in a relationship.
- Patients should be referred to GUM for a full sexual health screen
- Contact tracing for current partners and those <6 months prior to symptoms is ideally done through a GUM clinic
- Advise to avoid intercourse until the partner is screened, treated, and had a test of cure (if gonococcal infection)

Follow-up

Inpatients should be reviewed daily.

Those treated as outpatients should have review 4 weeks after presentation to check:
- They were compliant with treatment
- Vaginal examination to assess response to treatment
- Contact tracing has happened

If swabs showed gonococcal PID, both partners will need test of cure repeat swabs at least 2 weeks after treatment has finished.

In pregnancy

- PID is rare except in cases of septic abortion
- PID is associated with increased maternal and fetal morbidity, so IV antibiotic treatment is indicated. Although none is proven as safe in pregnancy, the benefit outweighs the risk
- In very early pregnancy, up to day 10 after fertilization and probably before the woman discovers she is pregnant, treatment may result in failed implantation

Further reading

Ness RB et al. Effectiveness of inpatient and outpatient treatment strategies for women with pelvic inflammatory disease: results from the Pelvic Inflammatory Disease Evaluation and Clinical Health PEACH Randomised Trial. *American Journal of Obstetrics and Gynaecology* 2002; **186**:929–37.

RCOG. *Management of Acute Pelvic Inflammatory Disease.* Green top guideline No 32, 2003. www.rcog.org.uk

Recommendations arising from the 31st Study Group: the prevention of pelvic infection. In: Templeton, A. (ed.) *The Prevention of Pelvic Infection*, pp. 267–70. London: RCOG Press, 1996.

> **◎ Box 3.1 Regimens for outpatient treatment**
>
> - IM injection of ceftriaxone 250 mg stat or cefoxitin 2 g stat with oral probenecid 1 g, followed by oral doxycycline 100 mg BD and oral metronidazole 400 mg BD for 14 days
> *or*
> - Oral ofloxacin 400 mg BD plus oral metronidazole 400 mg BD for 14 days

> **◎ Box 3.2 Regimens for inpatient treatment**
>
> - IV cefoxitin 2 g TDS and IV doxycycline 100 mg BD followed by oral doxycycline 100 mg BD and oral metronidazole 400 mg BD for 14 days
> *or*
> - IV clindamycin 900 mg TDS plus IV gentamicin (2 mg/kg loading dose followed by 1.5 mg/kg TDS) followed by oral clindamycin 450 mg QDS for 14 days or oral doxycycline 100 mg BD and oral metronidazole 400 mg BD for 14 days
> *or*
> - IV ofloxacin 400 mg BD plus IV metronidazole 500 mg TDS for 14 days
> *or*
> - IV ciprofloxacin 200 mg BD plus IV or oral doxycycline 100 mg BD plus IV metronidazole 500 mg TDS for 14 days

> **→ Box 3.3 Landmark research**
>
> PEACH study. In women treated with cefoxitin and then doxycycline, the pregnancy rates after 3 years were similar or higher than that of the general population (Ness et al. 2002)

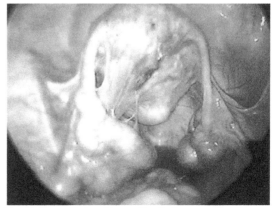

Fig. 3.8 Bilateral hydrosalpinges with adhesions caused by PID.

3.10 Hepatitis virus

Hepatitis A

Hepatitis A is caused by a picorna virus, an RNA virus, and is more commonly found in the developing world. There were 784 cases in England and Wales reported in 2004. Transmission is faeco-oral, mainly via food, water or close personal contact. Outbreaks have been reported in men who have sex with men, associated with oro-anal or digital–rectal contact. Vaccination may be offered to individuals at risk.

Other viruses which can cause hepatitis and may be sexually acquired include cytomegalovirus and Epstein–Barr virus (EBV).

Hepatitis B

Pathophysiology and demographics

Hepatitis B is caused by a hepadnavirus, a DNA virus. It is endemic worldwide, with high carriage rates (20%) in South East Asia, southern Europe, Central and South America, and Africa. In 2002, 1072 cases were notified in England and Wales, and 1000 new cases of hepatitis B were diagnosed in the UK in 2007. Transmission is by:

- Sexual contact (18% infection rates for heterosexual couples where one partner has acute hepatitis B)
- Parenteral—needlestick injuries, drug users sharing needles
- Vertical transmission from mother to child

Acquisition in adults: The incubation period is 40–160 days. It can result in an acute hepatitis, chronic hepatitis, chronic carriage, and cirrhosis. Liver carcinoma risk is increased. Of those infected, 90% will clear virus and gain lifelong immunity.

Hepatitis D is an incomplete RNA virus that requires hepatitis B outer coat. Diagnosis is by anti-HDV antibody test or HDV-RNA test. It is only found in patients with hepatitis B, largely injecting drug users and their partners. It can cause the acute hepatitis to be more severe and chronic liver disease to be rapidly progressive. There is a high rate of progression to cirrhosis. Response to antiviral treatment is poor.

Clinical assessment

History
- Asymptomatic in 10–50% of adults in the acute phase, especially if HIV co-infection
- Prodromal phase of flu-like symptoms
- Icteric phase with jaundice, anorexia, nausea, and fatigue

Examination
- No signs in prodromal phase
- Jaundice with pale stools and dark urine. Dehydration, liver enlargement, and tenderness can be found in icteric phase
- No signs in chronic infection
- Signs of chronic liver disease after many years, e.g. spider naevi, finger clubbing, jaundice, hepato-splenomegaly, ascites, liver flap, and encephalopathy

Investigations
- Serology (see Box 3.3)

Liver function tests in acute infection:
- Serum aminotransferases: ↑ALT and AST
- ↑Bilirubin
- ↑Alkaline phosphatase
- Coagulation tests—prothrombin time >5 suggests hepatic decompensation
- Exclude other causes of acute hepatitis
- In chronic infection there may be mildly raised ALT (<100 iu/l). In severe late-stage liver disease, the liver function tests are deranged
- Disease activity correlates with HBV-DNA levels

Management
- Full STI screen
- Advise protected sexual intercourse until non-infectious
- Advise to vaccinate partner and household contacts
- Partner notification
- Notifiable condition
- In the icteric phase, rest and oral hydration
- Hospital admission for supportive therapy may be indicated if severe. Mild to moderate acute disease can be managed as an outpatient
- Referral to specialist
- Treatment options include lamivudine, adefovir, and alpha-interferon. If patients respond they have reduced risk of liver damage and liver carcinoma in the long term
- Liver biopsy may be necessary to assess chronic disease
- Avoid alcohol
- Follow-up for acute infections with icteric phase should be weekly, with blood tests until LFTs normalize
- Serology should be repeated in acute infection in 6 months to assess possible chronic infection
- Follow-up for chronic infection should be yearly

Complications
- Fulminant hepatitis in <1%
- Chronic infection in 5–10% (higher if HIV, chronic renal failure, immunosuppressive therapy)
- Immunosuppressive treatment can reactivate hepatitis B
- Concurrent hepatitis C infection can lead to fulminant hepatitis, more aggressive chronic disease, and increased risk of liver hepatocellular carcinoma
- Mortality rate is <1% for acute cases
- Of chronic carriers, 10–50% develop cirrhosis, leading to premature death in 50% of those
- Ten per cent of those that develop cirrhosis develop liver hepatocellular carcinoma

Prophylaxis
- Hepatitis B immunoglobulin 500 iu may be administered to a non-immune contact after a single episode of unprotected sex or parenteral exposure, e.g. needlestick. This needs to be given <7 days post-exposure and works best <48 h
- Vaccination should be given to sexual and household contacts (up to 6 weeks after exposure offers protection). Accelerated regimens are: 0, 7, 21 days or 0, 1, 2 months with a booster at 12 months. If serology shows response (anti-HBs titres >10 iu/l) protection for 10 years or more

In pregnancy and breast feeding
See Section 6.7.

Hepatitis C

Pathophysiology and demographics

Hepatitis C is caused by an RNA virus in the flaviviridae family. It has high prevalence rates in South and East Asia and Eastern Europe. In the UK, prevalence rates vary from 0.06% in blood donors to 60% in intravenous drug users. A total of 5917 cases were reported in England and Wales in 2002. There were 1200 new cases diagnosed in the UK in 2007.

Transmission is by:
- Parenteral route, mainly, for example shared needles
- Sexual transmission (risk 1–11%)
- Vertical transmission (risk 5%, but higher if HIV-positive)

The incubation period is 4–20 weeks for acute hepatitis to develop, which is uncommon. Serology can take up to 9 months to convert.

Clinical assessment

History
- >90% asymptomatic
- Acute icteric hepatitis similar to hepatitis B

Examination
- Acute and chronic signs as hepatitis B

Investigations
- First test—enzyme linked immunoassay (ELISA)
- If the first is positive, a second test—a recombinant immunoblot assay (RIBA) or polymerase chain reaction (PCR)—is done
- A PCR test will be positive after 2 weeks
- Antibody tests can take 3 months to be positive
- To test for chronic carriage, a repeat test is needed after 6 months
- Other tests for liver function are indicated as for hepatitis B

Management
- Notifiable condition
- Referral to specialist
- Full STI screen
- Partner notification
- Condom use for sexual intercourse but, unless there is HIV co-infection, the transmission rates are low
- Follow-up is the same as for hepatitis B
- Vaccinate against hepatitis A and B as prognosis is worse if co-infection (there is no vaccination for hepatitis C)
- Interferon treatment may be indicated in the acute or chronic phase if active virus replication or liver disease
- Advise to avoid alcohol in acute disease
- Advise against donating blood or organs

Complications
- Less than 1% result in fulminant hepatitis
- Between 50–85% become chronic carriers; of these, 35% may have significant liver disease with normal LFTs
- Between 1–30% of chronic carriers progress to severe liver disease after 20 years
- Increased risk of liver carcinoma of 1–4%, but up to one-third of those with cirrhosis

In pregnancy and breastfeeding
- Pregnancy does not affect the clinical course of HCV
- Acute hepatitis is associated with miscarriage and premature labour
- Vertical transmission is 1–3% if HCV-RNA-negative and 4–6% if HCV-RNA-positive. No prevention currently available
- Transmission is increased with high titres of HCV-RNA and if there is co-infection with HIV
- Main fetal risk is the development of chronic liver problems in the long term, such as cirrhosis and hepatocellular carcinoma
- No need to deliver by CS unless co-infection with HIV
- Avoid fetal blood sampling, fetal scalp electrode, and instrumental delivery
- Breastfeeding is safe but avoid if nipples cracked or bleeding. It may be contraindicated with high viral load. The risk of transmission is thought to be same as in pregnancy itself
- Refer to gastroenterology for follow-up

Further reading
www.hepatitis.org.uk (Hepatitis C support website).

www.britishlivertrust.org.uk

⊙ Box 3.4 Hepatitis B serology

Stage of infection	HBsAg (surface Ag)	HBeAg (e Ag)	IgM anti-core Ab	IgG anti-core Ab	Hep B virus DNA	Anti-HBe	Anti-HBs
Acute (early)	+	+	+	+	+	–	–
Acute (resolving)	+	–	+	+	–	±	–
Chronic (high infectivity)	+	±	–	+	+	±	–
Chronic (low infectivity)	+	–	–	+	–	±	–
Immune (90%)	–	–	–	+	–	±	±
Post-vaccination	–	–	–	–	–	–	+

Ag, antigen; Ab, antibody.

Human immunodeficiency virus (HIV)

Demographics

By the end of 2007, the United Nations estimated that 33.2 million adults and children were living with HIV and AIDS. In the UK, by 2008 there were approximatly 37, 400 cases of HIV reported. There are currently 79, 000 living with HIV in the UK and another 18 000 undiagnosed individuals. In the UK, 79% of those infected are men. The prevalence of HIV is higher in men who have sex with men and in injecting drug users. Heterosexual transmission also occurs and is an increasing proportion of those diagnosed.

Pathophysiology

HIV was first detected in 1983 in a patient with acquired immunode-ficiency disorder (AIDS). Transmission can be sexual (↑risk with anal sex), vertical, and parenteral, e.g. sharing needles. The natural history is that HIV infection, when chronic, causes immune dysfunction as it infects T helper cells. Eventually, the immune deficiency leads to diseases which are an indicator of AIDS.

The virus attaches to CD4 molecules on the T cells and enters them. There are co-receptors for HIV entry which determine the susceptibility of the CD4-bearing cell to infection. This causes inhibition of lymphocyte growth and enhanced apoptosis. As the virus is a retrovirus, on entry to the cell the viral reverse transcriptase enzyme makes a DNA copy of the viral RNA genome. This proviral DNA is integrated into the host cell's DNA, and viral replication occurs as RNA transcripts are produced from the incorporated proviral DNA. New virus particles are assembled and released by budding.

HIV infection was classified into stages by the Centers for Disease Control depending on symptoms and CD4 count. AIDS is a clinical diagnosis. Details can be found on the BHIVA website.

The mortality rates from AIDS are decreasing and the time before AIDS develops is increasing owing to highly active antiretroviral therapy (HAART). Without therapy, about 75% of those infected with HIV will develop symptomatic disease within 10 years.

Clinical assessment

Acute infection

- At seroconversion, there may be a 'flu'-like illness with fever, malaise, lymphadenopathy, pharyngitis, and a rash
- An aseptic meningoencephalitis can also occur
- Asymptomatic
- Development of antibodies to the core protein p24 and surface proteins GP 41, 120, 160 develop within 2–6 weeks. This seroconversion can take up to 3 months

Chronic infection

- Asymptomatic in early stages
- One-third of patients have persistent generalized lymphadenopathy of >1 cm in over two extrainguinal sites
- Later in the infection, as CD4 count decreases, non-specific symptoms develop, e.g. diarrhoea, night sweats, fevers, weight loss. Patients develop minor opportunistic infections, e.g. oral candidiasis, herpes zoster, recurrence of herpes simplex, folliculitis. This stage is classified as symptomatic non-AIDS (CDC stage B)
- A CD4 count of <200×10⁶/l and the presence of stage B symptoms are associated with risk of progression to AIDS

Acquired immunodeficiency syndrome

AIDS is a clinical illness, not a serological diagnosis, and is defined by one or more indicator diseases which include oesophageal candidiasis, Kaposi's sarcoma, *Pneumocystis carinii* (now *jiroveci*) pneumonia, cerebral toxoplasmosis, HIV encephalopathy, etc.

Clinical assessment

Investigation

- Enzyme immunoassays to detect antibodies
- PCR to detect viral RNA—a high concentration is normal at the time of infection. If high later in disease, it is associated with a rapid decline in CD4 count and a quicker progression to symptomatic disease.
- A positive test must be repeated to rule out false positive
- Full sexual health screen

Pre-test discussion

Before offering an HIV test, it is important to discuss the reasons for the test, possible results, benefits, and impact of the test if positive. It is no longer recommended that this always be done by a specially trained individual. However, if the patient is at high risk, the following should be discussed for proper consent:

- The benefits of testing
- The health benefits of current treatments
- Knowing HIV status can allay anxiety
- A positive test may motivate people to decrease risk activities
- The opportunity to decrease the risk of transmission of the infection to others, e.g. infants, sexual partners
- A risk assessment, including date of last risk activity
- The 'window period'
- Implications of testing for mortgages, insurance, occupational risks, and confidentiality
- Details of how the result will be given
- If appropriate, explore support and coping mechanisms
- Obtaining informed consent for the test
- Information about HIV transmission and risk reduction

At GUM clinics, HIV testing is routine unless patients opt out.

Management

- BHIVA advise treatment if symptomatic or CD4 count is < 350×10⁶/l
- Antiretroviral therapy inhibits viral replication and reduces viral load. It cannot eradicate HIV as there are virus reservoirs in resting T cells and other long-lived cell populations
- Three types of drugs are used in current practice:
  1. Nucleoside reverse transcriptase inhibitors (inhibit the enzyme that produces the proviral DNA from the viral RNA), e.g. zidovudine
  2. Non-nucleoside reverse transcriptase inhibitors (mode of action as 1), e.g. nevirapine
  3. Protease inhibitors (inhibit post-translational processing of viral proteins), e.g. lopinavir
- Triple therapy is used—local guidelines should be used via the local specialist centre
- The aim of treatment is to reduce viral load to <50ml
- Failure of treatment or non-compliance is associated with emergence of viral genotypic mutations with reduced drug susceptibility
- HAART can be highly toxic, e.g. lactic acidosis, hepatitis, peripheral neuropathy, pancreatitis, effect on lipid metabolism, rash, etc. Close follow-up is necessary at a specialist centre
- Side effects such as nausea, diarrhoea, and lethargy are common and some treatments can be given
- Advice regarding protection for partners
- Partner notification

Complications

- Kaposi's sarcoma—widespread involvement of skin, mucous membranes, visceral, and lymph node disease. Nodules can occur in the lungs. It is aetiologically associated with a herpes virus. Prior to HAART, the median survival time was 2 years
- Non-Hodgkin's lymphoma—B cell tumours, extranodal disease is common, difficult to treat
- Opportunistic infections—*Pneumocystis carinii* pneumonia, *Mycobacterium tuberculosis*, candida, both oral and oesophageal, cryptosporidiosis, CMV causing hepatitis, and atypical mycobacterial infections
- Neurological complications—meningoencephalitis, myelopathy, peripheral neuropathy in acute infection. AIDS-related dementia, chronic subcortical encephalitis is seen in 90% of those dying of AIDS. CMV retinitis and cerebral toxoplasmosis also occur

In pregnancy, breastfeeding, and the neonate

This is discussed in detail in Section 6.7.

Post-exposure prophylaxis (PEP)

This is the use of triple HAART for a period of a month after an episode of exposure to HIV in a non-infected individual. Indications include needlestick injury, sexual assault, and sexual exposure. Evidence of the benefit is limited, and most comes from data on needlestick injury. Treatment with PEP should be available at emergency departments and started as soon as possible; within 72 h of exposure, ideally within 1 h. Follow-up should be in a specialist centre. HIV testing is indicated at both 3 and 6 months as the use of HAART may delay seroconversion.

Further reading

www.bashh.org British Association for Sexual Health and HIV —useful guidelines.

www.medfash.org.uk Medical Foundation for AIDS and Sexual Health.

www.bhiva.org.uk British HIV Association.

www.dh.gov.uk Government website on HIV policy.

www.hpa.org.uk Health Protection Agency Website for latest epidemiological data.

RCOG. *Management of HIV in Pregnancy*. Green top guideline No. 39, 2004. www.rcog.org.uk

Victims of sexual assault may disclose for the first time in the setting of the emergency department, a GU clinic or a GP surgery.

The law

Until 1976, rape was defined in common law as sexual intercourse with a woman without her consent, by force, fear or fraud. Oral penetration was only considered an indecent assault. The law was misleading and has been amended several times since.

Under the Sexual Offences Act 2003, rape is defined as a male intentionally penetrating the vagina, anus or mouth of another person with his penis without consent. The prosecution needs to establish lack of consent and this is often contested.

Epidemiology

Men, women, and children can all be victims of sexual assault. A high proportion of assailants are known to the victim, with coexistent domestic violence.

A large number of victims are vulnerable young people; 44% of victims of sexual assault are under 18 years; about one-third of victims currently seen in the London Haven sexual assault centres are under 18. It is thought that men are less likely to report sexual assault owing to the stigma surrounding male rape.

Globally, it is thought that one in five women have experienced at least one episode of rape or sexual assault. It is considered to be the most under-reported crime. In the year 2007–2008 there were 2,189 reported cases of rape in London.

With regard to date rape and drug-facilitated sexual assault, a recent study found the most commonly found drug was alcohol. Very few women had ingested substances they did not know about; of those that had, benzodiazepines were the most common.

The government wishes to improve reporting and conviction rates for rape. In many areas, the police who deal with victims are specially trained plain clothes officers who work entirely on sexual assault (e.g. in London they are called Project Sapphire Teams).

The first Sexual Assault Referral Centre (SARC) was set up in 1986 at St Mary's, Manchester. Victims are seen either via police referral or in some cases self-referral for examination, forensic samples or to give information anonymously to the police. The aim is to improve the care and quality of forensic examination. Medical aftercare is often available. Examples include The Havens in London, Reach in Tyne and Wear, and the Safe Centre in Preston.

Presentations

A woman (or man) may present through:

- The emergency department—with or without injuries
- A GU clinic—with concerns about sexual health
- The GP
- O&G—sexual assault may be disclosed during a consultation and can present with chronic pain, sexual dysfunction, unwanted pregnancy, fear of vaginal delivery, etc.

An approach—useful tips

- Do not panic if you are the first person to be told
- Find out if the police are involved or s/he wants this
- Take a simple history of where, when, who, and what. Write clearly, date and time the entry, and sign and print your name
- If the patient is bleeding heavily, go ahead and examine as the patient's health comes before forensic evidence
- If the patient is stable, do not do an internal examination
- Contact the local police with consent. They will send appropriate officers. Get advice from a forensic medical examiner. If the police are already involved, they will organize the forensic medical examination with consent

- If the patient does not want to involve the police, there may be a service for anonymous forensic examinations at a SARC in the area. Ask the emergency department or GU clinic about this
- Advise the patient not to wash before a forensic examination
- Advise the patient to 'drip dry' rather than using toilet paper to wipe after passing urine before the examination
- If there are injuries which warrant an examination in theatre, then coordinate with the forensic medical examiner to come and take forensic samples with consent
- Always consider medical aftercare (see section below)

Forensic examination

A forensic examination is a top-to-toe examination.

- Full history
- Take forensic samples
- Document all injuries, non-genital and genital

The process varies but usually takes several hours. Examinations of children should be done by an experienced practitioner (often the designated doctor for child protection).

Timings

An acute forensic examination includes taking forensic samples to test for drugs, assailant DNA, etc. The timings are based on evidence of persistence of spermatozoa.

- For vaginal rape DNA can be found up to 7 days after the assault
- For anal rape DNA can be found up to 3 days
- For prepubescent children DNA can be found up to 3 days
- DNA may be found orally up to 2 days (most likely <6 h)
- Skin—up to 3 days depending on how often washed
- Clothing—DNA may be present even after washing

Forensic samples

Usually a buccal swab or blood sample is taken to eliminate the complainant's DNA. A urine and/or blood sample may be taken if alcohol or drug use is known or suspected to have been given unknowingly.

Skin swabs from contact with the assailant may be taken if <24 h and washing has not yet occurred. Vaginal swabs are taken, starting with the outer vulva and working inwards, with an endocervical swab being the last swab, to avoid DNA contamination. The same approach is applied to the perianal, anal, and rectal swabs. In cases of vaginal rape, DNA from sperm has been found in the rectum owing to drainage and vice versa.

Findings

Many women who have been raped have no genital injuries owing to tissue elasticity and natural lubrication. The commonest site for injury is the posterior fourchette. The most significant injuries are often to the rest of the body. It is important to document bruises, lacerations, and abrasions meticulously.

Medical considerations on presentation

- Emergency contraception—Levonelle® or IUCD
- Hepatitis B vaccination—a super-accelerated course
- HIV post-exposure prophylaxis (PEP) is only recommended where the assailant is known to be at high risk or HIV-positive. With an unknown assailant, it is recommended in anal rape, multiple assailant rape, and those with genital injuries. If a victim of rape is keen to take PEP with an unknown source, a month's course is needed, with 6-month follow-up
- Tetanus vaccination
- Antibiotic prophylaxis if bitten during assault
- Hepatitis A vaccination in anal rape

- Antibiotic prophylaxis with azithromycin and cefixime can be considered in those unlikely to return for follow-up. This may treat pre-existing infection

Aftercare

Follow-up care is very important, either through a GU clinic or SARC.

Screening for STIs should be carried out at least 10 days after the assault. Completion of hepatitis B vaccination courses should be encouraged. Patients on PEP should have a baseline HIV test and then again at both 3 and 6 months. This is to allow for the 3-month window period and for the theoretical delay in seroconversion. PEP medications can have serious side effects, and liver and renal function should be monitored.

Long-term effects

- Infections
- Effect on sexual function
- Increased risk of further assault (owing to victim vulnerability)
- Post-traumatic stress disorder

Contacts
- Victim support 0845 30 30 900
- Samaritans 08457 909090
- Suzy Lamplugh Trust 020 8876 0305

Further reading

www.rapecrisis.org.uk

www.met.police.uk/sapphire/advice.htm

www.thehavens.co.uk

www.opsi.gov.uk Information re Sexual Offences Act.

www.forensic.gov.uk

Dalton M (ed.) Forensic Gynaecology—towards better care for the female victim of sexual assault. London: RCOG Press, 2004.

3.13 Psychosexual dysfunction in women

Women may present psychosexual problems to a health professional in a number of circumstances or with an entirely unrelated symptom. If the clues are not picked up, repeated consultations for seemingly minor or non-specific complaints may result.

Allow patients a non-judgemental confidential consultation to discuss their concerns.

Problems for women include:

- Loss of sexual interest
- Dyspareunia—superficial and/or deep
- Orgasmic dysfunction
- Vaginismus—severe pain on penetration of the vagina and an involuntary spasm of the pelvic floor muscles on penetration
- Chronic pelvic pain

It is always important to rule out an organic cause first.

Clinical assessment

Examination

- General appearance
- Secondary sexual characteristics
- BP, pulse, and urinalysis
- General examination—cardiovascular, central nervous system, abdomen, and external genitalia
- Assess stress incontinence
- Digital and speculum examination

Investigations

Consider investigations to rule out an endocrine cause if menstrual irregularity or symptoms of oestrogen deficiency:

- FSH and LH
- Oestradiol
- Prolactin to exclude pituitary prolactinoma
- Thyroid function tests (hypothyroidism or hyperthyroidism can cause dysfunction in sexual drive and libido)

Common times of presentation

- At start of sexual activity
- During pregnancy, after termination or birth
- At times of stress or illness
- After surgery, commonly gynaecological, breast or abdominal
- Around the menopause

Causes

There are many causes, and a detailed history may avoid over-investigation.

- Medical conditions, e.g. arthritis, multiple sclerosis, spina bifida, cirrhosis, general chronic illness
- Drugs, e.g. hormones such as COCP, cytotoxic drugs, tranquillizers, and antidepressants can all affect libido
- Lack of information about normal anatomy and function—myths leading to concerns
- Anxiety, shame about sex and sexuality—often related to upbringing and culture
- Stress and lack of time owing to other commitments
- Relationship problems, e.g. discrepancies in desire, abuse in the relationship, infidelity
- Previous abuse
- Depression or anxiety
- A change in body image around childbirth and the puerperium, e.g. breasts for feeding rather than pleasure

Management

- Allow patients time to disclose concerns—they may do this gradually at each consultation
- Concerns may worsen the sexual dysfunction and the cycle continues, so allowing patients to express their concerns may break this cycle and help
- Dispel misperceptions and take time to explore the reasons, as these may be due to a lack of understanding of normal anatomy or function, e.g. after a hysterectomy, what is at the top of the vagina? Using diagrams of the body can be helpful
- Basic advice, e.g. lubricant use during sex; spending time as a couple without having sex, then gradual week-by-week reintroduction; self-masturbation to increase awareness of sexual arousal
- Referral may be necessary to local services, e.g. psychosexual counselling or psychology.

Useful tip: the earlier vaginismus is recognized, the better the outcome

Prevention

Doctors carrying out intimate examinations are in a position of power. How the examination is carried out will affect how the woman perceives being examined in the future and, for example, the likelihood of her returning for her cervical smears.

Always respect the wishes of the patient with regard to the gender of the doctor, and offer a chaperone (see Section 1.2).

Explain to the patient exactly what the examination will entail and if there will be discomfort. Use simple language and check understanding. Ask if similar examinations have caused pain in the past and reassure. Ask if she has any concerns.

During the examination, listen to the patient. Be slow and gentle. Tell the patient what is about to happen. An examination may not always be necessary and, in patients with vaginismus, minimizing the number of examinations is important.

Useful tips

If a woman is very tense, ask her to think about trying to push the speculum out of her vagina using her muscles—this may relax the area and make the examination easier.

Offer women to insert the speculum themselves or to guide your hand to retain control.

Patients with a history of abuse or sexual dysfunction need extra time and explanation regarding what happens in labour. Some hospitals offer specialist clinics for the counselling of these patients and vaginal examinations may not be required.

Always take time to talk after labour and delivery. There are myths about the vagina and stitches, and reassurance may help. This may also apply to the partner, who is often affected by observing a traumatic delivery.

Further reading

www.basrt.org.uk British Association for Sexual and Relationship Therapy.

www.ipm.org.uk Institute of Psychosexual Medicine.

Hite S. The Hite Report—a nationwide study of female sexuality. New York: Seven Stories Press, 2004.

Chapter 4

Contraception

Contents

Covered elsewhere

4.1 General principles of contraception

Fertility

Between 80–90% of sexually active women would become pregnant if they did not use contraception for a year.

This section examines ways to prevent pregnancy. However, natural family planning can help couples trying to conceive to learn about their fertile time of the month and when best to try to conceive.

An approach

Faced with a number of options, it can be difficult to choose the most suitable. A useful approach is to consider the following.

- Is she **wishing to conceive?**
- **How devastating** would it be for the woman to conceive, or is the aim to space out pregnancies?
- **How reversible** does the method need to be—is she not likely to want to get pregnant ever again, or in the next 5 years, or in a few months?
- Which methods seem **acceptable** to her? Some women do not want hormonal contraception at any cost; their concerns should be explored
- Are there any absolute or relative **contraindications** to the method?

Always discuss the risk of sexually transmitted infections (STIs) and using condoms to protect against them.

Offer information leaflets. Be prepared for patients to take time to decide and try different methods before finding the one that works for them.

Pregnancy testing

Human chorionic gonadotrophin (HCG) is a glycoprotein, produced by the trophoblast after implantation, which prevents involution of the corpus luteum.

A pregnancy test detects HCG by a monoclonal antibody test. A urine pregnancy test can be positive at a level of 25 mIU/ml. At the time of the first missed period, this level can be detected. The levels double every 48 h in early pregnancy (between days 21–30 post-ovulation), peaking at 10–12 weeks. A test can be positive from day 5 after fertilization; a test 3 weeks after the episode of unprotected sexual intercourse gives a definitive result.

After a pregnancy has ended, the test can stay positive for 1–60 days. This depends upon initial levels, individual clearance rates, completeness of tissue removal, method of ending pregnancy, and clinical status of the pregnancy.

History (all types of contraception)

- Age
- Current contraception
- Past contraception including likes, dislikes, myths
- Pregnancy—numbers, pregnancy-induced problems, types of delivery, whether currently lactating
- Past major illness and operations—specifically hypertension, thromboembolic disease (TED), ischaemic heart disease or stroke, abnormalities of lipid metabolism, valvular or septal heart defect, migraine, liver disease, gallbladder disease, breast disease, sickle cell, diabetes and, if so, any complications
- Allergies
- Regular medication (including herbal remedies)
- Menstrual history, including LMP (normal or not), length of cycle, regularity, symptoms
- Previous gynaecological history and any other symptoms, e.g. postcoital bleeding
- STIs and sexual history, including last unprotected sexual intercourse
- Smoking
- Cervical smear history
- Family history—cardiovascular disease in a first degree relative aged <45 years, hyperlipidaemia, TED

Child protection

Young people under 18 years old will seek advice regarding contraception. It is important to encourage discussion. Young people need to access health services and be assured that consultations will be confidential. If they do not seek help, the result may be an unwanted teenage pregnancy. Ideally, special clinics have dedicated young persons support workers alongside health professionals.

Fraser competence, the ability to understand the implications and alternatives (see Section 1.11), should be assessed, including details about current and past relationships, non-consensual sex, and risk-taking behaviour, e.g. drug taking. If the young person is at risk or is being taken advantage of, there is a duty of care to involve other services. This should be done with consent where possible. If consent is not given, then the concerns must be expressed, and any breach of confidentiality explained and documented.

Sex with a child under 13 years is classed as rape, and the child should be treated and local child protection officers informed.

Even if there are no concerns, young people should be encouraged to discuss sex and contraception with carers or adults with whom they feel safe to talk. If there are concerns regarding a child, it is always best to seek advice, for example via social services.

When giving contraceptive advice, the health professional should ensure that:

- The young person understands the advice
- She is likely to continue having sex with or without contraceptive advice
- Her health may suffer unless she receives contraceptive advice
- It is in the patient's best interest to have advice
- The young person is encouraged to inform the adult with parental authority

Further reading

www.ffprhc.org.uk Faculty of Family Planning and Reproductive Health Care, UK. *Selected practice recommendations for contraceptive use.* London, UK: FFPRHC, 2002.

Guillebaud J. *Contraception—your questions answered.* Edinburgh: Churchill Livingstone, 2004.

4.2 Oral hormonal contraception—Part I

Mechanism of action

COCPs provide blood levels of synthetic oestrogen and progestogen which prevent ovulation by inhibiting the pituitary release of FSH and LH. They also thicken the cervical mucus, which prevents sperm penetration, and thin the endometrium, which reduces receptiveness to implantation.

COCPs can be monophasic (all pills contain the same dose), biphasic (two phases of pills with differing doses during the month), or triphasic (three phases of pills with differing doses) (see Figure 4.1).

The first seven pills in a COCP packet inhibit ovulation, and the remaining 14 maintain anovulation. During the seven pill-free days (or placebo pill days if using an every day preparation), the endometrium is shed and there is a withdrawal bleed. Contraceptive protection is maintained during the pill-free interval so long as the pills in the week prior to and after the interval are taken correctly.

Combined hormonal contraception can be given in the form of patches.

Demographics

COCPs are the commonest form of contraception; use peaks between the ages of 20 and 24 years in the developed world.

Efficacy

Pregnancy rates are 0.1% when fully compliant. For typical use (user and method failure accounted for), the failure rate is 5%.

Clinical assessment

History
See Section 4.1.

Investigations
Before prescribing the COCP:
- BP
- BMI: weight (kg)/height^2 (m)
- Internal and breast examination not routinely indicated
- Women should be encouraged to be breast aware, examine themselves monthly, but should be reassured that most lumps are benign
- No blood tests unless a specific problem is identified

Blood tests which may be indicated include:
- Liver function—if there is a query about liver disease. If results are abnormal, COCP use is contraindicated
- Lipid levels—only if the family history indicates a first degree relative who developed arterial disease <45 years or atherogenic disorder. Treating women for high cholesterol levels prior to starting the pill is not effective, as raised cholesterol levels in young, asymptomatic women only weakly predict coronary heart disease
- Thrombophilia screen—if there is a history of venous thromboembolism (VTE) in a first degree relative <45 years old

Contraindications and risks

Guidelines for the medical eligibility of patients are listed on the Family Planning website. There are four categories:
- Unrestricted use
- Benefits generally outweigh the risk
- Risks generally outweigh the benefit (relative contraindication)
- Unacceptable health risk and should not be used (absolute contraindication)

A woman having two of the conditions listed in the benefits outweigh the risk section should be counselled. There may be a cumulative effect, meaning that the COCP is contraindicated.

Absolute contraindications to the COCP are:
- Breastfeeding and <6 weeks' postpartum
- Smoking and >35 years
- BMI >40
- Multiple risk factors for CVS disease
- BP ≥160/95
- Current or past history of VTE
- Major surgery with prolonged immobilization
- Known thrombogenic mutations
- Current and history of ischaemic heart disease (IHD)
- Stroke
- Valvular and congenital heart disease complicated by pulmonary hypertension, atrial fibrillation, subacute bacterial endocarditis
- Migraine with aura
- Trophoblastic disease when HCG is raised
- Current breast cancer
- Diabetes with complications
- Active viral hepatitis
- Severe cirrhosis
- Benign and malignant liver tumours
- Raynaud's disease with lupus anticoagulant and therefore thrombotic tendency
- Pregnancy

Age
The COCP can be used from the menarche to age 50 if there are no other risk factors.

Smoking
The COCP is associated with a small risk of myocardial infarction in non-smokers; this is increased further in smokers.

Smokers >35 years of age should not be prescribed the COCP. If the woman stops smoking for 1 year and has no other risk factors, she may be considered for the COCP.

Obesity
Use of the COCP in women with a BMI >35 is associated with an increased risk of myocardial infarction (MI) and VTE, and is not recommended.

There is an increased risk of MI and VTE with raised BMI.

Hypertension
Women with hypertension are at increased risk of MI and stroke. The use of the COCP has a negligible effect on blood pressure. However, a cross-sectional survey found that blood pressure was significantly increased in COCP users compared to non-COCP users.

Venous thromboembolism
The background risk is 5 in 100 000. The relative risk of VTE with COCP use can increase by up to 5-fold depending on the progestogen but in absolute terms the risk is still low. The risk is greatest in the first year of use and returns to normal within weeks of discontinuation.

Stroke
The annual incidence of ischaemic stroke in women <35 years is 3 per 100 000. There is a 2-fold increase in this risk with use of low dose COCP but no difference in mortality rates.

Migraine
The risk of ischaemic stroke is increased in migraine sufferers but it is still low (17–19 per 100 000). This risk is thought to be greatest if the migraine is with aura. Aura occurs prior to the onset of headache. Symptoms of aura can be visual disturbances such as scotoma

(flashing lights do not constitute aura), unilateral paraesthesia and/or numbness, unilateral weakness, aphasia or other speech disorder. Migraine with aura is a contraindication. In those with migraine without aura the benefit may outweigh the risk. The pill must be stopped if aura or focal migraine develop.

Breast cancer
Studies on the effect of COCP on breast cancer risk are contradictory. Any excess risk, likely to be small, increases quickly after starting, does not relate to the length of time a patient takes the pill, and returns to baseline within 10 years of stopping the COCP.

Cervical cancer
There is a 4-fold increase in risk for those using COCP long term and positive for HPV. COCP use for less than 10 years has negligible risk. Women should be encouraged to have routine smears and give up smoking.

Liver cancer
Primary liver cancer risk is increased but this is dependent upon length of use.

Useful tips
Three things to discuss when prescribing the COCP:
1. Drug interactions
2. Gastrointestinal symptoms
3. Missed pills

Drug interactions
Liver enzyme inducers (e.g. rifampicin, St John's Wort, some antiretrovirals) increase the metabolism of the COCP, which can decrease the contraceptive efficiency. Condoms should be used during and for 28 days after discontinuation of the medication. A combination of more than one pill, so increasing the dose, can be prescribed, but this should be done by a specialist. Shortening the hormone-free interval also reduces ovarian follicular activity and may lower failure rates.

Antibiotic use alters gut flora and reduces the enterohepatic circulation of ethinyloestradiol. The evidence is contradictory as to whether this alters efficacy, so caution is needed. Women should be advised to use condoms during the antibiotic course and for 7 days afterwards. If this is in the last week of the active pills in the packet, continue straight on with the next packet (i.e. no withdrawal bleed as no pill-free week).

Other drugs—the bioavailability of theophylline, ciclosporin, and lamotrigine are altered by the COCP.

Gastrointestinal symptoms
If the woman vomits within 2 hours of taking the pill, it is as if she has missed the pill. If she has diarrhoea she should use condoms for the duration of the illness and for 7 days afterwards. For both these situations, if the symptoms last for over 3 days she should follow the rules for missed pills.

Missed pills
For standard pills (30 μg of ethinyloestradiol):
- If one or two pills are missed at any time, take the pill as soon as she remembers; no extra cover is needed, continue to take pills as usual. **Do not stop**
- If three or more pills are missed in the first week, she needs emergency contraception if unprotected sex and should use condoms for the next 7 days
- If three or more pills are missed in the second week, she needs to use condoms for 7 days
- If three or more pills are missed in the final week, she needs to use condoms for 7 days and continue with the next packet without a break

For low dose, i.e. 20 μg pills; if two or more pills are missed, then apply the rules for missing three or more 30 μg pills.

If the woman misses any pills she may experience breakthrough bleeding. She should be advised not to be concerned but to carry on taking her COCP as normal.

The pill should, where possible, be started on day 1–5 of the menstrual cycle where it is immediately effective. If it is certain the woman is not pregnant, the pill can be started later in the cycle but condoms would need to be used for the first 7 days. The woman should take a pill once a day at about the same time for 21 days and then have a 7-day break (or take the placebo pills in the every day pill).

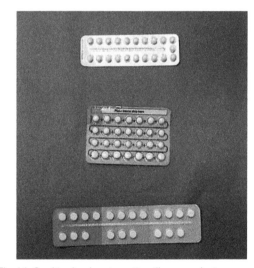

Fig. 4.1 Combined oral contraceptive pills—monophasic, continuous with placebo pills, and triphasic (from top to bottom).

Advantages of the COCP

- RCOG guidelines support the use of the COCP to decrease menstrual blood loss
- The COCP can also be used to diminish the symptoms of dysmenorrhoea
- Lower incidence of functional ovarian cysts and benign ovarian tumours
- Fifty per cent reduction in ovarian and endometrial cancer; the advantage continues for 15 years or more after stopping the COCP
- Lower risk of colorectal cancer
- Improvement in acne vulgaris. Dianette®, containing anti-androgenic cyproterone acetate, is a treatment option for women with severe acne who have not responded to oral antibiotics. There is a greater risk of VTE with this COCP. It should only be used for 3–4 months. Yasmin® may be as effective for mild to moderate acne
- Lower incidence of rheumatoid arthritis
- Less PID; may be because of the progestogen effect on the upper genital tract

Side effects and disadvantages of the COCP

Due to oestrogen (O) and progestogen (P)

Minor

- Spotting and unscheduled bleeding may be due to missed pills and can be common in the first few months of taking the pill (see missed pill section). If it continues to be a problem, a phasic pill can be tried
- Weight gain—there is no causal association with COCP
- Breast tenderness and bloating (O, P)
- Depression and loss of libido (O, P)
- Hair loss (P)
- Worsening of acne (P)
- Cramps and leg pains (P)
- Nausea when first starting (O)
- Dry vagina (P)
- Gingivitis
- Headaches (O)
- Vaginal discharge (O)
- Chloasma (O)
- Photosensitivity (O)
- Galactorrhoea (O)
- Superficial thrombophlebitis (P)
- Cervical ectopy (O)

If a woman finds these side effects intolerable, try reducing the dose of the pill or try another progestogen. For symptoms caused by oestrogen (O), try changing to a progestogen-dominant pill, e.g. Microgynon 30. For symptoms caused by progestogen (P), try changing to an oestrogen-dominant pill, e.g. Marvelon.

Major (see contraindications)

- VTE
- Stroke
- MI
- Cervical cancer
- Liver cancer

Follow-up

Ideally, follow-up should be 3 months after the first prescription and then every 6 months. Weight and blood pressure should be checked, along with reassessment of any change in medical problems or family history.

Risks if pregnancy conceived

In animal studies, sex steroids can be teratogens. The human literature is reassuring. The rates of birth defects are not increased with use of the COCP in early pregnancy.

Reversibility

Hormone levels should return to normal within a few weeks of stopping the COCP and there is no delay in return of fertility. In the past, women were advised to have two periods before trying to get pregnant. This was to aid dating of the pregnancy and is no longer routinely advised.

Progestogen-only pill (POP)

Mechanism of action

The POP works by causing cervical mucus to become viscous and hostile, preventing penetration of sperm into the uterus.

The POP also has the effect of thinning the endometrium, inhibiting implantation.

Ovulation is affected in 60% of women on POP; one-third do not ovulate, but the other two-thirds experience variable interference. Cerazette®'s main action is the inhibition of ovulation.

Efficacy

Efficacy increases with age as fertility declines. By 40 years, its failure rate is 0.5 per 100 000 women years, but this is likely to be higher in younger women. It is more likely to fail in women >70 kg. During breastfeeding, efficacy approaches 100%.

Demographics

The POP accounts for about 10% of the oral contraceptive use in the UK. POP is more commonly used by older women where it is more effective. POP may be used in women who cannot take the COCP, e.g. smokers >35 years, diabetics, and in those with sickle cell disease. The POP is suitable for breastfeeding; it does not inhibit lactation and milk contains only a minute amount.

Clinical assessment

History

See Section 4.1.

Investigations

No investigations are routinely necessary. It is good practice to check BP and weight (BMI).

Contraindications

Absolute contraindications for COCP are only relative for POP.

Absolute contraindications to POP use are:

- Pregnancy
- Undiagnosed vaginal bleeding
- Current breast cancer
- Trophoblastic disease where HCG is raised
- Severe arterial disease or a very high risk of this
- Previous ectopic pregnancy—POP should be avoided, as there is a small increased risk with this method
- Serious side effects experienced on COCP which cannot be attributed to oestrogen
- Acute porphyria

Tips for use

The POP must be taken every day with no break and within a 3 h window. It should be started on day 1–5 of the cycle (day 1 if the cycle is <23 days). If a woman is more than 3 h late taking the pill, it should be taken as soon as she remembers and then continue taking as normal. Condoms should be used for the next 2 days. The effect of progestogen on the cervical mucus wears off within 27–36 h, but builds up rapidly. (The 3-h rule increases to 12 h with Cerazette as its effect is primarily on the ovaries.) If the woman vomits within 2 h of taking the POP or has diarrhoea, then she must use condoms for the duration of symptoms and for 2 days afterwards. This is the equivalent to missing a pill.

Antibiotics have no effect on the POP.

Enzyme-inducing drugs may reduce the efficiency of the POP. Alternative contraception should be used if the medication is long term, or condoms should be used for the length of treatment and for at least 48 h afterwards, depending on the half-life of the drug.

Women who weigh >70 kg may have reduced contraceptive cover on the POP, and should be advised to take two POPs a day (off licence).

Advantages
- The POP can be used while breastfeeding
- Can be used if COCP is contraindicated
- May help with premenstrual tension
- Does not interfere with sex

Side effects and disadvantages
- Irregular bleeding is the commonest problem
- Increased risk of ectopic pregnancy
- Worsening acne
- Breast tenderness
- Weight gain
- Headaches
- Increased risk of benign functional ovarian cysts and pelvic pain (as interference with ovulation in 60%)

Follow-up
Six-month prescriptions can be given.

Risks if pregnancy conceived
The teratogenic risk is small. No cases of congenital abnormality have been reported. There is an increased risk of ectopic pregnancy. This may be because of the effect of progestogen on tubal function (contractility and the rate of ovum transport are decreased).

Reversibility
The effect of POP on cervical mucus is reversed after 36 h, and fertility will return to normal. If there has been an effect on ovulation, fertility may take a few weeks.

Further reading

Arowojolu AO et al. COC for treatment of acne. *Cochrane Database System Reviews* 2004; **3:**CD004425.

Baillargeon JP et al. Association between the current use of low dose oral contraceptives and cardiovascular arterial disease: a meta-analysis. *J Clin Endocrinol Metab* 2006; **90:**3863–70.

Collaborative Group on Hormonal Factors in Breast Cancer. Breast cancer and hormonal contraceptives: collaborative mpt analysis of individual data on 53 297 women with breast cancer and 100 239 women without. *Lancet* 1996; **347:** 1713–27.

Gallo MF et al. Combination contraceptives: effect on weight. *Cochrane Database System Reviews* 2003; **2:**CD003987.

WHO Collaborative Study of Cardiovascular Disease and Steroid Hormone Contraceptiion. *Lancet* 1995; **346:**1575–82.

4.4 Progestogen injections and implants

Mechanism of action

Both the injection and implant act in a similar way, the main mechanism of action being to inhibit ovulation. They both release progesterone and also have actions on cervical mucus and the endometrium. The injection is deep intramuscular, releasing progestogen gradually into the circulation. Etonorgestrel in the implant appears to inhibit LH, not FSH, and oestradiol is still produced.

Efficacy

Both are 99% effective. The pregnancy rate with injectables is <4/1000 over 2 years. The pregnancy rate with the implant is <1/1000 over 3 years.

Demographics

The most commonly used injection is Depo-Provera®, given every 12 weeks. Implanon (the currently used implant) lasts 3 years. Only 8% of 16–49 year olds who are using contraception use these methods.

Clinical assessment

History

See Section 4.1.

Investigations

No routine investigations are necessary. Blood pressure and weight (BMI) are good practice.

Diabetic patients need to monitor their blood glucose (BGs) as a slight reduction in glucose tolerance may occur with injectables.

Contraindications

- Liver adenoma
- Trophoblastic disease (active)
- Pregnancy
- Severe liver disease
- Undiagnosed vaginal bleeding
- Acute porphyria
- Liver enzyme-inducing drugs may cause inefficacy
- Current breast cancer
- Severe arterial disease or a very high risk of this
- Serious side effects experienced on the COCP which cannot be attributed to oestrogen
- Severe hypersensitivity to any component

The injection is suitable for women with previous ectopic pregnancy or ovarian cysts owing to its effect on ovulation.

The injection lowers HDL levels, so should be avoided in women with strong risk factors for arterial disease.

Useful tips

The injection

- Should be started on day 1–5 of the cycle with no need for barrier methods
- If started later (when pregnancy has been excluded), another method should be used for 7 days
- Do not give to a breastfeeding woman until 5 weeks' postpartum to allow the infant's enzyme system to develop (even though there are only trace amounts found in breast milk and no harm has been reported)
- If irregular bleeding is a problem toward the time when another injection is due, it can be given up to 4 weeks early
- Repeat injection can be given up to 2 weeks late without the need for added protection. Extra precautions and cover with emergency contraception should be discussed if later than 2 weeks

- If irregular bleeding is a problem throughout, women can be given a short course of oestrogen as HRT or COCP if not contraindicated
- Antibiotics do not affect efficacy
- Enzyme-inducing drugs may affect the metabolism of progestogen. If such a drug is required, the injection interval should be cut, though this is controversial
- Advise the woman not to touch the injection site as this will disperse the hormone more quickly
- Can be used if BMI>30

Implant

- Local anaesthetic is used to infiltrate and then a large-bore needle is passed subdermally and the implant introduced. The 40 mm × 2 mm rod is inserted into the non-dominant arm in between the head of the biceps and triceps
- Women should be told they will be able to feel the implant
- They should not touch it excessively
- It should be inserted on day 1–5 of the menstrual cycle and no extra precautions are needed
- It can be started later in the cycle if pregnancy is excluded; the woman must be told to use another method for 7 days after the implant has been inserted
- It can safely be used in those >70 kg
- Another form of contraception should be used for those taking regular enzyme inducers

Advantages

Injection

- Does not require day-to-day motivation
- Is non-intercourse-related
- Is very effective
- Can reduce menstrual symptoms
- May reduce premenstrual symptoms
- Is associated with reduced incidence of PID
- Can be used safely when breastfeeding
- Reduces risk of endometrial carcinoma
- Decreases risk of ectopic pregnancy
- Reduces functional ovarian cysts
- Associated with reduced risk of fits in epilepsy
- In sickle cell disease, reduces the number of crises and improves the haematological picture

Implant

- Longlasting (3 years for Implanon®)
- No interference with intercourse
- Can be used when breastfeeding
- Normal fertility returns without delay
- Decreases risk of endometrial cancer
- May reduce dysmenorrhoea or menorrhagia
- Amenorrhoea in 20% after the initial period of irregular bleeding
- Owing to its effect on ovulation, it can safely be used in those who have had a previous ectopic pregnancy

Side effects and disadvantages

Injection

- Galactorrhoea
- Non-reversible once the injection has been given

- Irregular bleeding, although if used continuously most women become amenorrhoeic within 1 year—this is perceived as a problem by some
- Weight gain up to 2–3 kg in a year
- Delay in return of fertility
- Research is not conclusive, but there may be an increased risk of developing osteoporosis if used in the long term in the young or over 40s. If there is a strong family history of osteoporosis, the woman needs to be counselled; another form of contraception may be preferable. This is because of the theoretical amenorrhoea. It is advisable to reassess a woman's risk every 2 years. The small loss of bone mineral density recovers when the injection is discontinued, and lifestyle advice should be given, e.g. weight-bearing exercise, stop smoking
- There may be a slight increased risk of breast cancer
- Small risk of infection at injection site

Implant

- Implants may be difficult to remove if they migrate or there is weight gain and may need specialist referral
- Irregular bleeding—oestrogen supplements may help relieve this symptom if not contraindicated. Fifty per cent will have prolonged or irregular bleeding
- Bruising or infection at the site of insertion; advise to keep dry for 3 days
- Acne
- Tender breasts
- Procedure required to fit and remove
- Keloid scar development at site of insertion and removal

Follow-up

Patients need appointments every 8 or 12 weeks for repeat injections. They should be given a reminder card for when they need the implant changing.

There is no follow-up required for the implant. An open door policy should be offered, as some women will need reassurance if they experience irregular bleeding.

Risks if pregnancy conceived

There is no increased risk of ectopic or miscarriage.

For both methods, there is a theoretical risk of masculinization of the female fetus (particularly enlargement of the clitoris) and possible hypospadias in males.

The teratogenic risks are very low with the low doses of progesterone. Studies associating Depo-Provera® exposure in early pregnancy with fetal growth retardation and increased perinatal mortality are likely to be related to confounding factors, e.g. social class.

Reversibility

For injection

There may be a delay of up to 10 months in the return of fertility. Women should be advised to stop 6 months prior to planning pregnancy and to use another form of contraception.

For implant

Once the implant is removed, blood hormone levels return to normal within a week, so there should be no delay in the return of fertility.

4.5 Barrier methods

Mechanism of action
There are four main barrier methods: male and female condoms, the diaphragm, and the cap. They work by preventing sperm reaching the ovum. In addition, they usually have spermicide which is lethal to sperm. They are made of latex or polyurethane. The male condom fits over an erect penis and should be worn throughout sexual intercourse. The female condom is put inside the vagina with a large ring left outside and fits loosely inside. The cervical cap is rarely used in the UK and is not considered in detail.

Demographics
Male condoms are most widely used. They protect against most STIs. Female condoms are expensive and bought over the counter which may be a disincentive. Diaphragms and caps are not widely used but can be very effective if the woman is motivated. They often suit older women and those spacing pregnancies.

Efficacy
Male condoms, if used according to instructions, are 98% effective. The failure rate is often much higher owing to user failure. For female condoms, the failure rate is 5%. For the diaphragm, the failure rate is 4–8/100 in 1 year (92–96% effective).

Clinical assessment
History
See Section 4.1.

Investigations
None.

Contraindications
Condoms (see Figure 4.2)
- Care needed if latex allergy or spermicide sensitivity

Diaphragms
- If unhappy to self-examine
- Septate vagina
- Uterovaginal prolapse
- Poor perineal muscle tone
- Inadequate retropubic ridge
- Acute vaginitis (treat first)
- Recurrent UTIs
- Rubber allergy
- Previous toxic shock syndrome

Useful tips
Condoms
General
- Always check expiry date and the British Standard Kitemark
- Care with nails and jewellery
- Water-based lubricants (e.g. KY® jelly) should be used. Petroleum jelly or oil-based products can damage the condoms
- If there is a failure, seek emergency contraception

Male
- Put a condom on prior to any touching of the vaginal area by the penis
- The tip of the male condom should be squeezed so that no air is trapped at the end while putting it on the erect penis; this prevents splitting
- The condom should be held on withdrawal then removed when clear of the vulva, wrapped, and disposed of in a bin

Female
- The female condom's outer ring should be held while the penis is inserted, and the penis should be guided in to prevent the

Femidom® being pushed inside or the penis slipping in between the female condom and the vaginal wall

Diaphragms
- Come in a variety of sizes
- Three types: flat spring, coil spring, and arcing spring
- The diaphragm must be fitted so it covers the cervix. Remind that it does not provide a sperm-tight fit
- Use with spermicide (10 cm of cream or jelly or one pessary—needs 10 min to dissolve)
- Insert before intercourse
- If intercourse does not occur within 3 h, then a top-up of spermicide is needed
- Leave in for 6 h after sex
- It can be left up to 24 h
- If intercourse again within 6 h, a spermicide top-up is required
- Rinse with warm soapy water and dry
- Yearly review to assess size and change diaphragm

Advantages
Condoms
- Only need to use during sex
- Protect against most STIs
- No medical side effects unless allergy to latex
- Easily available

Diaphragms
- Non-hormonal
- More independent of intercourse than condom
- No loss of sensation
- Provides some protection against some STIs

Side effects and disadvantages
Condoms
- Interrupt sex
- Latex or spermicide sensitivity (can get non-latex or without spermicide)
- Can break or come off inside the vagina
- Both partners need to be motivated—psychological barrier
- Female condoms can be noisy

Diaphragms
- Less effective
- Forward planning
- Messy
- Requires fitting
- UTI increased risk. To avoid, try a smaller size, advise emptying bladder before and after intercourse
- Discomfort—occasionally vaginal abrasions. Treat any infection, check the size, and try different spermicide
- Increased risk of candidiasis
- If incorrectly fitted, may lie in anterior fornix

Follow-up
Condoms
No follow-up needed.

Diaphragms
Learning the method requires two visits.

First visit:
- Counselling
- Pelvic examination

- Select size (use finger to estimate distance from behind cervix to pubic arch, and then size with practice diaphragms)
- Insert the appropriate size. Use largest size that is comfortable. If between two sizes on measuring, get woman to walk about and recheck
- Remove
- Get the woman to insert and remove it herself, having felt her cervix ('like the end of the nose')
- Woman goes home with practice device

Second visit:
- The woman should return with the device in place
- Check position and that she is happy to insert and remove

If a woman has a vaginal delivery or weight change >3 kg, the device will need to be refitted. The diaphragm should be checked regularly for holes and a new one issued yearly.

Risks if pregnancy conceived
No increased risks.

Reversibility
Immediately reversible.

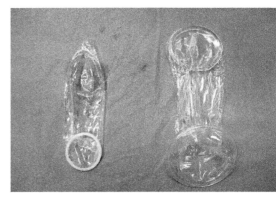

Fig. 4.2 Male and female condoms.

4.6 Intrauterine device and system

Mechanism of action

Intrauterine contraceptive device (IUCD)

This has copper in its core which acts by having a toxic effect on sperm and ova, and decreasing sperm motility. It also acts by impeding implantation. Different coils are licensed for different lengths of time, ranging from 5 to 10 years.

Intrauterine system (IUS)

This has a progestogen-releasing rod in its core which acts to thicken cervical mucus, prevent endometrial proliferation, and may affect ovulation in some women. The IUS is licensed for use as a contraceptive for 5 years and must be changed after this time (see also Section 12.4).

Demographics

Less than 8% of women using contraception use these methods. The IUS is being used by some women to treat gynaecological symptoms, with contraceptive effect as an added bonus. The IUCD has traditionally been recommended to older women in stable relationships.

Efficacy

Both are over 99% effective, with failure rates of about 0.2–2 per 100 woman years.

Clinical assessment

History

See Section 4.1.

Investigations

Prior to insertion, it is good practice to take a high vaginal swab, and endocervical swabs for chlamydia and gonorrhoea. If a woman is at low risk of STI, then this may not be necessary. If no facilities are available for screening, antibiotic prophylaxis against Chlamydia should be given prior to insertion.

Contraindications

To both methods

- Pregnancy
- Current STI or PID
- Unexplained genital tract bleeding
- Distorted uterine cavity, e.g. bicornate uterus
- Valvular heart disease

To IUCD

- Copper allergy
- Wilson's disease
- Heavy painful periods which are difficult to cope with

To IUS

- Hypersensitivity to levonorgestrel

Useful tips

(for insertion technique see Box 12.3 in Section 12.4)

General

- Easier to insert during menstruation
- Cervical shock is always a risk at the time of insertion; take a baseline pulse and blood pressure, and have resuscitation equipment available
- Be aware that if the woman is epileptic insertion may induce a seizure
- It can be fitted 4 weeks after a normal vaginal delivery or 6–8 weeks after CS
- The woman should be encouraged either to examine for the threads after each period or to come back at 6 weeks and 3 months, and then yearly for review

- Changing the IUCD or IUS needs to be performed during the period with no intercourse from day 1, or at any time if there has been no intercourse in the previous 7 days and a negative pregnancy test
- IUS—usually older women have a Mirena but this is also recommended in younger women with low risk of STIs

IUCD

- Can be inserted up to 5 days after the earliest expected day of ovulation (length of cycle minus 14) or at any time if no risk of pregnancy
- It is effective immediately
- If fitted in a woman over 40, it can be left in situ until she no longer requires contraception

IUS

- Insert on day 1–5 of cycle for immediate protection. It can be inserted if no risk of pregnancy and another method used for the following 7 days
- Should be changed every 5 years; if over 45 years it can remain until the woman no longer needs contraception

Advantages of IUCD and IUS

- Long term
- Do not need to worry about remembering
- Does not interrupt sex—partner should not be able to feel it
- No delay in return of fertility
- No interactions with other medications
- HIV-positive women can use it
- Nulliparous women can use it
- With the IUS, menstruation can be lighter (90%) and therefore reduce dysmenorrhoea

Side effects and disadvantages

IUCD

- Menstruation can be longer and heavier (30%)
- After insertion, spotting and intermenstrual bleeding (IMB) are common in the first few cycles; exclude other causes

IUS

- Irregular bleeding for up to 6 months after insertion; after this, up to 20% of women are amenorrhoeic, which may not be acceptable to the patient
- Acne

General

- In the first 3 weeks after insertion, there is an increased risk of pelvic infection
- There is no evidence that removing an IUCD is indicated in moderate or mild PID
- No protection against STIs
- Perforation at the time of insertion occurs 1:1000 (see Figure 4.4) and may be unnoticed. This may lead to the need for laparoscopy. Laparotomy may be required later to remove the intra-abdominal device as adhesions develop with time
- Expulsion (2–10 per 100 woman years); commonest in first 3 months
- Displacement
- If pregnancy occurs, 1:20 will be ectopic (higher rate than background 1:200 but decreased absolute risk since overall pregnancy rate is much lower). If there is a positive pregnancy test, the woman will need referral for a scan and the coil removing. A previous ectopic pregnancy is not a contraindication to IUCD/IUS insertion.

Follow-up

Women should be encouraged to examine themselves to check the coil strings after each period. If this is not acceptable to them, then follow-up for a coil check should be at 6 weeks and 3 months. All women should have one follow-up visit at 6 weeks and the chance to return to discuss concerns.

If the threads are lost:
- Exclude pregnancy
- Recommend alternative contraception
- Explore canal
- Refer for scan or X ray to locate and refer on as necessary

Risks if pregnancy conceived
- Exclude an ectopic pregnancy
- If coil remains in situ, there is an increased risk of mid-trimester miscarriage, pre-term delivery, and infection
- Ideally, remove the coil as soon as possible even if the woman is considering termination of the pregnancy; there is an increased risk of miscarriage, but this is higher if the coil is left in situ (50%), and is likely to occur during the second trimester with more complications
- No evidence of increased risk of fetal abnormality

Reversibility

There is no delay in return of fertility. The coil should be easily removed in clinic using sponge-holding forceps.

If it is not easy to remove or the strings are not visible or palpable on vaginal examination, then referral to a gynaecology clinic and removal under general anaesthetic ± hysteroscopy is sometimes necessary.

Actinomyces-like organisms (ALOs) and IUCD/IUS

Actinomyces israeli is a normal commensal of the gut and mouth. It can rarely cause pelvic actinomycosis, characterized by granulomatous pelvic and abdominal abscesses.

After 5 years, ALOs will be picked up on 20% of smears from IUCD and IUS users.

If the woman is asymptomatic and has no signs on examination, she should be informed of what symptoms to look out for (deep dyspareunia, pelvic pain, dysuria, IMB); the device may be left in situ and smears taken as directed.

If the woman has symptoms, an STI screen should be performed, the device removed, and sent to the laboratory to look for ALOs (making sure contraceptive needs are covered), and the woman should be offered treatment and review.

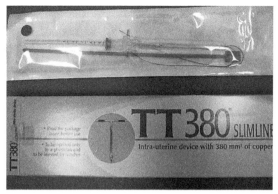

Fig. 4.3 Copper IUCD.

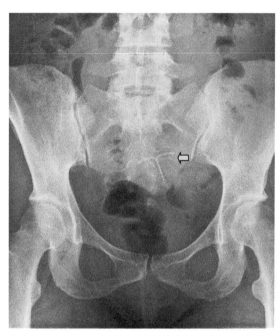

Fig. 4.4 X-ray of an intra-abdominal IUCD (⇦). (Kindly provided by Holly House Hospital.)

4.7 Natural family planning and emergency contraception

Natural family planning

This is a method which takes time to teach, generally about three or more cycles, and requires motivation by the couple.

It relies on the accurate identification of the fertile days of the woman's menstrual cycle, and the modification of sexual behaviour to abstain or use barrier methods.

Advantages

- Natural
- No side effects
- Efficient if well taught and motivated
- Low cost
- Not dependent on medical personnel once taught
- Promotes health awareness
- Encourages shared responsibility in a couple
- Ethically acceptable
- Can be used to prevent or plan pregnancy

Disadvantages

- Takes time to learn
- Difficulty charting
- Difficulty with abstinence
- Requires commitment
- More difficult at times of stress or hormonal change
- No protection against STIs
- Fertility monitoring devices, if used, are expensive

Physiology

FSH and LH have no observable signs and symptoms.

Oestrogen and progesterone from the ovaries form the clinical basis of fertility awareness methods:

- Before ovulation, oestrogen causes cervical mucus to become thinner and aids sperm penetration
- After ovulation, progesterone causes cervical mucus to become thick and hostile to sperm
- Cervical mucus becomes clearer, wetter, slippery, and stretchy during the most fertile time (spinbarkeit)
- The cervix changes from low, firm, and closed to high, soft, and open during the fertile time
- Sperm can fertilize an egg up to 6 days after ejaculation and an ovum can last up to 20 h. The fertile period is therefore about 8–9 days
- Progesterone causes basal body temperature to rise by 0.2°C after ovulation

Method

Women look for four things:

1. Their cycle
2. Consistency of cervical mucus (94% of women can detect the change, but it may be masked by seminal fluid, vaginal infections or spermicide)
3. Basal body temperature on first waking
4. Cervical position (may be difficult to determine)

From 6–12 previous menstrual cycle lengths

- Shortest cycle minus 20 days is the first fertile day
- Longest cycle minus 10 is the last fertile day
- For women whose cycles are 26–32 days, their fertile period is between days 6 and 22 of their cycle
- The failure rate using this alone is about 20%

From cervical secretions

- The fertile time starts from when a woman is first aware of any cervical secretions until the fourth morning after the day the secretions become sticky
- Using this alone failure rate is 20%

From basal body temperature

- The temperature chart does not identify the start of the fertile time, but the fertile time ends after three consistently high temperatures, higher than the preceding six. Readings must be taken prior to getting up, drinking, etc., and are not reliable for shift workers
- The failure rate is about 6% when used alone

Over-the-counter fertility kits are available which are useful both to prevent pregnancy and to assist conception

Withdrawal

This method is one of the oldest in history. It is still used by couples although it may not be openly discussed. If a couple is going to use this or nothing, then it should be discussed and their choice respected.

The failure rate of withdrawal of the penis prior to ejaculation has been quoted as being high. The chance of sperm in the pre-ejaculate causing fertilization is thought to be low as long as the man withdraws prior to the male orgasm.

It has been suggested that concurrent use of a spermicide may decrease the likelihood of pregnancy.

The method is free, always available, and non-hormonal. It may be unsatisfying to both partners.

There is no protection against STIs.

Emergency contraception (EC)

This is the prevention of pregnancy following unprotected sexual intercourse. There are two forms:

1. Oral hormonal method—levonorgestrel 1500
2. Copper intrauterine device

The hormonal method's action is not entirely understood. It is thought to inhibit ovulation by 5–7 days, therefore allowing any sperm present to lose their fertilizing capabilities.

The copper coil acts to prevent implantation (it does not cause a termination; legally, pregnancy starts at implantation not fertilization—the decision of a Government Judicial Review in April 2002). It is also toxic to sperm and ovum.

Emergency contraception is indicated in a large number of clinical situations. There is no time in the cycle when there is no risk of pregnancy, especially if the cycle is irregular or LMP uncertain.

The oral hormonal EC

- Should be taken as soon as possible
- Within 72 h—it is 95% effective in 24 h, 85% between 25 and 48 h, and 58% between 49 and 72 h (it can be considered up to 120 h but effectiveness is much reduced)
- 1.5 mg single dose
- Side effects—if the woman vomits (1%) within 2 h, repeat the dose; the next period may be early, delayed, heavy or light
- It can be used more than once per cycle, but stress the importance of a regular form of reliable contraception
- The only contraindications are pregnancy and ethical objections (though must refer on urgently)

- The woman may have three tablets (4.5 mg dose as a single dose) if taking enzyme-inducing tablets
- There may be an increased risk of ectopic pregnancy so, if the method fails, referral for an early scan is indicated

The copper IUCD:

- Within 5 days of unprotected sex
- High effectiveness of 99%
- 380 mm of copper has the lowest failure rate
- Screen for or treat for STIs prophylactically if high risk prior to insertion
- If the timing of ovulation can be estimated (length of cycle minus 14 days), then it can be fitted up to 5 days after this day even if multiple episodes of unprotected sex or if the event was over 5 days earlier
- IUCD is the preferred option if on liver enzyme-inducing drugs
- There is an increased risk of PID in the first 3 weeks after insertion

A pregnancy test should be carried out 3 weeks after the use of the EC or if the next menstruation is 7 days late.

Unplanned pregnancy

At least 30% of pregnancies are unplanned. Britain has one of the highest rates of teenage pregnancy in Europe. Patients should be counselled about their options:

- Continuing pregnancy
- Termination (see Section 5.9)
- Adoption

Useful numbers

- Sexwise for young people 0800 28 29 30
- Marie Stopes 0845 300 8090
- British Pregnancy Advisory Service 0845 7304030

4.8 Sterilization

Incidence

About 45% of UK couples aged betwen 40 and 44 years use this method.

Prerequisites

The couple must:
- Have completed their family
- Want a permanent method of contraception
- Have no other acceptable method
- Have explored regret (health of other children, breakdown of relationship)
- Plan interim contraception
- Choose which partner undergoes a procedure
- Explore woman's gynaecological symptoms and influences on her decision, e.g. menorrhagia

Female sterilization

Female sterilization is known as tubal occlusion. The Fallopian tubes are identified laparoscopically and a metal (Filshie™) clip is placed across each one. Photographic evidence should be taken (see Figure 4.5). Occasionally, for technical reasons, mini-laparotomy is required which extends hospital stay.
- The failure rate is 1:200, or more if done with CS or termination. (CREST study in America found higher failure rates than originally thought but did not look at Filshie™ clips)
- Sterilization does not interrupt sex and there is no need to think about contraception
- The method is not 100% reversible so the woman needs to be sure
- It offers no protection against STIs
- If it fails, there is a high risk of ectopic pregnancy (10%)
- Surgical risks include: damage to pelvic organs (3 per 1000) including bowel, bladder, and blood vessels; risk of general anaesthetic; risk of mortality (1 per 12 000)
- Those under 30 years should be discouraged from this method and other forms of contraception discussed
- Menstruation may be heavier but this may be subjective as periods return to 'normal' when, for example, COCP use is discontinued
- Use another form of contraception for cycle before operation or, ideally, abstain
- Always do a pregnancy test before the procedure
- Postoperatively it is usual to continue the current form of contraception until the next period

Newer methods are constantly being developed, including hysteroscopic methods.

Male sterilization

Male sterilization is known as a vasectomy. A small incision is made in the scrotum under local anaesthetic and a section of each vas deferens is tied and cut.
- The failure rate is 1:10 000
- Same advantages as female sterilization
- The method is not 100% reversible
- Risks include infection, haematoma, localized swelling and postvasectomy pain syndrome (3–8%). This syndrome is likely to be due to a granuloma. Symptoms improve with time
- It offers no protection against STIs

It may take up to 12 weeks until the ejaculate is free of sperm. Two semen samples must be negative for sperm at least 4 weeks apart prior to relying on it as a method of contraception.

Further reading

NICE. Hysteroscopic sterilisation by tubal cannulation and placement of intrafallopian implant. Guidance number IPG44, 2004. www.nice.org.uk

RCOG. Laparoscopic tubal occlusion. Consent advice 3, 2004. www.rcog.org.uk

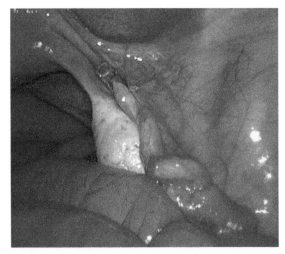

Fig. 4.5 Laparoscopic view of Filshie™ clip *in situ*.

Chapter 5

Starting and tentative pregnancy: preconception care, infertility, miscarriage, and termination

Contents

Covered elsewhere

- Polycystic ovary syndrome (PCOS) (see Section 12.11)
- The Abortion Act 1967 (see Section 1.11)

5.1 General preconception care

The aim of preconception care is to clarify, quantify, and minimize the risk to a pregnancy from any pre-existing medical conditions or lifestyle patterns of either partner that may affect reproductive outcome. It does not aim to identify those couples at high risk so that infertility treatment is denied to them.

Weight

- Women who have a normal BMI (20–25 kg/m^2) are more likely to conceive and have a healthy pregnancy
- Underweight women are likely to become anovulatory and amenorrhoeic. Ovulation can be induced in these women using pharmacological agents. However, any pregnancy is more likely to result in miscarriage and has an increased risk of a range of obstetric problems, such as fetal growth restriction (FGR). Children born in these circumstances are more likely to have long-term health issues, such as cardiovascular disease and diabetes
- Overweight women are also more likely to become anovulatory and amenorrhoeic. Fertility rates of 79% at BMI 25 drop to 12% if BMI is >35. The drop in fertility is more pronounced with coexisting polycystic ovary syndrome (PCOS). Any pregnancies in these women are also at higher risk of miscarriage and a range of obstetric complications, including gestational diabetes, pregnancy-induced hypertension, pre-eclampsia and medical interventions

Folic acid

- Folic acid preconceptually and in the first trimester reduces the risk of offspring having neural tube defects (NTD)
- A dietary supplement of 400 μg/day is recommended
- However, 5 mg/day is recommended if there is a history of epilepsy, NTD in a previous pregnancy or obesity (BMI>35 associated with higher incidence of NTD)

Exercise

- Regular, moderate exercise should be a part of general health maintenance
- Excessive exercise can lead to hypothalamic dysfunction in women and secondary amenorrhoea

Alcohol

- In men, alcohol has significant effects on Leydig cell function by reducing testosterone synthesis. Acetaldehyde is an alcohol metabolite that results in damage to the membranes of Leydig cells and subsequently induces formation of anti-Leydig cell antibodies
- Hypothalamic dysfunction can result from excessive alcohol intake and cause testicular dysfunction. Similarly, the hyperoestrogenic state that results in patients with cirrhosis can lead to further testicular dysfunction and impotence
- In women, alcoholism can lead to amenorrhoea. This is in part caused by hypothalamic dysfunction and in part caused by the associated general lifestyle and nutritional problems
- Excessive alcohol intake in pregnancy results in a recognizable fetal alcohol syndrome
- Women who are planning a pregnancy should be advised no more than 1–2 units of alcohol/week and avoid episodes of intoxication (or 'binge drinking'). Some clinicians advocate complete abstinence as the threshold intake for causation of fetal alcohol syndrome is unknown

Smoking

- Cigarette smoke metabolites are extremely toxic to gametes, causing morphological abnormalities in sperm and oxidative damage in oocytes and embryos
- In women, there is a direct correlation between the number of cigarettes smoked and the risk of infertility. A large population database study looking at 17000 women in the Oxford Family Planning Association database reported that 5 years after cessation of smoking 11% of women who smoked >20 cigarettes/day remained childless as opposed to only 5% of non-smokers
- Smoking may also have a direct bearing on ovarian function and reserve, as smoking brings forward the age of menopause
- Women undergoing IVF treatment are also almost 40% less likely to conceive if they continue smoking
- Smokers have a 20–30% risk of first trimester miscarriage (compared to 10–15% in the general population), a 50% increased risk of premature labour and twice the risk of a low birth weight baby compared to the general obstetric population
- Additionally, babies who live in a smoking household have a significantly increased risk of sudden infant death syndrome (SIDS/cot death)

Medical problems

Prompt referral prior to attempting pregnancy or infertility treatment is always preferable (see Chapter 7).

- To address medical problems prior to pregnancy
- To obtain accurate counselling
- To optimize maternal health before conception
- To avoid teratogenic medications
- To advise accurately about pregnancy risks
- To avoid multiple pregnancy where it would have a disproportionate risk to maternal life or health

5.2 Infertility

Definition
The definition of infertility is contentious, but may be defined as the inability to conceive after 1–2 years of regular, unprotected sexual intercourse in the absence of any known reproductive pathology. The cumulative spontaneous pregnancy rate is 85% after 1 year of trying and 92% after 2 years. Thus, although 7% of couples conceive spontaneously in the second year (half of the remainder), the initiation of investigations is justified.

Incidence
Infertility is becoming increasingly common and is currently estimated to affect at least 15% of couples. Of these couples, 70% will have primary infertility (no previous pregnancies) and 30% secondary (at least one previous pregnancy).

Aetiology in the female partner
Anovulatory infertility
Is the commonest cause of female infertility
Ovarian dysfunction
- Polycystic ovary syndrome (PCOS) is a condition of normogonadotrophic anovulation and is the commonest cause of anovulatory infertility (80%). Ovarian steroid hormone levels are usually normal and thus maintain the ovary–pituitary feedback loop (see Section 12.11)

Hypergonadotrophic hypogonadism
- Failure of the ovary to respond to pituitary gonadotrophin stimulation results. The absence of ovarian hormones (oestradiol and inhibin) results in loss of negative feedback to decrease pituitary secretion of gonadotrophins. Gonadotrophin levels rise excessively and reach menopausal levels (FSH>25, LH>15)
- Classically found in premature ovarian failure (where the pool of primordial follicles has been exhausted prematurely, i.e. <40 years). A variant of this is resistant ovary syndrome, where abnormalities in the FSH receptor cause increased FSH levels in the presence of a good reserve of ovarian follicles

Hypogonadotrophic hypogonadism
- Failure of the pituitary gland to produce FSH results in lack of stimulation to the ovaries. Usually this condition occurs in response to stress (e.g. excessive exercise, weight loss, anorexia nervosa, and psychological stress), which results in loss of pulsatile secretion of gonadotrophin-releasing hormone (GnRH)
- This may be a result of surgery or irradiation of the anterior pituitary, inflammation (e.g. sarcoidosis, tuberculosis), Sheehan's syndrome (postpartum pituitary necrosis), and, rarely, congenital deficiency (e.g. Kallmann's syndrome)

Other causes
- Hyperprolactinaemia
- Hypothyroidism

Tubal damage
Infection
- The principal cause of tubal damage is infection, usually as a result of pelvic inflammatory disease with *Chlamydia trachomatis* as the prime pathogen
- The Fallopian tubes may also be damaged secondary to pelvic infection as a result of appendicitis, septic miscarriage, tuberculosis, and other intra-abdominal inflammatory disorders such as Crohn's disease. Iatrogenic tubal damage can be the result of pelvic surgery

Endometriosis
- Inflammatory responses to the presence of endometriotic tissue may lead to adhesion formation and secondary tubal damage

Uterine factors
Intrauterine adhesions
- Results from postinflammatory scarring of the endometrial cavity following infection (endometritis) or trauma (excessive curettage). Asherman's syndrome describes amenorrhea due to cervical stenosis (see also Section 12.10)

Submucous fibroids
- The presence of fibroids that occlude the tubal ostia may lead to infertility. However, whether submucous fibroids in other locations are a cause of infertility remains uncertain (see Figure 5.1)

Congenital uterine anomalies
- The prevalence of congenital uterine anomalies in infertile women is the same as found in women with normal reproductive histories, 3%. Therefore, they are unlikely to be causal. However, their presence is associated with a significantly higher miscarriage rate, therefore surgery may be warranted

Aetiology in the male partner
Primary testicular dysfunction
Most cases of male factor infertility fall into this category; however, no predisposing cause is found in up to 50%.
- Failure of spermatogenesis may be secondary to trauma (e.g. torsion), infection (e.g. mumps orchitis), or neoplasm and subsequent chemotherapy
- Microdeletions on the Y chromosome are linked to azoospermia (absence) and severe oligospermia (↓ number)
- Azoospermic and severely oligospermic men should have a karyotype to identify rare chromosomal disorders, i.e. Klinefelter's syndrome, and to assess the risk of transmission to the offspring

Obstructive
Results in azoospermia.
- Congenital—congenital absence of vas is causal in 10%
- Iatrogenic (vasectomy)
- Infective
- Bilateral congenital absent vas is seen classically with cystic fibrosis (CF), and men should be screened for CF mutations

Endocrine
- Hypogonadotrophic hypogonadism
- Hyperprolactinaemia leads to impotence but does not affect sperm count

Autoimmune
- Twelve per cent have anti-sperm antibodies which may decrease sperm motility and affect sperm–egg interaction adversely. They are associated with vasectomy reversal

Drugs
- Recreational drugs, e.g. tobacco, alcohol, and marijuana adversely affect sperm function and production
- Anabolic and corticosteroids, sulfasalazine, and antifungal agents can affect spermatogenesis reversibly
- Erectile dysfunction can be secondary to beta-blockers and antidepressants
- Chemotherapy destroys germ cell lines and leads to irreversible azoospermia

Environmental
- Occupational exposure to heat, radiation, and chemicals can affect spermatogenesis

- Worldwide, there is some evidence of an overall decline in sperm count; the exact cause remains unknown but is thought to be environmental

Varicocele

Abnormally tortuous veins in the pampiniform plexus of the spermatic cord.

- More common on the left owing to the direct insertion of the spermatic vein into the renal vein
- May also be found incidentally in fertile men (11%), but the overall prevalence is higher in infertile men (25%)
- Surgical correction does not improve the sperm count or conception rates but is indicated if symptomatic

Unexplained

- If all the basic investigations are normal, this is termed unexplained (idiopathic) infertility
- Accounts for 40% of female infertility and 8–28% of infertility in couples.
- In these couples, expectant management will result in a per cycle pregnancy rate of around 2%. Up to 60% of couples with unexplained infertility of <3 years' duration will conceive spontaneously within 3 years
- A significant contributing factor to unexplained infertility is the increase in the mean age at which women seek to conceive, which leads to a drop in natural fertility

Further reading

David Adamson G, Baker V. Subfertility: causes, treatment and outcome. *Best Practice & Research Clinical Obstetrics & Gynaecology* 2003; **17(2):** III–X.

NICE clinical guideline for fertility: assessment and treatment for people with fertility problems, 2004. www.rcog.org.uk

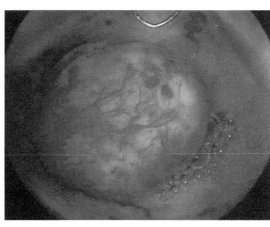

Fig. 5.1 Hysteroscopic view of a submucous fibroid.

5.3 Infertility assessment

Infertility usually affects a couple, hence they should be seen together. However, each partner should have the opportunity to be seen separately and confidentially to discuss personal issues or concerns, e.g. STIs, domestic violence, ambivalence, distress.

General investigations

- Rubella immunity status (female only)
- Opportunistic screening, e.g. cervical cytology, if not current
- HIV, Hepatitis B and C status—usually only required prior to commencement of assisted conception treatment (both partners)

Female partner

History

- Age—delay in childbearing is increasingly common in women today. Advancing age results in progressive reduction of ovarian reserve and poorer quality oocytes, thereby increasing the chances of a chromosomally abnormal pregnancy and failure of implantation or miscarriage
- Menstrual history—irregular cycles, oligomenorrhoea, and amenorrhoea are all signs of anovulatory cycles. In amenorrhoea, weight gain or loss, symptoms of hyperprolactinaemia, hypothyroidism, and the menopause should be checked.
- Obstetric history—ask about the time taken to achieve any previous pregnancy and any miscarriage ± surgical evacuation of uterus. Additionally, obstetric problems such as severe postpartum haemorrhage (PPH) may result in Sheehan's syndrome. It is important to note that women with previous CS also report reduced fertility
- Contraception—long-acting progestogen contraception, e.g. depot preparations, may result in delay in resumption of ovulation. The use of an IUCD may be associated with pelvic infection and increased risk of intrauterine adhesions and tubal damage
- Medical problems—poorly controlled medical problems (e.g. diabetes) have an adverse impact on fertility and should be addressed if identified. Similarly, some medications may interfere with reproductive function (i.e. some antidepressants may increase prolactin secretion and result in anovulation)

Examination

Physical examination may yield little extra information. However, certain aspects remain important.

- BMI—may indicate a weight-related cause for amenorrhoea
- Signs of endocrine disorders—acne, hirsutism, balding (polycystic ovary syndrome), acanthosis nigricans (diabetes), virilization (congenital adrenal hyperplasia), visual field defects (pituitary tumour and secondary hyperprolactinaemia), and signs of thyroid disease
- Vaginal examination—an enlarged uterus may indicate uterine fibroids. Fixed retroversion of the uterus or/and the presence of nodules in the posterior fornix and over the uterosacral ligaments may indicate severe pelvic endometriosis

Investigations

Ovarian reserve

Early follicular phase (day 2–5) gonadotrophin (LH, FSH), and oestradiol concentrations provide an assessment of ovarian reserve. An FSH level <10 and oestradiol <70 is considered normal and is prognostic of success with assisted conception treatment.

Ovulation

Regular cycles are indicative of ovulation. However, biochemical evidence is obtained by demonstrating a progesterone level >30 nmol/l in the midluteal phase of the cycle. A record should be made of the time of the next period as the midluteal phase occurs 7 days before the onset of menstruation. Additionally, commercially available LH testing kits detect the preovulatory surge accurately, and blood should be tested 7 days after.

Tubal patency

Conventional tubal patency tests not only confirm patency but can also give an indication of additional relevant pathology (see Section 5.4). However, the Fallopian tubes are more than just a passage for sperm and egg (enabling fertilization and early development as well). It should be remembered that patency does not equate to normal function.

- Hysterosalpingography (HSG) involves injection of radio-opaque dye through the cervix, into the uterus, and through the Fallopian tubes whilst an X-ray is taken (see Figure 5.3 in Section 5.4). It is usually performed in the first 10 days of a cycle. It may outline filling defects in the uterine cavity (indicating fibroids, endometrial polyps, a uterine septum or adhesions). Women should be screened and treated for pelvic infections, as the risk of procedure-related PID is estimated at 4%
- Laparoscopy and dye—methylene blue dye is instilled through the cervix, into the uterus, and through the Fallopian tubes and is visualized laparoscopically (see Figure 5.4 in section 5.4). Concomitant treatment of adhesions and endometriosis may also be possible
- HyCoSy (hysterosalpingo contrast sonography)—ultrasound is used to visualize medium injected into the uterine cavity, exiting via the Fallopian tubes

Ultrasound

The advent of high resolution transvaginal ultrasound probes has been a significant advance in gynaecology. Ultrasound is the principal tool for identification of uterine fibroids, polyps, adhesions, etc. When suspected, a hysteroscopy is warranted to confirm diagnosis and plan treatment. HSG may also indicate filling defects which should then be investigated by hysteroscopy. Ultrasound also enables the diagnosis of a range of pelvic pathologies such as polycystic ovaries, endometriosis, hydrosalpinges (see Figure 5.6), and pelvic adhesions. The role of 3D ultrasonography is being evaluated.

Male partner

Semen analysis

There is a large biological variation in sperm quality. Repeat tests in the same man can be highly variable. Semen analysis is performed according to World Health Organization (WHO) criteria (see Table 5.1)

Terminology

- Asthenozoospermia—reduced sperm motility
- Oligozoospermia—sperm concentration <20 ×10^6
- Teratozoospermia—abnormal sperm morphology
- Hypospermia—reduced volume of ejaculate

Severe abnormalities in semen analysis results warrant further investigation to determine if the defect is a primary testicular cause or outflow obstruction. Gonadotrophin levels should be tested to differentiate between the different causes.

Gonadotrophins

- Normal FSH and normal testosterone = obstructive
- ↑ FSH and normal testosterone = failure of spermatogenesis
- ↑ FSH and ↓ testosterone = complete testicular failure
- ↓ FSH and ↓ testosterone = hypogonadotrophic hypogonadism

Karyotype
- Several genetic syndromes (including cystic fibrosis) are associated with severe abnormalities in semen analysis

Testicular biopsy
- May indicate if any sperm are available for ICSI (intracytoplasmic sperm injection)

Table 5.1 WHO criteria for semen analysis	
	Normal range
Volume	>2 ml
pH	>7.2
Sperm concentration	$>20 \times 10^6$/ml
Total sperm number	$>40 \times 10^6$ per ejaculate
Morphology	>15% normal
Motility	>50% motile *or* >25% progressive motility

Management
General principles
- Normalization of BMI
- Smoking cessation
- Cut alcohol intake
- Regular unprotected sexual intercourse
- The effectiveness of complementary therapies for fertility problems has not been clinically evaluated and further research is needed before they can be recommended

Anovulation
The aim of treatment is to induce ovulation from a single follicle. Medical treatments carry a risk of multiple pregnancy and ovarian hyperstimulation syndrome (OHSS).
- Hypergonadotrophic hypogonadism—ovulation induction is not possible as either there are no follicles left or the ovary will not respond to gonadotrophins. Ovum donation should be considered
- Hypogonadotrophic hypogonadism—ovulation induction with either daily gonadotrophin injections or pulsatile infusion of GnRH
- Polycystic ovary syndrome (PCOS) (see also Section 12.11)—weight reduction alone will achieve resumption of ovulation in obese women (40–60%). Medical ovulation induction can be achieved using clomifene citrate (+ metformin if BMI>25), daily injection of gonadotrophin or pulsatile GnRH. Surgical treatment is also possible with laparoscopic ovarian drilling (see Figure 5.2). The surgical option involves destroying ovarian cortex and follicles, and may have long-term consequences. However, it does decrease the risks of multiple pregnancies and of OHSS and is cheaper overall

Tubal factor
- Some tubal obstructions may be amenable to surgical correction, with success rates as high as 70% for patency and pregnancy rates of 30%. Tubal surgery carries an increased risk of ectopic pregnancy but obviates risks associated with IVF
- If surgery is not possible, then IVF is the only option

Endometriosis (see Section 13.2)
- Medical management is not indicated in infertility as it results in anovulation, risks teratogenicity, and delays conception
- Surgical treatment of mild-to-moderate endometriosis improves natural conception rates postoperatively
- Surgical treatment of severe endometriosis may improve success at IVF

Uterine factors
The impact of these problems remains debatable and therefore any decision to treat should be made on a case-by-case basis.
- Submucous fibroids—hysteroscopic resection
- Uterine septum—hysteroscopic division
- Intramural fibroids—myomectomy; even removal of small (i.e. <5 cm) intramural fibroids has been shown to confer benefit to pregnancy rates after IVF
- Adhesions—hysteroscopic division and insertion of copper IUCD

Unexplained infertility
- Expectant management—60% of women with secondary unexplained infertility become pregnant within 3 years of investigations. This is probably more suitable when the female partner is younger (i.e. < 35 years)
- Controlled ovarian stimulation (COS)—using clomifene citrate or gonadotrophin injections, up to three oocytes are induced to develop. Subsequently, either timed sexual intercourse or intrauterine insemination (IUI) is carried out. This aims to give a pregnancy rate of 10–15% per attempt. Overall, COS–IUI is more cost-effective and less demanding, emotionally and physically, for the couple, than IVF
- IVF should be recommended if there is no success after three cycles of COS–IUI

Further reading
NICE clinical guideline for fertility: assessment and treatment for people with fertility problems, 2004. www.rcog.org.uk

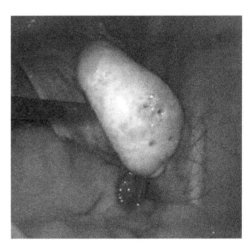

Fig. 5.2 Ovarian drilling. Note the diathermy points on the ovary (Kindly provided by Mr F. Odejinmi).

- Tubal factors account for 30–40% of female infertility cases
- The increasing incidence of pelvic infection continues to be a significant aetiological factor in tubal pathology, as demonstrated by the direct correlation between the number of episodes of pelvic inflammatory disease (PID) and risk of infertility (see Table 5.2)
- Tubal damage may also be secondary to endometriosis or iatrogenic following surgical sterilization

Table 5.2 Correlation between episodes of PID and risk of infertility

Number of previous episodes of PID	Incidence of tubal infertility (%)
1	12
2	23
3	54

Tubal surgery

Tubal surgery is a demanding procedure and requires a highly skilled gynaecologist. Success rates depend on surgical expertise and careful patient selection. In general, the more severe the tubal damage, the less likely tubal surgery is to succeed, and these women should be referred directly for IVF

Advances in minimally invasive surgery and microsurgery have provided improved ability to perform tubal reconstruction in selected cases with reduced morbidity. The fecundity rate following surgical treatment of tubal infertility is lower than per cycle IVF pregnancy rate. However, tubal surgery for infertility offers other advantages over IVF, including:

- Corrects pathology and may improve other symptoms concurrently, e.g. pain
- Couples may then have unlimited attempts to conceive—a cheaper option
- No increased risk of multiple pregnancies or ovarian hyperstimulation syndrome (OHSS)
- Less stress

General considerations

- Patient selection—the site and degree of tubal damage will significantly affect the outcome of reconstruction
- Microsurgical principles—minimize tissue trauma and handling, use fine non-absorbable sutures, use intraoperative magnification, repair all peritoneal surfaces, avoid desiccation of tissue, and maintain meticulous haemostasis

Tubal investigation

The aim is to provide information on the likely aetiology, severity of damage, and prognosis with surgery. Poor prognostic factors include luminal adhesions, a large hydrosalpinx (>2 cm), thick-walled hydrosalpinx, dual blockage (proximal and distal tubal obstruction), and loss of significant length of tube. Women who have indicators of poor prognosis should be referred for IVF.

Hysterosalpingogram

- Hysterosalpingogram (HSG) provides information on the patency of the Fallopian tubes and also the uterine cavity (outlining any filling defect such as submucous fibroids, polyps or adhesions) (see Figure 5.3)
- HSG not only provides information on patency but also location of obstruction (distal obstruction is associated with a hydrosalpinx), the state of the tubal lumen (preservation of rugae), and the

presence of peritubal adhesions (loculation of dye or abnormal orientation of the tube)
- Salpingitis isthmica nodosa (SIN), a consequence of previous PID, is identified by multiple small diverticular collections of contrast around the tube

Laparoscopy and dye (see Figure 5.4)

- May show an obvious hydrosalpinx (see Figure 5.5), pelvic and peritubal adhesions (see Figure 3.8 in Section 3.9); SIN appears as nodules over the cornual surface of the tube
- Dye may not enter the Fallopian tube (proximal block) or may fill the tube but not spill (distal block)
- Enables treatment as well as diagnosis
- Laparoscopy provides little information on the luminal aspect of the Fallopian tube

Management

Proximal disease

- Accounts for 25% of tubal disease
- Obstruction may be secondary to mucus plugs, polyps, synechiae or endosalpingosis (endometriosis). However, the most common cause is SIN, which indicates localized tubal disease only
- Microsurgical reconstruction achieves pregnancy rates of up to 60% and ectopic pregnancy rates of 10%
- Transcervical catheterization and tubal recanalization offers an alternative approach. However, pregnancy rates are lower (36%)

Distal disease

- Any inflammatory condition can lead to occlusion of the distal end of the Fallopian tube and accumulation of fluid within it, leading to a hydrosalpinx
- There are several grading systems for hydrosalpinges that involve assessment of the tubal mucosa, presence of peritubal adhesions, and wall thickness. By severity, hydrosalpinges can be divided into:
  - Hydrosalpinx simplex—thin-walled tube with flattened mucosal folds and without mucosal adhesions
  - Hydrosalpinx follicularis—thin-walled tube with adhesions
  - Hydrosalpinx with thick walls
- Assessment of tubal mucosa may be indirectly possible at HSG. However, salpingoscopy is the method of choice. There is a poor correlation between the state of the tubal serosa and mucosa
- Hydrosalpinx may be opened via:
  - Salpingostomy—opening the distal end of the tube
  - Neosalpingostomy—making a new distal opening
  - Fimbrioplasty—removing fibrous tissue and opening the fimbrial end of the tube
- The most successful of the procedures is fimbrioplasty, with success rates of up to 55% pregnancy rate. Salpingostomy has a pregnancy rate of around 25%, with a 16% ectopic pregnancy rate. Bilateral salpingectomies for hydrosalpinges improve IVF success rates

Peritubal adhesions

- Laparoscopic adhesiolysis to free adnexal adhesions has been shown to result in cumulative pregnancy rates of up to 60%
- Additionally, the procedure may have non-reproductive benefits such as reduction in pelvic pain

Reversal of sterilization

- Not available on NHS
- Highest success rates after Filshie clip sterilization, with pregnancy rates of up to 85% and ectopic pregnancy rates <10%
- Most women who conceive will do so in the first year after surgery

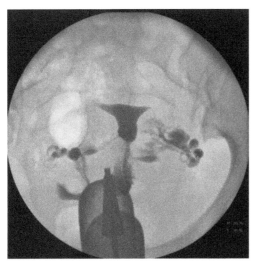

Fig. 5.3 Normal HSG demonstrating a normal uterine cavity with bilateral Fallopian tube fill and spill. (Kindly provided by Holly House Hospital.)

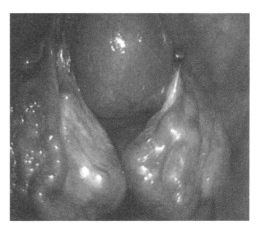

Fig. 5.5 Bilateral hydrosalpinges. (Kindly provided by Dr F. Odejinmi.)

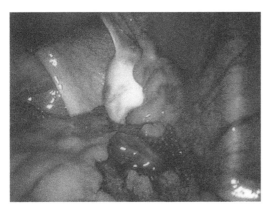

Fig. 5.4 Laparoscopy and dye test. Note the fill and spill of dye from the Fallopian tube.

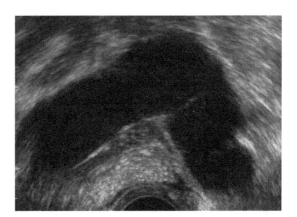

Fig. 5.6 Transvaginal ultrasound image of a hydrosalpinx.

5.5 Assisted conception

The first IVF baby was born in 1978 from a natural cycle egg collection. Since then, there have been significant advances in assisted reproduction technology (ART), and several techniques are now available depending in part on the indication.

Treatments

Ovulation induction

- Aims to develop a single follicle in women with anovulatory infertility
- Follicular development achieved with clomifene, gonadotrophin injection or gonadotrophin pump
- The addition of metformin may improve response to drugs
- Some studies suggest that metformin alone results in unifollicular ovulation in women with polycystic ovary syndrome (PCOS), with conception rates up to 8%
- Follicle development tracked using US and timed sexual intercourse at ovulation. If follicle tracking is unavailable, laparoscopic ovarian drilling is recommended in PCOS as there is equal efficacy without the risk of multiple pregnancy
- Ovulation timed either by urinary LH kit or HCG administration

Controlled ovarian stimulation + intrauterine insemination (COS+IUI)

- Aims to induce the development of up to three follicles by administration of clomifene or gonadotrophins
- Follicle development is tracked by US scan and the partner's washed, prepared sperm inserted into the uterine cavity (IUI) at ovulation
- Pregnancy rates are 10–15% per cycle

In vitro fertilization

- Aims to induce development of several follicles by administration of gonadotrophins
- The ovaries are 'downregulated' using gonadotrophin-releasing hormone (GnRH) agonists or antagonists. This prevents release of endogenous LH which can result in premature ovulation before egg collection
- Follicle development is tracked by ultrasound until at least three are >16 mm in size
- HCG is then given to 'trigger' re-entry into meiosis and expel the first polar body
- The follicles are aspirated 36–38 h later before ovulation can take place. Ninety per cent of follicles will yield an oocyte. Follicle aspiration is done using a needle guided by transvaginal ultrasound
- The oocytes and sperm are incubated overnight and if fertilization occurs then the embryos are incubated further
- Embryo transfer is performed 2 days after fertilization, and one or two embryos are usually placed in the uterine cavity under ultrasound guidance. Improvements in IVF success rates have meant that single embryo transfer (with additional embryos frozen and transferred in subsequent cycles) now gives equivalent pregnancy rates to routine two-embryo transfer; this has the additional benefit of a significant reduction in multiple pregnancy rates
- Luteal support is given by either HCG injections or vaginal progesterone

Intracytoplasmic sperm injection (ICSI)

- Indicated when there is severe male factor infertility
- After collection of oocytes (as with conventional IVF), sperm are directly injected into the oocyte. Fertilized embryos are replaced as per IVF
- Sperm can also be used from testicular aspiration (TESA–testicular sperm aspiration) or epididymal aspiration. (PESA–percutaneous epididymal sperm aspiration) and is used in men with previous vasectomy or vas deferens obstruction. The extracted sperm can be frozen and used when oocytes are available

Gamete intrafallopian transfer (GIFT)

- Only possible if Fallopian tubes are patent
- Oocytes collected and mixed with washed sperm and placed inside the Fallopian tubes

Indications for IVF

Tubal factor

- If not possible to correct surgically or no pregnancy 6 months after surgical correction

Unexplained

- If not pregnant despite COS+IUI (see Section 5.3)

Endometriosis

- Moderate or severe disease

Anovulation

- If not pregnant despite ovulation induction

Donor insemination (DI)

- If not pregnant after repeated cycles of DI

Oocyte donation

- Women with premature ovarian failure, poor ovarian response to ART or carriers of genetic disease

Surrogacy

- Women with normal ovaries who do not have a uterus or with medical contraindications to a pregnancy

Male factor

- Mild male factor may be suitable for IVF
- Moderate or severe male factor is an indication for ICSI

Prognostic factors

- Maternal age significantly affects outcome of IVF pregnancies, and older women (>35 years) have a poorer chance of pregnancy compared to younger women
- Duration of infertility has a significant impact on ART success as the longer the duration the worse the prognosis
- Number of previous cycles—the best chances of success with ART are in the first cycle
- A previous successful pregnancy (spontaneous or ART) improves the chances of success with ART
- BMI 19–30
- ↑ Success in non-smokers
- Salpingectomy before IVF if hydrosalpinges present will significantly improve outcome

Complications of assisted reproduction

Multiple pregnancy

- Current UK law (see Section 1.11) allows transfer of two embryos unless there are exceptional circumstances, e.g. age >40 years. Selective single embryo transfer is now being practised in order to reduce multiple pregnancy rates
- Any embryos not used in the treatment cycle can be frozen and used subsequently
- Multiple pregnancies carry significant risks to babies (miscarriage, prematurity, perinatal mortality and cerebral palsy) and mothers (pre-term labour, CS, pre-eclampsia, postpartum haemorrhage etc.)

Ovarian hyperstimulation syndrome (OHSS)

OHSS is a systemic disease resulting from vasoactive products released by hyperstimulated ovaries. It is characterized by increased capillary permeability, leading to leakage of fluid from the vascular compartment and accumulation within the third space. This leads to intravascular dehydration.

The incidence of OHSS varies between 0.6 and 33% depending on the definition. In its severe form, it can be life-threatening. It develops in response to luteinization of follicles either by LH or HCG.

Risk factors

- Young age (<30 years)
- Lean physique
- PCOS
- HCG administration
- Superovulation; >20 oocytes retrieved
- High or rapidly rising serum oestradiol
- Multiple pregnancy
- Previous OHSS

Prevention

- Identification of the higher risk patient
- Cycle cancellation—withholding HCG injection if excessive number of follicles develop
- Withholding embryo transfer (elective cryopreservation)
- Luteal phase support with progesterone (not HCG)

Clinical syndrome

- Mild—abdominal distension, mild pain, ovarian size <8 cm
- Moderate—mild OHSS plus US evidence of ascites, nausea, vomiting and diarrhoea, and ovarian size 8–12 cm
- Severe—any one of the following features constitutes severe OHSS: clinical ascites, hydrothorax, haemoconcentration (HCT >45%), electrolyte disturbance, oliguria and ↑ creatinine, ovarian size >12 cm
- Critical—tense ascites or large hydrothorax, HCT >55%, white cell count >25 10^9/L, oliguria or anuria, thromboembolism, acute respiratory distress syndrome (ARDS)

Management

Aims

- Reassurance and symptomatic relief
- Prevent or correct haemoconcentration
- Prevent thromboembolism
- Maintain cardiorespiratory and renal function

Outpatient management

- Suitable for mild OHSS
- Suitable for motivated patients who are able to monitor urine output and general observations
- Daily liaison or review by IVF centre

Inpatient management

- In moderate, severe, and critical OHSS
- Strictly adhere to local protocols
- General observations—4-hourly pulse, BP, and temperature; daily weight and abdominal circumference
- Urinary output—either measure voided samples or catheterize
- Strict fluid balance chart
- Blood investigations—FBC (including haematocrit), urea and electrolytes
- US—monitor ovarian size and ascites
- CXR—if suspected pleural effusion
- Low molecular weight heparin for thromboprophylaxis (especially if HCT >45%)

Consider drainage of third space, i.e. tense ascites, pleural and pericardial effusions. Colloid infusion might be necessary if large volume of fluid is drained.

In cases of severe or critical OHSS, a multidisciplinary approach involving the ITU/anaesthetists, haematologists, and renal physicians is advisable.

Further reading

NICE clinical guideline for fertility: assessment and treatment for people with fertility problems, 2004. www.rcog.org.uk

RCOG. Green Top guideline No 5. The Management of Ovarian Hyperstimulation Syndrome, 2006. www.rcog.org.uk/

HFEA Code of Practice. www.hfea.gov.uk

Miscarriage

Definition

- Loss of a pregnancy before 24 completed weeks gestation
- Expulsion of fetus or embryo weighing less than 500 g

Incidence

- Between 10 and 15% of clinically recognizable pregnancies will end in miscarriage

Aetiology

- Genetic—50% of clinically identifiable first trimester miscarriages are chromosomally abnormal. The risk of chromosomal abnormality falls with advancing gestation (50% at 8–11 weeks and 12% at 20–23 weeks). The most common is trisomy, followed by monosomy X and triploidy
- Infection—rare, but several organisms have been implicated in miscarriage, including *Listeria monocytogenes*, *Campylobacter*, *Brucella*, *Mycoplasma hominis*, cytomegalovirus, rubella, and coxsackie
- Second trimester miscarriages may be associated with uterine abnormalities, cervical incompetense, bacterial vaginosis, and multiple pregnancy
- Unexplained—25% of miscarriages have no identifiable cause

For further, rarer, causes see below under recurrent miscarriage.

Clinical presentation

- Threatened miscarriage—any vaginal bleeding, painful or painless, <24 completed weeks' gestation constitutes a threatened miscarriage. All women in this situation should be assessed clinically and viability determined by ultrasound. The management of miscarriage is then dependent on ultrasonography as the majority of these women will have a viable pregnancy
- Speculum and vaginal examination should be performed in all cases of threatened miscarriage. This also excludes local causes of bleeding. The presence of trophoblastic tissue passing through the cervical os confirms the diagnosis of miscarriage. Additionally, an open cervical os is highly indicative of miscarriage
- The passage of tissue through the cervical os may cause vagal shock and collapse leading to loss of consciousness, hypotension, and maternal bradycardia. This is in contrast to collapse secondary to hypovolaemia where there is a tachycardia. The treatment is prompt evacuation of the tissue from the cervical os using sponge forceps
- Septic miscarriage—occasionally, retained products of conception may become infected. These women will present with general malaise, offensive vaginal discharge, and fever. These cases should be admitted for intravenous antibiotics and surgical evacuation of the uterus

Types of miscarriage

- **Missed miscarriage** (early embryonic demise)—this occurs when the embryo has died or has not developed normally. The diagnosis is made on ultrasound when there is a gestation sac >20 mm in diameter with no identifiable embryo or there is no embryonic heartbeat when the crown–rump length is >6 mm. This may be entirely asymptomatic
- **Incomplete miscarriage**—this occurs when some of the products of conception have been passed and some are left in the uterine cavity. The diagnosis is made clinically if tissue is seen passing through an open cervical os or on ultrasound
- **Complete miscarriage**—this is the endpoint of all miscarriages and implies that all products of conception have passed. The diagnosis is made clinically when bleeding stops and pregnancy symptoms disappear or on ultrasound when the uterine cavity is empty

Ultrasound and miscarriage

- The main purpose of ultrasound is to identify normal, viable pregnancies, and reassure women as the majority of women with bleeding do not have a miscarriage
- US is also important to confirm that the pregnancy is intrauterine. It should never be forgotten that all women with a positive pregnancy test, abdominal pain, and vaginal bleeding may potentially have an ectopic pregnancy
- The identification of a viable pregnancy decreases the risk of miscarriage for a woman despite her symptoms, i.e. 15% chance of miscarriage at 6 weeks, falling to <5% at 9 weeks when a live embryo is seen
- Heterotopic pregnancy—rarely, an intrauterine pregnancy may coexist with an ectopic. Reported occurrence is 1:15–40 000 pregnancies. There is an increased incidence in assisted conception pregnancies when multiple embryos are replaced
- Molar pregnancy (see Section 5.8)

Management

Options

The management options are expectant, medical or surgical.

Several studies exist that demonstrate that in selected women, both expectant and medical management compare favourably with surgical evacuation of the uterus with no increase in the risk of infection or severe haemorrhage. Women choosing expectant or medical management should have access to an early pregnancy unit and/or A&E to seek medical attention should they experience heavy bleeding or become unwell.

Expectant management

This entails waiting for the uterus to expel the products of conception spontaneously. The woman should be advised that she is likely to have bleeding that is comparable to a heavy period associated with cramping lower abdominal pain. Simple analgesia is usually adequate, with follow-up 2 weeks later and an ultrasound scan to confirm complete miscarriage. Overall, >70% of women will complete their miscarriages within 3 weeks.

Medical management

This entails administering oral uterotonic agents (i.e. misoprostol) to facilitate evacuation of the uterus. Similar to expectant management, it is associated with pain and bleeding. An ultrasound scan should be arranged to confirm completion of the miscarriage.

Surgical management

ERPC (evacuation of retained products of conception under general or local anaesthesia) allows immediate removal of all tissue from the uterine cavity using a suction curette. It is associated with risks, including infection, bleeding, damage to the uterus, and incomplete evacuation of the uterus. However, many women prefer this option as it is associated with a predictably shorter duration of bleeding and less pain overall.

Anti-D immunoglobulin (Ig) should be given to all non-sensitized RhD-negative women with threatened or spontaneous miscarriages >12 weeks' gestation irrespective of the management and all miscarriages where the uterus is evacuated surgically (**B**).

Anti-D Ig may be given if there is heavy or repeated bleeding and bleeding associated with pain in gestations approaching 12 weeks.

Antibiotics—there is insufficient evidence to recommend routine antibiotic prophylaxis for all women prior to surgical evacuation of the uterus (**A**). Antibiotic therapy should be given if clinically indicated.

Recurrent miscarriage

Definition
- Three consecutive pregnancy losses <24 completed weeks' gestation

Incidence
- One per cent of women suffer from recurrent miscarriage
- This is higher than the statistical prediction of three consecutive miscarriages (calculated as 0.4%)

Aetiology
- Unexplained—the majority of couples will have no identifiable cause for their miscarriage
- Age—there is an increased risk of chromosomal abnormalities with advancing maternal age and an increased risk of miscarrying such a pregnancy. These women may also suffer infertility owing to diminished ovarian reserve
- Abnormal parental karyotype—3–5% of couples will have one partner who carries a chromosomal abnormality. In 60% of cases this is a balanced reciprocal translocation and 30% have a Robertsonian translocation (where the long arms of two chromosomes join and the short arms are lost)
- Antiphospholipid antibody syndrome—this affects 15% of women. There is a well recognized association between recurrent miscarriage and antiphospholipid antibodies, lupus anticoagulant, and anticardiolipin antibodies. The mechanism of pregnancy loss may be related to abnormal placentation
- Genetic thrombophilia—up to 5% of women will have hereditary thrombophilias, including activated protein C resistance (factor V Leiden mutation), antithrombin III deficiency, protein C and S deficiencies, which may be associated with pregnancy loss
- Congenital uterine anomalies—this affects 6% of women. The subseptate uterus is classically associated with recurrent first trimester miscarriage. The mechanism of pregnancy loss remains uncertain

Clinical assessment
Investigations
- Karyotype both partners
- Early follicular phase FSH and oestradiol
- Pelvic US
- Antiphospholipid syndrome screen—antiphospholipid antibodies should be elevated on two occasions >6 weeks apart: lupus anticoagulant (dilute Russell's viper venom time is the best test), anticardiolipin antibodies
- Thrombophilia screen—activated protein C resistance, antithrombin III, protein C and S levels

Management
- Parental chromosomal abnormality—refer to geneticist for counselling and to discuss prognosis. No treatment of the condition is available. However, prenatal diagnosis or preimplantation genetic screening may be offered.
- Antiphospholipid antibody syndrome (see Section 7.26)—first trimester low molecular weight heparin and low dose aspirin have been shown to increase the chances of a live birth significantly (70% versus 10% if untreated). Treatment commences when an embryonic heartbeat is seen on scan (6 weeks). Risks of long-term heparin use include osteoporosis (predominantly with unfractionated heparin) and heparin-induced thrombocytopenia
- Congenital uterine anomalies—hysteroscopic metroplasty has been shown to improve live birth rates significantly. However, this data comes from retrospective observational studies only
- Unexplained—the chance of a live birth following three consecutive miscarriages is still 70% with no treatment, so a positive attitude with reassurance is important

Further reading

RCOG. Greentop guideline No. 22. The use of anti-D immunoglobulin for Rh prophylaxis, 2002. www.rcog.org.uk

RCOG. Greentop guideline No. 17. The investigation and treatment of couples with recurrent miscarriage, 2003. www.rcog.org.uk

RCOG. Greentop guideline No. 25. The management of early pregnancy loss, 2006. www.rcog.org.uk

Sawyer E, Jurkovic D. Ultrasonography in the diagnosis and management of abnormal early pregnancy. *Clinical Obstetrics and Gynecology* 2007; **50(1):** 31–54.

5.7 Ectopic pregnancy

Definition

Implantation and development of a pregnancy in any site other than the endometrial cavity. Over 95% are in the Fallopian tube. Ectopic pregnancy is the most significant cause of maternal death in the first trimester.

Incidence

The incidence is increasing, and is currently around 20 in 1000 pregnancies. The rising incidence may be caused in part by improved detection following the availability of high resolution vaginal ultrasound. Additionally, the increased prevalence of pelvic infection and of assisted reproduction technology have contributed.

Classification

- Tubal (>95%)—ampullary (55%), isthmic (25%), fimbrial (17%), and interstitial (2%)
- Other (<5%)—cervical, ovarian, Caesarean scar
- Heterotopic—an ectopic pregnancy in combination with an intrauterine pregnancy. Occurs in 1:15–40 000 spontaneous pregnancies and up to 1% of pregnancies following assisted reproduction treatment

Pathophysiology

- Tubal factors—any condition or procedure (pelvic surgery) that potentially damages the Fallopian tubes increases the risk. However, pelvic infection, specifically with chlamydia, remains the most important cause, and ectopic pregnancy is up to 10 times more common in women with previous pelvic infection
- Chromosomal—chromosomally abnormal pregnancies are more likely to implant in the Fallopian tube
- Exogenous hormones—progesterone decreases smooth muscle contractility and is thought to predispose to ectopic pregnancy. Between 4–6% of pregnancies occurring in women taking the progesterone-only pill are ectopic
- IUCD—may be better at preventing intrauterine pregnancies than ectopic ones. If IUCD failure occurs an ectopic pregnancy should be suspected. Additionally, the IUCD itself may be associated with salpingitis and secondary tubal damage

Clinical presentation

Any woman of reproductive age presenting with a positive pregnancy test and pelvic pain has an ectopic pregnancy unless proved otherwise.

- Pain—unilateral or generalized pelvic pain. Subdiaphragmatic irritation from intra-abdominal blood results in shoulder tip pain
- Bleeding—mild vaginal bleeding occurs in up to 75% of cases and is a result of decidual shedding. A decidual cast is occasionally passed and may be mistaken for products of conception
- Collapse—depends upon the amount of intra-abdominal bleeding

Signs

- Acute abdomen—peritonism from haemoperitoneum may cause guarding. Cervical excitation may be present when there is blood in the pelvis
- Adnexal mass—an adnexal mass may be palpable if the ectopic pregnancy is large
- Cardiovascular compromise

Initial management

- Resuscitate—although most women are clinically well and haemodynamically stable, the nature of their condition is unpredictable and they may deteriorate quickly. Therefore all women should have large bore IV access (at least 14–16 G IV cannula)

- Blood should be sent at this time (see below)
- If haemodynamic compromise (i.e. tachycardic and/or hypotensive or feeling unwell), call for senior support, crossmatch blood (at least 2 units), and begin fluid resuscitation with colloids. It would be wise to alert anaesthetic and theatre staff of the situation

Investigations

- Urine pregnancy test
- Full blood count
- Group & save serum or crossmatch blood
- US scan (see Figures 5.7 and 5.8)

Inconclusive ultrasound scan

- The proportion of ectopics visualized varies with the expertise of the ultrasonographer, the quality of the ultrasound scan, and the ability to exclude an early normal intrauterine pregnancy
- Between 10–50% of scans for clinically suspected ectopic pregnancy will be inconclusive (depending on the ultrasonographer's expertise) i.e. 'an ectopic pregnancy cannot be excluded'
- All cases of inconclusive scans should be managed clinically primarily. In those deemed to be stable, i.e. no cardiovascular compromise and no significant free fluid in pelvis seen on scan, two serum HCG levels should be done 48 h apart
- Serial HCG levels serve two purposes:
  - To determine when the ultrasound scan should be repeated. Above a cut-off level of 1500 iu all pregnancies should be visualized. If not, consider laparoscopy
  - To monitor the rate of rise of HCG. In normal pregnancies this will at least double every 48 h. However, one-third of ectopic pregnancies show normal doubling of HCG

The ultrasound scan should then be repeated when the HCG is >1500 iu and if the pregnancy is not visualized on scan a laparoscopy should be considered

- A serum progesterone level may be helpful in the management of a suspected ectopic following an inconclusive scan. A low progesterone level (<20 mmol/l) is suggestive of a failing pregnancy irrespective of its location. Conversely, a high level (>60 mmol/l) is suggestive of an 'ongoing' pregnancy irrespective of its location

Further management

Expectant

- Some ectopic pregnancies may resolve spontaneously. However, determining which are suitable for conservative management can be problematic
- A serum progesterone level of <20 mmol/l is suggestive of an ectopic pregnancy that should resolve spontaneously

Medical

- Methotrexate (a folate antagonist) destroys proliferating trophoblastic tissue
- Success rates of 90% have been quoted; however, in many of these cases the diagnosis of ectopic pregnancy is not made with certainty
- This is generally suitable for small (<3 cm) ectopic pregnancies with no evidence of haemoperitoneum and HCG <3000 iu (Grade B recommendation)
- The dose depends on patient's body surface area; generally 50 mg/m^2
- A follow-up HCG level is taken to ensure resolution—this should fall by >15% between days 4 and 7 after injection
- Methotrexate is contraindicated in women with abnormal liver and renal function tests

Surgical

- Laparoscopy or laparotomy—laparoscopic management (see Figure 5.9) is the gold standard; however, laparotomy is used if the patient is significantly compromised or laparoscopic surgery is not feasible (**A**)
- Salpingectomy—removal of ectopic pregnancy and Fallopian tube
- Salpingotomy—linear incision on antimesenteric border of tube and extraction of ectopic pregnancy. There is a risk of residual trophoblast. Resolution should be ensured by follow-up HCG. In the presence of damage to the contralateral tube and desire for further pregnancies, this should be the first line (**B**)

Future reproductive performance

- 70% of women will have an intrauterine pregnancy after an ectopic pregnancy
- Risk of recurrence of ectopic pregnancy depends on the state of the remaining Fallopian tube, but is generally around 10% (higher if a salpingotomy is performed)
- All women who have had a previous ectopic pregnancy should have an early pregnancy scan to confirm location in a subsequent pregnancy

Further reading

RCOG. Greentop guideline No. 21: the management of tubal pregnancy, 2004. http://www.rcog.org.uk/

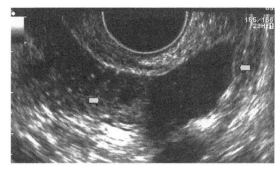

Fig. 5.7 Transvaginal ultrasound of a tubal ectopic pregnancy. Tubal ring (⇨); ovary (⇦).

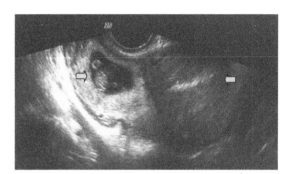

Fig. 5.8 Transvaginal ultrasound of a live ectopic pregnancy. Gestational sac with yolk sac, amniotic sac, and embryo (⇨); uterus (⇦).

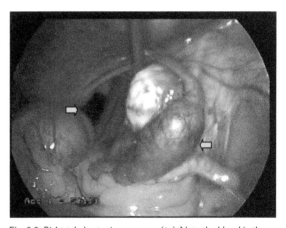

Fig. 5.9 Right tubal ectopic pregnancy (⇦). Note the blood in the pouch of Douglas (⇨).

These are unique tumours that develop from an abnormality at fertilization and are entirely fetal in origin.

They are composed of both syncytiotrophoblast and cytotrophoblast, and express a unique and characteristic tumour marker, HCG.

They are highly sensitive to chemotherapy.

Additionally, persistent GTD refers to a molar pregnancy that occurs after a normal pregnancy (this is very sensitive to chemotherapy).

Epidemiology
- The prevalence varies with geographical location but this may in part be caused by under reporting
- In the UK, the incidence is 1 per 714 live births; in the Far East it is double this
- Women of Asian or Far Eastern descent have a significantly higher risk

Risk factors
- Extremes of reproductive age: 20-fold ↑ if <15 years; 10-fold ↑ if >40 years
- Previous GTD significantly increases risk (0.6–2.6%)
- Diets deficient in protein, folic acid, and carotene
- Women of blood group A with blood group O partners have a 10-fold ↑ risk compared to women whose partners are group A
- Women who are blood group AB have a worse prognosis if diagnosed with GTD

Pathophysiology
- Complete moles are always euploid, of paternal origin, and sex chromatin-positive (46 XX or 46 XY).
- Complete moles arise when an empty ovum is fertilized by 2 haploid sperms
- A partial mole is triploid (69 XXY—70%; 69 XXX—27%; 69 XYY—3%) and arises when an ovum with an active nucleus is fertilized by a duplicated or two haploid sperm

Clinical assessment
Findings
The majority of women present with irregular bleeding (>90% have vaginal bleeding in the first trimester and present as threatened miscarriage) or with suspicious findings at routine US. The following are seen less often:
- 14–32% present with hyperemesis gravidarum
- A large-for-dates uterus—complete mole
- 15–30% of women have theca lutein cysts of the ovary. These may cause pain and surgical treatment may be required if rupture, torsion or haemorrhage occur. Women with theca lutein cysts are at higher risk of developing malignant sequelae to GTD
- 10% of women have biochemical hyperthyroidism
- 10–12% will have first or second trimester pre-eclampsia

Investigations
Ultrasound
- Complete moles have a characteristic US appearance of a multiple hypoechoic cystic structure that fills the uterine cavity, often described as a 'snowstorm' appearance (see Figure 5.10)
- Partial moles are often found in conjunction with a missed miscarriage. The placenta may have cystic spaces. However, the diagnosis is often made incidentally when products of conception are sent for histology after a miscarriage
- Choriocarcinoma often fills an enlarged uterus with a highly vascular mass that may invade through the myometrium. The mass may have irregular cystic areas of necrosis

Blood tests
- Serum HCG is detectable in urine and serum. Its level correlates closely with the tumour load. It is useful for diagnosis in conjunction with US and also for monitoring treatment and follow-up

Management
Surgical evacuation
- When diagnosed, the management of choice for molar pregnancy is suction curettage. This should be done by an experienced operator using a large 12-mm suction curette
- All women should have a CXR, FBC, group and save serum, liver and renal function tests, and electrolytes prior to surgery
- Medical termination of pregnancy is not advised as there is a theoretical risk of disseminating GTD tissue by the use of potent oxytocic agents
- All tissue should be sent for histology to confirm the diagnosis

Complications
- Excessive intraoperative bleeding secondary to uterine atony or perforation—all women should be made aware of the risk of transfusion and possible hysterectomy. Uterotonics may be used, e.g. single dose of oxytocin after complete evacuation
- Persistent trophoblast tissue—see below
- Pulmonary oedema—secondary to high output cardiac failure from severe pre-eclampsia, hyperthyroidism, anaemia or excessive fluid overload from resuscitation
- Trophoblast embolus—breach of the materno–fetal barrier and entry of trophoblast tissue into maternal circulation may result in disseminated intravascular coagulopathy (DIC) and acute respiratory distress syndrome (ARDS)

Follow-up
- All women diagnosed with a molar pregnancy should be registered at one of the three trophoblast treatment and screening centres (Charing Cross Hospital in London, Weston Park Hospital in Sheffield, Ninewells Hospital in Dundee).
- Follow-up is organized by the centre, with serial blood and urine analysis for at least 6 months post-evacuation
- Persistent GTD following a complete mole occurs in 15% of women and in 0.5% of cases after a partial mole. All cases should be managed in collaboration with a GTD screening and treatment centre

Future pregnancies
- Women should be advised not to conceive for 6 months after their serum HCG is undetectable
- The vast majority (98%) of women who fall pregnant after one GTD pregnancy have entirely normal reproductive and obstetric prognosis
- The COCP is an acceptable form of contraception after serum HCG levels are undetectable. However, if used prior to this, it may increase the risk of treatment failure and persistent GTD
- Follow-up is needed after all subsequent pregnancies with urine or blood samples for HCG. This is done via the local trophoblast treatment centre

Useful tip
If a woman gives a clear history of a miscarriage outside the hospital but there are no available products to be sent for histology, advise the patient to perform a pregnancy test (urinary HCG level) in a few weeks. A negative result is a simple way to exclude molar pregnancy.

Further reading

RCOG. Greentop guideline No. 38: the management of gestational trophoblastic neoplasia, 2004. www.rcog.org.uk

International society for the study of trophoblastic diseases. www.isstd.org

---

◎ Box 5.1 Classification of GTD

WHO classification

Premalignant

- Partial hydatidiform molar pregnancy
- Complete hydatidiform molar pregnancy

Malignant

- Invasive mole (chorioadenoma destruens)
- Choriocarcinoma
- Placental site trophoblastic tumours (PSTT)

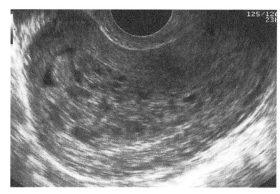

Fig. 5.10 Transvaginal ultrasound of a complete mole. Note the 'snowstorm' appearance of the material filling the uterine cavity.

5.9 Termination of pregnancy

The decision to end an unplanned pregnancy is one of the most difficult decisions a woman may have to make. Historically abortion services have been legalized and provided as the 'lesser of two evils'—to avoid maternal death and morbidity which occurs with self-administered and illegal techniques (see Section 1.11 for the Abortion Act 1967).

Advances in both surgical and medical technology have made termination of pregnancy an increasingly safe procedure, with minimal risk of long-term damage to any woman's general or reproductive health. However, any quality termination of pregnancy service should provide good pre-abortion care that provides counselling, a discussion on the alternatives to abortion with access to social services, and the use of contraception in the future.

Incidence
Women choose termination in one in five pregnancies (53 million terminations worldwide per year). In the UK 90% are carried out prior to 13 weeks and 98% before 20 weeks.

Initial medical assessment
- History—certainty of menstrual dates, symptoms suggestive of ectopic pregnancy, coexistent medical conditions that may influence method of termination and anaesthetic used
- Urine pregnancy test—confirm pregnancy
- US—date pregnancy and exclude miscarriage or ectopic pregnancy
- FBC, blood group, and Rhesus status

Methods of termination
Vacuum aspiration
- Usually employed from 7 to 12 weeks' gestation
- May require preoperative cervical preparation with 400 μg misoprostol PV at least 1 h before operation to enable ease of dilatation of cervix and decrease risk of traumatic complications (cervical trauma which increases the risk of future cervical incompetence, formation of false passage and perforation). Not usually needed if the woman is multiparous
- Usually done under general anaesthetic, but can be performed under local

Medical termination of pregnancy
- Usually employed for early (<9 weeks) or late (>15 weeks) abortion. *Tip:* In Scotland, used for all cases >12 weeks
- Gemeprost and misoprostol are prostaglandin E1 analogues that cause strong uterine contractions and result in expulsion of pregnancy
- Mifepristone is usually given to 'prime' the uterus. The antiprogesterone action causes the uterus to contract and also become more responsive to uterotonics
- Mifepristone and a prostaglandin analogue will result in complete abortion in 95% of cases. There are various regimens. The prostaglandin analogue is usually given 36–48 h after mifepristone

Dilatation and evacuation (D&E)
- Usually performed >15 weeks' gestation
- Requires cervical preparation
- Requires an experienced surgeon
- Advances in medical methods for termination of mid trimester pregnancies have resulted in fewer D&E operations

Termination after 20 weeks
This is uncommon and may involve an injection to stop the heart of the fetus (feticide) followed by either a medical termination or a surgical D&E

Complications
- Retained products of conception—1% need evacuation. Higher estimates are derived from US follow-up studies
  Manage clinically—if bleeding is significant or the patient chooses, then offer surgical evacuation of uterus (usually vacuum aspiration). Alternatively, if the bleeding is not significant, offer expectant management and rescan in 1 week (antibiotic cover may be considered)
- Bleeding—3 out of 1000 procedures
  It is usually controlled by evacuating the uterus and using uterotonics. However, women should be informed that a blood transfusion may be required albeit rarely. The risk of hysterectomy to control bleeding is very rare
- Uterine perforation – 1.5 out of 1000 procedures
  If this is suspected, then a laparoscopy should be performed to confirm and guide further management
- Infection—5%
  Prophylactic metronidazole and doxycyline for all women undergoing termination of pregnancy

Follow-up
- All Rhesus-negative women should be given anti-D immunoglobulin
- All women should be screened, or given prophylaxis, for chlamydia if having a surgical termination of pregnancy
- Contraception should be discussed and encouraged. Issues regarding previous contraceptive failure should be explored and alternatives offered. All hormonal and implantable methods (including IUCD) can be started immediately after a termination. An IUCD can be inserted after surgical abortion. Sterilization at the time of abortion should be discouraged as there is a high regret rate and also a higher risk of failure
- It is always important to talk about psychological support. This may be via the GP, a private clinic or informally by disclosing to close family or friends. Women should be reassured that grieving and guilt are normal reactions to having to make a difficult decision and support of their decision should be provided
- All women having an abortion should be offered and encouraged to take up an appointment either with the clinic or referring clinician (usually GP). This provides an opportunity to explore any psychological issues and go over the choice of contraception to improve compliance

Useful numbers
- Marie Stopes 0845 300 8090
- British Pregnancy Advisory Service 08457 304030

Further reading
NICE guideline: the care of women requesting induced abortion. www.rcog.org.uk

Chapter 6

Routine care and screening in pregnancy

Contents

Covered elsewhere

- Preconceptual care (see Section 5.1)

6.1 The normal physiological changes of pregnancy—cardiovascular and respiratory

Introduction

The body undergoes many changes during pregnancy that ensure fetal respiration, nutrition and excretion, as well as protecting the mother at birth.

Physiological changes are outlined below and how these manifest as some of the particular symptoms of pregnancy.

The key changes are cardiovascular, but respiratory, renal, haematological, gastrointestinal metabolic, and endocrine systems are all affected.

Cardiovascular changes

- Stroke volume (SV) increases by 10–30% and heart rate (HR) increases from the normal 70 to 80–90 bpm
- Cardiac output (CO), calculated as SV × HR, rises from 4 l/min at week 10 to 6 l/min by week 24
- Mean arterial BP falls by 6–19 mmHg. This reflects the reduction in peripheral vascular resistance which is characteristic of normal pregnancy
- Systolic BP falls slightly (4–6 mmHg) and diastolic BP falls more (8–15 mmHg), starting in the first trimester, with a nadir in the second trimester and returning towards non-pregnant levels by term (see Figure 6.1)
- When there are aberrant changes in the uteroplacental circulation, the expected decrease in BP may fail to occur, signalling pregnancy-induced hypertension or pre-eclampsia
- The hyperdynamic circulation of pregnancy increases the frequency of functional murmurs and accentuates heart sounds. A systolic ejection murmur is present in about 90% of pregnant women. A third cardiac sound is also commonly heard
- Premature atrial and ventricular beats are common during pregnancy
- Paroxysms of atrial tachycardia occur more frequently in pregnant women and may require treatment
- The increase in CO results in hypertrophy of the cardiac ventricles (left more than the right)
- The heart is enlarged and pushed up by the growing uterus. The aorta unfolds and the heart is rotated upwards and outwards. X-ray examination may show the heart displaced into a horizontal position, rotating to the left, with increased transverse diameter (see Figure 6.2)
- The ECG can change normally in pregnancy owing to cardiac strain and rotation of the heart (including atrial and ventricular ectopics, Q waves in leads I, II, and III, inverted T waves in lead III, ST segment depression and T wave inversion in inferior and lateral leads and left axis deviation—see Figure 6.3). However, changes must be interpreted in the context of the clinical picture and prior probability of cardiac or pulmonary event
- The enlarging uterus also compresses various abdominal vessels, including the iliac veins and inferior vena cava. Lying supine accentuates this venous compression. Venous compression can lead to a fall in venous return and CO and subsequently a fall in BP. Resulting symptoms include nausea, dizziness, even syncope (known as supine hypotensive syndrome)

Respiratory changes

The respiratory changes in pregnancy are less marked than the cardiovascular changes so many respiratory conditions remain stable.

Metabolic rate increases by 15%, leading to an oxygen consumption increase of 20%.

- The increase in blood volume and CO results in an increase in pulmonary blood flow
- Progesterone acts as a respiratory stimulant. Increased levels result in:
  - Bronchodilatation
  - Direct stimulation of respiratory centre
  - Increased respiratory centre sensitivity to CO_2
  - Concentrates carbonic anhydrase in RBCs, leading to more pCO_2 converted to bicarbonate (excess excreted by kidney)

Ventilation increases by 40% (physiological hyperventilation). There is no change in the vital capacity or the respiratory rate. However, women breathe more deeply, increasing their tidal volume from 500 to 700 ml, thus increasing the inspiratory capacity. This maternal hyperventilation results in higher pO_2 level and lower pCO_2 level with a compensatory fall in serum bicarbonate. This pO_2/CO_2 gradient facilitates efficient gas exchange between the mother and the fetus

- In late pregnancy, diaphragmatic elevation (see Figure 6.2) and increased intra-abdominal pressure results in a decrease of the residual lung volume. This leads to a decrease in total lung capacity of 200 ml. However, an increase in diaphragmatic excursion and use of accessory muscles means that the vital capacity remains unaltered
- Measurements of respiratory function remain unaltered in pregnancy. Peak flow rate (PFR) and forced expiratory volume in 1 second (FEV_1) remain unchanged

Respiratory alkalosis is normal in pregnancy—a normal pregnant woman has a compensated respiratory alkalosis and a diminished pulmonary reserve. Hyperventilation and increased pulmonary blood flow result in increase pulmonary gas transfer.

- There is ↑ pO_2, ↓ pCO_2, ↓ serum $[HCO_3]$ and ↑ arterial pH
- Normal arterial blood gases in pregnancy are: pH=7.44, pCO_2 = 30 mmHg (4.0 kPa), pO_2 ≥100mmHg (>13 kPa), bicarbonate = 18–22 mmol/l
- Breathlessness of pregnancy is experienced by over 75% of women owing to diaphragmatic elevation/movement and physiological hyperventilation

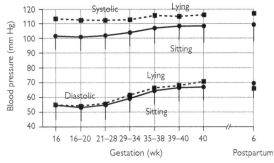

Fig. 6.1 Graph of blood pressure changes in pregnancy.

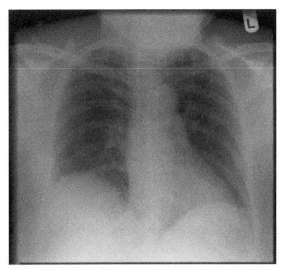

Fig. 6.2 CXR features in a pregnant woman: increased pulmonary vascular markings, pulmonary venous distension, and elevated right hemidiaphragm.

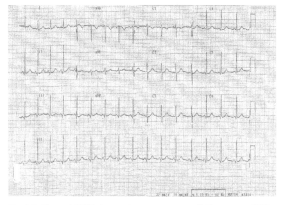

Fig. 6.3 Normal ECG changes in pregnancy: small Q waves and ST segment changes (anterior leads, C1, C2, C3).

6.2 The normal physiological changes of pregnancy—haematological, gastrointestinal, renal, metabolic, and endocrine

Haematological changes

- Total blood volume increases by 40% above non-pregnant levels
- Plasma volume rises from 6 weeks' gestation and stabilizes by 32–34 weeks
- RBC mass increases from early in the second trimester to 20–35% above non-pregnant levels by term

The disproportionate rise in plasma volume compared with the RBC mass results in haemodilution and decreased haemoglobin and haematocrit count. There is a physiological fall in Hb. An abnormal Hb <10.5 g/dl requires investigation. If iron stores are adequate, the haematocrit rises from the second to the third trimester

- Total WCC increases in pregnancy
- Platelet count decreases but stays within normal limits

Pregnancy alters the balance within the coagulation system to favour clotting which is assumed to be in preparation for controlling bleeding at the time of delivery.

- Concentrations of certain clotting factors—factors VIII, IX, and X increase, as does fibrinogen, with levels increasing by up to 50%
- Fibrinolytic activity is decreased, with a fall in concentrations of endogenous fibrinolytics such as antithrombin and protein S
- The tests of coagulation, activated partial thromboplastin time (APTT), prothrombin time (PT), and thrombin time (TT), remain normal

This hypercoaguable state is exacerbated by the compressive effect of the gravid uterus on the iliac vessels, causing venous stasis in the lower limbs. This is more marked on the left as the left iliac vein is compressed by the iliac and the ovarian arteries. On the right, the iliac artery does not cross the vein

This predisposition for clotting results in the increased risk of venous thrombosis associated with pregnancy.

Gastrointestinal changes

- Changes in gastrointestinal motility during pregnancy are caused by the effect of progesterone on the smooth muscle of the gastrointestinal tract. The result is decreased lower oesophageal pressure, decreased gastric peristalsis, and delayed gastric emptying. This predisposes to reflux, indigestion, and constipation
- Gastric acid secretion is reduced and may explain why peptic ulcer disease commonly improves in pregnancy
- Pregnancy affects bile transport. Oestrogen increases serum cholesterol and this is translated into increased bile salt synthesis. Progesterone also reduces gallbladder emptying so predisposing to gallstone formation
- Routine liver function test values remain normal during pregnancy apart from alkaline phosphatase which may be two to three times normal at term. The increase is because of placental production of this enzyme

Renal changes

Anatomical changes

- Renal blood flow mirrors cardiac output. Renal blood flow and glomerular filtration rate (GFR) increase by about 80% above non-pregnant levels in the second trimester. GFR reduces to 45% above prepregnancy levels by term
- Increased renal blood flow leads to increased bipolar renal length by 1 cm
- The renal calyces, ureters, and bladder become dilated under the influence of progesterone acting on smooth muscle and in later pregnancy owing to compression from the gravid uterus. The physiological dextrorotation of the uterus during pregnancy owing to the sigmoid colon on the left causes further dilatation of the right renal system
- Renal hydronephrosis is considered normal up to a pelvi-calyceal diameter of 5 mm on the left, 15 mm on the right, and dilatation of the ureters to 2 cm in the third trimester. This is evident on renal ultrasound from 10 weeks and can persist up to 16 weeks after delivery
- Urinary stasis predisposes to UTI and pyelonephritis
- Increased vascular tortuosity occurs in the bladder trigone which can lead to microscopic haematuria

Renal tubular function changes

- All physiological changes are maximal late in the second trimester and then start to return to prepregnancy level
- The increase in GFR leads to increased creatinine clearance and a lower serum creatinine and urea level in pregnancy. 'Normal' creatinine levels in pregnancy may indicate renal disease
- With prepregnancy serum creatinine ≥2.3 mg/dl (200 μmol/l), there is no increase in GFR in pregnancy
- The increase in GFR may overwhelm the ability of the renal tubules to reabsorb, leading to glucose and protein losses in the urine, hypercalciuria (300% increase), and bicarbonaturia (which compensates for respiratory alkalosis)
- Mild glycosuria and/or proteinuria can occur in normal pregnancy. The upper limit of normal for protein excretion is 300 mg in 24 h. 10% of normal pregnancies exhibit glycosuria
- A random urine protein (mg):creatinine (mmol) ratio of ≥30 is a good predictor of significant proteinuria
- Increasing proteinuria is common in pregnancies with underlying renal disease
- Serum albumin decreases by 5–10 g/dl
- Serum cholesterol increases by 50%
- Total body water increases by 6–8 l and plasma osmolality falls. There is a compensatory increase in renin and aldosterone levels so there is a predisposition to retain sodium (and water) during pregnancy as there is increased tubular reabsorption of sodium.

Renal endocrine function changes

- Increased renin and aldosterone secretion
- Increased erythropoietin production leads to an increase of red cell mass by 25%
- Increase of active vitamin D production

Metabolic changes

- Pregnancy is a diabetogenic state. Cortisol, progesterone, oestrogen, and human placental lactogen are all insulin antagonists
- In the first trimester there is a low insulin requirement and hypoglycaemia

- During the second and third trimesters there is increasing insulin resistance owing to increasing levels of insulin antagonists
- Insulin secretion increases to counter insulin resistance
- Glucose crosses the placenta by facilitated diffusion
- Increased nutrient availability to the fetus results in:
  - Increased postprandial peak blood glucose (BG)
  - In the fasted state, BG falls below prepregnancy level, with maternal reliance on lipolysis and ketogenesis (accelerated starvation)
  - Fasting glucose is lower in pregnancy
  - Owing to the above physiological changes, women with an already reduced pancreatic reserve develop glucose intolerance (see Section 7.15)
- Glycosuria occurs in 10% of normal pregnancies owing to reduced tubular glucose reabsorption and increased GFR
- There is no correlation between urinary and plasma glucose levels

Endocrine changes

- There is a relative maternal iodine deficiency. This is caused by a 2-fold increase in renal loss (↑ GFR + ↓ reabsorption), and active transport of iodine to the fetus
- Uptake of plasma iodide into the thyroid is increased by 3-fold. Insufficient dietary iodine leads to cellular hyperplasia and goitre
- Increased thyroid-binding globulin (TBG) hepatic synthesis leads to an increase in total thyroxine (T4) and an increase in total tri-iodothyronine (T3), but free T4 (FT4) levels remain unchanged
- First trimester—increased HCG (which is similar structurally to TSH) leads to decreased TSH and increased T4
- Second and third trimesters—T4 decreases
- Third trimester—TSH increases

Further reading

Chamberlain G, Broughton-Pipkin F (eds) *Clinical Physiology in Obstetrics*, 3rd edn. Blackwell Scientific Publications Oxford, 1998.

Nelson-Piercy C. *Handbook of Obstetric Medicine*, 3rd edn. Taylor and Francis, London, 2006.

Table 6.1 Haematology and biochemical values in pregnancy and prepregnancy (Adapted from Nelson-Piercy C. *Handbook of Obstetric Medicine*, 2006)

	Prepregnancy	First trimester	Second trimester	Third trimester
Full blood count				
Hb (g/dl)	11.5–15		11–14	
WBC x10⁹/l	4–11		6–16	
Platelets x10⁹/l	150–400		150–400	
MCV (fl)	80–100		80–100	
CRP (g/l)	0–7		0–7	
Renal function tests				
Urea (mmol/l)	2.5–7.5	2.8–4.2	2.4–4.1	2.4–3.8
Creatinine (µmol/l)	60–125	52–68	44–64	55–73
K (mmol/l)	3.5–5.2		3.3–4.1	
Na (mmol/l)	135–145		130–140	
Uric acid (mmol/l)	0.11–0.35	0.14–0.23	0.14–0.29	0.21–0.38
24-h urine protein (g)	<0.15		<0.30	
Liver function tests				
Bilirubin (µmol/l)	0–17	4–16	3–13	3–14
Total protein (g/l)	64–86		48–64	
Albumin (g/l)	35–45		28–37	
AST (iu/l)	7–38	10–28	12–29	11–30
ALT (iu/l)	0–38		6–32	
GGT (iu/l)	11–50	5–37	5–43	3–41
ALP (iu/l)	30–130	32–100	43–135	133–418
Bile acids (µmol/l)	0–14		0–14	
Thyroid function tests				
Free T4 (pmol/l)	11–23	10–24	9–19	7–17
Free T3 (pmol/l)	4–9	4–8	4–7	3–5
TSH (mu/l)	0–4	0–1.6	0.1–1.8	0.7–7.3

6.3 The first antenatal appointment

Introduction

The aims of antenatal care are to promote the wellbeing of the mother and her developing baby, to monitor the pregnancy, and identify any problems so that appropriate action can be taken. Antenatal care includes providing information, advice, and reassurance about pregnancy, childbirth, and motherhood as well as monitoring, screening, and treating problems where necessary.

In the UK, the majority of antenatal care is delivered by midwives. Maternity care, as a whole, is delivered by a team of professionals, including midwives, GPs, and obstetricians. Clear care pathways between health professionals for women experiencing any problems during the antenatal period are essential to deliver a safe and effective service.

Overview

The first appointment in pregnancy should be early (before 12 weeks' gestation) so that women can be provided with information to allow them to make decisions about a range of issues, including the pattern of care they wish to receive, choices about antenatal screening, and early discussions about planned place of birth. Women can also be provided with information on their lifestyle which help to optimize their health during pregnancy, e.g. diet, exercise, smoking, drugs, alcohol, working patterns.

In addition, the first appointment is usually the earliest opportunity (in the absence of preconception assessment) for the healthcare provider to undertake a number of baseline measurements, such as blood pressure, and to make an assessment of risk for the remainder of pregnancy. Although risk assessment in early pregnancy does not identify all women who will develop problems later in pregnancy, it will identify a number of women who may benefit from additional care.

At the first visit, it is recommended that the following occur:
- Take detailed history; this will identify women who may need additional care. The first visit history (or booking history) must include: detailed past obstetric history, medical and surgical history, family history (congenital problems), history of present pregnancy, drug history (prescribed and illicit), and social history
- Measure BMI, weight (kg)/height (m²), blood pressure (BP) and test urine for proteinuria
- Offer and give written information on topics such as diet and lifestyle, pregnancy care services in the community, maternity benefits, and information on screening tests
- A good source of information is The Pregnancy Book, available free to all first time pregnant women
- Check blood group and rhesus D (RhD) status
- Offer screening for anaemia, red cell alloantibody, hepatitis B virus, HIV, rubella, and syphilis status
- Offer screening for asymptomatic bacteriuria
- Offer early ultrasound scan for gestational age assessment. This is often called the dating or first trimester scan. It is performed between 10 and 13 weeks

All of the above have advantages for the mother and her developing child.

The next two tests below are screening tests for fetal abnormality and are *different in kind*. They provide information about her child which may be beneficial even if affected, but may also raise questions about continuing the pregnancy (or termination).
- Offer screening for Down's
- Offer ultrasound screening for structural anomalies (20 weeks)

The following list is not exhaustive. If any of the conditions below are present the woman should be considered for additional care:
- Pre-existing hypertension, cardiac or renal disease
- Pre-existing endocrine disease, epilepsy or psychiatric disorder
- Pre-existing disease, e.g. sickle cell disease or trait, previous venous thrombosis, previous cerebrovascular disease, autoimmune diseases, cancer, HIV, diabetes
- Age under 18 years or over 40
- BMI ≤18 or ≥35
- Previous CS or uterine surgery, e.g. myomectomy
- Previous pre-eclampsia, eclampsia or haemolysis, elevated liver enzymes, low platelets syndrome (HELLP)
- Three or more miscarriages under 12 weeks
- Previous preterm birth or mid-trimester loss
- Previous puerperal psychosis
- Previous neonatal death or stillbirth
- Previous baby with congenital abnormality
- Previous baby ≤2.5 kg or ≥4 kg at term
- Family history of genetic disorder

Other problems that may need early specialist input:
- Female genital mutilation (FGM)
- A history of domestic violence
- Illicit drug use

Lifestyle issues

- Prescriptions and dental treatment are free during pregnancy and for a year after the birth
- Women should be given information about maternity rights and benefits
- The majority of women can be reassured it is safe to continue working during pregnancy. Certain exposures are associated with teratogenicity, such as exposure to X-rays for healthcare workers, and adequate protection should be implemented
- Physically demanding work and prolonged standing is associated with poor pregnancy outcomes in terms of preterm birth, hypertension, and growth restriction. Pregnant women and their employers should assess the significance of this risk and adjust occupational exposure accordingly during the pregnancy
- Give advice on dietary intake and avoiding food-acquired infections (listeriosis, salmonella, and toxoplasmosis)
- Advise dietary supplementation with 400 µg of folic acid before conception and up to 12 weeks' gestation. This reduces the risk of neural tube defects (NTD). If a previous baby has being born with an NTD, a higher dose of folic acid, 5 mg should be given for 3 months preconception and for up to 12 weeks
- Advise women that few complementary therapies have been shown to be safe and beneficial in pregnancy and some Chinese herbal therapies are toxic
- Exercise started or maintained in pregnancy has not been associated with any adverse outcome. Women should avoid potentially dangerous activities, especially those that can result in abdominal trauma, and scuba diving which may result in fetal birth defects and fetal decompression disease
- Sexual intercourse in pregnancy is not known to be associated with any adverse outcomes, e.g. premature delivery
- Advise women that excess alcohol in pregnancy has an adverse effect on the fetus, including low birth weight, learning difficulties or, with heavy and prolonged drinking, fetal alcohol syndrome. Current advice limits alcohol intake to no more than 1–2 units per

week. One unit of alcohol is a single measure of spirit, one small glass of wine, half a pint of regular strength beer, lager or cider

- Smoking is associated with adverse pregnancy and prenatal outcomes, e.g. placental abruption, preterm prelabour rupture of the membranes, growth restriction, preterm birth and sudden infant death (SIDS). Women should be encouraged to stop or reduce smoking. Effective interventions include regular verbal and written advice at each antenatal visit, group sessions, and behavioural therapy. Women can also be directed to the NHS pregnancy smoking helpline
- Women should be discouraged from using cannabis or other illicit drugs
- Live vaccines are contraindicated in pregnancy. Killed or inactivated vaccines and toxoids can be administered

Subsequent antenatal appointments

The comprehensive 2008 NICE guideline for routine antenatal care for the healthy pregnancy women recommends 10 scheduled appointments for nulliparous women and seven for multiparous women with an uncomplicated pregnancy history.

The needs of each woman should be assessed at each visit and the activities detailed in Table 6.2 should be checked, as a minimum, at each visit.

What should not happen for healthy women at antenatal appointments?
The following interventions are *not* recommended as part of routine antenatal care, either because there is no evidence that they confer any benefit or because there is evidence that they are harmful.

- Repeated maternal weighing
- Breast examination
- Pelvic examination
- Screening for postnatal depression using the Edinburgh Postnatal Depression Score
- Iron supplements
- Screening for other infections—*Chlamydia trachomatis*, cytomegalovirus, hepatitis C, group B streptococcus, toxoplasmosis, bacterial vaginosis
- Screening for preterm birth by use of cervical length assessment or using fetal fibronectin
- Formal fetal movement counting
- Antenatal electronic cardiotocograpy (CTG)
- Ultrasound scanning after 24 weeks
- Umbilical artery Doppler ultrasound
- Uterine artery Doppler ultrasound to predict pre-eclampsia

Useful points to remember at antenatal visits
- Always check current gestation with the expected date of delivery (EDD) derived from the first trimester ultrasound scan
- Review latest blood test results and scans if needed
- Always check BP and urinalysis for proteinuria
- Check symphyseal fundal height (SFH)—see Section 6.9 and Figure 6.6)
- Check presentation at 36 weeks. If breech is detected, and confirmed on ultrasound, offer external cephalic version at 37 weeks' gestation (see Section 8.27)

Further reading

Mozurkewich EL, Luke B, Avni M, Wolf FM. Working conditions and adverse pregnancy outcome: a meta-analysis. *Obstetrics and Gynecology* 2000;**95**: 623–35.

www.dh.gov.uk Publications DH_074920. *The Pregnancy Book*. London: Health Promotion England, 2007.

The NHS Pregnancy Smoking Helpline 0800 169 9 169.

www.nice.org National Collaborating Centre for Women's and Children's Health commissioned by NICE, July 2008. Guideline CG62 Antenatal care: routine care for the healthy pregnant woman.

Table 6.2 Recommended schedule of antenatal visits in an uncomplicated pregnancy		
Antenatal visit	Nulliparous	Multiparous
16 weeks • Review results of all screening tests • Investigate Hb<11 g/dl and treat if necessary • Check BP and urinalysis for protein	✓	✓
18–20 weeks • Anomaly scan • If placenta found to be covering internal os, arrange scan at 36 weeks	✓	✓
25 weeks • Measure symphyseal–fundal height (SFH) • Check BP • Urinalysis for protein	✓	✗
28 weeks • Measure SFH • Check BP • Urinalysis for protein • Hb check and atypical red cell alloantibody • First dose of anti-D to Rhesus-negative women	✓	✓
31 weeks • Measure SFH • Check BP • Urinalysis for protein • Review test results • Investigate Hb<10.5 g/dl and treat if necessary	✓	✗
34 weeks • Measure SFH • Check BP • Urinalysis for protein • Second dose of anti-D to Rhesus-negative women	✓	✓
36 weeks • Measure SFH • Check BP • Urinalysis for protein • Check fetal presentation	✓	✓
38 weeks • Measure SFH • Check BP • Urinalysis for protein	✓	✓
40 weeks • Measure SFH • Check BP • Urinalysis for protein	✓	✗
41 weeks • Measure SFH • Check BP • Urinalysis for protein • Offer membrane sweep and offer date for induction of labour	✓	✓

6.4 Managing common symptoms in pregnancy

Many of the common symptoms of pregnancy arise as a result of the normal physiological changes of pregnancy described in Sections 6.1 and 6.2.

Reassurance that many of these symptoms are not harmful to the mother or fetus may be all that is needed. However, when symptoms are severe or might represent serious pathology, investigation or treatment is required.

Nausea and vomiting

Incidence
Between 80–85% of women experience nausea during the first trimester. Fifty-two per cent of women will also experience some degree of vomiting. Nausea and vomiting is more common in multiple pregnancy, Afro-Caribbean women, previous history in prior pregnancy, and molar pregnancy.

Pathophysiology
The cause of nausea and vomiting is still unclear, but it is strongly linked to the rise in HCG. Intractable vomiting may lead to hyperemesis gravidarum (see below).

Most cases of nausea and vomiting will stop by 16–20 weeks of gestation. Women should be reassured that this is not associated with a poor pregnancy outcome.

Clinical relevance
Nausea and vomiting can cause great disruption to daily activities, impairing the ability to function fully at work and in the home.

Management
- Reassurance to the pregnant woman that this phase will improve often alleviates great anxiety
- Antiemetics may be necessary
- Ginger and P6 acupressure (see Figure 6.4) are non-pharmacological treatments that have been shown in randomized controlled trials (Ia and Ib) to reduce the duration and severity of nausea and vomiting in pregnancy, and currently appear safe for the fetus

Hyperemesis gravidarum

Definition
Prolonged vomiting and nausea, leading to dehydration, ketosis, electrolyte derangement, and in severe cases weight loss

Incidence
Affects 1:1000 pregnancies

Risk factors
- Younger maternal age
- Non-smoker
- First pregnancy
- Multiple pregnancy
- Gestational trophoblastic disease

Clinical relevance
Hyperemesis gravidarum may lead to recurrent hospital attendances or admissions, adding to further disruption. This can lead to depression in up to 60% of women, with some electing to terminate the pregnancy. Serious but rare complications include oesophageal rupture, Wernicke's encephalopathy or central pontine myelinolysis

Investigations
Investigations may be normal or show signs of intravascular volume and electrolyte depletion, including hypernatraemia, hypokalaemia, low serum urea, hypochloraemic alkalosis, ketonuria, elevated haematocrit, abnormal liver function tests, and a biochemical thyrotoxicosis.

The last is transient and usually resolves by 18 weeks' gestation (a result of the thyrotropic action of HCG).

In suspected cases of hyperemesis the following investigations should be performed.
- Full blood count (FBC)—haematocrit will confirm severity of dehydration
- Urea and electrolytes (U&E)—provide a baseline assessment and guide intravenous hydration
- Thyroid function tests (TFT)—only if clinical suspicion of hyperthyroidism
- Urine dipstick and culture—confirm ketosis (dehydration) and exclude infection
- Liver function tests (LFT)—protracted vomiting leads to transient and reversible derangement
- Ultrasound (US)—confirm intrauterine pregnancy, number of fetuses, and exclude gestational trophoblastic disease

Management
- Exclude other causes of vomiting such as pyelonephritis, gestational trophoblastic disease, degeneration of fibroid, acute appendicitis, diabetic ketoacidosis, gastritis, peptic ulcer disease, gastroenteritis, hepatitis, pancreatitis, hyperthyroidism or a neurological cause (e.g. raised intracranial pressure from tumour)
- Admission to hospital if significant clinical dehydration
- Fluid replacement—intravenous fluids should be commenced with Hartmann's solution or 0.9% saline with either 20 mmol or 40 mmol of potassium chloride added guided by the investigation results. Dextrose or dextrose saline must not be used because glucose may further decrease the plasma potassium concentration and may precipitate Wernicke's encephalopathy (see below)
- Correction of hypernatraemia should be done cautiously and slowly. Too rapid correction can lead to maternal and fetal pontine myelinolysis (identified initially by a fixed gaze palsy)
- Thiamine supplementation should be given to all women in this situation. The inability to eat can lead to thiamine deficiency which results in Wernicke's encephalopathy and subsequent Korsakoff's psychosis. Supplementation should be commenced initially as IV Pabrinex®
- Antiemetics—first line antiemetics are promethazine and cyclizine; second line antiemetics are metoclopramide and prochlorperazine; third line treatment includes domperidone. In intractable cases, a short course of steroids can be used (5mg TDS for 5 days)
- The absence of urinary ketones is useful in management as it indicates that the body is no longer in catabolic metabolism and that the ketosis from dehydration is resolving
- Consider thromboprophylaxis

Heartburn

Definition
- A burning sensation or discomfort felt behind the sternum or throat or both, which can be associated with an acid regurgitation

Incidence
- Heartburn is a more frequent complaint with increasing gestation (up to 70% of women in the third trimester)

Pathophysiology
- Cause unclear but associated with the relaxing effect of progesterone on smooth muscle

Clinical relevance
- It is not associated with any adverse maternal or fetal outcomes

Diagnosis
- Based on history elicited without any abdominal findings on clinical examination. Heartburn and epigastric pain associated with pre-eclampsia can coexist, but checking maternal BP and urine for proteinuria will aid in diagnosing the latter

Management
- Advise women on simple measures before offering treatment, e.g. maintaining an upright posture especially after meals, eating small frequent meals, avoiding irritants such as caffeine or other trigger foods
- Safe first line treatments include Gaviscon® or magnesium trisilicate. If these do not work, ranitidine, an H_2 receptor blocker, can be considered. In intractable cases, where other measures have failed, a proton pump inhibitor (PPI) such as omeprazole can be used, but caution is advised due to toxicity shown in animal studies. Women should stop or be switched to an alternative if they are on a PPI prior to pregnancy

Constipation
- Constipation in pregnancy is made worse with iron
- Increasing wheat or bran fibre content in the diet is frequently effective
- Treatment with laxatives is best avoided. Stimulants such as bisacodyl, senna, and sodium docusate are more effective than bulk-forming laxatives such as ispaghula husk (Fybogel®) in women who do not respond to bran or wheat fibre supplementation

Haemorrhoids
- Dietary modification and reassurance that haemorrhoids will resolve after delivery is often all that is required
- Standard topical haemorrhoid cream can be used if anal itching, anal pain, and anorectal bleeding persist
- Rarely, thrombosed prolapsed haemorrhoids require surgical removal

Varicose veins
- Varicose veins are common and not harmful
- They are not associated with increased risk of deep vein thrombosis (DVT) in pregnancy
- Compression stockings (below- and above-knee) improve symptoms but do not prevent varicose veins

Backache
- Backache in pregnancy is very common
- It is associated with the increased lordosis of the lumbar spine and increased laxity of the back muscles due to relaxin
- Regular exercise in water, massage therapy, group or individual back care classes alleviate backache
- Symptoms of nerve involvement warrant a thorough clinical examination

Symphysis pubis dysfunction (SPD)
- SPD is a collection of signs and symptoms of discomfort and pain in the pelvic area, including pelvic pain radiating to the upper thighs and perineum and classically tenderness on palpation of the pubic bones.
- Symptoms are exacerbated with movement, e.g. walking, climbing stairs, etc. and are relieved with rest
- Symptoms are most common in the second and third trimesters
- Symptoms can become very debilitating, resulting in some women using crutches or a wheelchair for mobility
- No good effective treatments exist. Simple pain relief, pelvic support, and reassurance appear to offer some relief

Carpal tunnel syndrome
- Oedema of pregnancy may contribute to median nerve compression within the carpal tunnel in the hand
- Symptoms are localized to the radial half of the hand and include numbness, burning sensation, and tingling that may impair sensory and motor hand function
- There is no good evidence of effectiveness of any treatments. Wrist splints with analgesia may help. Corticosteroid injections are sometimes used in severe cases

Itching
One in five pregnant women experience some itching in pregnancy. This can be caused by:
- Pre-existing skin conditions, such as eczema
- Coincidental conditions which have occurred during the pregnancy, such as scabies or vulvovaginal candidiasis
- A number of pregnancy-associated conditions

The majority is due to pruritus gravidarum, with the itching commencing in the second or third trimester.

Pruritus gravidarum is itching without any evidence of a rash or any of the above causes being identified. The itching is often localized to the abdomen, palms, soles or is widespread. It rapidly resolves after delivery and treatment, if needed, is symptom-based.

Itching may also be due to obstetric cholestasis (see Section 8.22) which is a diagnosis of exclusion.

If the itching is associated with a rash, consider one of the pregnancy-associated dermatoses (polymorphic eruption of pregnancy, prurigo of pregnancy, pruritic folliculitis, pemphigoid gestationis—see Section 8.23).

Vaginal discharge
- Increase in vaginal discharge is a common physiological change in pregnancy
- Further investigation is warranted if it is associated with malodour, soreness, itching or dysuria
- Vulvovaginal candidiasis can be treated with topical imidazole. Oral therapy should be avoided in pregnancy

Further reading
Norheim AJ, Pedersen EJ, Fonnebo V, Berge L. Acupressure treatment of morning sickness in pregnancy. A randomised, double-blind, placebo-controlled study. *Scandinavian Journal of Primary Health Care* 2001; **19**:43–7.

Vutyavanich T, Kraisarin T, Ruangsri R. Ginger for nausea and vomiting in pregnancy: randomized, double-masked, placebo-controlled trial. *Obstetrics and Gynaecology* 2001; **97**:577–82.

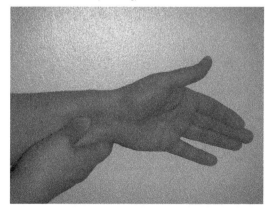

Fig. 6.4 P6 acupressure point (used in hyperemesis).

6.5 Screening for haematological conditions

Anaemia: iron and folate deficiency

Definition
Anaemia is a decrease in the number of red blood cells, haematocrit or haemoglobin (Hb) level. Acceptable Hb levels depend on gestation. Up to 12 weeks' gestation, Hb ≥11 g/dl is usual. Up to and over 28 weeks' gestation, Hb ≥10.5 g/dl is acceptable.

Pathophysiology
Rising plasma volume and maternal red cell mass cause a normal physiological fall in Hb level. Mean corpuscular volume (MCV) or corpuscular haemoglobin concentration (MCHC) usually remain the same. If they are abnormal, consider other causes of anaemia, e.g. haemoglobinopathies. In the UK, the most common cause of anaemia is iron deficiency, followed by folate deficiency. Iron and folate deficiency are usually caused by dietary deficiency. Iron requirements increase in pregnancy from 2.8 to 4 mg/day. A good diet supplies 14 mg per day of which only 2 mg is absorbed.

Clinical relevance
Treatment reduces symptoms and postpartum blood transfusion.

Diagnosis
Check ferritin levels (<30 μg/l indicates inadequate iron stores). Folate deficiency results in a macrocytic anaemia. A raised MCV may be normal in 25% of pregnancies but also consider drugs, e.g. azathioprine or alcohol. Check serum and red cell folate.

Management of low Hb
Routine iron supplementation in pregnancy has no measurable benefits on maternal or fetal outcomes. Side effects include nausea, constipation, and diarrhoea. More importantly, there appears to be a possibile increase in the risk of perinatal death. Iron therapy, oral or parenteral, can increase Hb by 0.8 g/dl/week.

The standard oral preparations of ferrous sulphate 200 mg twice a day or Pregaday® (which also contains 350 μg of folate) are suitable for the prevention and treatment of iron deficiency in pregnancy. Absorption is increased by ascorbic acid (vitamin C) and reduced by phytic acid and tannins found in tea and coffee.

The parenteral route should only be considered for those women intolerant to oral preparations.

Women at risk of folate deficiency include those taking any anticonvulsant drugs or folate antagonists, e.g. sulfasalazine or who have underlying haematological conditions, e.g. haemolytic anaemia, sickle cell disease, thalassaemia, hereditary spherocytosis. Folic acid 5 mg/day must be recommended throughout pregnancy for such women.

Blood group and red cell alloantibody

Definition
Serological testing identifies blood group type (ABO) and the presence of any antibodies. Rhesus D (RhD) is the most common red cell antibody.

Incidence
Fifteen per cent of the population are RhD-negative.

Pathophysiology
RhD incompatibility is the most common and most clinically relevant. The Rh factor is a molecule that occurs on the surface of RBCs. Blood is Rh-positive if RBCs have the Rh factor and Rh-negative if not. If the fetus is Rh-positive and its RBCs enter the maternal circulation, the woman's immune system may recognize them as foreign and produce Rh antibodies to destroy them. The process of antibody formation is termed Rh sensitization. If Rh antibodies cross the placenta to the fetus they will destroy fetal RBCs, resulting in fetal jaundice, anaemia, heart failure, hydrops, and death.

Rh sensitization is rare in a first pregnancy, as significant amounts of fetal blood do not usually enter the maternal circulation until delivery. However, once sensitized, problems are more likely with each subsequent Rh-positive pregnancy as women produce Rh antibodies earlier and in larger amounts.

Clinical relevance
Identification of blood group, RhD status and antibodies is important to prevent haemolytic disease of the newborn (HDN) and to identify women at risk of blood transfusion problems. Rh-negative women can be offered antenatal and postnatal immunoprophylaxis.

Diagnosis
Made on blood testing. The main antibodies causing severe HDN are anti-D, -C, and -Kell. Of lesser importance but still capable of causing HDN are anti-e, -Ce, -Fya, -Jka, and -Cw.

Management
All women should be screened at booking and 28 weeks to check group, Rh status, and the presence of antibodies.

RhD-negative women should be offered prophylactic anti-D at 28 and 34 weeks' gestation.

The management of affected pregnancies depends on the antibody detected and the titre, but ultimately, intrauterine fetal blood transfusion may be required.

Sickle cell and thalassaemia

(see also Sections 7.22 and 7.23)

Pathophysiology
Sickle cell anaemia is an inherited autosomal recessive condition, characterized by sickle-shaped RBCs and chronic anaemia.

Thalassaemias are a group of inherited anaemias characterized by defective haemoglobin synthesis. Different phenotypes result from unbalanced haemoglobin synthesis caused by decreased production of at least one globin polypeptide chain (α, β, γ, δ).

Demographics
Sickle cell trait is most prevalent among West Africans (20–25%), black Caribbeans (4–11%), Indians and Cypriots (0.75–1%).

Thalassaemia is most prevalent in Mediterranean, Middle and Far East populations, and less prevalent in Indians and Africans.

Clinical relevance
- α-thalassaemia major causes hydrops incompatible with life
- β-thalassaemia major is survivable with regular transfusions
- Sickle cell disease requires long-term medical input
- Sickle, α- and β- traits are important in order to quantify the genetic risk of the baby having a disease depending on the partner's genotype

Diagnosis
Screening and diagnosis of sickle cell and thalassaemia in pregnancy is made by haemoglobin electrophoresis.

Management of abnormal results
The aim of screening is to identify women at risk (preferably preconceptually or in early pregnancy). If the mother is a carrier, then the partner should be offered screening. A screen-positive couple should be offered prenatal diagnosis (by chorionic villus sampling (CVS), amniocentesis, or fetal blood sampling) so that timely and informed reproductive choices can be made.

National universal screening of newborn babies for sickle cell disorders began in April 2003 in England and Wales.

Symptomatic sickle cell disease or thalassaemia should be supervised by a multidisciplinary team of obstetricians, haematologists, midwives, and nurses (see Sections 7.22 and 7.23).

Platelet disorders

(see also Sections 8.14 and 8.15)

Although there is no explicit national screening programme for other haematological conditions, platelets are routinely measured at booking and may be high ($\geq 450 \times 10^9$/l) or low ($< 150 \times 10^9$/l).

Essential thrombocythaemia is a rare myeloproliferative disorder with isolated thrombocytosis. Other causes include infection, inflammation, and postsurgical acute phase response. Women with thrombocythaemia are at increased risk of growth restriction, possibly secondary to placental thrombosis. Platelet count $>600 \times 10^9$/l can be treated with aspirin 75 mg/day to reduce platelet aggregation and hence thrombosis.

A low platelet count may be caused by gestational thrombocytopenia, immune thrombocytopenic purpura (ITP), pre-eclampsia, HELLP syndrome, systemic lupus erythematosus, antiphospholipid syndrome, bone marrow suppression, HIV infection, other infections, drugs, haemolytic uraemic syndrome, thrombotic thrombocytopenic purpura (HUS-TTP). It may be a spurious result due to clumping.

Further reading

Murray NA, Roberts IAG. Haemolytic disease of the newborn. *Archives of Disease in Childhood, Fetal Neonatal Edition* 2007; **92**:83–88.

RCOG. Greentop guideline No. 22. Use of anti-D immunoglobulin for Rh prophylaxis, 2002. www.rcog.org.uk

NHS Sickle Cell and Thalassaemia Screening Programme www.sct. screening.nhs.uk

> ### ⊙ Box 6.1 Key points
>
> - Offer screening for anaemia at booking and 28 weeks. This allows time for treatment
> - Hb levels <11 g/dl at booking and <10.5 g/dl in the third trimester need investigation and treatment
> - Offer testing for blood group, RhD status, and red cell antibodies at booking and 28 weeks
> - Routine antenatal anti-D prophylaxis should be offered to all non-sensitized Rh-negative pregnant women. Offer screening for haemoglobinopathy
> - Clear care pathways should exist for women found to be haemoglobinopathy carriers
> - Low platelets need thorough investigation (see Section 8.15)

Current UK guidelines recommend screening for a number of infections which have an adverse impact on maternal and/or fetal outcomes where there are effective interventions to modify or eliminate these effects.

The infections which are routinely screened for are:

- Asymptomatic bacteriuria
- Rubella
- Hepatitis B
- HIV
- Syphilis

Other infections (including varicella zoster, herpes simplex, cytomegalovirus and toxoplasma) are discussed in Sections 8.24, 8.25, and 8.26. Although encountered in the UK population they are not routinely screened for. Some booking blood is always stored for later virological analysis if required.

Asymptomatic bacteriuria (ASB)

Definition
ASB is the bacterial colonization of the urinary tract system in the absence of clinical symptoms of urinary tract infection.

Incidence
In the UK, ASB is found in 2–5% of pregnant women.

Clinical relevance
Untreated ASB can result in pyelonephritis with a higher risk of preterm birth (up to 12.8%).

Diagnosis
Midstream urine culture is the gold standard for identification of ASB and it also allows for antibiotic sensitivity to be determined. Rapid testing is based on using a urine reagent strip that tests for one or more of nitrite, protein, and leukocyte esterase. Urine reagent strips will detect 50% of women with ASB if the strip tests positive for > trace protein, > trace blood, positive for nitrite or positive for leukocyte esterase.

Management
There is no urgency to treat asymptomatic women before MSU result returns with culture and sensitivity.

Treatment with antibiotics reduces persistent bacteriuria in pregnancy, reduces risk of preterm delivery or low-birth weight babies, and reduces risk of pyelonephritis.

Evidence suggests that screening and treating ASB reduces maternal and infant morbidity.

Rubella

Rubella (German measles) is a contagious viral infection.

Incidence
The susceptibility to rubella in pregnancy varies with parity (2% in nulliparous women versus 1.2% in multiparous women) and ethnicity (Oriental 8%, Asian and Black 5%, Mediterranean 4%, and Caucasian 2%). This is because of successful childhood and postnatal vaccination programmes in the UK.

However, 1–2% of young adult women have not had childhood infection or immunization and are therefore susceptible. With MMR vaccine uptake falling in the UK, more young children will be susceptible, making rubella in pregnancy more frequent. The overall risk of rubella infection in susceptible women is 2 per 1000.

Pathophysiology
Rubella can be transmitted from asymptomatic contacts or those with rash (10 days before until 15 days after the onset of rash). Congenitally infected infants may transmit rubella for many months after birth. Rubella is thought to invade the upper respiratory tract, with subsequent viraemia and dissemination of the virus to different sites, including the placenta.

The fetus is at highest risk for developmental abnormalities when infected during the first 16 weeks of gestation, particularly the first 8–10 weeks. Early on, the virus is thought to establish a chronic intrauterine infection with endothelial damage to blood vessels, direct cytolysis of cells, and disruption of cellular mitosis.

Clinical relevance
Rubella infection causes serious neonatal congenital abnormality depending on the gestation of infection. There may be no effects, multiple anomalies, or death *in utero*.

The most frequent abnormalities include intrauterine growth restriction, meningoencephalitis, cataracts, retinopathy, hearing loss, cardiac defects (patent ductus arteriosus and pulmonary artery stenosis), hepatosplenomegaly, and bone radiolucencies. Others are thrombocytopenia with purpura, dermal erythropoiesis resulting in bluish red skin lesions, adenopathy, and interstitial pneumonia.

After birth, observation is needed to detect subsequent hearing loss, mental retardation, or abnormal behaviour.

Diagnosis
Symptoms and signs
Rubella is suspected in a pregnant woman who presents with characteristic adenopathy and rash.

A 1–5 day prodromal illness precedes; it is usually mild, consisting of fever, malaise, and lymphadenopathy of the suboccipital, postauricular, and posterior cervical glands. The rash lasts 3–5 days and is less extensive than that of measles, beginning on the face and neck, and quickly spreading to the trunk and extremities (see Figure 6.5). A blanching, macular erythema appears on the face. Petechiae can form on the soft palate, coalescing into papules. This is Forschheimer's sign, occurring in 20% of cases and, if present, is diagnostic.

The detection of rubella IgG antibody early in pregnancy means women are immune to rubella (seropositive). In seronegative women who develop symptoms or signs of rubella, the diagnosis is made by seroconversion or a greater than 4-fold rise between acute and convalescent titres.

Diagnosing whether the baby has congenital rubella can be done by serology and viral culture of amniotic fluid or fetal blood sample. The gestational age of infection and the risk associated with diagnostic techniques should be considered when deciding whether to confirm infection in the fetus.

Management
Treatment for the mother is symptomatic in the acute phase. The vaccine is contraindicated in pregnancy as it carries a risk of toxicity as it is a live-attenuated vaccine, but it can be given following delivery. There is no treatment for the fetus, and termination is offered dependent on the risk of abnormality related to the gestation of infection. Prevention is by routine vaccination on delivery.

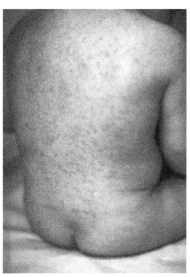

Fig. 6.5 Child with rubella rash. Rash of rubella typically described as pink dots under the skin which disappear without any evidence on the skin. (Kindly provided by the Public Health Image Library of the Centres for Disease Control and Prevention.)

Box 6.2 Risk of affected fetus with rubella depending on gestation

Risk of intrauterine rubella transmission
<11 weeks 90%
11–16 weeks 55%
>16 weeks 45%

Risk of adverse fetal outcome
<11 weeks—90% risk of microcephaly, severe developmental delay, profound sensorineural deafness, blindness, congenital cataracts
11–16 weeks—20% risk of all the above
16–20 weeks—minimal risk of deafness only
>20 weeks—no increased risk

Group B streptococcus (GBS)

Group B streptococcus is a bacterium, *Streptococcus agalactiae*.

Incidence
Approximately 20% of pregnant women in the UK are colonized with GBS in their vagina or rectum regardless of age or parity. The incidence of early onset GBS neonatal sepsis is 0.5/1000 births (or 340 affected babies annually).

Pathophysiology
GBS coexists in the genital and gastrointestinal tract, causing no disease or symptoms in the mother. Transmission to the fetus occurs during labour or where ruptured membranes allow for ascending infection from the vagina.

GBS infection arises from an initial focus of infection in the baby (which can be in the paranasal sinuses, middle ear, lungs or GI tract) that may later disseminate to meninges and kidneys. Sepsis in the neonate is the most common presentation for GBS infection.

Clinical relevance
GBS infection is the most common cause of severe early onset infection in the newborn, with a high mortality rate of 6% in term infants and 18% in preterm infants.

Diagnosis
GBS is best cultured from low vaginal and rectal swabs. It can also be cultured from urine.

Management
Universal screening for GBS carriage in pregnant women is not practised in the UK, unlike the USA, as the balance of risk and benefits associated with screening remain uncertain. In the UK, the incidence of neonatal infection with GBS is as low as the USA where universal screening and intrapartum antibiotic prophylaxis are practised.

It is recommended that intrapartum antibiotic prophylaxis for GBS should be offered if the woman has had a previous baby with neonatal GBS disease or if GBS is incidentally detected in urine or on a vaginal swab during the current pregnancy. There are a number of other risk factors which increase the likelihood of neonatal sepsis. These include preterm birth, prolonged ruptured membranes (>18 h), and intrapartum fever. For women with these risk factors (particularly if there are multiple risk factors), intrapartum antibiotic prophylaxis should be considered (such as benzylpenicillin or, if allergic to penicillin, clindamycin).

Box 6.3 Key points

- Women should be offered routine screening for ASB with an MSU early in pregnancy. Treatment reduces risk of preterm delivery
- If rubella antibody is not detected in pregnancy, vaccination should be given after delivery. Vaccination whilst pregnant is contraindicated
- Routine screening for GBS should not be offered because identification and treatment has not been shown to lower the risk of neonatal infection

---

Further reading

Morgan-Capner P, Crowcroft NS. Guidelines on the management of, and exposure to, rash illness in pregnancy. *Communicable Disease and Public Health* 2002; **5(1)**:59–71. (Includes consideration of relevant antibody screening programmes in pregnancy). www.hpa.org.uk

www.rcog.org.uk Prevention of early onset neonatal Group B Streptococcal disease Guideline No. 36, November, 2003.

Syphilis (see also Section 3.6)

Syphilis is one of a group of diseases caused by the spirochaete organisms of the genus *Treponema*. Sexually acquired syphilis is caused by *T. pallidum*. Other related treponemes cause non-venereal treponematoses such as bejel (*T. pallidum endemicum*), yaws (*T. pallidum pertenue*), and pinta (*T. carateum*).

Incidence

The incidence of infectious syphilis is low in the UK. The prevalence in pregnant women is estimated to be 0.068 per 1000 live births.

Pathophysiology

Syphilis is caused by *T. pallidum*, which is a spirochaete that enters through the mucous membranes or skin, reaching the regional lymph nodes, and then disseminating throughout the body. Syphilis is sexually transmitted and occurs in primary, secondary, and tertiary stages with long latent periods in between the stages. The risk of transmission is about 30% from a single sexual encounter with a person with primary syphilis. Prior infection does not confer immunity against re-infection.

Congenital infection is transplacental. Transmission in the latent or tertiary stage of syphilis is uncommon.

Clinical relevance

Early untreated syphilis will result in congenital infection in 70–100% of neonates and stillbirth in 30%. Early fetal signs include hydrocephalus, characteristic skin lesions, lymphadenopathy, hepatosplenomegaly, failure to thrive, meningitis, seizures, mental retardation, osteochondritis, and pseudoparalysis. The neonate may not show signs of infection up until 2 years of age. Maternal syphilis infection has long-term co-morbidity if untreated. Treatment is almost always curative in both mother and baby without any adverse maternal or fetal outcomes.

Diagnosis

Serological tests for syphilis are classified into two groups.

- **Non-treponemal** tests detect non-specific treponemal antibody. These include the Venereal Diseases Research Laboratory (VDRL) and rapid plasma reagin (RPR) tests
- **Treponemal** tests detect specific treponemal antibody. These include the *Treponema pallidum* haemagglutination assay (TPHA), the fluorescent treponemal antibody-absorbed test (FTA-abs) and enzyme immunoassay (EIA) tests

Current screening for syphilis involves a two-step approach. Firstly, the detection of treponemal antibody by a screening test, followed by confirmation of a reactive screening test result by further testing. The confirmatory test should ideally have equivalent sensitivity and greater specificity than the screening test and be independent methodologically, so as to reduce the chance of coincident false positive reactions. Serology cannot distinguish between the different treponematoses (syphilis, yaws, pinta, and bejel), so positive tests should be interpreted with caution.

Management

Any positive test result should be referred to a genitourinary medicine specialist for confirmation of the disease, contact tracing, treatment with penicillin, and monitoring. Public health agencies must also be notified.

Hepatitis B virus (see also Section 3.10)

Incidence

The prevalence of hepatitis B surface antigen (HBsAg) in pregnant women ranges from 0.1 to 1% depending on country of birth. It is more prevalent in women who are indigenous to countries where it is endemic, e.g. Africa, Indian subcontinent. The prevalence of carriage of the 'e' antigen (with greatest risk of transmission) is much lower.

Pathophysiology

HBV is a DNA virus which infects and replicates within hepatocytes. It is excreted in bodily fluids—blood, saliva, vaginal fluid, and semen. Transmission can be sexual, vertical (mother to neonate) or via contaminated blood, e.g. blood transfusion, sharing needles in drug users.

Vertical transmission usually occurs at birth, primarily from maternal–fetal microtransfusions during labour or contact with infectious secretions in the birth canal. This accounts for 95% of neonatal HBV infection. The risk of transplacental transmission is thought to be much lower (<5%). The risk of transmission is highest from asymptomatic HBV surface antigen carriers with e antigen.

Neonatal HBV infection is usually asymptomatic and can result in chronic subclinical disease.

Clinical relevance

Eighty-five per cent of babies born to mothers who are positive for hepatitis e antigen (eAg) become HBV surface antigen carriers and subsequently chronic carriers, compared with 31% of babies born to mothers who are eAg-negative. Chronic carriers of HBV surface antigen are 22 times more likely to die from hepatocellular carcinoma or cirrhosis in adulthood. Mother-to-child transmission of hepatitis B can be reduced if the baby receives immunoglobulin and vaccination.

Diagnosis

All pregnant women should be offered serological testing for HBV surface antigen. There are no antenatal tests for the fetus.

Management

The risk of mother-to-child transmission is recognized. However, there is no good evidence to suggest that elective CS could further reduce mother-to-child transmission versus immunoglobulin and vaccination of the neonate at birth. Maternal hepatitis B infection is not an indication for CS.

Neonates whose mothers are HBV surface antigen-positive should be given both HBV immune globulin and their first dose of HBV vaccine within 24 h of birth. This is 95% effective at preventing HBV infection and thus the chronic carrier state. Once this immunization is initiated, mothers may breastfeed.

Women should be offered an appointment with a hepatologist for discussion of future significance and recommending testing and vaccination of partners should be considered. Breastfeeding is safe.

Human immunodeficiency virus (HIV)

(see also Section 3.11)

HIV (either HIV-1 or HIV-2) causes a multisystem chronic infection that leads to progressive immunological deterioration, opportunistic infections, and malignancies. The end stage is acquired immunodeficiency syndrome (AIDS).

Incidence

HIV-1 causes most cases in Europe, Asia, Central, South, and East Africa. HIV-2 appears less virulent and causes most cases in parts of West Africa. In certain areas of West Africa, both organisms are prevalent and may co-infect patients. Epidemic global spread began in the late 1970s and AIDS was recognized in 1981. More than 40 million people are infected worldwide. Of the 3 million annual deaths and 14 000 new daily infections, 95% occur in the developing world, half in women, and 15% in children <15 years.

Prevalence in pregnancy varies geographically. Surveillance shows a rate of ~0.5% in London and 0.03% outside London. About 300 HIV-infected women give birth annually in the UK.

Pathophysiology

HIV attaches to and penetrates host T lymphocyte cells via surface CD4+ molecules. This allows integration and multiplication of the HIV viral DNA with each cycle of the host cell's division. Infected CD4+ lymphocytes produce >98% of plasma HIV virions.

The main consequence of HIV infection is damage to the immune system, specifically loss of CD4+ T lymphocytes, which are involved in cell-mediated and, to a lesser extent, humoral immunity. CD4 lymphocyte depletion may result from direct cytotoxic effects of HIV replication, cell-mediated immune cytotoxicity, and thymic damage that impair lymphocyte production.

HIV is transmitted by sexual, parenteral or perinatal means by contact with body fluids (specifically blood, semen, vaginal secretions, breast milk, saliva, exudates from wounds or skin and mucosal lesions) that contain free virions or infected cells. Transmission is more likely with higher concentrations of virions, which can be very high during primary infection, even if asymptomatic. HIV is not transmitted by saliva or droplets produced by coughing or sneezing, or by casual contact.

HIV is transmitted from mother to offspring by transplacental or perinatal routes in 30–50% of affected cases, thus justifying screening in pregnancy. HIV is excreted in breast milk, thus breastfeeding can also transmit HIV.

HIV virion concentrations in plasma are measured by nucleic acid amplification assays and expressed as HIV RNA copies/ml.

Antibodies to HIV are measurable usually within a few weeks after primary infection. Vertical transmission is greatest if the viral load is high and/or the CD4 count is low.

Diagnosis

All pregnant women are offered screening for HIV status early in pregnancy. Detection is by the presence of HIV antibody in maternal serum. Maternal antibodies against HIV-1 or HIV-2 are detectable in 95% of women within 3 months of exposure.

As maternal HIV antibody may persist for up to 18 months in the infant, detection of the HIV virus is used for diagnosis.

Managment

HIV infection in the mother and the neonate can become a chronic health and social problem. Without intervention, the risk of mother-to-child transmission is 30–50% but risk is related to viral load.

Avoidance of breastfeeding is the single most effective, and safest, intervention. With antiretroviral treatment this can be reduced to <8%. Not breastfeeding, antiretrovirals, and CS combined reduce vertical transmission to 1% or less.

Newer highly active antiretrovirals (HAART) may reduce viral load to negligible levels (thus avoiding the need for CS and intrapartum interventions), but longer term effects are still unknown.

Invasive diagnostic procedures, instrumental delivery, fetal scalp electrode, and fetal blood sampling in labour should all be avoided if possible in women who are HIV-positive.

> **Box 6.3 Key points**
> - All pregnant women should be offered screening for HBV so effective postnatal intervention can be offered
> - All women should be offered screening for HIV as rates of mother-to-child transmission are significantly reduced with antiretroviral drugs, not breastfeeding, and elective CS
> - Routine screening for syphilis is recommended, as effective treatment is available, reducing transmission

Further reading

www.nice.org.uk Antenatal care: routine care for the healthy pregnant woman. National Collaborating Centre for Women's and Children's Health, commissioned by NICE, July 2008, Guideline CG62.

www.nsc.nhs.uk National Screening Committee. A useful website for all UK screening programmes.

www.bhiva.org British HIV Association. Management of HIV infection in pregnant women 2008.

6.8 Screening for clinical conditions

Diabetes mellitus—gestational and pre-existing

(see also Section 7.15)

Definition

At present there is no consensus on the definition, management or treatment of gestational diabetes mellitus (GDM), which is defined as 'carbohydrate intolerance resulting in hyperglycaemia of variable severity with onset or first recognition during pregnancy'.

Incidence

Varies depending on definition. In the UK it is estimated to affect around 2% of pregnancies versus 3–10% in other developed countries.

Pathophysiology

Pathophysiology is based on disorders of insulin metabolism. Insulin reduces serum glucose levels by increasing cellular uptake. Glucagon and cortisol increase glucose production. The placenta produces insulin antagonists (human placental lactogen (HPL), progesterone, and HCG) as well as cortisol, all of which increase glucose production. This is beneficial to the growing fetus which uses glucose as its primary metabolic substrate. If the pancreatic β-cells are unable to produce sufficient insulin to balance this increase or if there is maternal insulin resistance, then a state of hyperglycaemia develops.

Antenatal screening

The rationale for screening for GDM is that this allows clinicians to intervene to improve perinatal outcome. This has recently been confirmed in the large Australian Carbohydrate Study in Pregnancy (ACHOIS) randomized trial from Australia. Worldwide, however, there is huge variation in the method used for screening.

Most UK centres undertake some form of screening for GDM. This can be risk factor assessment followed by specific laboratory-based screening for women judged to be at 'high-risk'. Some centres use universal laboratory-based screening.

An example of selective screening would be to perform a random blood glucose, both in early pregnancy and then at 28–32 weeks (or with a formal oral glucose tolerance test, OGTT), but only in women with a risk factor. An abnormal result is likely to be ≥7 mmol/l.

Alternatively, universal screening for all women may be undertaken between 28 and 32 weeks with a random glucose test. If this is high, then a formal OGTT is performed for diagnosis.

In the UK, NICE recommends a screening policy based on risk factor assesment. Risks include:

- BMI >30
- Previous macrosomic baby (>=4.5 kg)
- Previous GDM
- Diabetes in a first-degree relative
- Ethnic origin with a high prevalence of diabetes (eg South Asian, black Caribbean and Middle Eastern)

If a risk factor is present then an oral GTT at 24–28 weeks (16–18 if previous GDM) should be performed.

NICE does not recommend screening for gestational diabetes using fasting or random plasma glucose, glucose challenge test or urinalysis for glucose.

Management

For women with pre-existing diabetes, antenatal care involves a higher awareness of the increased risk of congenital and cardiac anomaly; fetal growth restriction may occur as well as macrosomia, increased incidence of pre-eclampsia, and polyhydramnios.

Once GDM is diagnosed, good glucose control is important either with diet alone or combined with insulin. Increasingly, oral hypoglycaemics are used in pregnancy, though their safety and effectiveness is uncertain.

Management of GDM is similar to established diabetes mellitus (see Section 7.15).

Pre-eclampsia

(see also Sections 8.11–8.14)

Definitions

Pre-eclampsia is defined as hypertension (BP≥140/90 mmHg on at least two occasions taken at least 4 h apart or one reading of >170/110 mmHg) manifesting after 20 weeks of gestation that is associated with new onset proteinuria which resolves after delivery.

Pregnancy-induced hypertension (PIH) is defined as hypertension developing after 20 weeks' gestation that resolves after delivery but is not associated with proteinuria.

Chronic hypertension is defined as hypertension that predates a pregnancy or appears prior to 20 weeks of gestation.

Risk factors

Recognized risk factors for pre-eclampsia include nulliparity, age ≥40 years, sibling or maternal history of pre-eclampsia, history of previous pre-eclampsia, BMI ≥35 at booking, multiple pregnancy, pre-existing vascular disease, diabetes, hypertension, SLE.

Antenatal screening

Measurement of BP and urine analysis for proteinuria is an effective screening tool for hypertensive disorders.

- **BP** should be measured in a consistent manner. An automated machine, suitable for pregnancy, or manual sphygmomanometer, is recommended using the correct size cuff for the upper arm. The woman should be sitting or semi-reclined with the upper arm at the level of the heart, using Korotkoff V for diastolic pressure
- **Urine analysis** is significant if 1+ or more of protein is detected and a 24-h urine protein measurement should be performed. If there is >300 mg/24 h, this confirms the diagnosis of pre-eclampsia. Levels of proteinuria >500 mg/24 h are linked to more adverse maternal and fetal outcomes
- **All women should be educated** about the symptoms of pre-eclampsia (such as headaches, visual disturbances, blurring or flashing before the eyes, pain below the ribs or vomiting) and asked to report them

For management of pregnancy-induced hypertension and pre-eclampsia see Sections 8.10–8.14.

Placenta praevia

(see Section 8.3)

Antenatal screening

Maternal and fetal mortality and morbidity are increased with placenta praevia, thus providing the rationale for screening.

Screening for the position of the placenta is routine at the 20-week anomaly scan and identifies a low lying placenta. A re-scan should be arranged at 36 weeks for an asymptomatic minor placenta praevia or at 32 weeks for an asymptomatic major placenta praevia. This will determine the placental position and aid with third trimester management (**C**).

Transvaginal ultrasound (TVS) has been found to be safe and more accurate than transabdominal ultrasound (TAS) in identifying a low lying placenta, especially when posterior (**B**). Therefore, the RCOG has recommended that all women with a low lying placenta identified at the TAS anomaly scan should have a TVS (**C**).

Preterm birth

(see also Sections 8.18–8.20)

Clinical relevance

Predicting, preventing, detecting, and treating preterm birth are important, not as an end in themselves, but as a means of reducing adverse events for the child. Preterm birth is the most important single cause of perinatal mortality, with most mortality and morbidity experienced under 30 weeks. In addition, it accounts for the majority of severe childhood disability (varying degrees of cerebral palsy, chronic lung disease, and neurodevelopment delay).

Pathophysiology

With preterm delivery, it is not clear whether infection or inflammation is the cause or the effect of preterm delivery.

Antenatal screening

Identification of women at high risk remains paramount, and is best done at the first appointment. Risk factors include, primarily, a previous preterm delivery, recurrent cervical dilatation, second trimester termination of pregnancy, trachelectomy, repeated cone biopsy (see also Box 8.12 in Section 8.18).

Advances in screening and predicting preterm birth include measurement of fetal fibronectin (FFN) in vaginal secretions and transvaginal US scan of cervical length.

Cervical length as a screening tool is reserved for women with a previous preterm delivery (early or late). The consensus cervical length taken at 23 weeks should be ≥25 mm. Serial measurements can also be performed to assess for the degree of shortening, if at all, and the presence of funnelling, which is a predictor of poor outcome (see Section 8.20).

Presence of FFN (see Box 6.4) taken as a high vaginal swab in the late second or early third trimester increases the likelihood of delivery before 34 weeks by a factor of four in both high and low risk women. The absence of FFN is strongly associated with prolongation of the pregnancy for an indeterminate length of time. New evidence suggests using FFN solely for high-risk women at 24 weeks is a helpful predictor of subsequent preterm delivery, giving a likelihood ratio of 11.8 and 0.48 for a positive test and a negative test respectively. Currently, use of FFN is limited to clinical trials and specialist units.

Routine screening for preterm birth is not recommended practice in the UK. Nevertheless, it is common practice to offer screening to high-risk women.

Management (see also Section 8.19)

The mainstay of management of high risk women involves:

- Insertion of a cervical suture
- Treatment for symptomatic bacterial vaginosis with vaginal clindamycin or oral metronidazole. In some studies this has being shown to reduce the rate of preterm prelabour rupture of membranes (PPROM) and delivery
- Treatment with progesterone—the consensus is that progestagenic agents reduce the risk of preterm labour in some high-risk women

The Health Technology Assessment (HTA) Programme has commissioned a systematic review on predictive factors for preterm labour.

⊘ Box 6.4 Fetal fibronectin (FFN)

- A glycoprotein found in amniotic fluid and placenta
- Is detected in cervicovaginal secretions <16 weeks' gestation (before fusion of the fetal membranes) and late in pregnancy before labour. It is not normally detected between 22 and 37 weeks' gestation
- In threatened preterm labour, it is thought that disruption of the chorionic–decidual interface leads to detection of FFN in the cervicovaginal secretions
- A bedside test is available for detection of FFN
- The sensitivity, specificity, positive, and negative predictive values of FFN for predicting delivery within 14 days in symptomatic women were 65%, 93%, 43%, and 97% in a recent study
- A woman with a negative FFN is unlikely to go into labour within 14 days
- However, the decision to withhold corticosteroids ± tocolysis must be decided on an individual basis. It is difficult to withhold corticosteroids in a symptomatic woman when they confer much benefit

---

Further reading

Chatterjee J, Guilam J, Vatish M, Thornton S. The management of preterm labour. *Archives of Disease in Childhood, Fetal Neonatal Edition* 2007; **92:**88–93.

Confidential Enquiry into Maternal and Child Health: Pregnancy in Women with Type 1 and Type 2 Diabetes in 2002–03, England, Wales and Northern Ireland. London: CEMACH, 2005.

Crowther CA, Hiller JE, Moss JR, et al. Effect of treatment of gestational diabetes mellitus on pregnancy outcomes. N Engl J Med 2005; 352(24): 2477–2486. ACHOIS Trial Group

NICE. Diabetes in Pregnancy. Clinical Guideline. National Collaborating Center for Women's & Children's Health. London: RCOG Press, 2008. www.nice.org.uk

Health Technology Assessment commissioned research. Screening to prevent pre-term birth—systematic reviews of accuracy and effectiveness literature with economic modelling. June 2008. www.hta.ac.uk

www.rcog.org.uk RCOG. Green top guideline No. 27. Placenta praevia and placenta praevia accreta: diagnosis and management, 2005.

Shennan A, Jones G, Hawken J et al. Fetal fibronectin test predicts delivery before 30 weeks of gestation in high risk women, but increases anxiety. *British Journal of Obstetrics and Gynaecology* 2005; **112:**293–6.

World Health Organization. Definition, diagnosis and classification of diabetes mellitus and its complications. Report of a WHO consultation, 1999.

One aim of antenatal care is to detect abnormalities of fetal growth and to ensure fetal wellbeing. Methods for this include both informal and formal maternal observation of movements, abdominal palpation, symphyseal–fundal height (SFH) measurement, auscultation of the fetal heart, cardiotocography (CTG), and ultrasound.

Each time a pregnant woman is seen antenatally, some assessment of fetal growth and wellbeing should be undertaken.

Monitoring of fetal movement

The simplest, cheapest, and most continuous test of fetal wellbeing remains the mother's perception, and her concerns should always be taken seriously.

The role of routine counting of fetal movements (FM) to indicate fetal wellbeing and prevent late fetal deaths has been explored in large randomized controlled trials and did not show a reduction in perinatal mortality. Therefore, routine formal fetal movement counting is not recommended.

Mothers are still encouraged to report early if they notice changes in the usual pattern or diminished fetal movements (e.g. none by noon or <10 by the evening).

Abdominal palpation

Abdominal palpation can be used to assess fetal size, presentation, and engagement of the presenting part. Palpation alone is not accurate in estimating fetal growth.

At 36 weeks, the presenting part should be determined. If it is not cephalic, an ultrasound scan should be performed to check the presentation and lie, and any obvious cause for malpresentation. This allows external cephalic version (ECV) to be offered to appropriate women with a breech presentation.

Symphyseal–fundal height

For measurement of SFH see Figure 6.6.

SFH is used clinically as a more objective way of indicating whether the baby is small or large for dates, when compared with abdominal palpation. Discrepancy can arise if there are errors in the expected date of delivery (EDD), with polyhydramnios, multiple pregnancy, fibroid uterus or maternal obesity.

SFH should be plotted on a growth chart in the notes. Some maternity units employ a customized SFH chart as a screening method to detect fetal growth problems based on the mother's weight, height, parity, and ethnicity. The benefit of these charts compared with conventional charts remains uncertain.

Auscultation of the fetal heart

Auscultation has formed an integral part of antenatal care and can be done with either a Pinnard or a hand-held Doppler ultrasound.

Hearing the fetal heart (FH) confirms that the fetus is alive but has no predictive value on any measure of fetal outcome. There is therefore no real clinical value associated with routine antenatal auscultation.

Less maternal self-reliance and extra anxiety may even be created (e.g. by hearing entirely normal ectopic beats).

Cardiotocography

The use of antenatal CTG for routine fetal assessment in normal pregnancies is not recommended as it has not been shown to improve perinatal morbidity or mortality. See Section 9.8 for CTG interpretation.

Ultrasound scan

The value of ultrasound scan (US) for routine fetal assessment in the third trimester for normal pregnancies is uncertain. However, it may be useful for monitoring fetal growth and wellbeing for women where risk factors are present.

US assessment of growth and fetal wellbeing includes:

- Measurement of liquor volume
- Fetal growth pattern and weight estimate from biometric measurements

Other tests can include:

- Fetal breathing, movements, and tone
- Doppler assessment of umbilical artery

Interpretation of ultrasound scan

Fetal growth

The fetus grows from a mean of 500 g at 24 weeks, 1 kg at 28 weeks to 3.5 kg at 40 weeks. There is rapid weight gain from 27 to 37 weeks and then growth velocity slows.

Individual biometric measurements for the fetal abdominal circumference (AC), biparietal diameter (BPD), head circumference (HC), and femur length (FL) are plotted on centile charts. Combining the parameters results in an estimated fetal weight (EFW). The AC is the most sensitive predictor of fetal weight (thought to reflect glycogen stores of the liver).

As there is substantial operator-dependent error in fetal biometry, the recommended frequency for growth scans to determine growth velocity is no less than 2-weekly. A discrepancy of as much as 15% may exist between EFW and actual fetal weight, so care must be taken not to over-interpret the measurement in isolation.

Individual biometric measurements are less predictive of important intrauterine growth restriction than the overall fetal growth velocity. If consecutive measurements show that the fetal growth is crossing centiles, is <10th centile or >95th centile, there is enough cause for concern to consider other tests of fetal wellbeing.

Liquor volume assessment

The main source of amniotic fluid is fetal urine after 20 weeks' gestation. Any disruption to fetal urine production, passage, or swallowing can alter the volume. The normal amount of amniotic fluid is 500 ml at 18 weeks, rising to a maximum of 800 ml at 34 weeks and falling to 600 ml at term.

A sonographer can describe the volume subjectively but this is not reliable. Objective measurements include maximum vertical pool (MVP), which measures the largest single pool of amniotic fluid, or the amniotic fluid index (AFI), which is the sum of the measured largest pool of amniotic fluid in each quadrant of the uterus.

Oligohydramnios is defined as MVP <2 cm or AFI <5th centile (see Box 6.5) and is the best single predictor of poor outcome.

Box 6.5 Amniotic fluid index

<5 cm	Oligohydramnios
5–10 cm	Reduced
10–17 cm	Normal
17–25 cm	Increased
>25 cm	Polyhydramnios

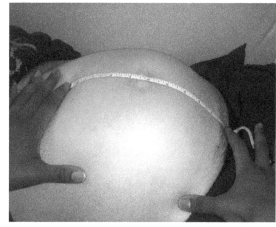

Fig. 6.6 Correct method of measuring SFH. Measurement should start at the fundus (variable point) and continue in a longitudinal axis to the outer most point of the symphysis pubis using a non-elastic tape. Note that the doctor is measuring with the centimetre side of the tape facing down to avoid biased measurement.

Fetal growth restriction and small for gestational age

Small for gestational age (SGA) is a description of a fetus or infant that is below a specific biometric or estimated weight threshold. The commonly used threshold is the 10th centile for estimated fetal weight (EFW) or postnatal birth weight.

Fetal (or intrauterine) growth restriction (FGR or IUGR) refers to an antenatal disease process where a fetus fails to achieve its expected genetic growth potential.

SGA fetuses are a heterogeneous group containing those that have failed to achieve their growth potential and others that are constitutionally small (or 'normal small'). Abdominal circumference (AC) and EFW are the most accurate measures of SGA. Approximately 50–70% of infants with a birth weight <10th centile are constitutionally small.

Growth-restricted fetuses are at greater risk of stillbirth, iatrogenic prematurity, perinatal asphyxia, neonatal complications, and impaired neurodevelopment.

Symmetrical and asymmetrical growth restriction are often described as separate entities but in clinical practice the differentiation is less clear. Symmetrical FGR describes a fetus whose biometric parameters for head circumference (HC) and AC are similar, whereas asymmetrical growth restriction describes a fetus where the AC is small compared to the HC, i.e. there is head sparing. This situation probably reflects progressive disruption of the uteroplacental circulation, resulting in a fetus with poor liver glycogen stores. For causes of FGR see Box 6.6.

Assessment of the growth-restricted fetus should include a detailed structural ultrasound examination, as up to 19% have some form of congenital abnormality. Fetal karyotyping and viral studies should be considered in early onset or symmetrical growth restriction.

Doppler

Doppler ultrasound has been used to examine fetal, placental, and uterine circulations. Measurements of velocity and flow are unreliable because of the small diameter of the vessels. However, the flow velocity waveform can be measured and analysed to assess downstream resistance in the peripheral vessels.

Umbilical artery Doppler has been shown to improve fetal outcome, primarily in high-risk pregnancies. Various indices (resistance index, RI or pulsatility index, PI) can be used. There is normally a decrease in umbilical artery impedance/resistance with advancing gestation (i.e. less opposition to blood flow) and so diastolic flow increases relative to systolic (see Figure 6.7). Consequently, Doppler measurements from the umbilical artery fall with increasing gestation. Raised umbilical artery resistance may indicate a problem downstream in the placenta. This can lead to the observation of absent or even reversed end-diastolic flow, which are indicative of marked fetal compromise.

The interval between the first occurrence of absent or reversed end-diastolic flow in the umbilical artery and the development of an abnormal CTG and/or biophysical profile ranges from 1 to several weeks.

Umbilical artery Doppler measurement has become a routine part of scanning and its predictive role is clear for the growth-restricted fetus in a high-risk pregnancy. It has been demonstrated that measurement of the umbilical artery Doppler in a low-risk pregnancy does not reduce perinatal morbidity or mortality.

In sick fetuses with early onset growth restriction, closer observation using fetal Dopplers is used to time delivery judiciously by assessing compensation–decompensation (e.g. middle cerebral 'brain-sparing', ductus venosus 'A' waves, umbilical vein pulsation,

umbilical artery absent or reverse end-diastolic flow), and end-organ damage (e.g. echogenic bowel, enlarged heart, ventricular haemorrhage).

Outcome, of death or long-term damage, depends on gestation, size and sickness, and close liaison is required between fetal medicine and neonatology.

Biophysical profile

Physiology

The principle underlying the measurement of the biophysical profile (BPP) is that the fetus, when exposed to chronic hypoxia, will have a depressed central nervous system. This will manifest as reduced heart rate variability, decreased movement, decreased tone, and fewer than usual breathing movements. If the degree of cardiovascular compensation to protect vital organs (such as the brain and heart) is severe, depressed renal blood flow also results in oligohydramnios.

Clinical use

Measurement of the BPP in high-risk pregnancies has not been shown to improve perinatal outcome in randomized controlled trials. However, there is some evidence from uncontrolled observational studies that a BPP in high-risk women may have good negative predictive value, i.e. fetal death is rare with a normal BPP (see Box 6.7).

BPP is not recommended for routine monitoring in low-risk pregnancies or for primary surveillance in growth restriction. However, when the umbilical artery Doppler is found to be abnormal, BPP may be useful given its negative predictive value. This is further supported by evidence that, in high-risk women, the BPP is rarely abnormal when Doppler findings are normal.

The optimal surveillance strategy in fetuses with absent or reversed end-diastolic flow is unclear. The only management option available in these situations is timed early delivery, and the balance between prevention of intrauterine death versus neonatal death or complications of iatrogenic prematurity is complex. Options include daily CTG or BPP and/or fetal venous Doppler with delivery when the CTG becomes pathological (decelerations with reduced variability) or the BPP becomes abnormal (≤4) or there are changes in the blood flow patterns in other fetal blood vessels such as the ductus venosus or middle cerebral artery.

Macrosomia

Macrosomia is a postnatal diagnosis, defined in several ways, as a birth weight >4 kg, or >4.5 kg, or >90th centile for gestation corrected for sex and ethnicity. It can be constitutional, genetic (e.g. Beckwith-Wiedemann syndrome) or secondary to diabetes.

The importance of recognizing fetal macrosomia is that the risk of shoulder dystocia increases with increasingly severe macrosomia. The four methods of estimating fetal weight antenatally are all unreliable, but more significant if congruent; maternal assessment (in relation to whether larger, smaller or the same size as a previous baby), clinical palpation, SFH, and US EFW (which is only accurate ±500 g at term).

On ultrasound, if the EFW is >4000 g (or above the 95th centile) or the AC is above the 90th centile, macrosomia may be inferred, especially if other parameters are within normal range. Early induction of labour (IOL) and elective CS are postulated but unproven means of preventing shoulder dystocia.

It is important to document 'watch for shoulders' so that birth attendants are alert and ready to deal with any emergency.

Further reading

Edmonds DK (ed.) *Dewhurst's Textbook of Obsterics and Gynaecology*, 7th edn. Blackwell Publishing.

Twinning P, McHugo JM, Pilling DW. *Textbook of Fetal Abnormalities*. London: Churchill Livingstone, 2000.

www.rcog.org.uk Investigation and management of small-for-gestational-age fetus. Greentop guideline No. 31, 2002.

⊕ Box 6.6 Causes of fetal growth retardation

Symmetrical

- Constitutional
- Chromosomal abnormality (e.g. trisomy 13 and 18, triploidy)
- Fetal infection (e.g. cytomegalovirus, toxoplasmosis, rubella)
- Structural abnormality

Asymmetrical

- Unknown
- Hypertension
- Diabetes
- Lupus
- Recurrent antepartum haemorrhage
- Multiple pregnancy
- Smoking
- Substance abuse
- Malnutrition

◎ Box 6.7 Biophysical profile

A score of 2 is given for each component if the criterion is met or 0 if it is not. Each score is added to make a total score. Scores of 10 or 8 are reassuring, 6 or 4 are equivocal, and 2 or 0 are ominous.

- Fetal breathing movement
- Fetal gross body movement
- Fetal tone
- Amniotic fluid
- Reactive fetal heart rate pattern (on CTG)

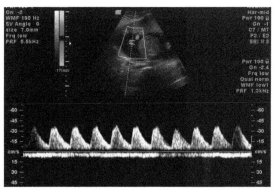

Fig. 6.7 Umbilical artery Doppler. Normal umbilical artery Doppler ultrasound (upper channel). This shows forward flow at the end of diastole (trough of the waveform). There is continuous flow in the umbilical vein (lower channel). (Kindly provided by Dr Meekai To).

Clinical relevance

Twins and higher order pregnancies account for 1% of all pregnancies. They are at a greater risk of antenatal and peripartum complications compared to singleton pregnancies. This includes a higher perinatal morbidity and mortality rate; therefore closer monitoring antenatally and intrapartum are essential to reduce the risks to the mother and her babies.

Incidence

- One in 90 naturally conceived pregnancies are twins
- Naturally occurring triplet births occur in approximately 1 per 7000–10 000 births
- Naturally occurring quadruplet births occur in 1 per 600 000 births

Zygocity and chorionicity

Dizygotic ('non-identical') twins

Incidence

- Seventy per cent of twin pregnancies are dizygotic (DZ)
- They constitute 11 out of 1000 deliveries in North America and Europe. The rate is highest in Africa (up to 40 per 1000 deliveries in Nigeria) and lowest in Japan (6.7 per 1000 deliveries)
- Increasing because of assisted reproductive techniques (ART). Clomiphene increases the risk of twins by 5–10% and ovulation induction by 20–30%

Physiology

- Polyovulation can be hereditary and is associated with increasing age (over 35 years) and parity (four or more pregnancies)
- Two ova will each be fertilized by one sperm to form two genetically different pregnancies
- Each baby will have their own placenta and amniotic sac, i.e. dichorionic (DC) diamniotic (DA)

Monozygotic ('identical') twins

Incidence

- Thirty per cent of twin pregnancies are monozygotic (MZ)
- No regional variation: 3–4 per 1000 births
- ART increases the incidence of MZ twins 4-fold

Physiology

- Early splitting of one fertilized ovum to form two genetically identical pregnancies

Timing determines chorionicity

- Thirty per cent split within 3 days of fertilization, forming a DCDA twin pregnancy; each twin will have their own placenta
- Seventy per cent split after 3 days, forming a monochorionic (MC) twin pregnancy, whereby the twins share one placenta. If this is before day 9, each fetus will have its own amniotic sac; termed monochorionic diamniotic (MCDA)

- One per cent split between days 9 and 12, forming monochorionic monoamniotic (MCMA) twins. They share both a placenta and amniotic sac
- Splitting after day 12 results in conjoined twins who share parts of their body to varying degrees (see Figure 6.8)
- MC twins can only be monozygotic

Determination of chorionicity

Chorionicity is the main factor in determining pregnancy outcome and not zygosity.

In MC twins, vascular anastomoses in the placenta give rise to a shared circulation. These increase further the risks of an MC pregnancy versus a DC one. Thus, MC and DC pregnancies are managed differently, which highlights the importance of determining chorionicity early in pregnancy by ultrasound.

- US at 10–14 weeks is nearly 100% effective in determining monochorionicity
- Chorionicity is harder to determine later in pregnancy
- In a MCDA pregnancy, two amnions separate both pregnancies. A thin membrane is seen on US which forms a 'T' shape as it meets the placenta (see Figure 6.9)
- In a DCDA pregnancy, two chorions and two amnions separate the pregnancies, and this is seen as a thicker separating membrane. As this membrane meets the placenta, a 'lambda' sign is seen (see Figure 6.10)
- In MCMA pregnancies, no dividing membrane is seen, and the fetus and umbilical cords can be seen intertwined
- Same sex twins can be MC or DC
- Different sex twins are always DC

General management principles

Assessment of fetal growth and wellbeing in multiple pregnancies uses the same tools as for singletons. Such pregnancies are at increased risk of a range of maternal and fetal problems (see Sections 8.28 and 8.29). There are several issues to consider when assessing multiple pregnancies.

- Some mothers can distinguish the movements of the fetuses and this is reassuring between visits
- The SFH measurement will always be larger than expected and bears no relationship to fetal growth
- Auscultation of the FH, if done, should detect two FHs separated by at least 10 bpm
- Where facilities for portable US are present, detection of two viable FHs is preferable

Increased surveillance of all twin pregnancies is recommended. There is no universal agreement, but good practice is that for MC twins, fortnightly growth scans and review should be initiated from 16 weeks. For DC twins, monthly growth scans from 28 weeks is practical. See Box 6.8 for a summary of general antenatal care for twin pregnancies.

- US at 11–14 weeks to determine chorionicity, measure nuchal translucency and confirm dates
- Oral iron and 5 mg folate supplements to prevent anaemia
- Detailed anomaly and cardiac scans
- Gestational diabetes screening
- Regular growth scans (4-weekly for DCDA twins, 2-weekly for MC twins)
- Monitor for signs of twin-to-twin transfusion in MC twins
- Regular BP and urine checks to identify pre-eclampsia
- Corticosteroids if preterm delivery anticipated
- Discussion antenatally regarding mode of delivery
- The woman should understand symptoms and signs of preterm labour and know to attend the hospital promptly if they develop

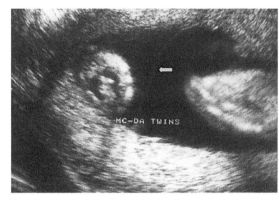

Fig. 6.9 Monochorionic diamniotic twins demonstrating the 'T' sign (⇦).

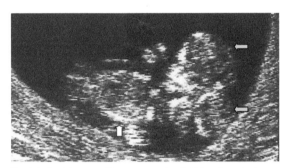

Fig. 6.8 Conjoint twins. There are two heads (⇦) and one body (⇧), i.e. this is a dicephalon/thoracopagus twin. (Kindly provided by Panayiota Papasozomenou).

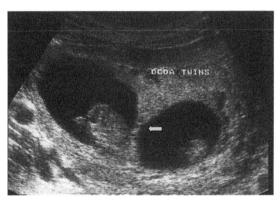

Fig. 6.10 Dichorionic diamniotic twins demonstrating the 'lambda' sign (⇦).

6.12 Screening for fetal chromosomal anomalies

Background

Chromosome abnormalities are common causes of miscarriage, intrauterine death, and congenital abnormality.

Screening for fetal anomalies using ultrasound scan assessment and maternal serum screening aims to detect structural or chromosomal abnormalities that are either incompatible with life, associated with a high morbidity and long-term disability, or where there is potential for treatment *in utero* or immediately postpartum.

Although women should be provided with clear information about all screening tests undertaken in pregnancy, this is particularly important in relation to screening for fetal anomalies as, unlike tests for maternal benefit, there are implications that may not be in her self-perceived best interest.

The absolute risk of a couple having an affected child is increased if risk factors are present. These include a family history of an inherited condition (e.g. cystic fibrosis, sickle cell disease, Duchenne muscular dystrophy, myotonic dystrophy), consanguinity, or if the woman has had a previous affected child. Structural abnormalities are increased if there is a significant maternal medical history such as diabetes, thyrotoxicosis, autoimmune disease and epilepsy, especially if teratogenic drugs are used.

Chromosome anomaly

Unlike structural abnormalities, chromosomal abnormalities are much more difficult to identify on ultrasound screening alone. Even if identified they are not diagnostic.

Many chromosomal abnormalities are incompatible with life. However, those that are not have major implications for the child and the family, which is why so much attention has focused on screening for Down's syndrome. Ultrasound measurement of the thickness of nuchal fluid behind the neck at 11–13 weeks' gestation is one feature which indicates the risk of Down's syndrome (see Figure 6.11).

Screening for Down's syndrome

Down's syndrome (trisomy 21) is caused by an extra chromosome 21 and is the most common congenital syndrome (incidence 1:600–800 of all births).

It results in a range of problems for the affected child; primarily intellectual impairment (80% severe versus 20% mild or none), increased mortality and morbidity due to congenital malformations, e.g. cardiac defects, increased risk of leukaemia, thyroid disorder, epilepsy, and Alzheimer's disease.

The risk of Down's syndrome increases with maternal age (see Figure 6.12). The level of serum markers vary with gestation (see Table 6.3). Therefore, algorithms which calculate the increased risk associated with changes in maternal serum markers are critically dependent on maternal age as well as an accurate estimate of gestational age.

One of the most frequent reasons for a falsely high screening test result is uncertain, or inaccurately recorded, gestational or maternal age.

Current Down's screening strategies in the UK include a mixture of nuchal translucency (NT) screening (at 11–13 weeks' gestation); screening with serum markers (usually at about 16 weeks' gestation); and a combination of the two approaches, with NT screening in the first trimester combined with first or second trimester serum screening in a combined or integrated approach. The latter has the advantage of increased sensitivity and specificity, but the acceptability has not been well evaluated.

In the UK, all national screening programmes, including Down's syndrome screening, are controlled by the National Screening Committee (NSC).

The NSC recommends that all maternity units should offer all women a test for Down's syndrome screening which provides a detection rate of >75% and a false positive rate <3% (see Table 6.4).

The serum markers used to indicate an increased risk of Down's syndrome are pregnancy associated plasma protein A (PAPP-A) and β-human chorionic gonadotrophin (HCG), both of which are produced by the placental syncytiotrophoblast; alpha fetoprotein (AFP), produced by the fetal yolk sac and fetal liver; unconjugated oestriol (uE3) produced by the placenta and fetal adrenals, and inhibin A produced by the placenta (see Table 6.3).

Screening tests can only provide a woman with a risk assessment of how likely she is to carry a pregnancy affected by Down's syndrome.

The only method for diagnosis involves an invasive test and karyotyping of fetal cells.

Prenatal diagnosis

The screening tests used for Down's syndrome only indicate whether the pregnancy is at an increased risk of Down's syndrome.

Confirmation of whether the fetus is affected requires invasive diagnostic procedures such as amniocentesis or chorionic villous sampling, both of which have a 1–2% pregnancy loss rate (of what is usually a wanted and normal pregnancy).

Similarly, the options available to couples with a diagnosis of a severe structural fetal anomaly are usually limited to termination of pregnancy or postnatal treatment.

If the postnatal treatment is not required immediately after birth, the advantages of knowing about the condition in advance may not be sufficient for all women to accept screening.

Prenatal diagnosis may be offered to women in the following situations:

- Screen-positive (usually defined as a calculated risk of >1:250)
- A previous pregnancy affected by a genetic disorder
- One or more relatives affected by a genetic disorder
- US has detected a structural abnormality known to be associated with a chromosomal abnormality (e.g. exomphalos and trisomy 18)

See Section 6.14 for details of invasive testing.

Box 6.9 Examples of congenital abnormalities

Genetic disorders

- Trisomy 21 (Down's syndrome)
- Trisomy 18 (Edward's syndrome)
- Trisomy 13 (Patau's syndrome)
- Triploidy
- Sex chromosome abnormalities
- XXX
- XYY
- XXY (Klinefelter's syndrome)
- XO (Turner's syndrome)
- Single gene disorders, e.g. fragile X, Huntington's chorea, Tay–Sachs disease, cystic fibrosis

Structural disorders (see Section 6.13)

- Congenital heart disease
- Neural tube defects, e.g. anencephaly, encephalocele, spina bifida
- Abdominal wall defects, e.g. exomphalos, gastroschisis
- Genitourinary anomalies, e.g. renal dysplasia, polycystic kidneys, Potter's syndrome
- Lung disorders, e.g. pulmonary hypoplasia, diaphragmatic hernia

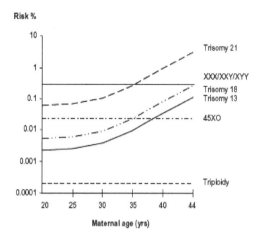

Fig. 6.12 Maternal age-related risk of Down's syndrome and other chromosomal anomalies at the time of the 11–13-week scan. (Kindly provided by the Fetal Medicine Foundation.)

Table 6.3 Maternal serum markers and the changes with gestation and Down's syndrome

Serum marker	Taken first trimester	Taken second trimester	Serum level change with gestation	Serum level change in Down's syndrome
PAPP-A	✓	✗	↑	↓
HCG	✓	✓	↓	↑
AFP	✗	✓	↑	↓
uE3	✗	✓	↑	↓
Inhibin-A	✗	✓	↓ Until 17 weeks, then ↑	↑

Table 6.4 Screening tests for Down's syndrome that reach the NSC standard for screening

Test	Gestation (weeks)
Combined NT + HCG + PAPP-A	11–14
Quadruple HCG + AFP + uE3 + inhibin A	14–20
Integrated NT + PAPP-A and then HCG + AFP + uE3 + inhibin A	11–14 and then 14–20
Serum integrated (As integrated but no NT)	11–14 and 14–20

Further reading

www.nsc.nhs.uk. UK National Screening Committee. Useful for all UK screening policies.

www.library.nhs.uk National Library for Health. Useful for all UK antenatal and neonatal screening tests.

www.fetalmedicine.com Fetal Medicine Foundation.

www.nscfa.web.its.manchester.ac.uk Fetal anomaly screening programme.

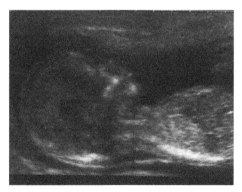

Fig. 6.11 Midsagittal view of head, neck, and upper thorax of a fetus with an increased NT of 3 mm (+ calipers) at 12 weeks. Karyotyping diagnosed trisomy 21.

6.13 Screening for fetal structural anomalies

Ultrasound scan of the fetus

Structural abnormalities are best seen on ultrasound scan (US) and may be detected during the first trimester scan but more usually at the anomaly scan during the second trimester.

Many structural abnormalities are associated with genetic abnormalities. Identification may lead to an invasive diagnostic test being offered (see Section 6.14).

Fetal medicine is a specialist tertiary referral service underpinned by subspecialty training and working in conjunction with genetics, paediatrics, pathology and other laboratory specialties.

Serological screening

The presence of specific fetal markers can be quantified in maternal serum and used to indicate an increased risk of two abnormalities: neural tube defects (including spina bifida) and trisomy (particularly Down's syndrome).

Alphafetoprotein (AFP) is raised in open neural tube defects, but US is more sensitive so serum screening for this purpose is no longer used (see Figure 6.13).

Soft markers

US not only identifies major structural abnormalities but also a number of 'soft markers'. These are structural features which do not, of themselves, pose any major problem for the fetus.

Soft markers are found in approximately 5% of all pregnancies and include:

- Choroid plexus cyst
- Mild renal pelvis dilatation
- Echogenic bowel
- Echogenic cardiac foci
- Mild cerebral ventricule dilatation

These are variants from normal which change the likelihood ratio of an abnormality (from the background risk, usually related to age) (see Table 6.5).

Multiple 'soft markers' increase the risk of an underlying chromosomal abnormality.

Structural abnormalities

Birth defects occur in 2–4% of pregnancies.

The most common structural abnormalities are found in the brain, heart, gastrointestinal system, renal tract, and limbs.

Some anomalies (e.g. anencephaly, see Figure 6.14) have a high rate of detection, while others (e.g. cardiac or facial; see Figure 6.15) require higher degrees of technical skill (see Table 6.6).

Each abnormality has a specific relationship to underlying aetiology and chromosome risk. For example, spina bifida (Figure 6.13) has no chromosome association, gastroschisis (Figure 6.17) is related to young age, whereas exomphalos (Figure 6.18) is related to concurrent cardiac abnormality and is highly associated with chromosome anomaly (approximately 30%).

Some anomalies regress *in utero* (e.g. congenital cystic adenomatoid malformation (CCAM); Figure 6.20), some are amenable to corrective paediatric surgery (e.g. gastroschisis, exomphalos and cleft lip; Figures 6.17, 6.18, and 6.15), and others are untreatable (e.g. acrania; Figure 6.14).

Table 6.5 Incidence of major and minor defects or markers in the second trimester scan in trisomy 21 and chromosomally normal fetuses

	T21	Normal	Positive LR	Negative LR	LR for isolated marker
Nuchal fold	107/319 (33.5%)	59/9331 (0.6%)	53.05 (39.37–71.26)	0.67 (0.61–0.72)	9.8
Short humerus	102/305 (33.4%)	136/9254 (1.5%)	22.76 (18.04–28.56)	0.68 (0.62-0.73)	4.1
Short femur	132/319 (41.4%)	486/9331 (5.2%)	7.94 (6.77–9.25)	0.62 (0.56–0.67)	1.6
Hydro-nephrosis	56/319 (17.6%)	242/9331 (2.6%)	6.77 (5.16–8.80)	0.85 (5.16–8.80)	1.0
Echogenic focus	75/266 (28.2%)	401/9119 (4.4%)	6.41 (5.15–7.90)	0.75 (0.69–0.80)	1.1
Echogenic bowel	39/293 (13.3%)	58/9227 (0.6%)	21.17 (14.34–31.06)	0.87 (0.83–0.91)	3.0
Major defect	75/350 (21.4%)	61/9384 (0.65%)	32.96 (23.90–43.28)	0.79 (0.74–0.83)	5.2

From these data the positive and negative likelihood ratios (LR) (with 95% confidence interval) for each marker can be calculated. In the last column is the likelihood ratio for each marker found in isolation. From Nicolaides KH. Screening for chromosomal defects. *Ultrasound Obstet Gynecol* 2003; **21**: 313–21.

Table 6.6 Detection rates for structural abnormalities at different gestational ages

Abnormality	% Detection at 12–14 weeks scan (no. detected/total)	% Detection at 15–22 weeks scan (no. detected/total)[1]	% Detection at 18–22 weeks scan (no. detected/total)[2]
Anencephaly	80 (8/10)	100 (6/6)	100 (43/43)
Spina bifida	9 (1/11)	67 (8/12)	92 (80/87)
Major cardiac anomalies	2 (1/58)	15 (8/52)	61 (11/18)[+]
Diaphragmatic hernia	0 (0/3)	50 (2/4)	62 (5/8)
Gastroschisis	50 (2/4)	80 (4/5)	100 (31/31)
Exomphalos	50 (1/2)	60 (3/5)	92 (11/12)
Bilateral renal agenesis	0 (0/2)	100 (2/2)	85 (17/20)

[+]Major cardiac abnormality (hypoplastic left heart); [1] Saltvedt *et al* 2006; [2] Smith and Hau 1999.

Further reading

Saltvedt S, Almström H, Kublickas M, Valentin L, Grunewald C. Detection of malformations in chromosomally normal fetuses by routine ultrasound at 12 or 18 weeks of gestation—a randomised controlled trial in 39 572 pregnancies. *British Journal of Obstetrics and Gynaecology* 2006; **113(6)**:664–74.

Smith NC, Hau C. A six year study of the antenatal detection of fetal abnormality in six Scottish health boards. *British Journal of Obstetrics and Gynaecology* 1999; **106**:206–12.

www.nscfa.web.its.manchester.ac.uk Fetal anomaly screening programme. Screening information, professional information and Down's syndrome education and training.

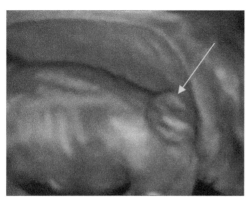

Fig. 6.13 3D US image of lumbar spina bifida (arrow). (Kindly provided by Dr Meekai To.)

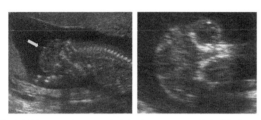

Fig. 6.14 Fetus with acrania (⇨) leading to anencephaly. (Kindly provided by Dr Meekai To.)

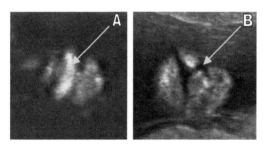

Fig. 6.15 A Fetal lips (coronal plane) demonstrating intact upper lip (arrow). B Fetal lips (coronal plane) demonstrating right-sided cleft lip (arrow). (Kindly provided by Dr Meekai To.)

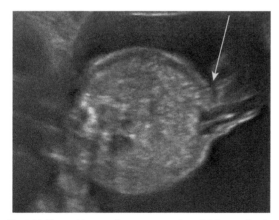

Fig. 6.16 Normal image of transverse section of abdomen showing cord insertion (arrow). (Kindly provided by Dr Meekai To.)

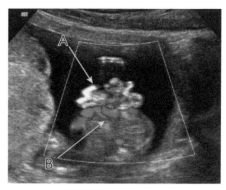

Fig. 6.17 Gastroschisis. Free-floating loops of bowel (A) seen arising lateral to cord insertion (B). (Kindly provided by Dr Meekai To.)

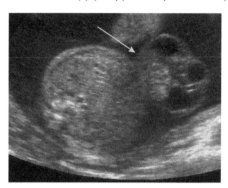

Fig. 6.18 Transverse section of abdomen showing exomphalos (arrow) containing liver and bowel. (Kindly provided by Dr Meekai To.)

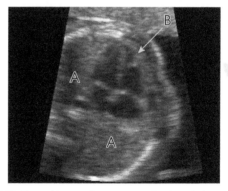

Fig. 6.19 Normal image of transverse section through chest demonstrating lungs (A) and four-chamber view of heart (B). (Kindly provided by Dr Meekai To.)

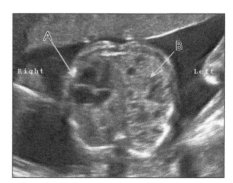

Fig. 6.20 Congenital cystic adenomatoid malformation of the lung (CCAM) causing right mediastinal shift (A) and replacing left lung tissue (B). (Kindly provided by Dr Meekai To.)

6.14 Invasive tests

Prenatal diagnostic tests

Prenatal diagnostic tests are offered to women identified as being at high risk of having an affected pregnancy based on the results of the screening test (see Table 6.4). This is done by culturing fetal cells obtained by an invasive method. These methods include amniocentesis, chorionic villus sampling and fetal blood sampling.

Amniocentesis is the most common invasive prenatal diagnostic procedure undertaken in the UK. It is performed to obtain amniotic fluid for karyotyping of fetal cells and the majority of these procedures are undertaken from 15 weeks (15+0) onwards.

Chorionic villus sampling (CVS) is usually performed between 12 and 14 weeks' gestation, and involves aspiration of placental tissue. CVS can be performed using either a transabdominal or transcervical approach. Both tests carry a risk of miscarriage and other complications (see Box 6.10 and Table 6.7).

Two types of laboratory test can be used to examine the fetal chromosomes.

Full karyotype—checks all the chromosomes. Results from this test are usually ready within 2–3 weeks as fetal cells are cultured in a growth medium.

Rapid test—FISH (fluorescent *in situ* hybridization) or PCR (polymerase chain reaction) techniques check for specific chromosomes. The disorders that can be detected by the rapid test include Down's (trisomy 21), Edwards' (trisomy 18) and Patau's syndrome (trisomy 13) and, if requested, sex chromosome disorders. Results are usually available after 3 working days. The limitation of FISH and PCR is that not all possible chromosomal abnormalities will be detected, but results are available sooner than conventional culture.

Fetal blood sampling (FBS) is performed from 18 weeks onwards when blood can be aspirated from the umbilical vein. Although occasionally used in prenatal diagnosis, the main use of FBS is to determine haematocrit to guide red cell transfusion in Rhesus and other blood group incompatibilities. The risks and complications are similar to CVS and amniocentesis.

All invasive tests are relatively contraindicated in HIV-infected women, and consideration of pre-exposure prophylaxis must be discussed. The risk of mother-to-child transmission associated with invasive diagnostic procedures is thought to be low in hepatitis B and C.

All Rh-negative women need anti-D following invasive testing.

Further reading

www.rcog.org.uk RCOG Greentop guideline No. 8. Amniocentesis and chorionic villus sampling, 2005.

✚ Box 6.10 Risks of CVS and amniocentesis

Maternal
- Miscarriage—1% with amniocentesis, 1–2% with CVS
- Chorioamnionitis
- Haemorrhage
- Haematoma
- Rhesus sensitization
- Uterine contractions

Fetal
- Fetal infection (higher for bloodborne diseases such as HIV, <1:1000 for bacteria)
- Fetal injury
- Rupture of membranes
- Oromandibular limb hypoplasia (specific to CVS performed at <10 weeks' gestation)

Table 6.7 Differences between CVS and amniocentesis

	CVS	Amniocentesis
What does it involve?	Taking a small amount of placenta under ultrasound guidance	Taking a small amount of amniotic fluid under ultrasound guidance
When is the safest time to have the procedure?	After 10 weeks of pregnancy. Transcervical CVS is usually done at 11–13 weeks, transabdominal after 12 weeks	After 15 weeks of pregnancy
What is the risk of miscarriage?	About 1–2%	About 1%
What is involved in ending the pregnancy?	Termination of pregnancy, either surgically or medically	Termination, usually by induction of labour

Chapter 7

Medical problems prior to pregnancy

Contents

Covered elsewhere

General management

Importance of identification

- A major cause of indirect maternal death (33 suicide and 22 drug overdoses; CEMACH, 2007)
- Associated with many deaths from other causes

The greatest risk of developing psychiatric disorders in women is during the reproductive years. Many develop these for the first time during pregnancy or the puerperium.

Women with psychiatric disorders have increased risk of:

- Inadequate contraception and unplanned pregnancy
- Substance abuse, including tobacco and alcohol
- Relapse during and after pregnancy
- Inadequate antenatal care and poor outcome

Prepregnancy counselling and early booking visit:

- Discuss the risk of relapse
- Advise the importance of good nutrition
- Check substance abuse (tobacco, alcohol, drugs)
- Review treatment options

Professional interpreters: instead of relatives or friends.

Early antenatal care: refer to tertiary centres if the complication is outside the experience of the local obstetrician.

Multidisciplinary care: an integrated care plan and regular communication between specialties (obstetrician, psychiatric liaison, midwife, GP, and health visitor) are important.

Termination of pregnancy: if potentially life-threatening.

Delivery in a consultant-led obstetric unit: plans for management in labour should be made in advance.

Postpartum: multidisciplinary follow-up.

General treatment options

First line therapy—attend to psychosocial stressors and non-pharmacological, e.g. psychotherapy, counselling, and relaxation.

Women who relapsed after stopping a medication should remain on it during pregnancy. Maintain minimum doses. Monotherapy is better than polytherapy.

Discuss risks of medication:

- Lack of data in pregnancy and breastfeeding
- Fetal risks may include teratogenicity, neonatal toxicity or withdrawal, and long-term behaviour problems
- Avoid antifolates in early pregnancy as links with neural tube defects (carbamazepine and valproate)
- Birth defects occur in 2–4% of the general population, regardless of prenatal medication exposure

Major depression

Major depression is the commonest psychiatric disorder in reproductive age women.

Incidence in pregnancy

1st trimester: 7%, 2nd trimester: 13%, 3rd trimester: 12%.

Pregnancy has no effect on its onset or recurrence.

Diagnostic criteria are that 5 of 9 symptoms below are present over a 2-week period. *Symptoms must be present for diagnosis:

- *Depressed mood most of the day, nearly every day
- *Marked ↓ interest or pleasure in activities (anhedonia)
- Major change in appetite or weight
- Decrease or increase in sleep
- Psychomotor agitation or retardation

- Fatigue
- Feelings of worthlessness or excessive inappropriate guilt
- Diminished ability to think or concentrate; indecisiveness
- Recurrent thoughts of death or suicide

Screening pregnant women for depression

- Most pregnant women do not seek treatment
- Identification depends on screening during antenatal visits
- Women with risk factors for depression should be targeted for screening as this increases the efficiency

Risk factors for depression in pregnancy

- Past history of depression (5-fold ↑ risk)
- Family history of mood disorder
- Marital conflict
- Younger age
- Limited social support with greater numbers of children
- Tobacco or alcohol abuse
- Unemployed
- Lower educational attainment

Effect of depression on pregnancy

- Maternal risks: substance abuse, postpartum depression, pre-eclampsia
- Fetal risks: low birthweight and spontaneous preterm birth
- Long term behavioural effects: developmental delay, antisocial behaviour, and criminality

Treatment for depression in pregnancy

- Depends on severity and woman's preferences
- Interpersonal or cognitive behavioural psychotherapy is effective for mild depression
- Antidepressants are recommended when psychotherapy fails, with severe symptoms or marked functional impairment
- Selective serotonin reuptake inhibitors (SSRI) or serotonin and norepinephrine reuptake inhibitors (SNRI) are effective agents
- Counsel about risk of relapse in up to 75% of patients if antidepressant is discontinued in pregnancy.

Paroxetine use >25 mg/day in the first trimester is associated with a risk of congenital heart defect of 2%, largely minor. However, in some cases, the benefits of continuing paroxetine may outweigh the potential risk to the fetus. It is associated with neonatal toxicity: lethargy, hypotonia, anticholinergic symptoms, and withdrawal syndromes (irritability, tachypnoea, tachycardia, feeding difficulties).

Postnatal

- Observe for postpartum depression
- If on antidepressant, observe for neonatal toxicity or withdrawal syndrome

Bipolar disorder

Prevalence

- 1% of the population
- Onset: up to 40% of women with bipolar disorder have their first episode after the birth of their first child

Diagnosis

- Mania: abnormally and persistently elevated or irritable mood for ≥1 week, with ≥3 of the following, and resulting in functional impairment:
  Inflated self-esteem or grandiosity, reduced need for sleep without daytime fatigue or lowered energy, ↑ talkativeness, flight of ideas, distractibility, increase in goal-directed activities, disinhibited

behaviour, excessive involvement in pleasurable activities with high potential for painful consequences
- Hypomania: less severe form of mania, shorter duration, and often associated with less functional impairment

Effect of mania on pregnancy
There is an increased risk of poor outcome, mainly because of high risk behaviour, poor nutrition, drug use (alcohol, tobacco), and lack of antenatal care.

Management
- Multidisciplinary: involve obstetricians, psychiatric liaison officers, midwives, general practitioners, and health visitors
- Check for substance abuse
- Encourage attendance for antenatal care

Treatment
Lithium: effective but increases the risk of fetal heart defects, including Ebstein anomaly.

Anticonvulsants: carbamazepine and valproate are effective for the control of aggressive behaviour and mood stabilization but are associated with increased risk of neural tube defects.

Atypical antipsychotics: limited safety data in pregnancy.

The lowest effective dose should be used in pregnancy.

In severe cases, electroconvulsive therapy is effective for the treatment of depression and mania in pregnancy.
- Detailed anomaly scan at 20 weeks, especially if on medication
- Monitor fetal growth with serial ultrasound scans

Postnatal management
- Observe for relapse, as risk after delivery is 25–30%
- Psychotic relapse requires prompt admission to a psychiatric facility, preferably to a mother and baby unit

Careful examination of the neonate to exclude abnormality.

Schizophrenia
A chronic brain disorder characterized by psychosis and profound disruption in cognition and emotion; affecting language, thought, perception, affect, and sense of self.

Prevalence
- 1% of population
- Age of onset: mainly late adolescence to early adulthood. Relatively less common <14 years or >35 years

Diagnostic criteria for schizophrenia
Requires ≥2 of the following over ≥1 month:
- Hallucinations
- Delusions
- Disorganized speech
- Catatonic behaviour
- Negative symptoms, i.e. lack of motivation, self-neglect, inappropriate emotion, inability to experience pleasure, unable to pay attention or show facial expressions, or start or complete tasks

Social or occupational dysfunction for ≥6 months.

Exclusion of schizoaffective or mood disorder.

Exclusion of drug abuse or other conditions (temporal lobe epilepsy, intoxication or cerebral damage).

Relationship to pervasive developmental disorder: the additional diagnosis of schizophrenia is made in autism or pervasive developmental disorder only if delusions or hallucinations are also present for ≥1 month.

Effect of pregnancy on schizophrenia
- Severity of illness during pregnancy varies
- Postpartum psychosis in 16%, perhaps due to oestrogen withdrawal

Effect of schizophrenia on pregnancy
- Increased risk of stillbirth
- Low birth weight
- Small for gestational age and prematurity

This is mainly due to lack of self-care and antenatal care, poor nutrition, and drug use (alcohol, tobacco). Offspring have a genetic predisposition to schizophrenia.

Treatment
Pharmacological therapy is essential.

First generation antipsychotics
- Chlorpromazine, fluphenazine, haloperidol, mesoridazine, perphenazine, thioridazine, trifluoperazine
- Interfere with dopamine transmission
- Side effects: extrapyramidal symptoms, tardive dyskinesia, sedation, cognitive impairment, weight gain, diabetes, hyperprolactinaemia, seizures, postural hypotension, dry mouth, constipation, and urinary retention

Second generation (atypical) antipsychotics
- Risperidone, olanzapine, quetiapine, ziprasidone, aripiprazole, clozapine
- Side effects: obesity and increased risk of diabetes

Effect of antipsychotics on pregnancy
- Older class of antipsychotics: reduce fertility due to hyperprolactinaemia. This may change with the newer antipsychotics that do not cause hyperprolactinaemia
- Phenothiazines: increase the risk of congenital abnormalities by an extra 4 per 1000

Management
- Involve full multidisciplinary team
- Check for substance abuse
- Continue treatment in pregnancy
- Stopping treatment can lead to relapse
- Reduce to the lowest effective dose
- Avoid depot preparations (neonatal extrapyramidal side effects)
- Offer psychosocial support and encourage antenatal care
- Psychotic relapse requires prompt admission to a psychiatric facility, preferably a mother and baby unit
- Assess the patient's ability to care for a baby and need for additional psychosocial support
- Monitor fetal growth with serial ultrasound scans

Safety of psychotropic drugs
FDA (Food and Drug Administration) pregnancy categories:
A. Controlled studies in women show no risk
B. Animal studies show no risk but no controlled studies in humans; or animal studies show adverse effect that has not been confirmed in human studies
C. Animal studies show risk but no controlled studies in humans; or no available studies in animals or humans
D. There is evidence of risk in humans, but the drug may have benefits that outweigh the risk
E. Risk outweighs any benefit

Most psychotropic medications are in Category C (human studies unavailable). Category B is not safer than Category C.

Further reading
www.cemach.org.uk Saving Mothers Lives 2003–2005 report. London: CEMACH, 2007.

Hendrick V. *Psychiatric disorders in pregnancy and the postpartum: principles and treatment.* New Jersey: Humana Press, 2006.

7.2 Substance abuse

Alcohol abuse in pregnancy

- Outside pregnancy, 90% of women in the UK drink alcohol.
- The frequency and quantity of alcohol consumption by women of reproductive age is increasing.
- Infertility associated with endometriosis and anovulation is commoner among women who drink alcohol.
- Binge drinkers (≥5 drinks/session) are at increased risk of sexually transmitted diseases and unplanned pregnancy.
- One-third of women will stop drinking when pregnant:
  - Older, parous, higher social class women tend to drink more but reduce intake in pregnancy
  - Adolescents are more likely to binge but less likely to reduce intake in pregnancy
- Women who abuse alcohol tend to smoke, have poor diet, other substance abuse, and poorer outcomes.

Effects of alcohol abuse on pregnancy

- Increased risk of spontaneous miscarriage (2 or 3-fold)
- Risk of preterm birth is controversial (may be caused by poor nutrition and other substance abuse)
- Fetal alcohol syndrome (FAS)—diagnostic criteria:
  Level 1—confirmed maternal alcohol exposure
  Level 2—dysmorphic features: short palpebral fissure, flattened upper lip, philtrum, and midface
  Level 3—fetal growth restriction (FGR): ≥1 of the following
  - Low birth weight for gestational age
  - Failure to thrive not due to nutrition
  - Disproportionally low weight to height
  Level 4—CNS involvement: ≥1 of the following
  - Reduced cranial size at birth
  - Structural brain abnormalities (microcephaly, corpus callosum agenesis, cerebellar hypoplasia)
  - Neurological signs (impaired fine motor skills, neurosensory hearing loss, poor tandem gait, poor hand–eye coordination)
- Other FAS disorders:
  - Mental retardation most common and serious deficit
  - Congenital heart disease: atrial or ventricular septal defect
  - Renal hypoplasia, hydronephrosis or bladder diverticula
  - Short stature and skeletal deformities
- Neonatal effects:
  - Withdrawal symptoms—irritability, hypotonia, tremors
    Neonatal jaundice
- Long-term effects on children:
  - Increased risk of neglect and abuse
  - Attention and memory deficits, hyperactivity
  - Learning disabilities (arithmetic and reading diffculties)
  - A dose–response relationship between alcohol intake (especially first trimester) and reduced height and weight in children
  - Increased risk of aggressive behaviour, psychiatric disorders, and substance abuse

Fetal alcohol syndrome

- Incidence 1:1000 births
- Four per cent in heavy drinkers
- Up to 33% in women who drink ≥18 units/day
- Not seen consistently in babies of heavy drinkers
- Thought to be multifactorial and reflect interplay of genetics, nutrition, smoking, other drugs, and alcohol

Management

Antenatal management

Advise all pregnant women:

- Prenatal alcohol exposure is the commonest cause of preventable mental retardation
- There is no 'safe' level in pregnancy. Drinks per session is more important than units per week. Limit alcohol intake to one standard drink per day
- Effects of alcohol can occur throughout pregnancy

T-ACE questionnaire can be used to screen all pregnant women or target women with growth impaired fetus:

- **T** (tolerance)—how many drinks does it take to make you feel high? Tolerance if >two drinks (2 points)
- **A** (annoyed)—have people annoyed you by criticizing your drinking? (1 point)
- **C** (cut down)—have you ever felt you ought to cut down your drinking? (1 point)
- **E** (eye opener)—have you ever had a drink first thing in the morning to steady your nerves? (1 point)

Score ≥2 identifies >70% of heavy pregnant drinkers
T-ACE questionnaire is more effective than markers of heavy intake (blood alcohol, gamma glutamyl transferase (γGT), mean corpuscular volume (MCV), thiocyanate)

Counselling and support

- Advise withdrawal has no adverse effects
- Provide a telephone contact number and specialist treatment referral for women with alcohol problems

Maternal nutrition

- Alcohol decreases gastric absorption and placental nutrient transfer (amino acids, glucose, zinc, and folic acid)
- Advise the importance of good nutrition
- High protein supplementation can minimize some effect

Check for other substance abuse

- Smoking—advise increased risk of low birth weight and mental retardation even at low alcohol intake. Effect of smoking on weight is three times the effect of alcohol

Domestic violence

- Alcohol abuse is associated with domestic violence
- Detection is increased using repeated and structured screening questionnaire, and asking direct questions
- Non-judgemental care, confidentiality, and clear documentation (not in the hand-held notes) are important
- Offer to inform the police
- Give information about local support services (Women's Aid Federation and Refuge)

Intrapartum management

- High doses of analgesia may be required
- Induced liver enzymes interact with general anaesthesia

Postpartum management

- Alcohol withdrawal occurs after 48 h
- Mother may be violent, have problems caring for her baby, and underlying stress, depression, and lack of social support
- Give sedatives and vitamin supplements, especially thiamine
- Most women restart drinking postpartum
- Breastfeeding should be discouraged in heavy drinkers as it may cause neonatal drowsiness, further damage, and aggravate

existing maternal nutritional problems. Alcohol may also interfere with milk production

- Careful follow-up from social services

Smoking in pregnancy

Prevalence

In the UK, smoking in pregnancy has fallen from 23% in 1995 to 19% in 2000 to 17% in 2005

This reduction is partly due to the NHS Stop Smoking Services which began in 1999, and in line with the Department of Health Priorities and Planning Framework 2003–2006, which contains a target to reduce the proportion of pregnant women who smoke by 1% per year to a target of 15% by 2010. This framework focuses on smokers from disadvantaged groups.

Of women who smoked:

- 10% stopped just before pregnancy
- 20% stopped during pregnancy
- 4% cut down before pregnancy
- 33% cut down during pregnancy
- 20% of former smokers relapsed during pregnancy
- Most women who stop in pregnancy relapse postpartum

Factors associated with higher prevalence of smoking in pregnancy:

- Social—material deprivation, single status, high parity
- Psychosocial—depression, stress, domestic violence
- Inherited and environmental—commoner in women whose mother also smoked, especially during pregnancy
- Fear of weight gain in pregnancy

Associated with increased risks

- Spontaneous miscarriage
- Ectopic pregnancy
- Placental complications—praevia, abruption, insufficiency, low birth weight (<2500 g). Most of the adverse effects of smoking are produced through placental damage
- Preterm prelabour rupture of membranes, very preterm birth (<32 weeks) and perinatal death
- Lower rates of initiation, and reduced duration, of breastfeeding
- Reduced arousal reflexes in the baby and sudden infant death syndrome
- Attention deficit and learning difficulties in early childhood
- Long-term effects—criminal behaviour in the male offspring
- Maternal mortality (2-fold) due to smoking-related diseases

Management

Antenatal management

Smoking cessation programmes should be implemented in all maternity care settings as they are effective in reducing smoking in pregnancy.

These programmes include:

- Educating mothers on the risks of smoking to the fetus and infant, and the benefits of smoking cessation
- Advising mothers that smoking cessation reduces preterm birth and low birth weight by up to 20%, and increases mean birth weight
- Recommendations to cease smoking and set a quit date. Smoking cessation by midpregnancy improves outcome
- Teaching cognitive behavioural strategies for cessation
- Provision of reward, social or peer support
- Nicotine replacement therapy—this is not more effective than other types of intervention and possible adverse effects of nicotine on the fetus

A routine part of antenatal visits should include attention to smoking behaviour, support for smoking cessation, and relapse prevention. There is a tendency to underreport smoking cessation failure and relapse

Intrapartum management

There is no specific intrapartum management but the risk of general anaesthesia is increased in women who smoke

Postpartum management

- Encourage breastfeeding
- Advise that parental smoking can lead to acute respiratory illness (including asthma) in children, middle ear infections and cot death
- Give contraceptive advice. Smokers ≥35 years should avoid combined oral contraception

Further reading

www.rcog.org.uk RCOG greentop guidelines. Statement No. 5. Alcohol consumption and the outcomes of pregnancy, 2006.

www.cdc.gov Centres for Disease control and prevention. Fetal alcohol syndrome. Guidelines for referral and diagnosis, 2004.

Lumley J, Oliver SS, Chamberlain C, Oakley L. Interventions for promoting smoking cessation during pregnancy. *Cochrane Database of Systematic Reviews* 2004; No. CD001055. www.cochrane.org

Walker JJ, Walker A. Substance abuse. In: James DK, Steer PJ, Weiner CP, Gonik B (eds). *High Risk Pregnancy Management Options*, Elsevier Saunders: Philadelphia, 2005: 721–41.

7.3 Illicit drug abuse

General
- 90% of women in drug treatment services are 15–39 years
- In women <35 years, 50% have experimented with drugs, and 40% of 15–16-year-olds have used cannabis, LSD or amphetamines
- One in six are regular drug users and 3% have a drug problem
- Most users abuse more than one substance
- Cannabis is the commonest drug used
- In deprived <25-year-olds, heroin and benzodiazepines are more prevalent

Morbidities associated with illicit drug use
- Alcohol and tobacco abuse ⇒ poor fetal growth
- Poor nutrition ⇒ underweight, anaemia
- Use of needles ⇒ cellulitis, phlebitis, superficial thrombosis. Deep venous thrombosis often follows use of femoral veins. Subcutaneous tissue damage, abscesses, necrotizing fasciitis. Systemic endocarditis, septic osteomyelitis, septicaemia. Risk of hepatitis B and C, HIV. Hepatitis C is found in 40–60% of injecting drug users

Management
Antenatal management
Multidisciplinary care—involve obstetricians, midwives, dietician, addiction services, social workers, and neonatologists.

There should be a contract of management guaranteeing non-judgemental care and confidentiality.

Factors which contribute to poor outcome include inadequate antenatal care, poor nutrition, smoking, and/or alcohol.
- Encourage patients to attend all appointments. Ideally, provide transport service to and from hospital
- Provide supportive environment and follow-up
- Emphasize the importance of good nutrition
- Encourage patients to keep a drug diary
- Check for other substance abuse

Users of cannabis or benzodiazepines:
- No specific management problems in pregnancy
- Encourage ceasing drug use and warn against progression to more harmful drugs

Heroin users:
- Explain fetal risks, especially use of street heroin
- Discuss the benefits of a drug substitute
- Convert heroin to methadone and review dose
- Regular urine toxicology may assist dose adjustment
- Advising cessation of heroin is often not useful

Cocaine users:
- Educate about fetal risks, especially with bingeing as same perinatal complications as with daily use
- Sudden cessation not associated with adverse fetal effects
- There is no drug substitute

Screen for HIV, hepatitis B, and hepatitis C.

Urine toxicology testing to screen for other drug use.

Fetal anomaly scan at 18–22 weeks' gestation.

Monitor fetal growth with serial ultrasound scans.

Intrapartum management
- If on methadone maintenance treatment (MMT)— this should be continued during labour
- Continuous fetal heart rate (FHR) monitoring during labour
- Difficult venous access may need liaison with anaesthetists and possible central line insertion

- High doses of analgesia may be required. Epidural analgesia should be offered
- Take precautions for hepatitis B, hepatitis C or HIV
- Alert paediatricians of impending delivery

Postpartum management
- Observe baby for withdrawal symptoms
- In heroin or MMT users—avoid naloxone in babies as this may cause severe neonatal withdrawal
- Neonatal narcotic abstinence syndrome (NAS) may be treated with morphine or methadone. However, <50% of babies require treatment. Phenobarbitone may be used for convulsions
- Encourage breastfeeding if mothers are HIV-negative and not injecting drug users
- Give contraceptive advice
- Continued support after delivery is required, especially with childcare. Many women return to heroin or cocaine after delivery. Mother and baby should stay in hospital until all agencies are aware of discharge plan

Specific drug problems

Heroin addiction
- Processed from morphine, highly physically addictive
- Taken by injection, snorting or smoked
- Effect—euphoria, drowsy, CNS depression resulting in reduced social interaction and loss of motivation
- Pregnancies are difficult to date owing to prenatal amenorrhoea and late booking

Fetal effects (non-teratogenic):
- Acute placental infection, FGR, preterm birth, stillbirth
- Crosses blood–brain barrier leading to a fast 'high' of the fetus. During abstinence, fetal activity, and oxygen demand increases. If this coincides with labour or placental insufficiency, fetal death may result. Thus, heroin reduction should be done slowly

Neonatal narcotic abstinence syndrome
- Characterized by CNS hyperirritability (less marked in premature), high-pitched cry, sneezing, respiratory distress, poor feeding, gastrointestinal dysfunction, and fits
- Often normal at birth but develop NAS within 48 h
- Severity of NAS increases with street heroin and FGR
- As methadone is stored in fetal lung, liver and spleen, NAS can be delayed until 2 weeks of age. Severity of NAS is worse with methadone compared with heroin
- Multiple drug use may influence NAS: benzodiazepine and cocaine delay the onset, cocaine may reduce the severity
- Symptoms often resolve within few days, although irritability and tremors may persist for 3 months

Long-term effects:
- Increased risk of SIDS (3-fold)
- No long-term neurological or cognitive deficits directly associated with heroin or methadone in pregnancy
- Mothers often have childcare problems. There are more behavioural problems and delayed cognitive development among offspring. Children who are adopted at an early age develop normally

Methadone maintenance treatment
Women on MMT have a history of regular heroin use, withdrawal symptoms and positive urine toxicology.

Benefits:
- At therapeutic doses, MMT is compatible with normal lifestyle. Does not cause euphoria, sedation, and no adverse effects on motor skills, mental capacity or employability
- Reduction in illicit heroin use, infection transmission and overdose death
- Improves health, birth weight, prolongs gestation

Dose:
- Depends on amount of heroin used and is titrated slowly to the lowest dose that prevents withdrawal symptoms. Risk of NAS lower with low MMT dose
- The goal is risk reduction—90% of women on MMT continue to use street heroin and this affects morbidity. MMT is less effective if maintenance dose is reduced or women are pressurized to abstain. Supportive environment is more successful than the amount of MMT dose used
- The dose is the same as outside pregnancy. As the metabolism of methadone rises in pregnancy it may need to be split into twice daily

Buprenorphine may be an alternative to MMT but at present its safety in pregnancy has not been established.

Cocaine addiction

Snorted as hydrochloride salt (coke), smoked or injected in the free-base form (crack).

Cocaine addiction is mainly psychological. Regular use is associated with exhaustion, dehydration, and poor nutrition.

Fetal effects:
- Potent vasoconstrictor, may lead to fetal vascular disruption. Teratogenic effect less common with cocaine than alcohol use
- Transplacental passage is greatest in first and third trimesters with freebase usage. Vasoconstriction of uterine, placental, and umbilical artery limits placental transfer so that there is less gas and nutrient change
- Increased risk of placental abruption, thick meconium-stained liquor, premature rupture of membranes, fetal hypoxia, FGR, preterm birth, and stillbirth
- Intestinal atresia, limb reduction defects, aplasia cutis
- Classically restricts head circumference growth
- Prune-belly syndrome, hydronephrosis, hypospadias, heart defects, and gastroschisis have been reported
- Poor nutrition, alcohol and tobacco abuse ⇒ low birth weight
- Cocaine bingeing is associated with preterm birth, placental abruption, and stillbirth

Neonatal effects:
- Cocaine withdrawal symptoms may peak at 3 days of life and persist for 3 weeks (irritability, tremors, mood alterations, hypertonia)
- Increased risk of mild intracranial haemorrhage in babies with low birth weight
- Reduced numbers of oligodendrocytes and prolonged auditory brainstem response latencies consistent with disturbed myelin synthesis. These changes persist for up to 6 months

Long-term effects on children:
- Reduced head circumference
- Increased risk of developmental delay
- Reduced Stanford–Binet Intelligence Scale verbal and visual reasoning
- More likely to live with relatives or foster homes
- More likely to be aggressive

Marijuana or cannabis
- Commonest illicit drug used in pregnancy

Effect on pregnancy and offspring:
- Reported to improve appetite and relieve nausea
- Associated with increased incidence of gastroschisis
- No evidence of abnormal developmental outcome at 1 month
- Negative effect on performance present at 3 years

No management problems with cannabis use, but users should be warned against progression to more harmful drugs.

Benzodiazepines
- Outside pregnancy, commonly used as anxiolytics and sedatives
- No adverse fetal effects. Meta-analyses showed no evidence of cleft lip or palate
- Neonatal withdrawal—hypotonia, poor feeding, apnoea
- No management problems in pregnancy, but users should be encouraged to cease drug use

Amphetamines
- Synthetic amines similar to adrenaline (epinephrine)
- Taken orally, sniffed or injection
- Do not cause physical dependence

Effect—stimulatory, exaggerate normal reaction to stress and may cause aggressive and violent behaviour. These have been used to counteract fatigue and improve athletes' performance. Recovery is associated with fatigue and depression

Maternal risks:
- Increased risk of hypertension and pre-eclampsia

Fetal risks:
- Increased risk of cleft palate and gastroschisis
- Vasoconstriction may lead to fetal hypoxia, FGR, stillbirth, placental abruption, and preterm birth

Neonatal withdrawal:
- Hyperactivity, tremors, disordered sleep pattern, poor feeding

Effect on children born to mothers on amphetamines
- 80% of children brought up in stable foster homes
- Impaired long-term growth
- Poor school performance with significant deficiency in mathematics and language

Management in pregnancy:
- Multidisciplinary care
- Encourage to stop drug use. No drug substitute
- Check blood pressure and urinalysis frequently
- Monitor fetal gowth with serial ultrasound scans
- Continuous fetal heart monitoring during labour
- Alert paediatricians of impending delivery

Further reading

www.drugrehab.co.uk

www.drugscope.org A reading list of substance misuse and pregnancy is available.

Walker JJ, Walker A. Substance abuse. In: James DK, Steer PJ, Weiner CP, Gonik B (eds). *High Risk Pregnancy Management Options*, Elsevier Saunders: Philadelphia, 2005: 721–41.

7.4 Chronic hypertension

BP measurement

- Automated BP recording systems can systematically underestimate BP. Values should be compared at the beginning of antenatal care, using conventional sphygmomanometers
- Woman seated and appropriate cuff size
- Use Korotkoff phase V (disappearance) instead of IV (muffling) as it is more reproducible and better correlated with the true diastolic BP in pregnancy
- In late pregnancy, the gravid uterus may obstruct venous return when supine (supine hypotension), thus measure BP with woman sitting up or lying on her side

Definitions

- Hypertension—a blood pressure (BP) of ≥140/90 mmHg on two consecutive occasions, at least 4 h apart
- A change in BP from the booking level is no longer included in the definition owing to a lack of relation to adverse outcome
- Severe hypertension—BP ≥160/110 mmHg
- Chronic hypertension—persistent hypertension before 20 weeks of gestation or beyond 6 weeks postpartum, in the absence of a hydatidiform mole

Incidence

Hypertension a very medical disorder in pregnancy.

- Affects 10% of pregnancies
- Accounts for 25% of antenatal admissions

Chronic hypertension:

- Affects 3% of pregnancies
- Accounts for 25% of hypertension in pregnancy
- Incidence may increase as age and obesity rise

Classification of chronic hypertension:

- 95% of cases are essential hypertension (idiopathic)
- 5% of cases are secondary hypertension

Pathophysiology of secondary hypertension

Renal: glomerulonephritis, polycystic kidneys, chronic pyelonephritis, tubulointerstitial disease, and renal artery stenosis.

Endocrine: Cushing's syndrome, Conn's syndrome, phaeochromocytoma, thyrotoxicosis, diabetes with vascular involvement.

Vascular: coarctation of the aorta.

Effects of pregnancy on hypertension:

- Vasodilatation causes a reduction in BP, mainly diastolic, with a mean drop of 10 mmHg by midpregnancy
- A nadir in BP is reached at 22–24 weeks' gestation. Then a gradual rise to prepregnancy levels at term
- Up to 60% of women with chronic hypertension become normotensive by the second trimester. Differentiating undiagnosed chronic from pregnancy-induced hypertension (PIH) is difficult. The diagnosis is often made retrospectively
- BP usually falls immediately after delivery, then increases over the next 5 days, peaking on days 3–6
- Women with no history of chronic hypertension who were normotensive thoughout pregnancy may also develop transient postpartum hypertension

Effects of hypertension on pregnancy

- The risk of adverse outcomes is not increased in patients with mild, uncomplicated hypertension

Maternal risks:

- Pre-eclampsia occurs in 20% of cases, and in up to 50% of those with severe chronic hypertension
- Placental abruption occurs in 2% of mild hypertension and 10% of severe hypertension

- Other complications—cerebrovascular haemorrhage, congestive heart failure, acute renal failure, liver failure, disseminated intravascular coagulation, and death
- Higher risks if severe hypertension, hypertension for >15 years, age >40, diabetes, renal disease, coarctation of aorta, cardiomyopathy or connective tissue disease

Fetal risks depend on the severity of hypertension:

- Superimposed pre-eclampsia or abruption, and poor uteroplacental perfusion may lead to fetal growth restriction (FGR) and death
- Iatrogenic preterm birth and its complications

Pre and antenatal management

Early antenatal care

Establish the cause, duration, and severity of hypertension. Women with chronic hypertension first diagnosed in early pregnancy should be investigated for secondary causes.

Detail history and perform physical examination.

Initial investigations

- Urinalysis and serum U&E to identify renal disease and Conn's syndrome
- Blood glucose and ECG, with age, smoking, and family history to assess cardiovascular risk. Perform echocardiogram if long history of hypertension or left ventricular hypertrophy on ECG

Additional investigations

Only if there is a suspicion of other underlying causes:

- Past history of early onset pre-eclampsia, FGR, placental abruption or fetal death, ± proteinuria—consider pre-eclampsia. Check uric acid, liver function tests (LFT), and platelet count. Check for antiphospholipid antibodies if suspicious, e.g. second trimester pre-eclampsia
- Past history of renal disease, presence of proteinuria, haematuria, or raised creatinine—consider renal disease. If there are palpable kidneys, consider polycystic kidneys. Perform 24-h urine collection for creatinine clearance and protein, and renal ultrasonography
- Headache, sweating, palpitations, panic—consider thyrotoxicosis, phaeochromocytoma. Check thyroid function, 24-h urine for catecholamines, metanephrine and vanillylmandelic acid levels
- Tetany, muscle weakness, polyuria, hypokalaemia—consider Conn's syndrome. Perform adrenal scan
- Appearance suggestive of Cushing's syndrome—perform plasma and 24-h urinary cortisol, and adrenal scan
- Chest pain or delayed femoral pulse—consider coarctation of the aorta. Perform CXR, echocardiogram
- Abdominal or loin bruit—consider renal vascular disease

Counsel patients:

- Usual antihypertensives are non-teratogenic
- Discuss the maternal and fetal risks of chronic hypertension and use of antihypertensives
- Bed rest or dietary changes are not proven to be beneficial

Review medication:

- Women on treatment may discontinue medication if normotensive. This is usually temporary, and treatment should be resumed when necessary
- Angiotensin-converting enzyme (ACE) inhibitors may be teratogenic. Preconception, they should be substituted

Monitor for the development of pre-eclampsia:

- Frequent review for BP checks and urinalysis
- Serum urea and electrolytes, uric acid, LFT, platelets

- Doppler assessment of uterine arteries at 20–24 weeks. Abnormal Dopplers predict a 50% risk of pre-eclampsia and women should be monitored more frequently
- Development of significant proteinuria in the absence of renal disease indicates superimposed pre-eclampsia
- Monitor fetal growth with serial ultrasound scans

Moderate hypertension (140/90–159/109 mmHg):
- It is unclear whether or not treatment is worthwhile
- Treatment halves the risk of developing severe hypertension, regardless of the type of drug used, and reduces the risk of miscarriage. β-blockers are more effective than methyldopa in preventing severe hypertension
- However, treatment does not significantly affect the incidence of pre-eclampsia, abruption, perinatal mortality, preterm birth rate or small for gestational age (SGA)

Women with severe hypertension (≥160/110 mmHg):
- Treatment is required immediately as there is an increased risk of direct arterial damage which may lead to cerebrovascular haemorrhage, renal, and liver failure
- Stroke is the single commonest cause of maternal death with pre-eclampsia. A lower threshold for treatment may be advisable if the overall clinical picture suggests rapid deterioration (e.g. signs and symptoms such as hyper-reflexia, severe headache, sudden onset of epigastric pain, or lowered platelets) (CEMACH, 2007)
- Avoid sudden drops in BP and do not overtreat (maintain BP ≃140/90 mmHg), as increased risk of fetal distress and SGA possibly caused by placental hypoperfusion

Acute severe hypertension (see Section 8.13):
- Once BP is controlled, deliver if at, or near, term
- If very preterm, the BP responds and there are no other complications, then pregnancy may be continued to improve fetal outcome
- IM corticosteroids should be given to accelerate fetal lung maturity if likely to deliver <34 weeks

Intrapartum management
- Aim for vaginal delivery
- Maintain BP ≥140/90 and ≤160/110 mmHg
- Provide effective pain relief. Offer regional analgesia
- Continuous electronic fetal monitoring
- Avoid or limit maternal bearing down if severe BP
- Avoid ergometrine in third stage as it can worsen BP

Postpartum management
- Prepregnancy antihypertensives should be resumed. Avoid diuretics in breastfeeding owing to increased thirst
- 10% of maternal deaths due to hypertension occur postpartum. Women with severe hypertension should be treated and monitored for ≥48 h as they are at increased risk of renal failure, pulmonary oedema, and hypertensive encephalopathy
- If treated, there is little data on whether one antihypertensive agent is preferable to another
- Drugs with minimal milk to maternal plasma ratios make breastfeeding acceptable: methyldopa, β-blockers with high protein binding, ACE inhibitors and nifedipine

Contraceptive advice
Avoid the COCP in mild hypertension. Contraindicated in moderate-to-severe. POP should be prescribed instead.

Lifestyle advice
To prevent cardiovascular disease, avoid smoking and maintain a healthy weight.

Antihypertensives
There is no clear evidence that one antihypertensive is preferable. The choice is dictated by fetal safety. Magnesium sulphate (used to prevent fits), high-dose diazoxide, ketanserin, nimodipine, and chlorpromazine have serious disadvantages and should not be used for treating severe hypertension.

Methyldopa
- Centrally acting α-agonist inhibits vasoconstriction
- Safe in pregnancy. Long-term use is not associated with adverse effect in the offspring
- Side effects—depression, sedative effect, tiredness and may increase liver transaminases in 5% of women
- Avoid postpartum owing to the risk of depression

Nifedipine
- Calcium-channel blocker inhibits the influx of calcium ions to vascular smooth muscle, causes arterial vasodilatation
- Safety in pregnancy has been established
- Avoid sublingual route as risk of sudden maternal hypotension, placental hypoperfusion, and fetal distress
- Concomitant use with magnesium sulphate may cause abrupt hypotension and increased risk of magnesium toxicity
- Side effects—flushing, nausea, vomiting
- Amlodipine has been used but lacks safety data

Hydralazine
- Vasodilator with a direct relaxing effect on blood vessel smooth muscle, predominantly in the arterioles
- Safety in pregnancy has been established
- Usually given as an infusion for acute severe hypertension with colloid to reduce reflex tachycardia and abrupt hypotension due to vasodilatation
- Side effects—headaches, flushing, palpitations, nausea, light-headedness. Lupus-like syndromes have been reported. Can precipitate pulmonary oedema

α- and β-adrenergic blockers
- β-blockers block adrenoceptors in the heart, peripheral blood vessels, airways, pancreas, and liver
- Labetolol is an α- and β-blocker that has an additional arteriolar vasodilating action lowering peripheral resistance but is usually classed with β-blockers. Side effects include flushing, light-headedness, palpitations, and scalp tingling
- β-blockers, particularly atenolol, were thought to cause FGR, but meta-analyses show that FGR is related to fall in mean arterial pressure
- β-blockers are more effective in preventing severe hypertension, and better tolerated than methyldopa
- Generally safe in breastfeeding. Small risk of transient neonatal bradycardia, hypotension, and hypoglycaemia

Angiotensin-converting enzyme inhibitors
- First line antihypertensive agent outside pregnancy
- Act on renin–angiotensin–aldosterone system
- May be teratogenic
- Contraindicated in later pregnancy as associated with fetal hypotension, renal failure, oligohydramnios, and FGR
- Change to a different drug, preferably prepregnancy, or early in the first trimester to allow stabilization of the new drug
- Safe for use when breastfeeding

Diuretics (thiazides and furosemide)
- Increase renal excretion of salt and water, reduce blood volume
- Not recommended during pregnancy for hypertension but used in heart failure and pulmonary oedema
- Thiazides increase the risk of neonatal thrombocytopenia and hypoglycaemia
- Safe for use when breastfeeding

7.5 Endocrine causes of hypertension

Cushing's syndrome

This comprises the symptoms and signs associated with prolonged exposure to elevated levels of free plasma glucocorticoid.

Incidence

Rare. Most patients have anovulatory infertility.

Pathophysiology

In pregnancy, most are caused by benign adrenal adenomas (44%) or adrenal carcinomas (12%).

Outside pregnancy, 80% are caused by pituitary adenomas (Cushing's disease).

Clinical features

- Central weight gain, excessive purple striae, acne, hirsutism
- May present with early onset hypertension, pre-eclampsia and/or glucose intolerance
- Discriminating feature is proximal myopathy

Effect of pregnancy on Cushing's syndrome

Exacerbations during pregnancy have been reported.

Effect of Cushing's syndrome on pregnancy

Fetal and neonatal risks:

- ↑ risk miscarriage, FGR, prematurity, and mortality
- High maternal cortisol may suppress fetal corticosteroid secretion and cause neonatal adrenal insufficiency

Maternal risks:

- ↑ risk of mortality, congestive heart failure due to hypertension, preeclampsia, diabetes, wound breakdown, opportunistic infections, emotional lability and psychosis
- Women with treated Cushing's sydrome do well

Investigations

- Total and free plasma cortisol, cortisol-binding protein and urinary free cortisol all increase in pregnancy but the diurnal rhythm of plasma cortisol is preserved. Pregnancy-specific ranges for cortisol levels should be used
- Elevated 24-h urinary free cortisol level is diagnostic of Cushing's syndrome
- Low adrenocorticotrophic-releasing hormone (ACTH) level and failure to suppress cortisol with 8 mg dexamethasone test suggest adrenal cause
- If high ACTH, consider a pituitary cause
- Locate tumour with ultrasound scan, CT or MRI

Prepregnancy management

- Advise completing treatment before pregnancy
- Optimize blood pressure (BP) and blood glucose levels if patient is hypertensive or diabetic (see Sections 7.4 and 7.15)

Adrenal tumours

- First line treatment is surgery
- Adrenalectomy during pregnancy is safe. Significantly reduces fetal loss, prematurity, and maternal morbidity
- Ideal timing for surgery is second trimester. If diagnosis is made in third trimester, consider delivery first
- Immediately after surgery, initiate cortisol replacement therapy until the hypothalamic–pituitary–adrenal axis returns to normal. Weaning from replacement doses should not be attempted until after delivery
- Second line treatment is medical. There is limited experience with cyproheptadine, metyrapone or ketoconazole in pregnancy. Metyrapone has been associated with progression to pre-eclampsia, and ketonazole is teratogenic in animal studies

Pituitary tumours

Trans-sphenoidal surgery is the gold standard treatment.

Intrapartum and postpartum management

- Owing to poor wound healing, vaginal delivery is preferable
- Monitor mother and baby for cortisol withdrawal problems

Conn's syndrome/primary hyper-aldosteronism

Incidence

This condition comprises 0.7% of all hypertensive patients, but is a rare cause of hypertension in pregnancy.

Normal physiology

- Sympathetic stimulation (acting via β_1-adrenoceptors), renal artery hypotension, and reduced sodium delivery to the distal tubules stimulate the release of renin by the kidney
- Renin acts on angiotensinogen, which undergoes proteolytic cleavage to form the decapeptide angiotensin I
- Angiotensin-converting enzyme (ACE), found in vascular endothelium, mainly in the lungs, cleaves off two amino acids from angiotensin I to form the octapeptide, angiotensin II
- Angiotensin II acts on the adrenal cortex to release aldosterone
- Aldosterone acts on the kidneys to ↑ sodium and fluid retention
- Hyperaldosteronism suppresses the release of renin

Physiological changes in pregnancy

- Plasma renin and angiotensin II levels rise 2–3-fold
- Plasma and urinary aldosterone levels rise 3-fold in the first trimester and 10-fold by the third trimester

Pathophysiology

- Adrenal aldosterone-secreting tumour
- Adrenal carcinoma
- Bilateral adrenal hyperplasia

Clinical presentation

- Hypertension
- Hypokalaemia (<3 mmol/l). Symptoms are often absent, but include lethargy, muscle weakness, thirst, polyuria, and nocturia
- Increased urine potassium levels

Diagnosis

- Plasma levels of aldosterone increase and renin decreases, when compared to the normal pregnancy-specific range
- In pregnancy, prolonged upright posture results in a modest increase in plasma renin levels. If the renin activity remains suppressed, consider hyperaldosteronism
- Hypokalaemia—urinary potassium loss can be less than that in non-pregnant patients with Conn's syndrome because of the antagonizing effect of progesterone
- The presence of hypertension and hypokalaemia is an indication for an adrenal scan

Before making a biochemical diagnosis:

- Correct hypokalemia as it suppresses aldosterone
- Discontinue diuretics for at least 2 weeks
- β-blockers ↓ renin release, so reduce doses
- Avoid calcium channel blockers for 2–3 h

Management

- Manage as for chronic hypertension in pregnancy
- Treat hypokalaemia with potassium supplement or potassium-sparing diuretics. Amiloride is safe to use in pregnancy

- Treatment used outside pregnancy, such as ACE inhibitors and spironolactone, is contraindicated in pregnancy. Spironolactone is a potassium-sparing diuretic with anti-androgen properties which may cause feminization of a male fetus
- Adrenalectomy cures the disease. It may be performed in the second trimester or deferred until after delivery

Glucocorticoid-remediable aldosteronism

- A hereditary form of primary hyperaldosteronism
- Characterized by the ectopic production of aldosterone in the cortisol-producing zona fasciculata, which is under the regulation of corticotrophin
- Presents from childhood onwards with hypertension and hypokalaemia
- In pregnancy, there is an increased risk of an exacerbation of hypertension and increased rate of CS (32%)

Phaeochromocytoma

Incidence

- Between 0.5 and 2/1000 of hypertensive patients (may be normotensive or have a labile BP)
- Half of cases are diagnosed at post mortem
- No sex or racial difference in the incidence
- Rare in pregnancy

Pathophysiology

- A catecholamine-producing tumour which arises from the chromaffin cells of the adrenal medulla or the sympathetic nervous tissue
- Excessive catecholamine production may cause life-threatening hypertension or cardiac arrhythmias but if the tumour is diagnosed, it is curable
- 10% are bilateral, 10% extra-adrenal, 10% malignant, 10% familial

Familial disease may be part of:

- Multiple endocrine neoplasia (MEN) types IIa and IIb—70% of phaeochromocytoma are bilateral
- Neurofibromatosis—phaeochromocytoma occurs in 1%
- Von Hippel–Lindau (VHL) syndrome—associated with phaeochromocytoma, renal cell carcinoma, and cerebellar haemangioblastomas

The tumour may secrete catecholamine constantly or intermittently. The familial type tend to produce mostly norepinephrine but the sporadic type produce mostly epinephrine. Dopamine may also be produced.

Clinical features

- Symptoms tend to occur intermittently but with time become more frequent and severe
- Commonest symptoms—headaches, profuse sweating, palpitations, and tremor

- Other symptoms—anxiety, blurred vision, dyspnoea, vomiting, abdominal pain, constipation, and convulsions
- Half of hypertension is paroxysmal and mainly occur before 20 weeks of gestation. There is no proteinuria
- A hypertensive crisis may be precipitated by childbirth, induction of anaesthesia, opiates, dopamine antagonists, decongestants (pseudoephedrine), drugs that inhibit catecholamine reuptake (tricyclic antidepressants, cocaine)

Effect of phaeochromocytoma on pregnancy

- Levels of urinary catecholamines, metanephrines and vanillylmandelic acid (VMA) are unaffected by normal pregnancy but are increased with phaeochromocytoma
- Hypertensive crisis in pregnancy may lead to cerebral haemorrhage or severe congestive heart failure
- Maternal mortality 55% when diagnosis is made postpartum, 11% when diagnosis is made antenatally

Management

- Avoid pregnancy until disease is treated
- Establish the diagnosis—24-h urinary collection will show increased levels of catecholamines, metanephrines and VMA excretion
- MRI—to locate the tumour

Medical management

- Control hypertension with α-blocker (phenoxybenzamine or prazosin)
- Control tachycardia with β-blocker

Surgical management

- In early pregnancy, tumour resection after α-blockade should be performed, even at the risk of miscarriage, because of the high maternal and fetal mortality
- Third trimester—the gravid uterus complicates surgery. α-blockage is used to await fetal maturity. CS delivery with simultaneous or delayed tumour resection by open or laparoscopic approach

Postpartum

- Monitor for recurrence

Further reading

Abalos E, Duley L, Steyn DW, Henderson-Smart DJ. Antihypertensive drug therapy for mild to moderate hypertension during pregnancy. *Cochrane Database of Systematic Reviews*, 2007. No. CD002252. www.cochrane.org

Duley L, Henderson-Smart DJ, Meher S. Drugs for treatment of very high BP during pregnancy. *Cochrane Database of Systematic Reviews*, 2006. No. CD001449. www.cochrane.org

Roberts JM, Pearson G, Cutler J, Lindheimer M. Summary of the NHLBI working group on research on hypertension during pregnancy. *Hypertension* 2003; **41**:437–45.

Walfisch A, Hallak M. Hypertension. In: James DK, Steer PJ, Weiner CP, Gonik B (eds). *High Risk Pregnancy Management Options*. Elsevier Saunders: Philadelphia, 2005: 772–97.

7.6 Cardiac disease

Physiological changes in pregnancy
See Section 6.1

Incidence
Serious cardiac disease complicates 1% of pregnancies. The incidence is rising because of maternal age, obesity, improved survival in congenital heart disease (CHD), ischaemic heart disease (IHD), cardiomyopathy (CM), Marfan's, and immigrants with undiagnosed disease.

Maternal deaths 2003–2005
- Cardiac disease is the leading cause of indirect maternal deaths
- Numbers are rising—35 (1997–1999), 44 (2000–2002), 48 (2003–2005)
- Death rate—2.3 per 100 000 maternities
- Commoner than deaths from thromboembolic disease (TED)
- Leading causes were myocardial infarction (MI) (related to IHD) and aortic dissection

Prepregnancy (or booking)
Prepregnancy service provision—all women with suspected or known cardiac disease should attend.
Multidisciplinary care—involve obstetricians, cardiologists and anaesthetists.
Independent interpreters—do not rely on relatives.
Identify risks of acquired disease
Age ≥35, obesity, hypertension, smoking, history of rheumatic fever, family history of heart disease.
Assess maternal risk—score 1 for each of the following

Past event:	Heart failure (HF), arrhythmia, cerebrovascular accident (CVA) or transient ischaemic attack (TIA)
Symptoms:	New York Heart Association (NYHA) class ≥III
Examination:	Cyanosis (SaO$_2$<90%)
CXR, ECG, Echo:	Left ventricle ejection fraction (LVEF) <40%

The risk of a cardiovascular event in pregnancy depends on the total: score 0, 5%; score 1, 27%; score ≥2, 75%

Discuss:
- Long-term prognosis of heart disease
- Effect of pregnancy on disease:
  - Risk of permanent deterioration
  - Maternal risk of morbidity and death (see Box 7.4)
- Effect of disease on pregnancy:
  - Fetal risks (see Box 7.6)
  - Maternal risks and pregnancy outcome
- Timing of pregnancy and contraceptive advice. Avoid pregnancy in high-risk patients (see Box 7.4)
- IVF—risk of ovarian hyperstimulation and multiple pregnancy
- Optimize cardiac function and minimize risk
- Avoid teratogens
- When to discontinue
- Pros and cons of anticoagulation (see Section 7.8)
- Consider surgery and arrhythmia ablation before pregnancy

General measures:
- Treat hypertension, diabetes, obesity, stop smoking
- Folic acid supplement
- Check rubella immunity

Management
Antenatal
All women should have a booking visit—if not seen prepregnancy, follow the management plan above.
Multidisciplinary care—involve obstetricians, cardiologists, anaesthetists, paediatricians, GPs, and midwives

Refer high-risk women to tertiary centres
- Develop an integrated care plan
- Regular communication between specialties
- Plan for management of labour in advance
- A system to check non-attenders immediately
- Advanced life support training for all doctors and midwives

Termination of pregnancy
- Advise in high-risk cases
- Should be easily accessible

Serial assessments
- Evaluate symptoms (NYHA class; see Box 7.2)
- Regular examinations
- Screen for arrhythmias (ECG)
- Evaluate for pulmonary hypertension (PH), ventricular and valve function (echo)

Fetal surveilance
- Offer anomaly scan
- Detailed fetal cardiac scan (see Box 7.5)
- Serial growth scans for fetus at risk of fetal growth restriction (FGR)

Elective admission
- For high risk or cyanotic patients who decline TOP
- Bed rest
- Oxygenation
- Thromboprophylaxis

Intrapartum
Plan for labour and elective delivery in advance.

Avoid aortocaval compression: left lateral or upright position.

Manage in intensive care environment (especially high risk):
- Full resuscitation facilities should be available
- Monitor HR (screen for arrythmias), BP, O$_2$ saturation
- Strict fluid balance—avoid fluid overload, systemic vasodilatation or falls in BP (caution with epidurals + oxytocin)
- Avoid ergotamine for the third stage (↑BP)
- Antibiotic endocarditis prophylaxis is not routinely required (see Box 7.9)
- Aim for vaginal birth (no evidence that CS ↓cardiac risk)

Shorten second stage with assisted delivery for patients with:
- High risk of morbidity or death (see Box 7.4)
- Cyanosis
- Cyanotic CHD

Elective CS in patients with:
- Recent MI (within 2 weeks of labour)
- Aortic root dilatation >4 cm (as risk of dissection in labour)

No evidence that general anaesthesia decreases cardiac risk.

Continuous fetal CTG monitoring.

Postpartum
- Multidisciplinary follow-up
- Maintain intensive care monitoring for high risk and cyanotic patients
- Encourage early mobilization
- Monitor BP
- Monitor fluid balance in PH, ejection systolic murmur (ESM), L→R shunt, ventricular dysfunction, unrepaired tetralogy of Fallot (ToF). Fluid shift may cause congestive cardiac failure (CCF)
- Screen newborn for CHD in mothers with CHD, coarctation of the aorta (CoA)
- Contraceptive advice

Incidence >90%

Benign murmurs secondary to hyperdynamic circulation:
- Early or mid-systolic, soft
- Highest intensity in left sternal edge (LSE), followed by aortic and pulmonary areas
- No investigation is required

Suspicious murmurs are associated with:
- History suggestive of cardiac disease
- NYHA class ≥II
- Loud or long—late systolic, pansystolic, diastolic
- Refer to cardiologist or arrange for an echocardiogram

Palpitations and arrhythmias

In normal pregnancy, heart rate (HR)↑, stroke volume (SV) ↑, cardac output (CO) ↑, and blood volume ↑.

Frequency and severity of arrhythmias ↑ in pregnancy.

Palpitations
- Poor correlation between symptoms and arrhythmia
- Most symptoms are benign; only 10% have arrhythmias
- Ix: ECG or 24-h Holter monitoring

Atrial and ventricular ectopics
- Occur in 50–60% of pregnancies
- No adverse effects, so no further investigation required
- Reassure. Advise to avoid caffeine, tobacco, and illicit drugs

Sinus tachycardia
- Ix underlying anaemia, infection, thyrotoxicosis, HF, PE
- No treatment is required if above causes are excluded

Arrhythmia
- Commonest complication in pregnancies with CHD
- Bradyarrhythmias—most are asymptomatic and benign, less common than tachyarrhythmias
- Ix: thyroid function tests (TFT) and echo (exclude structural heart defect)
- Treat if life-threatening, or frequent and symptomatic

Supraventricular tachycardia (SVT)
- Commonest arrhythmia in pregnancy
- Rx: vagal manouevres. Adenosine is safe in pregnancy and will reveal underlying atrial flutter, Wolff–Parkinson–White syndrome or terminate the SVT. If this fails, digoxin, verapamil, flecainide, esmolol or DC cardioversion

Atrial flutter (AFL) and atrial fibrillation (AF)
- Rare but occur in the presence of mitral valve disease
- Thromboprophylaxis required
- Rx: digoxin is safe in pregnancy and breastfeeding

Ventricular tachycardia (VT)
- Causes—electrolyte abnormality, CM, myocarditis, long QT syndrome, cocaine, alcohol, CHD, 'primary' VT
- Rx: unstable VT—DC cardioversion, stable VT—medical management
- Flecainide and lidocaine are safe in pregnancy and breastfeeding. Procainamide may cause maternal side effects (lupus-like syndrome, blood dyscrasia). Avoid amiodarone owing to fetal bradycardia, neonatal hypothyroidism and hyperthyroidism and FGR, but may be used in life-threatening VT

Long QT syndrome
- Particularly postpartum. Associated with syncope or cardiac arrest
- Rx: β-blocker

◎ **Box 7.2 New York Heart Association classification**

I	No limitations of physical activity
II	Slight limitation—ordinary physical activity causes symptoms (fatigue, palpitation, dyspnoea or angina)
III	Marked limitation—less than ordinary physical activity causes symptoms
IV	Unable to perform physical activity—symptoms at rest

◎ **Box 7.3 Classification of cardiac disease**

Congenital heart disease
Non-cyanotic
- Abnormal shunting: e.g. atrial septal defect (ASD), ventricular septal defect (VSD), patent ductus arteriosus (PDA)
- Outflow tract obstruction, e.g
  - Coarctation of the aorta (CoA)
  - Aortic stenosis (AS), pulmonary stenosis (PS)

Cyanotic
- Tetralogy of Fallot (ToF), pulmonary atresia
- Transposition of the great arteries (TGA)

Inherited conditions
- Mitral valve prolapse (MVP), Marfan's syndrome
- Hypertrophic cardiomyopathy (HCM)

Acquired disease
Rheumatic heart disease (RHD)
- Mitral stenosis (MS), Mitral regurgitation (MR)
- Aortic stenosis (AS), Aortic regurgitation (AR)

Myocardial infarction (MI)
Cardiomyopathies (CM)
- Peripartum (PPCM), dilated (DCM)

➕ **Box 7.4 Risk of maternal morbidity and death**

High risk (mortality >10%)—avoid pregnancy
- Pulmonary hypertension
- Coarctation of the aorta with valvular involvement
- Marfan's syndrome and aortic root dilatation >4 cm
- Ventricular dysfunction (past PPCM + residual disease)
- Severe mitral stenosis (or MS with NYHA ≥III)

Moderate risk (mortality 2–10%)
- MS and AF
- AS
- Prosthetic heart valve
- Past PPCM, no residual disease
- ToF: unrepaired or residual disease, and no PH
- Previous MI
- Marfan's syndrome and normal aorta

Low risk (mortality <2%)
- Successfully repaired CHD, CoA, ToF
- Unrepaired small septal defects or PDA
- Regurgitant valve disease
- Pulmonary or triscuspid valve disease
- MS with NYHA class <III
- MVP without MR

Ventricular septal defect

Incidence
Ventricular septal defects (VSD) comprise 30% of total cases of congenital heart disease (CHD). Rare in pregnancy as small VSDs close spontaneously, and the larger are corrected in childhood.

Aetiology
- Can be isolated abnormality
- Associated with Down's, Turner's, tetralogy of Fallot (ToF)
- Acquired following myocardial infarction (MI)

Clinical features (depends on size of VSD)
- Small—usually asymptomatic, Maladie de Roger (loud pansystolic murmur (PSM))
- Moderate to large—fatigue, dyspnoea, cardiomegaly, PSM in LSE, prominent apex beat, palpable systolic thrill
- Complications of large VSD: L→R shunt, ↑ load on right heart (RH), pulmonary hypertension (PH), Eisenmenger's syndrome (ES) or paradoxical embolization

Management
- Small or corrected VSDs: usually no adverse outcome
- Identify arrhythmia, evaluate for PH (echo)
- Consider surgical repair of uncorrected moderate or large VSD before pregnancy
- Avoid hypotension in labour to prevent shunt reversal

Patent ductus arteriosus (PDA)
Persistent patency of ductus arteriosus between descending aorta and pulmonary trunk or left main pulmonary artery.
- Associated with maternal rubella infection
- Usually corrected surgically in childhood
- Uncorrected patent ductus arteriosus (PDA) account for <5% of CHD in pregnancy

Clinical features
- Most are asymptomatic
- O/E: bounding pulse, thrill over clavicle/first rib, continuous machinery murmur as shunting in both systole and diastole
- ECG: left ventricular hyperplasia (LVH)

Complications
- Women with uncorrected PDAs are at risk of congestive cardiac failure (CCF)
- Large PDA may cause PH

Management
- Corrected PDA poses no problems in pregnancy
- Counsel with reference to 4% risk of CHD in offspring
- Uncorrected PDA:
  - Serial echos to evaluate for PH and size of PDA
  - Monitor fluid balance intrapartum and postpartum

Ostium secundum atrial septal defect
Intra-atrial septum defect at the level of fossa ovalis.

Incidence
Common CHD (up to 25%), affects women more than men.

Clinical features
- Most are asymptomatic. May have palpitations
- O/E: ejection systolic murmur (ESM) pulmonary area
- ECG: Right bundle branch block, RVH

Complications
- AF or supraventricular tachycardia (SVT) more common >40 years of age
- Small risk of paradoxical embolism
- L→R shunt may cause right heart failure (RHF). PH uncommon

Management
- Identify arrhythmia, evaluate for PH (NYHA class, echo)
- Routine antenatal care if no complications

Coarctation of the aorta (CoA)
Narrowing of the aorta, most commonly just distal to the origin of the left subclavian artery. Males> females.

Other abnormalities may be present:
- Bicuspid aortic valve (85% of patients), VSD
- Left-sided obstructive or hypoplastic heart defects
- Turner syndrome (35% have aortic coarctation)
- Aneurysms—circle of Willis, intercostal arteries or distal aorta

Complications
- Angina, hypertension, CCF, aortic dissection, sudden death
- If unrepaired, most women reach childbearing age. Less than 20% of patients survive to age 50 years
- If repaired <14 years, the 20-year survival rate is 91%. If repaired >14 years, the 20-year survival rate is 79%

Pregnancy
- In women with unrepaired CoA, the mortality rate is 3–8%
- Surgical repair reduces but does not eliminate the risk of aortic dissection, thus all pregnant women with a history of CoA should be considered high risk
- Significant stenosis of the aorta or involvement of the aortic valve is a contraindication to pregnancy

Diagnosis
- Clinical hallmark of CoA—differences in upper and lower extremity arterial pulses and blood pressures
- CXR—prominent aortic knob, the stenosed area may appear as an indentation of the proximal thoracic descending aorta in the shape of a number 3. Rib notching may be present (owing to persistent pulsation of dilated intercostal arteries)
- Confirm by echocardiography, pulsed-wave Doppler, and colour flow mapping

Management
- Uncorrected cases—advise surgical repair before pregnancy or termination if pregnant
- Screen for aneurysms (CT brain) and aortopathy (echo)
- Minimize risk by strict blood pressure control and β-blockade to decrease cardiac contractility
- Treat hypertension (see Section 7.4)

Transposition of the great arteries (TGA)
Aorta arises from RV, pulmonary artery arises from LV. Incompatible with life. Survivors have had the 'arterial switch/Mustard/Senning operation' in childhood.

Incidence
The incidence is 5–7% of all CHD.

Complications
Sinus node dysfunction with bradycardia, atrial arrhythmias, and systemic RV dysfunction.

Congenitally corrected TGA (ccTGA)

Systemic VR enters LV which ejects into PA. Pulmonary VR enters RV which ejects into the aorta. Thus, a systemic RV circulation.

Associations

Tricuspid valve abnormalities, VSD, PS, complete heart block, Wolff–Parkinson–White syndrome

Effect of repaired TGA and ccTGA on pregnancy

Pregnancy tolerated if normal RV function and no arrhythmia.

Effect of pregnancy on repaired TGA and ccTGA

Pregnancy may have a long-term adverse effect on the ventricular function of women with repaired TGA.

Management

Prepregnancy

Assess RV function, heart rhythm, exercise test to ensure the ability to accommodate ↑ HR + ↑CO.

Antenatal

- Serial assessment of RV and valve function
- Women with repaired TGA are at risk of thromboembolic disease (TED), thus thromboprophylaxis and low dose aspirin

Univentricular hearts and Fontan operations

- A single ventricle supports systemic circulation
- VR is diverted directly into the pulmonary circulation without a ventricle, driven only by systemic VR
- All patients have 'low CO status'
- 10-year survival rate: 60–80%

Complications

- Atrial arrhythmias common, may lead to deterioration
- Predisposed to thrombosis owing to sluggish blood flow
- Impaired ventricular function, especially if systemic RV
- May result in cyanosis

Specific management in pregnancy

- Risk of pregnancy depends on presence of arrhythmias, cyanosis, and ventricular function
- Evaluate arrhythmia, ventricular function, exercise test to check ability to ↑CO and maintain O_2 saturation
- Bed rest, anticoagulation, and low-dose aspirin

Tetralogy of Fallot (ToF)

Large VSD, RVH, RV outflow obstruction, and overriding aorta. Associated with DiGeorge syndrome (DGS) in 15% of cases. Without surgical repair, life expectancy is shortened.

Incidence

Incidence of 3.5% CHD, commonest cyanotic CHD

Surgical repair

- VSD closure
- Relief of RV outflow obstruction ± patching of PV annulus, which may lead to pulmonary regurgitation (PR) ⇒ RV dysfunction, VT and sudden death
- After repair—mild to moderate PR is tolerated well in pregnancy provided there is no ventricular dysfunction

Effect of pregnancy on unrepaired disease

↑ CO ⇒ ↑ VR to hypertrophic RV. Together with ↓ peripheral VR ⇒ ↑ in R→L shunt ⇒ ↓ oxygenation and worsening cyanosis

Effect of unrepaired disease on pregnancy

- Cyanosis ⇒ ↑ risk of fetal loss, fetal growth restriction, preterm birth
- Polycythaemia secondary to hypoxaemia ⇒ ↑ risk of TED
- Paradoxical embolism through R→L shunt ⇒ CVA

Management

- Prepregnancy—genetic test for DGS (50% recurrence)

> **Box 7.5 Indications for detailed fetal cardiac scan**
>
> *Maternal*
> - Family history or maternal CHD
> - Pre-existing diabetes mellitus
> - Autoimmune antibodies
> - Use of teratogenic drugs
>
> *Fetal*
> - Extracardiac anomalies (including aneuploidy)
> - Monochorionic twin pregnancy
> - Fetal arrhythmia
>
> *Ultrasound findings*
> - Nuchal translucency >3.5 mm
> - Suspicious cardiac scan
> - Two 'soft' markers suspicious of aneuploidy

> **Box 7.6 Counselling about fetal risk**
>
> **Autosomal dominant inheritance** (50% risk)—e.g. Marfan's syndrome, HCM
> **Cyanosis**—fetal loss, preterm birth, low birth weight
>
> | SaO_2 (%) | Chance of a live birth |
> | --- | --- |
> | >90 | 92% |
> | 85–90% | 45% |
> | <85% | 12% |
>
> **CHD recurrence**
> Baseline risk—0.8/1000, 85% of babies with CHD are born to mothers with no risk factors
> Overall risk in offspring of women with CHD is 2–5%
> Risk is ↑ if the mother rather than the father has CHD
> Risk of specific CHD in offspring:
>
> | Defect | CHD in father | CHD in mother |
> | --- | --- | --- |
> | ASD | 2% | 5% |
> | VSD | 2% | 6–10% |
> | AS | 3% | 13–18% |
> | CoA | 2% | 4% |
> | PS | 2% | 4% |
> | ToF | 2% | 3% |
>
> **Teratogenic drugs**
> Discuss **long-term paediatric follow-up** in affected babies

> **Box 7.7 Cardiac effects of drugs used in pregnancy**
>
> *Anticoagulants* (see Section 7.8)
> *Antihypertensives* (see Section 7.4)
> *Lithium* ↑ risk of Ebstein anomaly
> *Paroxetine* increases risk of CHD by 2%
> *Oxytocin* Vascular smooth muscle relaxant ⇒ ↓ BP, compensated by ↑ HR in normal pregnancies. Antidiuretic effect ⇒ ↓ Na, water retention ⇒ pulmonary oedema
> In cardiac disease, avoid rapid IV bolus or large doses
> *Ergometrine* ↑BP. Avoid in cardiac disease and hypertension
> *Misoprostol* No effect on HR, BP, PVR. Limited data
> *Ritodrine* β-agonist ⇒ ↑HR, pulmonary oedema. Avoid
> *Atosiban* No effect on HR, BP, PVR. Used for tocolysis

Mitral valve prolapse (MVP)

One or both MV leaflets prolapse into the left atrium (LA) during systole.

Prevalence
- Commonest cardiac problem, women > men
- Prevalence in women of reproductive age is up to 21%

Aetiology
- Possibly an inherited condition

Clinical features
- Most are asymptomatic
- Fatigue, palpitations, syncope, chest pain
- Auscultation—midsystolic click ± mid-to-late murmur
- Echocardiogram shows mitral valve prolapsing into LA

Complications
- MR (more likely >45 years of age), arrythmias (particularly supraventricular tachycardia (SVT)), bacterial endocarditis, cerebral ischaemia, sudden death

Management
- Echocardiogram to confirm the presence of MR
- Surgical correction of severe MR before pregnancy
- Observe arrhythmias—β-blocker, digoxin may be used

Mitral stenosis

In severe mitral stenosis (MS), the valve area is <1 cm^2.

Aetiology
- Over 50% of patients have had rheumatic fever
- Over 90% rheumatic valve disease affects the mitral valve (MV)

Complications
- LA outflow obstruction ⇒ slow filling of LV and fixed CO
- LA pressure ↑ to ↑ CO, resulting in left atrial hypertrophy (LAH) and dilatation, which may cause AF, ↑ pulmonary capillary pressure, pulmonary oedema, and eventual reactive pulmonary hypertension (PH) and right heart failure (RHF)
- There is an increased risk of bacterial endocarditis

Symptoms
- May be asymptomatic for many years
- Increase load on the heart or onset of AF ⇒ dyspnoea, palpitations, syncope, fatigue
- Increased pulmonary capillary pressure ⇒ cough, pink frothy sputum and haemoptysis

Examination
- Malar flush
- Pulse—low volume or irregularly irregular pulse (AF)
- Tapping apex beat, apical diastolic thrill, L parasternal heave
- Auscultation—loud S1, soft S2, loud P2, opening snap, low-pitched mid-diastolic murmur. May have functional pulmonary regurgitation (PR) and pulmonary oedema

Effects of pregnancy on mitral stenosis
- Increased HR result in ↓ LV filling, ↓ SV and ↓ CO
- This leads to ↑ LA pressure, ↑ pulmonary vascular resistance (PVR), pulmonary oedema, and arrhythmias
- Increased blood volume ⇒ further ↑ in LA pressure
- Most complications occur in the third trimester or labour
- Poorer prognosis with severe MS or NYHA ≥III

Management
Prepregnancy
- Assess cardiac function and degree of MS
- Advise to avoid pregnancy in severe MS or NYHA ≥III, until after correction (open, closed, balloon valvotomy, or valve replacement)

Antenatal
- In severe MS or NYHA ≥III, offer termination of pregnancy (TOP)
- Serial echocardiograms to assess cardiac function
- Avoid ↑HR by restricting physical activity
- β-blockers to ↓HR, ↑ LV filling time and to reduce the risk of pulmonary oedema
- In AF, treat with digoxin or DC cardioversion
- Pulmonary oedema—O$_2$, diamorphine, and diuretics
- Cardiac catheterization may be used to evaluate and treat refractory pulmonary oedema
- Balloon valvotomy for severe, non-calcified, MS in pregnancy has good maternal and fetal outcomes

Intrapartum and postpartum
- Pain control prevents ↑HR
- Epidural analgesia is safe, but avoid ↓BP
- Monitor fluid balance. Consider central venous pressure monitoring in severe MS

Aortic stenosis

Incidence
Aortic stenosis (AS) is generally a disease of men or the elderly (progesses with age).

Uncommon in pregnancy, accounting for 5–10% of left heart disease (LHD), usually in conjunction with MV disease

Aetiology
Congenital biscuspid valve, CoA, LHD, Marfan's syndrome, Ehlers–Danlos type IV, Turner's syndrome, atherosclerosis.

Symptoms
- Mild AS—usually asymptomatic
- Severe AS—exercise-induced angina, syncope, palpitations, and dyspnoea

Examination
- Pulse—slow rising, low BP
- Double apical impulse, systolic thrill (aortic area)
- Loud S1, soft S2, prominent S4, systolic ejection click mid-systolic murmur (aortic area, radiate to carotids)

Complications
- ↑pressure gradient ⇒ LVH, LVF, LA enlargement, ↑ RH pressure
- LVF ⇒ ↓ BP, ↓ CO, tachyarrhythmias & sudden death
- Increased risk of bacterial endocarditis

Effect of pregnancy on AS
- In severe AS, there is a restricted capacity to ↑ CO
- Resting tachycardia may indicate LVF, unable to maintain ↑SV

Effect of AS on pregnancy
- Mild-to-moderate AS is usually well tolerated
- Severe AS—cardiac complications occur in 10%
- Risk of fetal growth restriction (FGR) and ↑ risk of CHD

Box 7.8

	Valve area	Mean pressure gradient
Normal aortic valve	3–4 cm^2	0 mmHg
Mild to moderate AS	2 cm^2	30–50
Severe AS	1 cm^2	>50

Management

Prepregnancy

- Evaluate the degree of AS with echocardiogram and exercise test. Severe AS should be surgically repaired
- Indicators of risk—failure to achieve normal ↑ in BP and CO with exercise, impaired LV function or symptoms

Antenatal

- Restrict activity—β-blockers for symptom control
- Evaluate for arrhythmias and CCF
- Serial fetal growth scans
- Balloon valvotomy may allow temporary relief of severe AS and continuation of pregnancy

Intrapartum

- Monitor fluid balance. Avoid ↓BP and ↓ blood volume (BV)
- Caution with epidural. Fluid overload may ⇒ pulmonary oedema (if so, avoid rapid diuresis)
- O$_2$, morphine, and inotropes to maintain CO

Postpartum

- Monitor fluid balance. Avoid ↓ BP and ↓ BV
- Close follow-up as disease progresses

Prosthetic heart valves

Bioprosthetic valves

- Made of heterografts (bovine or porcine valves or pericardium) or homografts (human aortic valves)
- Do not require lifelong anticoagulation
- Valve failure requires replacement after 10–15 years. Pregnancy may accelerate valve failure

Mechanical valves

- Made of non-biological materials
- 8-fold increased risk of valve thrombosis or embolic events in non-pregnant women. Anticoagulation reduces this risk by 75%
- Lifelong anticoagulation is indicated
- Do not require replacement

Mechanical heart valves and pregnancy

- Anticoagulation must be continued throughout pregnancy
- Thromboembolic disease (TED) risk depends on type of valve:
  - The risk is higher with mitral valve than aortic valve
  - The risk is less with the newer bileaflet valves (St Jude, Carbomedics), compared with ball and cage valves (Starr–Edwards) or single-tilting disc (Bjork–Hiley)

Mechanical heart valves and anticoagulation in pregnancy

Warfarin

- Less risk of valve thrombosis compared with heparin
- Crosses placental barrier, ↑ fetal risk:
  - 6% risk of warfarin embryopathy when used 6–12 weeks, especially with doses >5 mg/day. Features include chondrodysplasia punctata, midface hypoplasia, short proximal limbs, short phalanges, scoliosis
  - Risk of miscarriage

- Risk of stillbirth and fetal intracerebral haemorrhage, especially if used within 2 weeks of labour
- Risk of low IQ and neurological dysfunction

Heparin

- Does not cross placental barrier, safe for fetus
- Unfractionated heparin—prolonged use increases maternal risk of heparin-induced osteoporosis, thrombocytopenia and skin allergy (injection site)
- Low molecular weight heparin (LMWH)—no significant effect on maternal bone mineral density or platelet count. Skin allergy is less when compared with unfractionated heparin

Three anticoagulant regimen choices in pregnancy

- Warfarin throughout pregnancy (maintain INR 2.5–3.5)
- Discontinue warfarin before 6 weeks' gestation. LMWH from 6–12 weeks' gestation, followed by warfarin again
- LMWH throughout pregnancy with regular anti-Xa monitoring (may be suitable for newer bileaflet valves)

The choice of anticoagulant regimen will depend on

- The type and number of mechanical valves
- Previous history of TED
- Dose of warfarin needed to maintain a therapeutic INR
- Patient choice

Specific management in pregnancy

- If bleeding or need to deliver urgently whilst on anticoagulant—reverse warfarin with fresh frozen plasma (FFP) and vitamin K, reverse heparin with protamine sulphate
- Stop warfarin and give heparin for 10–14 days before delivery
- Withold heparin on the day of delivery to prevent postpartum haemorrhage (PPH)
- Recommence heparin after delivery
- Delay restarting warfarin until 2–7 days postpartum to prevent secondary PPH
- Warfarin and heparin are safe during breastfeeding

Box 7.9 Cardiac conditions considered to increase risk of infective endocarditis

- Acquired heart disease with stenosis or regurgitation
- Valve replacement
- Structural congenital heart disease (including surgically corrected or palliated conditions, but excluding isolated ASD, fully repaired VSD or PDA, and closure devices judged to be endothelialized)
- Previous infective endocarditis
- Hypertrophic cardiomyopathy

NICE recommends that women with the above conditions do not require routine endocarditis prophylaxis. In the presence of suspected or confirmed infection, antibiotics that cover organisms that cause infective endocarditis should be used. (Prophylaxis against infective endocarditis. March 2008 Guideline no. 64. www.nice.org.uk/cg064). However, current consensus is that women with the above conditions (especially those with mechanical valves or previous endocarditis) should receive antibiotic prophylaxis if an operative delivery is undertaken.

7.9 Acquired heart disease

Dissection of thoracic aorta

An intimal tear in the aorta causes blood to track into the medial layer, which splits and forms a false channel.

- Type A—involves ascending aorta (mostly in pregnancy)
  Type B—involves aorta beyond the left subclavian origin
- 75% of dissections occur in those aged ≥40 years

Risk factors

Pregnancy, hypertension, Marfan's syndrome, Ehlers–Danlos syndrome type IV, coarctation of the aorta, Turner's syndrome, 'crack' cocaine use, bicuspid aortic valve.

Clinical features

Suspect in any pregnant woman with acute severe chest pain, particularly if interscapular radiation, ± hypertension.

Complications

- Depend on the arterial branches involved and compression of nearby organs
- Rapid blood loss and shock, cardiac tamponade, aortic regurgitation, thrombus formation, stroke, acute renal failure, myocardial infarction (MI), mesenteric ischaemia, paraplegia
- Mortality rate increases with delayed diagnosis. Outside pregnancy, mortality is 1% per hour for first 48 h

Diagnosis

- CXR may show mediastinal widening
- Confirm by echocardiogram, CT or MRI

Management

- Careful and rapid control of BP
- Type A dissection—cardiac surgery to replace the aortic root and expeditious delivery by CS

Marfan's syndrome

Autosomal dominant, connective tissue disorder, which affects the skeletal, ocular, and cardiovascular systems.

Clinical features

- ↑height, arm span > height, lens dislocation, high arched palate, arachnodactyly, depressed sternum, joint laxity
- Cardiac disease in 80%—MVP, mitral regurgitation (MR), and aortic root dilatation

Pathophysiology

- Mutations in the fibrillin-1 (*FBN1*) gene on chromosome 15q21.1. The glycoprotein fibrillin is a major building block of microfibrils
- Microfibrils serve as substrates for elastin in the aorta and other connective tissues

Abnormal microfibrils result in:

- Weakened aortic wall, leading to progressive aortic dilatation and eventual aortic rupture or dissection due to the tension caused by left ventricular ejection impulses. Risk increased in pregnancy owing to ↑ CO
- Reduced structural integrity of the lens zonules, ligaments, lung airways, and spinal dura

Effect of pregnancy on Marfan's syndrome

- Increased risk of maternal mortality owing to aortic rupture or dissection, even in women with normal aorta
- Higher risk if aortic root dilatation >4 cm (10% risk) or family history of aortic rupture or dissection

Specific management in pregnancy

- Counsel—those with cardiac lesion tend to have offspring with cardiac abnormalities
- Aortic root >4 cm, delay pregnancy until after surgery

- Serial echo every 6–10 weeks to observe aortic root size
- Strict BP control, β-blockers reduce rate of aortic root dilatation
- Restrict activity to minimize haemodynamic stress
- Adequate pain relief in labour; consider epidural
- Elective CS with epidural if aortic root >4 cm
- Risk of dissection persists for 6–8 weeks postpartum

Hypertrophic cardiomyopathy (HCM)

Hypertrophic cardiomyopathy (HCM) is left ventricular hypertrophy (LVH) without chamber dilatation or an identifiable cause.

Incidence

One in 500 of the population.

Aetiology

Autosomal dominant inheritance in 70%.

Clinical features

- Most are asymptomatic. Often diagnosed on family screening or investigation of heart mumur in pregnancy
- ↓ BP or ↓ BV ⇒ LV outflow obstruction ⇒ syncope, angina
- O/E—double apical pulsation (palpable S4)
- Auscultation—ejection systolic murmur (ESM) caused by LV outflow obstruction; pansystolic murmur (PSM) caused by MR

Complications

Ventricular tachycardia (VT), heart failure (HF), common cause of sudden death in young people.

Risk factors for sudden death

Family history of sudden death, previous syncope, VT.

Effect of pregnancy on HCM

- Well tolerated owing to ↑ BV and the ability to ↑ SV
- However, ↑ HR ⇒ ↓ diastolic filling time

Specific management in pregnancy

- β-blockers if symptomatic. Avoid ↑ HR. Caution with oxytocin
- Avoid vasodilatation, ↓ BP or ↓ BV. Caution with epidural
- Implantable cardiac defibrillators may be used

Peripartum cardiomyopathy (PPCM)

The development of HF and LV systolic dysfunction diagnosed by echo, between 8 months' gestation and 5 months' postpartum, with no identifiable cause and no previous heart disease.

Incidence

One in 5000–10 000 pregnancies.

Risk factors

Increased age, ↑BP, multiple pregnancy, multiparity, Afro-Caribbean.

Complications

HF, thromboembolism or arrhythmia.

Clinical features

- Symptoms of HF—dyspnoea on exertion (NYHA > II), orthopnoea, paroxysmal nocturnal dyspnoea, palpitations, abdominal discomfort caused by passive congestion of liver
- Signs of HF—↑HR, ↓BP, displaced apical impulse, gallop heart rhythm, arrhythmia, functional MR, pulmonary oedema, ↑jugular venous pressure (JVP), peripheral oedema
- Pulmonary embolism (PE)—↑HR, ↓BP, dyspnoea, haemoptysis
- Cerebral embolism—hemiplegia, aphasia, incoordination
- Acute MI secondary to coronary embolism
- Mesenteric artery occlusion—acute abdominal syndrome secondary to bowel infarction

Diagnosis (by echocardiography)
- Left ventricular ejection fraction (LVEF) <45%
- Fractional shortening <30%
- LV end-diastolic (LVED) pressure >2.7 cm/m². Dilatation of all four chambers of the heart is often seen

Management
- Antenatal—elective delivery
- Thromboprophylaxis
- Conventional treatment of HF: O_2 therapy, diuretics, vasodilators (hydralazine +/or nitrates), cardioselective β-blocker—bisoprolol or carvedilol (vasodilator), inotropes and ACE inhibitors in the postpartum
- Control arrhythmia—digoxin
- Consider immunosuppression if myocarditis on endo-myocardial biopsy, that fails to improve within 2 weeks of HF therapy.
- Intra-aortic balloon pumps, LV assist devices
- Cardiac transplant

Prognosis and recurrence
- Maternal mortality 25–50%. Most deaths occur close to presentation. Recent study—95% survival rate at 5 years
- 50% of patients make a spontaneous and full recovery. More likely if LVEF >30%, LVED <60 mm, FS >20%
- Recurrence depends on normalization of LV function
  - Full recovery—HF 20–25%, mortality rate 0%, persistent LV dysfunction in 10–14%
  - Residual disease—HF 45–50%, mortality rate 20–25%, persistent LV dysfunction in 30–40%

Subsequent pregnancy
- Avoid pregnancy, offer termination (TOP) with residual disease
- Thromboprophylaxis
- Admit for bed rest and O_2 therapy in third trimester
- Elective delivery

Myocardial infarction (MI)

Incidence
- Uncommon but rising as maternal age increases
- Usually third trimester and peripartum

Risk factors
Increased age, smoking, diabetes, obesity, ↑BP, hyperlipidaemia, family history of ischaemic heart disease (IHD).

Aetiology in pregnancy
- Commonly non-atherosclerotic conditions with acute presentation, e.g. coronary thrombosis or dissection
- MI due to atherosclerosis occurs in <50% of cases. Tends to present antenatally with risk factors of IHD
- 40% have no risk factors, 30% have normal coronary arteries
- Other—coronary artery aneurysm, spasm or embolism, congenital coronary anomalies, and cocaine abuse

Commonest site of infarction
- Anterior wall of the LV
- The territory of the left anterior descending artery

Diagnosis
ECG and troponin I.

Effect of MI on pregnancy
- Maternal mortality 20%, fetal outcome depends on mother

Management
- As for non-pregnant—heparin, β-blockers, nitrates, dopamine, calcium channel blockers can be used
- IV and intracoronary thrombolysis, percutaneous transluminal coronary angioplasty have been used

- Low-dose aspirin (75–150 mg/day) for secondary prophylaxis. In acute MI 150–300 mg/day may be given
- CS if labours within 2 weeks of MI as risk of mortality

Specific management of women with previous MI
- Prepregnancy—stress testing and echo. Residual LV dysfunction and continuing ischaemia are poor prognostic features
- Stop statins prepregnancy as ↑ risk of CNS and limb defects
- Secondary prevention—aspirin or clopidogrel and β-blockers
- Restrict physical activity in pregnancy
- Monitor for arrhythmias and congestive cardiac failure (CCF)

Pulmonary hypertension (PH)
Mean pulmonary artery pressure (PAP) ≥25 mmHg at rest or ≥30 mmHg during exercise.

Eisenmenger's syndrome (ES)
PH secondary to L→R shunt resulting in shunt reversal and cyanosis.

Pathophysiology
↑ PVR ⇒ ↑ right heart pressure (RHP) and inability to ↑ O_2. O/E—L parasternal heave, loud P2, soft murmur (↑RHP)

Aetiology of PH
- Primary—idiopathic disease of pulmonary vasculature
- Secondary—chronic ↑PAP in lung disease (cystic fibrosis), connective tissue disease (scleroderma), pulmonary veno-occlusive disease, ES

Effects of pregnancy on PH and ES
- Poor tolerance of changes in BV or CO, especially in labour, delivery and early postpartum. ↑CO, ↓BV, postpartum fluid shift or overload may lead to HF, MI, arrhythmias or sudden death
- Maternal mortality 30–50%. Most die postpartum
- Postoperative fluid shift during CS may ⇒ ↑ mortality
- TED aggravates PH and is usually fatal
- TOP is associated with mortality rate of up to 7%

Effects of PH and ES on pregnancy
- Chronic maternal hypoxia ⇒ FGR, fetal loss, preterm delivery
- Neonatal survival rate 90%

Specific management in pregnancy
- Avoid pregnancy, offer TOP
- Thromboprophylaxis
- Admit for rest and monitor O_2 saturation in the third trimester
- Aim for vaginal delivery with shortened second stage
- Monitoring PAP does not improve outcome
- Consider calcium channel blocker to improve CO
- Consider selective pulmonary vasodilators (inhaled nitric oxide, IV prostacyclin, bosantan)

Further reading
Silwa K, Fett J, Elkayam U. Peripartum cardiomyopathy. *Lancet* 2006; **368**:687–93.

Steer PJ, Gatzoulis MA, Baker P (eds) *Heart disease and pregnancy*. London: RCOG Press, 2006.

> **Box 7.10 Cardiac diseases and risk of thrombosis**
> - Mechanical heart valves
> - Pulmonary hypertension/Eisenmenger's syndrome
> - Cardiomyopathies
> - Arrhythmias, especially AF
> - Coronary artery disease
> - CHD

7.10 Respiratory disease

Physiological changes in pregnancy
See Section 6.1.

Dyspnoea

Incidence
- Seventy per cent report dyspnoea which is mostly physiological
- It is difficult to differentiate between benign and serious causes, i.e. asthma, infection, embolism, and heart disease

History
- Insidious onset, no associated cough, chest discomfort or acute exacerbation—consider physiological or anaemia
- Wheeze, cough, nocturnal worsening—consider asthma
- Insidious onset, cough, haemoptysis—consider TB
- Sudden onset ± chest pain or haemoptysis—consider pulmonary embolism (PE)
- Orthopnoea, paroxysmal dyspnoea—may be heart failure
- Palpitations ± chest pain—consider arrhythmia

Examination
- Pallor, cyanosis, dehydration, fever, oedema, ↑ JVP
- Pulse—rate, rhythm, volume
- Heart—murmur, added heart sounds
- Chest—respiratory rate, expansion, wheeze, crackles

Investigations
- O_2 saturation, arterial blood gas (ABG) if <95%
- ECG
- Haemoglobin

Additional investigations
- Peak expiratory flow rate (PEFR) or forced expiratory volume in 1 s (FEV_1) if history suggests asthma
- 24-h Holter monitoring if palpitations
- CXR with abdominal shielding if suspected consolidation, pneumothorax, PE, heart disease
- Ventilation–perfusion scan/CT angiogram if suspect PE
- Echocardiography if suspected heart disease
- Fetal monitoring in acute events or hypoxaemia

Asthma

Prevalence
- Commonest pre-existing medical condition in pregnancy, affecting 7% of women of reproductive age
- Rising prevalence is related to birth and rearing practices and atmospheric pollution
- Often undiagnosed or undertreated in pregnancy

Pathophysiology
Episodic partial obstruction of airflow in the small airways, by a combination of mucous plugging and bronchospasm.
- Caused by an allergic response to inhaled antigens or as a reflex response to cold air, solvents or other stimuli
- There is low grade chronic inflammation of the airways

Clinical features
- Symptoms—cough, dyspnoea, wheeze, chest tightness. These are variable, intermittent, tend to be worst at night, and provoked by triggers, including exercise. Symptoms may worsen after taking β-blockers or NSAIDs
- Triggers include pollen, animal dander, dust, exercise, emotion, upper respiratory tract infections, and cold air
- Signs—tachycardia, ↑ respiratory rate, bilateral expiratory wheeze, use of accessory muscles, and hyperinflation of the lungs in chronic asthma
- Personal or family history of asthma, eczema or allergic rhinitis

Complications
- **Chronic asthma**—persistent airway obstruction despite drug therapy. Chronic alveolar hypoventilation may lead to pulmonary hypertension and right ventricular hypertrophy
- **Status asthmaticus**—severe, prolonged attack of asthma that does not respond to bronchodilator therapy. May die from acute respiratory insufficiency

Effect of pregnancy on asthma
One-third each worsened, improved, and unchanged.

Presence of a female fetus is associated with worse maternal asthma.
- In severe asthma, the risk of an exacerbation requiring medical intervention is as high as 50%
- Between 11–18% of asthmatic mothers have acute exacerbation, and of these, 62% will require hospitalization

Severe symptoms mainly occur at 24–36 weeks' gestation, but are least likely to occur >36 weeks or during labour, possibly due to endogenous steroid production

Effect of asthma on pregnancy
Maternal risks
- ↑ risk of pre-eclampsia and maternal mortality
- In 2003–2005, there were 6 deaths due to asthma

Fetal risks
- Low birth weight—risk increases in asthma requiring hospitalization or in those not using inhaled corticosteroids
- Preterm birth—associated with the use of oral steroids and theophylline, or having a respiratory problem in pregnancy
- Perinatal mortality and neonatal hypoxia

Treatment improves outcomes for mother and fetus.

Side effects of oral corticosteroids include hypertension, reduced glucose tolerance, depression, and infections

Diagnosis and investigations (objective tests)
The characteristic feature of asthma is variability of PEFR and FEV_1, either spontaneously over time or in response to therapy. One of the following is highly suggestive of asthma:
- PEFR: >20% variability over ≥3 days in a week for ≥2 weeks
- FEV_1: ≥15% and 200 ml increase after short acting β_2-agonist (salbutamol 400 µg by metered-dose inhaler and spacer or 2.5 mg by nebulizer)
- FEV_1: ≥15% and 200 ml increase after a trial of steroid tablets (prednisolone 30 mg/day for 14 days)
- FEV_1: ≥15% decrease after 6 min of exercise (running)

Antenatal management of asthma
Early antenatal care
Multidisciplinary care—involve obstetrician, physician, midwives, and GP
Counsel
- Importance and safety of continuing asthma treatment
- Risk of adverse maternal or fetal outcomes with poorly controlled asthma is greater than the risk from using conventional medication

- If asthma is well controlled throughout pregnancy, there is little or no increased risk of poor outcomes
- Avoidance of asthma triggers
- Dangers of smoking to herself and the baby and give appropriate support to stop smoking
- In labour, asthma attack is rare but continue medication
- Risk of atopic disease in the infant is 1:10 if mother has asthma but 1:3 if both parents have atopic disease. Risk is reduced by breastfeeding

Management is the same as in the non-pregnant patient
- Optimize therapy and maximize lung function
- Inhaled corticosteroids reduce the risk of acute asthmatic attack and reduce the risk of readmission following exacerbation
- Check theophylline blood levels in those requiring therapeutic levels to maintain asthma control
- The safety of leukotriene antagonists (montelukast or zafirlukast) has not been proven in pregnancy but may be continued in women who had good asthma control with these agents before pregnancy
- Patients on oral steroids—monitor BP and blood glucose. Treat hyperglycaemia with insulin if necessary but do not reduce or discontinue oral steroid therapy

Intrapartum management
- Aim for vaginal delivery in absence of acute severe asthma. 90% have no symptoms during labour
- Theoretical risk of hypothalamic–pituitary–adrenal suppression if prednisolone >7.5 mg/day for >2 weeks. Give parenteral hydrocortisone 100 mg 6-hourly during labour
- Prostaglandin E2 may safely be used for induction
- All forms of pain relief in labour may be used safely
- Regional is preferable to general anaesthesia owing to the risk of chest infection and associated atelectasis
- Syntometrine may be used for PPH prophylaxis
- Ergometrine or prostaglandin F2α (carboprost) should be used cautiously for PPH due to uterine atony because of the risk of bronchospasm

Postpartum management
- Encourage breastfeeding
- Continue asthma medications as usual and reassure that these are safe for use in breastfeeding
- NSAIDs may be used with caution. Ask about sensitivity

Management of acute exacerbation of asthma
Admit.

Levels of severity of acute asthma exacerbations
Moderate—PEFR 50–75% best or predicted
Severe—one of: PEFR 33–50% best or predicted, respiratory rate ≥25/min, pulse ≥100 bpm, or inability to complete sentences in one breath
Life-threatening—severe asthma plus one of: PEFR <33% best or predicted, SpO_2 <92%, PaO_2 <8kPa, silent chest, cyanosis, feeble respiratory effort
Near fatal—raised $PaCO_2$ and/or requiring mechanical ventilation with raised inflation pressures

Relieve hypoxaemia
- Give O_2 (40–60%) with high flow mask (Hudson)
- Maintain oxygen saturation >95%
- ABG required if SaO_2 <95% or life-threatening asthma

Relieve bronchospasm
- Repeated inhaled β₂-agonists at 15–30-min intervals
- Salbutamol and terbutaline have the same efficacy

- If not life-threatening, give via metered-dose inhaler and a large volume spacer or by wet nebulization driven by O_2
- Life-threatening—O_2-driven nebulized route recommended. Continuous nebulization as effective as bolus β₂-agonists
- Reserve IV route for patients in whom inhaled therapy cannot be used reliably
- In severe asthma and those that respond poorly to an initial bolus dose of β₂-agonist, consider continuous nebulization using an appropriate nebulizer system

Steroid therapy
- Reduces mortality, relapses, subsequent hospital admission and requirement for β₂-agonist. Pregnant women with acute asthma exacerbation are less likely to receive oral steroids and thus this increases the risk of ongoing exacerbations
- The earlier it is given, the better the outcome
- Steroid tablets are as effective as injected steroids. Prednisolone 40–50 mg/day or parenteral hydrocortisone 100 mg 6-hourly are as effective as higher doses
- Continue steroid tablets for ≥5 days or until recovery
- After recovery, steroid tablets can be stopped without tapering provided the patient receives inhaled steroids

Ipratropium bromide (anticholinergic) therapy
- Nebulized ipratropium bromide 0.5 mg 4–6-hourly, should be added to β₂-agonist in acute severe or life-threatening asthma or those with a poor initial response
- Produces greater bronchodilatation than β₂-agonist alone, leading to a faster recovery and shorter stay
- Unnecessary in mild exacerbations or after stabilization

Intravenous magnesium sulphate
Consider a single dose (1.2–2 g IV infusion over 20 min) in acute severe or life-threatening asthma or those with poor initial response to inhaled bronchodilator therapy.

Rehydration and correction of electrolyte imbalance
β₂-agonist and/or steroids can cause hypokalaemia.

Continuous electronic fetal monitoring
CXR with abdominal shielding is recommended
Suspected consolidation, pneumothorax, life-threatening asthma, poor treatment response, if requiring ventilation

Other treatment
- IV aminophylline unlikely to result in more bronchodilatation
- Routine antibiotics are not indicated. Infections precipitating asthmatic exacerbations are often viral in type

Intensive care referral
Deteriorating PEFR, persisting hypoxia, hypercapnoea, acidosis, exhaustion, feeble respiration, drowsiness, confusion, coma, and respiratory arrest.

Further reading

www.sign.ac.uk/guidelines Scottish Intercollegiate Guidelines Network. British guideline on the management of asthma, 2005.

Murphy VE, Gibson PG, Smith R, Clifton VL. Asthma during pregnancy: mechanisms and treatment implications. *European Respiratory Journal* 2005; **25**:735–50.

Powrie R. Respiratory disease. In: James DK, Steer PJ, Weiner CP, Gonik B (eds). *High Risk Pregnancy Management Options*. Elsevier Saunders: Philadelphia, 2005.

7.11 Granulomatous disease

Tuberculosis in pregnancy

Incidence
- In 2007, the overall incidence in the UK was 15/100 000 population
- TB rate in the UK-born population has remained stable since 2000 but rate in the non-UK-born is increasing
- Most cases occur in young adults age 15–44 years
- In London in 2000, the incidence of TB in pregnancy was 143 in 100 000; all infected patients were recent immigrants without HIV

Aetiology
- *Mycobacterium tuberculosis* (commonest), *bovis*, and *africanum*
- *M. microti* does not cause human disease
- Spread from person to person via inhaled droplet nuclei

Clinical features
- 20% of infected pregnant women are asymptomatic, and others are more likely to have non-specific symptoms. Delay in diagnosis is more common
- Commonest site for TB in pregnancy is pulmonary
- There is a well established link between extrapulmonary TB and immigrants to the UK. Extrapulmonary TB also occurs in 60% of patients with concomitant HIV
- Symptoms—cough, weight loss, fatigue, fever, night sweats, haemoptysis, altered bowel habit, and lymph node swelling
- Have high index of suspicion in recent immigrant with non-specific symptoms

Effect of pregnancy on TB
- Pregnancy does not increase the risk of TB
- Prognosis similar to non-pregnant women provided no delay in diagnosis and treatment begun early

Effect of TB on pregnancy
Depends on site and time of diagnosis related to delivery

Site of TB
- Pulmonary—most problems, increased risk of low birth weight, preterm birth, and perinatal mortality
- Lymph node TB—no adverse outcome
- Genital tract TB—congenital TB infection
- Other—increased hospitalization and low birth weight

Time of diagnosis
- Maternal and fetal outcome improved by early diagnosis
- Preterm birth and perinatal mortality increased if diagnosed after first trimester
- Undiagnosed or untreated—infant and maternal mortality is 30–40%. Increased risk of congenital TB in baby
- Some studies report increased miscarriage, pre-eclampsia, and difficult labour requiring intervention

Investigations
- Tuberculin skin test (TST) such as Mantoux, using purified protein derivative (PPD) of *M. tuberculosis*, is valid and safe in pregnancy. Does not differentiate latent infection and active TB
- Intradermal PPD injection into an infected person provokes a cell-mediated delayed-type hypersensitivity reaction, and zone of induration.
    - 0–4 mm: negative test, do not give BCG (live vaccination) in pregnancy. Repeat TST after delivery
    - 5–10 mm: doubtful positive. Interferon-γ blood test may be performed if known recent exposure or HIV-positive. If no recent exposure, re-test after 3 months
    - >10 mm: positive test

- TB-specific immune-based blood tests (interferon-γ)— more sensitive and specific at detecting TB; a recent test and not available in all units. Use TST before the blood test, if needed
- CXR with abdominal shielding is indicated in women with positive TST and interferon-γ tests
- Sputum sample for smear, PCR testing, culture, and drug sensitivity test in women with positive TST and CXR suggestive of TB or pulmonary symptoms. Treatment should be started if sputum test is positive
- Extrapulmonary TB should be investigated in consultation with the local TB specialists

Treatment
- Uncomplicated TB in pregnancy: 2-month isoniazid, rifampicin, pyrazinamide, and ethambutol, followed by a 4-month course of isoniazid and rifampicin
- Isoniazid—hepatitis, peripheral neuropathy, skin reaction
- Rifampicin—hepatitis, fever, nausea, orange secretions
- Pyrazinamide—hepatitis, thrombocytopenia, nephrotoxicity, interstitial nephritis
- Ethambutol—peripheral neuropathy, retrobulbar neuritis
- Latent TB infection (positive TST but no active disease) —delay treatment until after delivery
- TB prophylaxis with isoniazid for a total of 6–9 months should be given to pregnant women who have
    - HIV infection and exposure to an active case of TB
    - HIV infection and a doubtful TST (≥5 mm)
    - Doubtful positive TST and exposure to active TB case

Management of TB in pregnancy
- Commonly used anti-TB drugs are not teratogenic and safe in pregnancy
- Untreated TB is associated with a greater risk to the mother and fetus than TB treatment
- In drug-resistant TB, fetal risks of second line anti-TB drugs are unknown

Perform contact tracing among family members and other close contacts to ensure that others are not infected.

Other tests
HIV testing, baseline liver function test (LFT), serum creatinine, platelet count, visual acuity, and red–green discrimination tests before starting treatment.

Treatment in pregnancy
- Pyridoxine (vitamin B6) supplement 25–50 mg/day should be given to pregnant or lactating women taking isoniazid
- Review monthly for LFT and sputum smear and culture until two consecutive negative specimens on culture
- Vitamin K from 36 weeks onwards to reduce the risk of haemorrhagic disease of the newborn
- No specific management for labour and delivery

Postpartum management
Encourage breastfeeding in HIV-seronegative women.
- The baby cannot be infected via breast milk. The exception is the rare tuberculous mastitis
- Small amounts of anti-TB drugs in breast milk do not cause newborn toxicity, nor are they effective treatment
- Continue pyridoxine supplements
- Baby should be given BCG as between 70–80% effective at reducing the risk of developing active disease (typically extrapulmonary lymph node and meningeal TB)

Infectious risk
- Only pulmonary TB is potentially infectious, particularly with a positive sputum smear
- Usually non-infectious after 2 weeks of rifampicin and isoniazid

Babies of sputum-positive mothers diagnosed near delivery should receive TB prophylaxis, followed by TST at 6–12 weeks.
- If negative TST, stop TB prophylaxis and give BCG
- If positive TST and child is well, treat for 6 months

Prepregnancy
Advise delay until TB treatment is completed.

Sarcoidosis

A multisystem granulomatous disease of unknown cause, characterized by non-caseating epithelioid granulomas.

Prevalence
- 20/100 000 UK population, females more than males
- Peak incidence in third and fourth decades of life
- Higher prevalence in Afro-Caribbean women (3–4-fold)

Clinical features
Many clinical patterns as may involve many systems.
- Main site—lung involment is visible on CXR in 85–90% of cases, with bilateral hilar lymphadenopathy and multiple shadows all over the lung fields. Symptoms include progressive dyspnoea, cough, chest pain, fever, fatigue, and weight loss. Clinically difficult to differentiate from TB

Other sites:
- Skin (34%): erythema nodosum, lupus pernio
- Eyes (27%): iridocyclitis, chorioretinitis, keratoconjunctivitis
- Extrarenal calcitriol synthesis $\Rightarrow$ hypercalciuria $\pm$ hypercalcaemia
- Brain (5%): affects pituitary and hypothalamus
- Heart: arrhythmia and cardiomyopathy
- Joint: arthropathy
- Jaundice, hepatomegaly, splenomegaly

Microscopic features
- Non-caseating epithelioid granuloma
- Giant cells, including Langhan's type
- Calcium-rich inclusions in some giant cells
- Asteroid bodies and conchoid (Schaumann) bodies

Investigations and diagnosis
- Hypercalcaemia may be present
- Normal FBC, ESR, LFT, alkaline phosphatase, phosphate
- Tuberculin skin test negative
- Kveim test—intradermal injection of sarcoid tissue extraction, followed by a skin biopsy 6 weeks later. A non-caseating granuloma in biopsy is diagnostic

Effect of pregnancy on sarcoidosis
- Pregnancy does not affect the course of disease

Effect of sarcoidosis on pregnancy
- Does not cause adverse maternal or fetal outcome unless there is pulmonary hypertension or fibrosis, or hypoxaemia
- Steroids may ↑ gestational hypertension and diabetes
- Chronic maternal hypoxia ⇒ fetal growth restriction (FGR), fetal loss, and preterm delivery
- Maternal hypercalcaemia leads to:
  - Suppression of fetal parathyroid gland and increased risk of permanent hypoparathyroidism in neonate
  - Delayed neonatal hypocalcaemia and tetany (usually 5–14 days after birth)

Treatment and prognosis
Depend on severity.
- Stage 1—bilateral hilar adenopathy
- Stage 2—bilateral hilar adenopathy + interstitial infiltrates
- Stage 3—interstitial disease with shrinking hilar nodes
- Stage 4—advanced fibrosis

Up to 75% of stage 1 and 2 disease self-resolve. Stage 3 and 4 disease require treatment with steroid therapy.

Management
Antenatal management
Reassure sarcoidosis does not cause adverse outcomes unless severe.

In *pulmonary hypertension*, advise to avoid pregnancy.

Assess cardiorespiratory status:
- Obtain O_2 saturation level at rest and with exercise
- Pulmonary function test (PFT), including a diffusing capacity for carbon dioxide (DL_{CO})
- CXR

Blood tests: FBC, LFT, urea and creatinine, calcium level (repeat blood tests each trimester).

Echocardiogram for pulmonary hypertension.

Review by *anaesthetists*.
- Monitor disease progression.
- Repeat the above blood tests each trimester

Initiate steroid therapy if significant disease progression.

Reassess cardiorespiratory status in patients complaining of worsening dyspnoea or development of other symptoms, with O_2 saturation levels, PFT, CXR, blood tests.

In *women with hypercalcaemia*:
- Advise ↑ fluid intake, ↓ oral calcium, avoid vitamin D or phosphate supplements and maintain electrolyte balance
- Calcitonin does not cross the placenta and has been used to lower calcium levels in pregnancy

In severe disease: *fetal surveillance* with serial growth scans.

Intrapartum management
- If prednisolone >7.5 mg/day for >2 weeks, there is a theoretical risk of hypothalamic–pituitary–adrenal suppression. Parenteral hydrocortisone 100 mg 6-hourly in labour
- Avoid inhalation anaesthesia if substantial parenchymal disease
- High block conduction anaesthesia may cause significant respiratory compromise

Postpartum management
- In women with hypercalcaemia: give calcium supplementation to the neonate and observe for neonatal tetany
- Encourage breastfeeding
- Contraceptive advice

Further reading

www.hpa.org.uk Health Protection Agency. Pregnancy and tuberculosis: Guidance for clinicians. TB4Pr/baby leaflet, 2006.

www.hpa.org.uk Focus on Tuberculosis. Annual surveillance report 2006 England, Wales and Northern Ireland. PublicationID= 62.

Llewelyn M, Cropley I, Wilkinson RJ, Davidson RN. Tuberculous diagnosed during pregnancy: a prospective study from London. *Thorax* 2000: **55**:129–32.

Powrie R. Respiratory disease. In: James DK, Steer PJ, Weiner CP, Gonik B (eds). *High Risk Pregnancy Management Options*, Elsevier Saunders: Philadelphia, 2005: 828–64.

7.12 Cystic fibrosis

Definition
Cystic fibrosis (CF) is an autosomal recessive, multisystem disorder caused by deranged chloride transport.

Incidence
- 1: 2000 live births
- 1: 20 Caucasians are heterozygous for the CF gene
- Rare in African and Chinese populations
- CF in pregnancy increasing as more survive to adulthood

Pathophysiology
- CF gene, on the long arm of chromosome 7, codes for 168-kDa CF transmembrane regulator protein (CFTR)
- CFTR is a complex chloride channel found in the lungs, pancreas, liver, biliary tract, gut, reproductive tract, choroid plexus, heart, and renal tubules
- CFTR influences cellular functions such as sodium transport across the respiratory epithelium, cell surface glycoprotein composition, and antibacterial defences
- There are >900 disease-related mutations of the CF gene. The commonest in Caucasians is ΔF508 (70% of cases)
- Deranged chloride transport ⇒ thick, viscous secretions and a high sweat sodium concentration

Lungs
- Disordered epithelium in nose, paranasal sinuses, and intrapulmonary conducting airways but normal alveolar function
- Airway surface is dehydrated and mucociliary clearance is reduced
- Changes in salt concentration and cell surface glycoproteins promotes bacterial colonization and reduces bacterial clearance, leading to inflammatory lung damage, bronchiectasis, and small airway narrowing
- Over 70% of CF adults have chronic chest infection with *Pseudomonas aeruginosa. Burkholderia cepacia* infection is associated with accelerated pulmonary deterioration
- Respiratory failure is the commonest cause of death

Pancreas
Normal synthesis of pancreatic enzymes. Dehydration of secretions. Stagnation in the pancreatic ducts with subsequent malabsorption, progressive destruction of the pancreas and Islet cells, resulting in insulin deficiency.

Biliary tract
Dehydrated bile leads to plugging, chronic local damage, biliary cirrhosis, and extrahepatic biliary stenoses.

Gastrointestinal tract
High sodium, viscous gastric secretions, and altered fluid movement across intestine, compounded by dehydrated biliary and pancreatic secretions, and alterations in the osmotic load in the lumen secondary to pancreatic exocrine failure ⇒ meconium ileus in neonates and distal intestinal obstruction syndrome in adults.

Reproduction
- All mutations linked with congenital absence of the vas deferens and male infertility
- Rarer mutations linked with isolated male infertility and no other evidence of CF disease
- Female infertility owing to malnutrition-related amenorrhoea and production of abnormal viscous cervical mucus

Diagnosis
Two abnormal sweat test results but molecular diagnosis is rapidly replacing this.

Effect of pregnancy on CF
Patients may become emaciated owing to the increased nutritional demands of pregnancy.

Effect of CF on pregnancy
- CF carriers are healthy, normal pregnancy outcomes
- CF disease outcomes depend on the severity of lung disease, pancreatic function, and presence of diabetes
- ↑ risk of maternal death with severe lung disease
- ↑ risk of gestational diabetes
- Chronic hypoxia ⇒ fetal growth restriction (FGR), fetal death, prematurity
- Malnutrition may lead to FGR

Management
Prepregnancy management
Refer for genetic counselling
- Information about ethnicity is important
- Genetic testing is appropriate if:
  - Either partner has CF
  - Two carriers are contemplating a pregnancy
  - Either partner is a CF carrier
  - A relative has CF or is a carrier of CF
- Identify the specific gene mutation
- Determine the partner's carrier status
- Advise patient that screening tests will identify 90% of CF mutations. A negative test does not completely exclude CF, especially in a non-Caucasian patient

Prenatal diagnosis
- If the mutation is identified, this may be performed with chorionic villus sampling or amniocentesis
- Counsel about the risk of miscarriage
- If the fetus has CF, there is no cure. The patient may opt for termination, although life expectancy has significantly increased with early diagnosis and modern treatments

Alternatives to prenatal diagnosis
- Artificial insemination using donor sperm
- Artificial insemination using egg donation fertilized with the father's sperm and embryo transfer
- Preimplantation genetic diagnosis

Assess and optimize nutritional status
- BMI <18 is a relative contraindication to pregnancy
- Give nutritional advice
- Give pancreatic enzyme replacement to aid absorption
- Review diabetic status with probable conversion to insulin if on oral hypoglycaemic agents

Assess cardiopulmonary status
- Advise against pregnancy if pulmonary hypertension or if FEV_1 <50% predicted
- Examine for pulmonary hypertension (↑ jugular venous pressure, left parasternal heave, loud second heart sound)
- Check O_2 saturation and arterial blood gas (ABG)
- Pulmonary function test
- Echocardiogram for pulmonary hypertension

Optimize lung function
- Physiotherapy to clear mucus from the lungs
- Antibiotics to control infection and lung damage

Antenatal management

- Multidisciplinary care, including chest therapists, nutritionists, and GPs. Inform paediatricians if offspring is at risk of CF and prenatal diagnosis was not performed or if the offspring has CF
- Assess cardiopulmonary status. Termination offered if pulmonary hypertension or FEV_1 <50% predicted
- Optimize nutritional and lung function. Enteral feeding may be required in hyperemesis or decreasing weight
- Counsel that:
  - Malnutrition may cause FGR
  - Pulmonary exacerbations may cause preterm birth
  - Bronchodilators are safe in pregnancy
- Screen for gestational diabetes and treat if diabetic (see Section 7.15)
- Pulmonary hypertension (see Section 7.9)
- Fetal surveillance: serial ultrasound scan for growth

Intrapartum management

- Aim for vaginal delivery
- Monitor O_2 saturation. Provide O_2 if required
- Central haemodynamic monitoring if pulmonary hypertension
- Assisted vaginal delivery for maternal exhaustion
- Avoid general anaesthesia

Postpartum management

- Monitor respiratory function
- Encourage breastfeeding
- Contraceptive advice
- Neonatal population screening for CF is offered as part of first week 'Guthrie test' in some areas. Test measures immunoreactive trypsin assays on blood spots
- A sweat test is used if the baby is >2 months old

Further reading

Powrie R. Cystic fibrosis. In: James DK, Steer PJ, Weiner CP, Gonik B (eds). *High Risk Pregnancy Management Options*. Elsevier Saunders: Philadelphia, 2005:845–8.

Warrell D, Cox TM, Firth JD, Benz EJ. Cystic fibrosis. In: *Oxford Textbook of Medicine*. Oxford University Press, 2004.

Myotonic dystrophy

Definition
Degenerative neuromuscular and neuroendocrine condition characterized by progressive distal muscle weakness and wasting.

Incidence
Pregnancy in severely affected women is rare.

Aetiology
Autosomal dominant inherited disorder.

Clinical features
- Progressive muscular dystrophy and muscle weakness
- Myotonia (delay in muscle relaxation after contraction)
- Myopathic facies
- Cardiac disease—conduction defects, arrhythmia, congestive cardiac failure
- Pneumonia and hypoventilation
- Frontal alopecia, cataracts
- Mental retardation

Effect of pregnancy on myotonic dystrophy
- May be asymptomatic, present for the first time in pregnancy, or have exacerbations, mainly third trimester
- Rapid improvement after delivery

Effect of myotonic dystrophy on pregnancy
- Increased risk of first and second trimester miscarriage
- Polyhydramnios (associated with an affected fetus)
- Preterm birth (polyhydramnios and myotonic uterus)
- Perinatal death
- Placenta praevia
- Postpartum haemorrhage (PPH), owing to uterine atony

Congenital myotonic dystrophy
- Only in babies of mothers with myotonic dystrophy
- Generalized hypotonia and weakness, no myotonia
- Difficulty breathing, sucking, and swallowing
- Talipes and arthrogryposis (multiple joint contractures caused by fetal akinesia)
- Mental retardation
- Poor prognosis with delayed developmental milestones

Management
Antenatal management
- *Genetic counselling*: discuss prenatal diagnosis using DNA linkage analysis. Discuss risk of chorionic villus sampling (CVS) or amniocentesis
- *Assess maternal cardiorespiratory status*: ECG, pulmonary function test and educate about symptoms of arrhythmia
- Encourage physical activity
- Serial ultrasound scan to assess amniotic fluid volume
- Referral to anaesthetists and inform paediatricians

Intrapartum management
- Uterine myotonia may result in dysfunctional labour
- Assisted vaginal delivery if significant maternal weakness
- Avoid general anaesthesia and non-depolarizing neuromuscular blocking drugs
- Avoid respiratory depressants such as opiates which may exacerbate pulmonary hypoventilation
- Anticipate PPH—active management of third stage
- Paediatrician to be present at delivery

Myasthenia gravis

Prevalence
The prevalence of myasthenia gravis (MG) is 2–10 per 100 000 population. Female:male = 2:1. Onset usually in the second or third decade of life.

Pathophysiology
Autoimmune disease affecting the nicotinic neuromuscular transmission, resulting in varying weakness of skeletal muscle.

Between 85–90% of patients have anti-acetylcholine receptor antibodies (anti-AchR) which block neuromuscular transmission at the postsynaptic level of the neuromuscular junction. 75% have thymic lymph follicle hyperplasia, and 15% have lymphoblastic or epithelial thymic tumours. Thymectomy results in remission in 35% and improvement in 50%.

Clinical features
- Disease is characterized by a relapsing–remitting course
- Diplopia, ptosis, dysphagia, fluctuating weakness of skeletal muscles without reflex loss, sensory loss, or poor coordination
- Worsened by stress, illness, fever, and certain drugs

Diagnosis
Tensilon test: administration of edrophonium chloride (short-acting anticholinesterase) transiently improves symptoms.

Effect of pregnancy on myasthenia gravis
- 40% deteriorate, 30% improve, 30% worsen postpartum
- Exacerbation less likely if prior thymectomy

Effect of myasthenia gravis on pregnancy and labour
- No difference in miscarriage and fetal death rates
- Increased risk of preterm birth and low birth weight
- First stage—no change as the uterus is smooth muscle
- Second stage—may be affected by weak maternal expulsive effort but no change in the average length of labour
- Transplacental anti-AchR passage may cause the following:

Neonatal MG (affects 10–20% neonates)
Hypotonia, weak cry, difficulty feeding, and respiration. Respond to edrophonium. Transient: onset in 48 h, resolves in 2 months.

Arthrogryposis multiplex congenita (rare)
Lack of fetal movement result in multiple joint contractures, pulmonary hypoplasia, and polyhydramnios.

Management
Prepregnancy
- Multidisciplinary consultation (obstetricians, paediatrician, neurologists, and anaesthetists)
- Recently diagnosed MG patients tend to progress from ocular to generalized skeletal muscle involvement over 1–2 years. Advise postponing pregnancy until remission
- Consider thymectomy in symptomatic patients
- Discuss the risk of exacerbation in pregnancy and postpartum, preterm birth, and neonatal MG

Antenatal
- Identify and treat infections promptly
- Treatment with anti-acetylcholinesterase (pyridostigmine, neostigmine). If increased dose is required, best done by reducing the dose intervals before increasing each dose
- In myasthenic crisis, assisted ventilation is required
- Cholinergic crisis (drug overdose)—nausea, vomiting, cramping pain, diarrhoea, excess salivation and sweating, severe weakness (depolarizing block), bradycardia, respiratory failure

- Some patients need immunosuppression with steroids, azathioprine and cyclosporin, which should be continued thoughout pregnancy and postpartum
- Plasmapharesis and IV IgG can be used if refractory
- Thymectomy is not recommended in pregnancy
- Fetal surveillance for arthrogryposis multiplex congenita
- Anaesthetic review

Intrapartum
- Aim for vaginal delivery
- Instrumental may be required to prevent exhaustion
- Parenteral treatment owing to delayed gastric emptying
- Safe—epidural anaesthesia, amide type local anaesthetics
- Avoid—aminoglycosides, magnesium sulphate, beta-blockers, beta-agonists, narcotics, and neuromuscular blockers

Postpartum
Review dosage and watch for neonatal MG.

Multiple sclerosis

Prevalence
- 1:1000 population
- Female: male = 2:1
- Rises with increasing latitude

Aetiology
- An autoimmune disease resulting in multifocal demyelination of the central nervous system (CNS)
- There are multiple areas of inflammation and demyelination in the brain and spinal cord, associated with an increased helper: suppressor T cell ratio
- There is a genetic element which is associated with specific human leukocyte antigens
- Concordance of MS among monozygotic twins is 30% and 2% among dizygotic twins

Clinical features
- May present with any CNS symptom
- Commonly, there is visual loss, diplopia, vertigo, paraesthesia, poor coordination, spasticity, tremors, bladder incontinence, and fatigue
- 85% have relapsing–remitting disease
- 15% have progressive disease from onset

Diagnosis
MS is a clinical diagnosis. No specific test.

Investigations to help confirm diagnosis include:
- MRI to detect lesions compatible with demyelination
- Lumbar puncture to evaluate cerebrospinal fluid for the presence of oligoclonal bands

- Serum IgM antibodies against myelin-based protein
- Visually evoked responses (EEG test for slowed reponse to flickering patterns in optic neuritis)

Most patients have a previous established diagnosis.

Effect of pregnancy on MS
- Pregnancy or breastfeeding have no effect on MS
- Relapse rate decreases, especially in third trimester, possibly because of decreased cell-mediated immunity and increased humoral immunity in pregnancy
- Between 20 and 40% of patients relapse during postpartum period

Effect of MS on pregnancy
- No adverse effect on pregnancy, labour, and delivery
- No effect on miscarriage, congenital anomaly or stillbirth
- Risk of developing MS in offspring: 3%

Management
Prepregnancy
- Joint consultation with obstetrician and neurologist
- Consider withdrawing treatment if in remission
- Discuss risk of exacerbation postpartum and the increased risk of offspring developing MS

Antenatal
- Monitor for relapse or worsening disease activity
- Identify and treat infections promptly. Patients with bladder symptoms should be screened regularly. Acute relapses may be treated with IV corticosteroids
- Long-term immunosuppression with azathioprine
- Avoid prophylaxis (beta-interferon, glatiramer)
- Physiotherapy and stretching exercises

Intrapartum
- Aim for a vaginal delivery. Instrumental vaginal delivery may be required to prevent exhaustion
- Give IV hydrocortisone in labour if antenatal steroids
- No contraindication to regional or general anaesthesia

Postpartum
Watch for relapse.

Further reading

Bennett KA. Pregnancy and multiple sclerosis. *Clin Obstet Gynecol* 2005; **48(1)**:38–47.

Flint Porter T, Ware Branch D. Autoimmune diseases. In: James DK, Steer PJ, Weiner CP, Gonik B, (eds). *High Risk Pregnancy Management Options*. Elsevier Saunders: Philadelphia, 2005:975–8.

Stafford IP, Dildy GA. Myasthenia gravis and pregnancy. *Clin Obstet Gynecol* 2005; **48(1)**:48–56.

7.14 Epilepsy

Definitions

Epileptic seizure—a sudden alteration of consciousness, motor, sensory, autonomic or psychic events owing to abnormal excessive or synchronous neuronal activity in the brain.

Epilepsy—a brain disorder characterized by a predisposition to generate two or more epileptic seizures, unprovoked by any immediate identifiable cause.

Status epilepticus—a single seizure lasting more than 30 min or recurrent seizures without recovery of consciousness between episodes.

Sudden unexpected death in epilepsy (SUDEP)—sudden, unexpected, non-traumatic, and non-drowning death in epileptic patient, with or without evidence of a seizure, and excluding status epilepticus, where post mortem does not reveal a toxicological or anatomical cause for death.

Classification of seizures
- Primary generalized (tonic–clonic or absence or myoclonic)
- Partial or secondary generalized (complex partial)
- Temporal lobe

Prevalence
- 1% of population; 0.5% of pregnancies
- Commonest neurological problem in pregnancy

Aetiology of epilepsy
Idiopathic (most cases)
- Most patients have a prepregnancy diagnosis
- 30% have a positive family history

Secondary epilepsy caused by:
- Previous trauma or surgery to the brain
- Antiphospholipid syndrome
- Intracranial mass lesions
- Pregnancy (gestational epilepsy)

Other causes of seizures in pregnancy/puerperium
- *Infections*—meningitis, encephalitis, brain abscess, cerebral malaria, tuberculoma, toxoplasmosis
- *Vascular disease*—eclampsia, hypertensive encephalopathy, stroke, subarachnoid haemorrhage, cerebral vein thrombosis, thrombotic thrombocytopenic purpura
- *Metabolic*—hyponatraemia, hypoglycaemia, hypocalcaemia, liver failure, renal failure, drug and alcohol withdrawal
- *Drug toxicity*—local anaesthetics, tricyclic antidepressants, amphetamines, and lithium
- **Postdural puncture**
- **Pseudoepilepsy**

Effect of epilepsy on pregnancy
- ↑ risk of fetal congenital anomaly, mainly secondary to the use of antiepileptic drugs in pregnancy
- ↑ risk of epilepsy in offspring: one affected parent = 4%, one sibling = 10%, both parents = 15%
- ↑ risk of fetal hypoxia with repeated or prolonged seizures
- No difference in miscarriage or obstetric outcomes
- Maternal death—there were 11 indirect deaths from epilepsy in the UK in 2003–2005, of which six were classified as SUDEP

Fetal and neonatal effects of anti-epileptic drugs (AED)
The background congenital anomaly rate is 2–3%.

Congenital anomaly rate is higher in babies born to:
- Epileptic mothers compared to non-epileptic mothers (II)
- Treated compared to untreated epileptic mothers (II). Congenital anomaly rate with a single antiepileptic drug (AED) use is 6–8%
- Mothers taking polytherapy compared to monotherapy (II)

Over 90% of mothers on AED have normal children.

A genetic predisposition may also be the cause of anomalies.

Major anomalies
- Neural tube defects—1–2% valproate, 1% carbamazepine
- Cleft lip/palate—phenytoin, phenobarbitone, carbamazepine
- Cardiac defects—phenytoin, phenobarbitone, valproate
- Urogenital defects—phenytoin, phenobarbitone, valproate
- Further studies from collaborative pregnancy registries are needed, but most published evidence suggests that valproate, especially at higher dose, is associated with an increased rate of congenital malformations compared to other AEDs
- An overlap exists in the AED type used and a particular congenital anomaly

Minor anomalies
- V-shaped eyebrows, epicanthal folds, hypertelorism, low-set ears, flat nasal bridge, long philtrum, microstomia, prominent lower lip, irregular teeth, hypoplastic nails, and/or distal digits

Non-teratogenic effects
- Neonatal withdrawal effects (poor feeding, seizures)
- Neonatal coagulopathies associated with raised level of prothrombin induced by vitamin K absence (PIVKA) (II)
- Early onset developmental delay with polytherapy (II)
- Increased childhood neuroblastoma (III)

Effect of pregnancy on epilepsy
- Seizure frequency—increased in 37% (highest risk in the peripartum period), decreased in 13%; no change in 50%

Increased seizure frequency may be caused by hormonal influence, ↓ serum AED level (vomiting, malabsorption, increased liver and renal AED clearance), emotional stress, sleep deprivation, non-compliance to AED owing to teratogenic fear and/or hyperventilation during labour.
- Unknown whether pregnancy increases SUDEP

Management
Prepregnancy management
- Joint counselling from obstetricians and neurologists
- Benefits of seizure control outweigh the risks of fetal anomalies, neurodevelopmental or cognitive outcomes
- Consider AED withdrawal if seizure-free for more than 2 years on minimal AED dose and negative EEG
- Risk factors for relapse/deterioration in pregnancy—seizure ≥1/month, multiple seizure types, tonic–clonic or prolonged seizures, juvenile myoclonic seizure (AED should be continued), positive EEG
- AED withdrawal should be done 6 months before pregnancy. The patient should not drive during this period
- If AED required, use monotherapy at the lowest dose needed to achieve seizure control. The lowest serum AED level that prevents seizure should be determined. Use divided AED doses or slow-release preparation to reduce fetal effects. Avoid valproate
- High-dose folic acid supplementation 5 mg/day

Antenatal management
- Women presenting already pregnant on AED should remain on their current medication

- Regular checks of seizure control. In women who have seizures, monitor serum AED levels in each trimester and the last month of pregnancy.
- Raise AED dose to maintain effective serum AED levels
- Safety advice:
  - Take showers rather than baths
  - Ensure that relatives/partners know how to place the woman in the recovery position during a seizure
- Assess for AED toxicity clinically: ataxia, drowsiness, slurred speech, vertigo, and nystagmus
- Continue folic acid supplementation throughout pregnancy owing to a small risk of folate-deficiency anaemia
- Prenatal screening for congenital anomalies:
  - Anomaly scan at 18–20 weeks
  - Fetal cardiac scan at 22 weeks
- In women on AED, commence oral vitamin K 10 mg/day from 36 weeks to prevent neonatal coagulopathies

Intrapartum management
- Epilepsy is not an indication for IOL or CS. Consider CS with uncontrolled epilepsy or status epilepticus for fetal reasons
- Between 1–2% will have seizures during labour. Women should deliver in hospital and should not be left unattended
- Limit the risk of seizure with early, effective pain relief

Postpartum management
- Give neonates vitamin K 1 mg IM to avoid coagulopathy
- Breasfeeding is not contraindicated with AEDs
- Watch for neonatal sedation and withdrawal with phenobarbitone or benzodiazepines
- Check serum AED. Physiological changes postpartum may cause raised AED level. If AED dose was raised in pregnancy, this should be gradually returned to pre-pregnancy dose (IV)
- Between 1–2% will have seizures on the first postpartum day
- Advise that new mothers:
  - Ask for extra help with sleep deprivation
  - Ensure supervision when bathing the baby
  - Feed and change the baby on the floor whilst sitting or leaning against a wall
- Check effective contraception before discharge home
- As the earliest documented ovulation after childbirth is 3 weeks, contraception should be used from 3 weeks
- Hepatic enzyme-inducing AEDs (phenytoin, primidone, phenobarbitone, carbamazepine) reduce contraceptive efficacy of oestrogens and progestogens, thus avoid low-dose progestogen-only pill or combined pill
- Consider medroxyprogesterone injections (Depot-Provera) 8-weekly instead of 12-weekly or subdermal implant (Implanon)
- Mirena IUS or intrauterine copper device are effective and may be inserted from 6 weeks postpartum

Status epilepticus
- Is a medical emergency
- Intubation and ventilation
- Intravenous phenytoin
- Involve physicians and neurologists
- If antenatal, deliver when stable

Box 7.11 Safety of common antiepileptic drugs
- FDA Category D (teratogenic)—phenytoin, primidone, phenobarbitone, carbamazepine, and sodium valproate
- FDA Category C (risk in animals)—vigabatrin and topiramate
- FDA Category B (no animal risk)—levetiracetam, gabapentin, and tiagabine

Box 7.12 Investigations of a first seizure in pregnancy
- Detailed neurological history and examination
- Take bloods for FBC, U&E, uric acid, LFT, glucose, calcium, clotting screen, blood film
- CT or MRI of the brain
- Lumbar puncture if infection suspected and an intracranial mass effect has been ruled out by imaging studies
- EEG

Box 7.13 What to do during a seizure
- **Call for help**—obstetricians, anaesthetists, midwives, porters. Involve consultants early
- **Avoid injury**—secure a safe environment around the patient, do not restrain patient
- **Recovery position** to prevent aspiration and aortocaval compression
- **Maintain airway**
- **Administer oxygen**—monitor O_2 saturation levels
- **Observe duration and type of seizure**
- **Control seizure**—think eclampsia until proven otherwise (see Section 10.3). Most seizures are of short duration.

If known epileptic and the seizure is not self-limiting, treat acutely with short-acting benzodiazepines rectally or intravenously (lorazepam, clonazepam, diazepam).

If epileptic frequency is increased despite taking AED, check serum AED level
- **Clinical observations**—pulse, BP, temperature, respirations, oxygen saturation, urinalysis, hourly urine output
- **Transfer to labour ward and monitor fetus**
- **Deliver** when stable if maternal or fetal compromise

Further reading
Perkin GD. Epilepsy in later childhood and adults. In: Warrell D, Cox TM, Firth JD, Benz EJ (eds). *Oxford Textbook of Medicine*. Oxford University Press, 2004.

www.cochrane.org Adab N, Tudur Smith C, Vinten J, Williamson PR, Winterbottom JB. Common antiepileptic drugs in pregnancy in women with epilepsy. *Cochrane Database of Systematic Reviews* 2004, No. CD004848.

Carbuapoma JR, Tomlinson MW, Levine SR. Neurologic disorders. In: James DK, Steer PJ, Weiner CP, Gonik B (eds). *High Risk Pregnancy Management Options*. Elsevier Saunders: Philadelphia, 2005:1061–97.

7.15 Diabetes in pregnancy

Physiological changes in pregnancy
See Section 6.2.

Pre-existing diabetes mellitus
Diabetes mellitus (DM) is a metabolic disease of hyperglycaemia owing to defects in insulin secretion, action, or both.

Prevalence
DM is becoming commoner: 0.4% of pregnancies.
- Type 1 (T1DM)—insulin-dependent: 0.3%
- Type 2 (T2DM)—non-insulin-dependent: 0.1%

Aetiology of type 1 DM (insulin deficiency)
- Autoimmune disease: presence of islet-cell antibodies
- Strong genetic component: HLA-DR3 and DR4
- Possible viral component with seasonal distribution

Aetiology of type 2 DM (insulin resistance)
- Less strong genetic component than T1DM
- Incidence ↑ with age and obesity

Complications of chronic hyperglycaemia
- Infections—candida, staphylococcus (skin)
- Macrovascular arterial disease—coronary, cerebral, peripheral
- Lower life expectancy as risk of stroke (2x) and MI (4x)
- Microvascular—retinopathy, nephropathy, neuropathy

Effect of pregnancy on pre-existing DM—maternal
Pregnancy risks are the same for T1DM and T2DM.

↑ Hypoglycaemic attacks
- More often in early pregnancy owing to ↑ insulin sensitivity, tighter blood glucose (BG) control or 'hypoglycaemic unawareness'
- Every 1% ↓ in HbA1c ⇒ 33% ↑ hypoglycaemic attacks
- All 3 DM maternal deaths 2000–2002 due to hypoglycaemia

↑ Insulin requirement, especially 28–32 weeks and T1DM.

Diabetic ketoacidosis may be caused by hyperemesis, infections, use of β-agonists or steroids for fetal lung maturity.

Progression in retinopathy (2-fold):
- May develop for the first time in pregnancy
- 10% risk of progression with mild retinopathy
- 50% risk of progression with proliferative retinopathy
- ↑ risk with hypertension and pre-eclampsia
- Related to insulin sensitivity in early pregnancy, tight BG control and ↑ retinal blood flow

Progression in nephropathy (see Section 7.19):
- Definition—proteinuria >0.3 g/day before 20 weeks
- ↑ proteinuria >20 weeks gestation
- No long-term effect with mild renal impairment
- If severe renal impairment (serum creatinine >177 μmol/l), the risk of end-stage renal disease is 33%
- Hypertension occurs in 30% with nephropathy. The risk of deterioration ↑ with hypertension

Autonomic neuropathy and gastric paresis progress.

Normochromic normocytic anaemia may only respond to treatment with recombinant erythropoietin.

Effect of pre-existing DM on pregnancy—fetal
↑ miscarriage related to poorly controlled DM
↑ major congenital abnormality 42/1000 births
- Congenital heart defects (3-fold ↑ risk)

- Neural tube defects (3-fold ↑ risk NTD)
- Situs inversus, renal anomalies—(agenesis, cystic kidney, duplex ureter), duodenal or anal atresia
- Sacral agenesis—rare but specific to DM

↑ risk of macrosomia (2-fold):
- Birth weight ≥4 kg or growth ≥90th centile for gestation
- Pedersen hypothesis—insulin is anabolic and growth-promoting. Maternal hyperglycaemia ⇒ fetal hyperglycaemia ⇒ fetal pancreatic β-cell hyperplasia and hyperinsulinaemia ⇒ macrosomia, organomegaly, and accelerated skeletal maturation
- No difference in birth weight between T1DM and T2DM
- 30% ↑ risk of macrosomia if mean postprandial whole BG >6.7. Birth weight is poorly correlated with HbA1c
- ↑ risk of traumatic delivery (10-fold ↑ Erb's palsy)
- Shoulder dystocia 8% versus 3% general population

↑ risk of preterm birth (5-fold)
- 2-fold increased risk of spontaneous preterm labour
- A 36% preterm birth rate (75% iatrogenic)
- ↑ risk of polyhydramnios ⇒ prelabour rupture of membranes and cord prolapse
- ↑ risk of neonatal admission: 30% of term babies, versus 10%

↑ risk of perinatal mortality and morbidity (4-fold)
- Attributed to maternal hyperglycaemia
- Babies of T1DM and T2DM have comparable risks
- 5-fold ↑ risk of stillbirth and 3-fold ↑ risk of neonatal mortality, mainly due to fatal congenital abnormalities
- Polycythaemia and jaundice as chronic hypoxia stimulates renal erythropoietin and delays HbF to HbA switch
- Risk of neonatal hypoglycaemia

↑ risk of unexplained stillbirth
- Possibly caused by chronic hypoxia/acidosis caused by fetal insulinaemia, increased fetal O_2 requirements, uteroplacental vasculopathy. Risk highest at term
- Maternal ketoacidosis has 20–50% stillbirth rate
- CTG, Doppler velocimetry or biophysical profiles do not predict or prevent unexplained stillbirth

Effect of pre-existing DM on pregnancy–maternal
↑risk of infection: urinary tract, kidney, respiratory, endometrial, wound, and vaginal candidiasis
↑ risk of hypertension
↑ risk of pre-eclampsia: 30% ↑ risk with hypertension and nephropathy related to glycaemic control at conception and first half of pregnancy. Each 1% increment in first trimester HbA1c ↑ the risk of pre-eclampsia by 60%. Each 1% fall in HbA1c before 20 weeks ↓ the risk by 40%

Outcome of nephropathy
Hypertension, 42%; pre-eclampsia, 41%; preterm birth, 22%; FGR, 15%; major anomalies, 8%; perinatal mortality, 5%

↑ risk of obstetric intervention
- Spontaneous vaginal delivery rate only 24%
- IOL rate of 39% versus 21% overall.
- Risk of CS (67%)
- IOL more likely to end with emergency CS (43%)
- Almost 50% of emergency CS caused by 'fetal distress'

Diagnosis of diabetes
A 2-h blood glucose after an oral glucose tolerance test (OGTT) with 75 g of anhydrous glucose intake (see Table 7.1).

Table 7.1

Blood glucose (mmol/l)	Fasting		2-h
Diabetes	≥7.0	**or**	≥11.1
Impaired glucose tolerance	<7.0	**and**	7.8–11.0

Table 7.2 Clinical and demographic features

	T1DM	T2DM
Median age onset	15 years	29 years
Ethnic group	90% white	50% white
Deprivation		Higher rates
Overweight	No	Usually
Symptoms	Thirst, polyuria	Asymptomatic

Management

Preconceptual management

Multidisciplinary care ideal

- Only 34% receive prepregnancy counselling
- Up to 40% of diabetic pregnancies may be unplanned

HbA1c used to measure long-term glycaemic control.

- Prepregnancy HbA1c is ↑ in fetal congenital abnormality, normally formed stillbirth, and neonatal death
- Risk of congenital abnormality is 5% with HbA1c <8%, and up to 25% with HbA1c >10%
- Good glucose control ↓ miscarriage and pre-eclampsia

Effective contraception advised until good glucose control.

Dietary advice: low-sugar, low-fat, high-fibre diet.

Folic acid: 5 mg/day up to 12 weeks' gestation to prevent NTD.

Retinal assessment: treat proliferative retinopathy.

Assess renal function (see Section 7.19):

- Check blood pressure, serum U&E, and urinalysis
- Quantify proteinuria with 24-h urinary collection
- ACE inhibitors if nephropathy until pregnancy confirmed
- Advise against pregnancy if serum creatinine ≥1.5 mg/dl (124 µmol/l) as 40% risk of rapid renal deterioration

Assess cardiovascular risks: stop statins before pregnancy.

Thyroid function: autoimmune disease associated with T1DM.

Counsel regarding risk of DM in offspring:

- Maternal T1DM: 2–3%, paternal T1DM: 6–9%, both parents T1DM: 20–30%

Pregnancy contraindicated: ischaemic heart disease, untreated proliferative retinopathy, severe gastroparesis, severe renal impairment (creatinine clearance <250 mmol/l).

Medication: switch women with T2DM to insulin. Avoid oral hypoglycaemic agents (sulphonylureas and biguanides) as these cross the placenta and cause fetal hypoglycaemia. Metformin has good safety data.

General measures: stop smoking, reduce weight if obese, check rubella immunity.

Antenatal management

Ultrasound scans. All diabetic women should be offered:

- First trimester scan for accurate dating
- Detailed anomaly scan at 18–22 weeks
- Serial growth scans in third trimester

In addition, should offer (depending on resources):

- Nuchal translucency scan at 11–14 weeks
- Detailed fetal cardiac scan at 22 weeks

Retinal assessment—in each trimester. Laser photocoagulation may be used to treat proliferative retinopathy.

Blood glucose monitoring—women should monitor BG levels regularly, preferably using glucose meters, and adjust their insulin dosage to achieve normal BG range. The targets are:

- HbA1c <7.0%
- Preprandial BG 3.5–5.9 mmol/l
- Postprandial BG <7.8 mmol/l. Pregnancy outcomes correlate better with postprandial BG level

Avoid starvation and severe calorie restriction because of the risk of ketoacidosis. Insulin should not be stopped during periods of illness or hyperemesis. The dose may need to be increased in the presence of infection.

Discuss hypoglycaemia

- Provide a glucagon kit and instructions to relatives and partners. Follow it by oral high glucose drink/food
- Ensure safe driving
- Women usually require a 'snack' mid-morning, mid-afternoon and before retiring at night

Check thyroid function in women with T1 DM.

Regular visits for BP and urinalysis to detect pre-eclampsia and UTI.

Nephropathy—regular U&E, creatinine clearance and 24-h urinary protein. Strict BP control to prevent ongoing renal damage.

Intrapartum management

Aim for spontaneous vaginal delivery by the EDD to minimize stillbirth risk if diabetes is well controlled and no pregnancy complications.

CS is recommended if estimated fetal weight (EFW) >4.5 kg. No evidence that IOL ↓ the risk of shoulder dystocia.

IV short-acting insulin and dextrose during labour:

- Follow agreed multidisciplinary protocol
- Separate giving sets to allow ↑ dextrose infusion and insulin cessation in the event of hypoglycaemia

Labour <34 weeks:

- Consider maternal corticosteroids
- β-agonists and corticosteroids ↑ insulin requirement
- Use insulin sliding scale to maintain BG
- Atosiban is preferable to β-agonists if tocolysis is required

Advise continuous CTG monitoring; FBS as per usual indications.

Postpartum management

- After delivery, insulin infusion should be halved
- Encourage breastfeeding
- Once eating normally, recommence insulin SC at the prepregnancy dose, or lower if breastfeeding
- Breastfeeding T2DM may need to continue insulin
- Check baby's BG by 4–6 h of age, before a feed
- Give contraceptive advice

Further reading

Ang C, Howe D, Lumsden M. Diabetes. In: James DK, Steer PJ, Weiner CP, Gonik B (eds). *High Risk Pregnancy Management Options.* Elsevier Saunders: Philadelphia, 2005.

www.cemach.org.uk. Pregnancy in women with type 1 and type 2 diabetes in 2003–2005.

Nelson-Piercy C. *Handbook of Obstetric Medicine.* Informa Healthcare, London, 2006.

NICE. Diabetes in pregnancy, 2008. www.nice.org.uk/cg063

Physiological changes in pregnancy
See Section 6.2.

Thyrotoxicosis
A state of excessive thyroid hormones. Hyperthyroidism occurs when thyrotoxicosis is caused by thyroid overactivity.

Incidence
Affects 0.2% of pregnancies.

Pathophysiology
95% of women have Graves' disease:
- An autoimmune disorder which produces thyroid-stimulating hormone (TSH) receptor-stimulating immunoglobulins (TSI), causing growth of thyroid gland and hyperthyroidism
- There is a genetic predisposition. Half of patients have a family history of autoimmune thyroid disease
- Environmental factors: smoking, high iodine intake, stress

In 5% there is toxic multinodular goitre, toxic nodule, subacute or acute thyroiditis (de Quervain's), iodine treatment, amiodarone, lithium, hyperfunctioning ovarian teratoma, TSH-producing adenoma, HCG-producing tumour, or thyroid cancer.

Clinical features
- If thyrotoxicosis occurs for the first time in pregnancy, it usually occurs late in the first or early second trimester
- Many symptoms overlap with pregnancy: heat intolerance, palpitations, vomiting, tachycardia, goitre, palmar erythema, and emotional lability
- Discriminatory symptoms: weight loss, tremor, lid lag, lid retraction, persistent tachycardia, prepregnancy symptoms or persisting beyond first trimester
- In Graves' disease, there is also a diffuse firm goitre and 50% of patients have ophthalmopathy

Diagnosis
- ↑ FT4 (free T4) or ↑FT3 (free T3), and ↓ TSH
- Most women already diagnosed and on treatment
- Difficult in first trimester because 60% of women with hyperemesis gravidarum have biochemical hyperthyroidism in absence of thyroid disease. Trophoblastic disease must also be excluded.
- Presence of TSI suggests true hyperthyroidism.
- Diagnostic radio-iodine scans are contraindicated.

Effect of pregnancy on thyrotoxicosis
- First trimester: exacerbation may occur owing to ↑ HCG or ↓ absorption of medication due to vomiting
- Second and third trimesters: relative immunosuppression ⇒ improvement in Graves' disease and ↓ TSI levels
- Pregnancy has no effect on Graves' ophthalmopathy
- Postpartum: exacerbation may occur, especially if there has been improvement during pregnancy

Effect of thyrotoxicosis on pregnancy
Maternal risks
- Pregnancy outcome is good with good control on medication or previously treated Graves' disease
- Poorly controlled disease may ⇒ hypertension, pre-eclampsia, placental abruption
- Heart failure and 'thyroid storm' have maternal mortality of 25%. Highest risk of 'thyroid storm' is at delivery
- Rarely, retrosternal extension of goitre may cause tracheal obstruction and problem if intubation required

Fetal risks
- Untreated or newly diagnosed in pregnancy: ↑ miscarriage, fetal growth restriction (FGR), preterm birth, and perinatal mortality
- Effect of antithyroid medication (thionamides):
  - High doses may cause fetal hypothyroidism
  - Carbimazole rarely causes aplasia cutis: patches of absent skin at birth, mainly on the scalp
- Transplacental TSI results in thyrotoxicosis in 1% of babies of women with Graves' disease, especially if:
  - Poorly controlled disease or high TSI titres
  - Active disease in the third trimester
  - May also occur in treated Graves' disease, following thyroidectomy or radioactive iodine
- Perinatal mortality without treatment is 25–50%

Management
Prepregnancy management
- Mutidisciplinary
- Advise regarding timing: avoid pregnancy for 4 months after radioactive iodine treatment. Women should be euthyroid for ≥3 months before pregnancy
- General measures: folic acid , stop smoking

Antenatal management
Continue medication in pregnancy:
- Most women are treated with thionamides, i.e. carbimazole or propylthiouracil (PTU), which competitively inhibit active thyroid hormone production
- Give lowest dose that maintains a euthyroid clinical state, with FT4 at the upper end of the normal range
- Avoid 'block-and-replace' regimens. High dose thionamides may cause fetal hypothyroidism. Thyroxine does not cross the placenta to protect the fetus

In the newly diagnosed patient:
- PTU is preferable as it crosses the placenta less readily than carbimazole. Women who are already stable on carbimazole should not change
- Initial treatment: high dose carbimazole (40 mg) or PTU (400 mg) daily for 4–6 weeks and reduce to lowest effective dose
- Treatment may take 3–4 weeks to take effect, when preformed T4 and T3 are depleted. Propanolol 40 mg TDS may be used to control sympathetic symptoms and reduce peripheral conversion of T4 to T3

Monitor the patient:
- Check thyroid function tests (TFT) monthly in newly diagnosed, and 3-monthly in stable patients
- Side effects of thionamides: nausea, vomiting, diarrhoea, urticaria, and agranulocytosis. Advise women to report any signs of infection, sore throat or fever
- Screen for agranulocytosis. If neutropenia occurs, consider an alternative treatment

Fetal surveillance
- Serial scans for growth, heart rate, and goitre. Suspect fetal thyrotoxicosis if FGR, tachycardia or goitre
- Measure maternal TSI titre early and late in pregnancy. If high, ↑ risk of fetal or neonatal thyrotoxicosis
- Cordocentesis for TFT may be necessary. In fetal thyrotoxicosis: ↑ maternal dose of thionamides. If mother already euthyroid, give thyroxine replacement as well
- Radioactive iodine is contraindicated because placental transfer may cause fetal thyroid ablation

- Thyroidectomy: rarely indicated, advocated if unsuccessful medical therapy, dysphagia or stridor due to a large goitre or suspected carcinoma. Postoperative complications: hypothyroidism (25–50%), hypoparathyroidism, and recurrent laryngeal nerve palsy

Intrapartum management
- Labour and delivery may precipitate 'thyroid storm', especially in undertreated patients
- Features include extreme symptoms of hyperthyroidism, fever, heart failure, and mental disorientation (seizures, psychosis, coma)
- Management includes: supportive therapy (IV fluids, oxygen, temperature and glycaemic control), high-dose PTU, iodide therapy, dexamethasone, and propanolol

Postpartum management
- Cord blood should be taken for TFTs
- Regular TFTs in babies of women with high titre TSI in late pregnancy or taking high doses of thionamides while breastfeeding
- Encourage breastfeeding. Carbimazole ≤15 mg or PTU ≤150 mg daily are safe in breastfeeding mothers
- Graves' disease may flare, especially if medication was reduced or discontinued during pregnancy. May need to reintroduce medication 2–3 months postpartum
- Distinguish Graves' disease flare (treatment required) from postpartum thyroiditis (not required):
  - Radioactive iodine scan shows ↑ uptake in Graves'
  - TSI is absent in postpartum thyroiditis
  - Stop breastfeeding for 24 h after radioactive scan
- Give contraceptive advice

Neonatal thyrotoxicosis
- Symptoms: weight loss, tachycardia, irritability, jitteriness, poor feeding, goitre, hyperexcitability, hepatosplenomegaly, stare and eyelid retraction, congestive cardiac failure
- Onset may be delayed for 14 days if the mother was on thionamides
- Transient condition, lasting 2–3 months, i.e. the time it takes for TSI to be cleared from the neonatal system
- Mortality rate is up to 15% if untreated. Antithyroid treatment should begin promptly but only short term

Hypothyroidism in pregnancy

Clinical hypothyroidism is uncommon in pregnancy because of its association with subfertility and menstrual disorders.

Incidence
1% of pregnancies.

Pathophysiology
Autoimmune disease: associated with thyroid peroxidase (microsomal) autoantibodies (TPA), which causes lymphoid infiltration, leading to fibrosis and atrophy of the thyroid gland.

There are two subtypes:
- Hashimoto's thyroiditis
- Atrophic thyroiditis

Iatrogenic: after radio-iodine, thyroidectomy or drugs (amiodarone, lithium, iodide, thionamides)

Secondary hypothyroidism: Sheehan syndrome (postpartum pituitary necrosis after postpartum haemorrhage (PPH)), lymphocytic hypophysitis, hypophysectomy

Transient: subacute de Quervain's or postpartum thyroiditis

Clinical features
- Many symptoms overlap with pregnancy: weight gain, lethargy, tiredness, hair loss, dry skin, constipation, carpal tunnel, fluid retention, goitre
- Discriminatory: cold intolerance, bradycardia, delayed relaxation of deep tendon reflexes (especially ankle)
- Women are more likely to have goitre with iodine deficiency or Hashimoto's thyroiditis (due to thyroid gland regeneration)
- If autoimmune, other diseases may be present: pernicious anaemia, vitiligo, type 1 diabetes mellitus

Diagnosis
- ↓ FT4 and ↑ TSH
- Most women diagnosed prepregnancy
- TPA confirms diagnosis but present in 20% of normal population (do not use in isolation)

Effect of pregnancy on hypothyroidism
- Pregnancy does not improve or exacerbate hypothyroidism

Effect of hypothyroidism on pregnancy
- Pregnancy outcome is good if women are euthyroid
- TPA does not affect the fetus
- Undertreated women have ↑ risk of miscarriage, pre-eclampsia, abruption, low birth weight, stillbirth, impaired neurological development and ↓ offspring IQ
- Thyroxine hardly crosses the placenta and does not affect the fetus

Management
Prepregnancy management
- Mutidisciplinary care
- Check TFT and optimize thyroxine doses prepregnancy
- Advise delay pregnancy until good control is achieved

Antenatal management
- Most patients are on maintenance doses of thyroxine (100–200 μg/day). Women who are euthyroid in early pregnancy do not usually require dose adjustments
- Iron or aluminium hydroxide antacids interfere with thyroxine absorption. Avoid taking simultaneously
- Women who require ↑ in thyroxine in pregnancy are likely to have pre-existing undertreatment rather than an increased demand due to pregnancy
- Newly diagnosed: should begin thyroxine immediately. 100 μg/day is appropriate. Introduce thyroxine at lower dose if history of heart disease
- Euthyroid women: check TFTs once each trimester. Following any adjustments in thyroxine dose, TFTs should be checked every 4–6 weeks
- In women on thyroxine replacement following the treatment of Graves' disease (radio-iodine therapy or thyroidectomy), TSI should be measured in early and late pregnancy to predict fetal or neonatal thyrotoxicosis
- Fetal surveillance: serial scans for growth and goitre if newly diagnosed or undertreated hypothyroidism

Postpartum management
- Check TFTs if thyroxine dose was adjusted
- Up to 75% with TPA develop postpartum thyroiditis
- Observe for postpartum depression, which is commoner in women with thyroid antibodies
- TSH is measured in all neonates with a Guthrie test

Subclinical hypothyroidism

- Definition: serum TSH above normal range and FT4 within normal range in an asymptomatic patient
- ↑ risk of clinical hypothyroidism within 5 years, especially if thyroid autoantibodies
- Offspring more likely to have psychomotor deficiencies age 2 and lower IQ scores age 7–9
- No studies show thyroxine influences outcome
- Routine screening and treatment not recommended

Thyroid nodules and cancer

Incidence
2% of pregnancies.

Aetiology
- de Quervain's thyroiditis
- Up to 40% of nodules in pregnancy may be malignant
- Commonest is papillary carcinoma
- 90% of thyroid cancers are nodules

Clinical features
Usually causes hyperthyroidism.
Features indicating malignancy:
- Previous history of radiation to the neck or chest
- Nodule: fixed, painless, rapid growth
- Lymphadenopathy, voice change, Horner's syndrome

Features indicating de Quervain's thyroiditis:
- History of viral infection before nodule appearance
- Nodule tenderness

Diagnosis
- Radioactive iodine scans are contraindicated
- US can distinguish cystic from solid nodules. Cystic nodules are usually benign, especially if <4 cm
- Fine needle aspiration or biopsy if rapidly enlarging nodule, cystic nodules >4 cm or solid nodules >2 cm
- TFT and thyroid antibody test to exclude a toxic nodule or Hashimoto's thyroiditis
- ↑ thyroglobulin titre (>100 µg/l) suggests malignancy

Effect of pregnancy on thyroid malignancy
No adverse effect.

Effect of thyroid malignancy on pregnancy
- Adverse effect depends on hyperthyroidism
- Retrosternal extension of disease may cause tracheal obstruction, a problem if intubation required

Management
Prepregnancy management
Avoid pregnancy until 1 year after high-dose radioactive iodine to prevent fetal congenital abnormality.

Antenatal management
- Multidisciplinary
- Biopsy (after delivery if nodule is found in the second half of pregnancy). If biopsy confirms malignancy, surgery should not be delayed unless very near term. If pathology borderline, can delay surgery until after delivery
- Treated thyroid cancer: continue thyroxine to maintain TSH suppression. Residual tumour or metastasis is usually

TSH-dependent. Give high dose thyroxine postoperatively to suppress TSH
- Radioactive iodine is contraindicated in pregnancy and should be delayed until after delivery

Intrapartum management
Particular care if intubation is required in patients with large goitre or retrosternal extension.
Suspect retrosternal extension in patients with stridor, dysphagia, vocal cord paralysis or Horner's syndrome.

Postpartum management
Breastfeeding contraindicated with radioactive iodine.

Postpartum thyroiditis

Incidence
Between 5–10% of pregnancies.

Pathophysiology
- A destructive autoimmune thyroiditis
- Occurs in up to 75% of patients with thyroid peroxidase (microsomal) autoantibodies (TPA)
- 25% have a first-degree relative with autoimmune thyroid disease
- Incidence is 3-fold higher in type 1 DM

Clinical features
- Usually presents 3–6 months after delivery
- Symptoms: usually vague and attributed to puerperium
- Biphasic: transient hyperthyroidism owing to ↑ release of preformed T4 (instead of ↑ production), followed by prolonged hypothyroidism as thyroid reserve depleted
- Monophasic: transient hyperthyroidism or hypothyroidism
- Small, painless goitre is present in 50%

Diagnosis
- TFTs to confirm hypothyroidism or hyperthyroidism
- Distinguish postpartum Graves' disease flare (needs treatment) from postpartum thyroiditis (does not)
  - Radioactive iodine scan shows ↑ uptake in Graves' disease and ↓ uptake in postpartum thyroiditis
  - TSI is absent in postpartum thyroiditis
- Stop breastfeeding for 24 h after radioactive scan

Management
- Most patients recover spontaneously within 1 year
- Need for treatment depends on symptoms not TFTs
- Hyperthyroidism: use β-blocker instead of thionamides
- Hypothyroidism: thyroxine replacement therapy
- Thyroxine may be withdrawn in some patients after 6–9 months. Repeat TFTs to ensure complete recovery. Advise patients to avoid conception during this time
- Permanent thyroxine replacement recommended with ↑ TSH level and thyroid antibodies as ↑ risk of overt hypothyroidism within 5 years. Long-term annual TFTs. Observe for postpartum depression, which is commoner in women with thyroid antibodies.

Recurrence and prognosis
- Between 3–4% of patients remain permanently hypothyroid
- Between 10–25% have recurrent postpartum thyroiditis
- Between 20–40% of patients with TPA will develop permanent hypothyroidism within 5 years

Table 7.3 Pregnancy-specific thyroid function tests (pmol/l)				
Trimester	First	Second	Third	Non-pregnant
FT4	10–24	9–19	7–17	11–23
FT3	4–8	4–7	3–5	4–9
TSH	0–1.6	0.1–1.8	0.7–7.3	0–4

7.18 Parathyroid disease

Calcium homoeostasis in pregnancy

Pregnancy is a relative hypocalcaemic state caused by:

- Active transport of Ca^{2+} to the fetus across placental:fetal gradient of 1:1.4, stimulated by fetal ± placental PTH
- ↑ renal loss due to ↑ glomerular filtration rate (GFR)
- ↓ serum albumin ⇒ ↓ protein-bound total calcium

To compensate:

- Maternal PTH ↑ ⇒ parathyroid hormone (PTH)-like effect on the kidney but inhibits bone reabsorption
- ↑ in renal synthesis of 1,25-dihydroxy vitamin D (two or 3-fold in third trimester) ⇒ ↑ intestinal Ca absorption

Free ionized calcium concentration is unchanged.

Maternal PTH levels vary and do not cross the placenta.

Placental supply of Ca^{2+} ceases at delivery which stimulates neonatal PTH + $1,25(OH)_2D_3$ production.

Hypercalcaemia

Aetiology: hyperparathyroidism, malignancy, immobilization, intoxication of vitamin D or A, sarcoidosis, familial hypocalciuric hypercalcemia, thiazide diuretics.

90% have hyperparathyroidism or malignancy.

Primary hyperparathyroidism

Definition

Pathological, self-regulated, overactive state of parathyroid gland, resulting in hypercalcaemia and hypophosphataemia

Incidence

- 3 times commoner in women than men. Third commonest endocrine disease after diabetes and thyroid
- 25% of cases occur during reproductive age
- Incidence in women of reproductive age 8:100 000

Aetiology

- 90% have solitary parathyroid adenoma
- Between 6–9% have generalized chief-cell hyperplasia
- Between 1–2% have parathyroid carcinoma

Clinical features

- 80% of pregnant women are asymptomatic. Diagnosis retrospective after neonatal hypocalcaemia and tetany
- Hypercalcaemic symptoms mimic normal pregnancy: fatigue, thirst, hyperemesis, constipation, depression

Complications

- Pancreatitis, renal calculi, end-organ calcification
- Renal impairment and ↑ phosphate level
- Cardiac arrhythmia
- Hypercalcaemic crisis ⇒ uraemia, coma, cardiac arrest

Diagnosis

- ↑ ionized Ca^{2+} levels. Normal or ↑ levels of PTH assay
- Ultrasound to locate adenomas (±CT scan or MRI) as 10% have ectopic adenomas in the thyroid, thymus, pericardium or behind oesophagus
- Radiolabelled scans are contraindicated in pregnancy

Effect of pregnancy on hyperparathyroidism

- Pregnancy improves hypercalcaemia
- ↑ incidence of renal calculi in pregnancy (24–36%), due to hypercalciuria ⇒ ↑ urinary tract infections (UTI) and pyelonephritis

- ↑ incidence of pancreatitis
- Postpartum exacerbation as fetal calcium drain ceases

Effect of hyperparathyroidism on pregnancy

- Maternal: hyperemesis, hypertension, and pre-eclampsia
- Miscarriage, intrauterine death, FGR, preterm birth
- Hypercalcaemia ⇒ suppression of fetal parathyroid gland and ↑ risk of permanent hypoparathyroidism
- Delayed neonatal hypocalcaemia and tetany (usually 5–14 days) occur in 50% of babies of untreated mothers

Management

Prepregnancy management

Parathyroidectomy before conception.

Antenatal management

- Multidisciplinary
- Asymptomatic with mild hypercalcaemia <12 mg/dl may be managed conservatively (↑ fluids, ↓ oral Ca, phosphate supplement), but still ↑ risk neonatal morbidity
- Symptomatic or Ca level >12 mg/dl: advise urgent parathyroidectomy, best performed in second trimester
- Calcitonin does not cross the placenta and has been used to lower calcium levels in pregnancy
- Fetal surveillance with serial growth scans

Postpartum management

- Calcium supplementation for neonates
- Mothers of babies with hypocalcaemia should have their serum calcium levels checked

Hypoparathyroidism

The commonest cause of hypocalcaemia. Absence of PTH impairs the metabolism of endogenous vitamin D to $1,25(OH)_2D_3$, which is required for intestinal Ca absorption.

Aetiology

Complication of thyroid surgery (1–2% after total thyroidectomy). May also be caused by autoimmune disease.

Clinical features

- Paraesthesia and numbness of the fingertips and perioral area, tetany, spontaneous muscle cramps
- Chvostek's sign: twitching of the ipsilateral facial musculature by tapping over cranial nerve VII at the ear
- Trousseau's sign: carpal spasm provoked by ischaemia, induced by inflation of BP cuff around the arm

Treatment

Oral calcium and vitamin D supplements

Vitamin D treatment is best with 1,25-dihydroxy cholecalciferol (calcitriol) as faster acting, more potent, and shorter half-life than other preparations. Titration of dose against serum Ca levels is possible. 1α hydroxy cholecalciferol (alfacalcidol) is a suitable alternative.

Effect of hypoparathyroidism on pregnancy

Untreated hypocalcaemia ↑ fetal loss, preterm labour, causes fetal hypocalcaemia leading to secondary hyperparathyroidism, bone demineralization, neonatal rickets, and seizures.

Diagnosis

↓ serum free calcium and ↓ PTH levels.

Management

- ↑Ca^{2+} demands in pregnancy require ↑ vitamin D dose

- Serum Ca^{2+} and $1,25(OH)_2D_3$ in low normal range to prevent teratogenic effects of vitamin D overdose, maternal hypercalcaemia or overmineralization of fetal bones
- Serum Ca^{2+} and albumin should be measured monthly
- ↓ vitamin D dose after delivery

Further reading

Kenyon AP, Nelson-Piercy C. Thyroid disease. In: James DK, Steer PJ, Weiner CP, Gonik B (eds). *High Risk Pregnancy Management Options*. Elsevier Saunders: Philadelphia, 2005:1005–17.

Schnatz PF, Curry SL. Primary hyperparathyroidism in pregnancy: evidence-based management. *Obs Gynecol Surv* 2002; **57(6):** 365–76.

7.19 Other endocrine disorders

Physiological changes in pregnancy
See Section 6.2.

Pituitary disease in pregnancy

Physiological changes in pregnancy
- Oestrogen stimulates lactotroph proliferation ⇒ anterior pituitary gland doubles in size in pregnancy. Postpartum involution is slower in breastfeeding women
- Serum prolactin ↑ by up to 10-fold
- Gonadotrophins (LH and FSH) ↓
- Basal growth hormone (GH) levels remain unchanged
- Thyrotropin levels remain unchanged
- Adenocorticotropic hormone (ACTH) levels ↑ throughout pregnancy but levels are lower than upper non-pregnant levels
- Oxytocin levels ↑ throughout pregnancy
- Placenta secretes ACTH, corticotropin-releasing hormone (CRH), human placental lactogen (hpL) which resembles GH and a variant of placental GH (hGH-v).

Prolactinoma
The commonest pituitary tumour in pregnancy.

Effect of pregnancy on prolactinomas
- Microprolactinomas (<1 cm): less than 3% of patients have symptomatic growth of tumour in pregnancy
- Macroprolactinomas (≥1 cm): 30% have symptomatic growth of tumour in pregnancy, with the highest risk in the last trimester. Risk of tumour growth is decreased to 4% if patients had surgery or radiotherapy before pregnancy

Effect of prolactinomas on pregnancy
There is no adverse effect on pregnancy outcomes.

Clinical features
- Menstrual disturbances, galactorrhoea, anovulatory cycles
- Most women require ovulation induction
- Tumour growth and pressure on adjacent structures:
  - Persistent severe frontal headaches
  - Visual field defects (bitemporal hemianopia), due to pressure on optic chiasma
  - Diabetes insipidus (DI)

Diagnosis
- ↑ serum prolactin level (not reliable in pregnancy)
- Visual field testing
- MRI of the sella turcica

Management
Prepregnancy management
- Multidisciplinary
- Avoid pregnancy until prolactinoma treated
- Give contraceptive advice
- Arrange for MRI to evaluate the size of prolactinoma
- Perform other pituitary function tests
- General measures: folic acid, stop smoking

Treatment
- Microprolactinoma: dopamine-receptor agonist (DA), i.e. bromocriptine or cabergoline suppresses prolactin
- Macroprolactinoma: trans-sphenoidal surgery
- Radiotherapy (contraindicated in pregnancy)

Antenatal management
- DA's are safe in pregnancy. Cabergoline has fewer side effects than bromocriptine, particularly less nausea
- Serum prolactin level is not useful in pregnancy
- Microprolactinoma: stop DA and review each trimester
- Macroprolactinoma: continue DA, review monthly
- Formal visual field testing is required if symptoms (headaches, visual loss, DI) or macroprolactinomas
- Symptomatic: MRI is needed to monitor tumour size.
- If tumour enlargement:
  - Elective delivery if fetus is mature
  - Medical treatment with DA if premature
  - Surgery if failed medical treatment
  - Radiotherapy delayed until after delivery

Intrapartum management
No different from the general obstetric population.

Postpartum management
- Breastfeeding OK. DA safe but may suppress lactation
- Arrange for MRI to monitor tumour size
- Check serum prolactin 2 months after breastfeeding
- Contraceptive advice

Acromegaly
A rare disorder due to excessive GH secretion.

Incidence
5 of 100 000 pregnancies. Most are infertile.

Aetiology
Commonest: acidophilic or chromophobic pituitary adenoma.

Clinical features and complications
Insidious onset, thus diagnosis usually 40–60 years of age
- Excessive sweating is the most prominent symptom
- Facial change: frontal bossing, ↑ mandible size
- Soft tissue swelling: broad nose, thick lips, macroglosia (may cause sleep apnoea and difficult intubation)
- Large hands and feet, carpal tunnel syndrome
- Headaches, tiredness, and lethargy
- Menstrual disturbance and infertility (40% have hyperprolactinaemia owing to prolactin secretion by adenoma or stalk compression ⇒ secondary hyperprolactinaemia, hypopituitarism, and ↓ gonadotrophins)
- Degenerative arthropathy
- Impaired glucose tolerance/diabetes. GH is insulin antagonist
- Goitre
- Cardiac arrhythmias, hypertension, and cardiomyopathy
- Visual field defects: tumour pressure on optic chiasma

Effect of pregnancy on acromegaly
Tumour growth may cause visual field defects.
Pregnancy does not alter the course of acromegaly.

Effect of acromegaly on pregnancy
No adverse effect on the fetus as GH does not cross placenta, thus measures to ↓ GH secretion in pregnancy are not warranted.
There does not appear to be an increase in the incidence of diabetes or hypertension in pregnancy.

Diagnosis

Difficult in pregnancy because standard radioimmunoassay cannot differentiate between pituitary GH and placental GH.

Insulin-like growth factor 1 (IGF-1) is secreted in the liver and other target tissues in response to, and mediates, the action of GH. IGF-1 levels are only useful for diagnosis outside pregnancy because levels increase in normal pregnancies.

Lack of suppression of GH to glucose tolerance test may help with diagnosis.

MRI of the sella turcica confirms presence of tumour.

Management

Prepregnancy management

Multidisciplinary involving obstetricians, endocrinologists, ophthalmologists, and surgeons before, during, and after pregnancy.

- Arrange for MRI to evaluate the size of tumour
- Perform other pituitary function tests
- Screen for diabetes, hypertension, and cardiomyopathy

First line treatment: trans-sphenoidal surgery.
Second line: radiotherapy, if GH high after surgery.
Bromocriptine or cabergoline may ↓ GH and prolactin.
Octreotide (somatostatin analogue) ↓ GH levels.
General measures: folic acid, stop smoking.
Treatment with vasopressin ⇒ ↑ urine osmolality but not as marked as neurogenic DI.

Antenatal management

- Octreotide has been used to ↓ GH levels in acromegalic pregnancy but safety not established
- In most patients, treatment can be delayed until after pregnancy, unless there is significant tumour growth
- Observe for symptoms of tumour growth (headaches, visual field defects, DI)

Intrapartum management

No different from general obstetric population.

Postpartum management

- Breastfeeding OK. DA safe but may suppress lactation
- Contraceptive advice

Diabetes insipidus

Normal physiology

- Posterior pituitary releases antidiuretic hormone (ADH) in response to ↑ plasma osmolality, ↓ blood pressure or stress. ↑ plasma osmolality stimulates thirst
- ADH conserves water from the renal tubules, and combined with thirst, maintains a plasma osmolality of 285–295 mOsmol/kg
- Urine:plasma osmolality ratio is normally >2:1, provided plasma osmolality is ≤295 mOsmol/kg

In pregnancy

- Serum ADH levels remain unchanged
- ↑ plasma volume and ↓ sodium concentration ⇒ ↓ plasma osmolality. The osmostat is reset at 275–280 mOsmol/kg. Thus, a ↓ threshold for ADH release
- Placental vasopressinase degrades ADH
- Vasopressinase level ↑ through pregnancy and declines postpartum. To compensate, ADH release is ↑ 4-fold

Definition of diabetes insipidus

Failure of the renal tubules to conserve water, resulting in dilute polyuria and polydipsia.

Incidence

Rare.

Clinical features

- Polydipsia, polyuria
- Dangerous dehydration if patient is unable to consume large quantities of fluid
- Seizures

Types of diabetes insipidus

Neurogenic (central)

- Deficiency of ADH
- Pituitary adenoma, craniopharyngiomas, skull trauma, neurosurgery, Sheehan syndrome
- Treatment with vasopressin ⇒ ↑ urine osmolality

Nephrogenic

- ADH resistance in the kidneys
- Chronic renal failure, inherited nephrogenic DI
- Vasopressin treatment ⇒ no effect on urine osmolality

Gestational

- Transient ADH deficiency in pregnancy or postpartum
- ↑ placental vasopressinase production (reported in multiple pregnancy) or ↓ hepatic degradation of placental vasopressinase (associated with pre-eclampsia, HELLP (haemolysis, elevated liver enzymes, low platelets) syndrome, acute fatty liver of pregnancy)
- Treatment with synthetic deamino-D-arginine vasopressin (DDAVP), which is more resistant to degradation by placental vasopressinase, ⇒ ↑ urine osmolality

Dipsogenic (psychogenic or primary)

- Found in up to 50% of DI
- Excessive water drinking

Diagnosis

- Exclude other causes of polyuria: diuretics, hyperglycaemia, hypercalcaemia, hypokalaemia, renal tubular
- Water deprivation test is used to differentiate neurogenic and nephrogenic DI. Not appropriate in pregnancy as dehydration may be hazardous
- Perform other pituitary function tests: prolactin level, TFTs
- Headaches and visual field defect suggest pituitary tumour: arrange MRI

Effect of pregnancy on DI

- Half with pre-existing DI deteriorate in pregnancy and improve postpartum
- Pregnancy may unmask subclinical DI owing to ↑ placental vasopressinase

Effect of DI on pregnancy

No significant adverse effect has been reported.

Management

- DDAVP is safe in pregnancy and breastfeeding
- DDAVP more effective than vasopressin in pregnancy
- In neurogenic DI, DDAVP dose needs to be ↑ in pregnancy and ↓ postpartum
- In nephrogenic DI: treatment is by correcting hypercalcaemia and hypokalaemia, and with thiazide diuretics
- New onset of DI in pregnancy or puerperium: exclude pre-eclampsia, HELLP syndrome, and acute fatty liver of pregnancy. DDAVP is treatment of choice
- Monitor DI clinically and regular serum electrolytes

7.20 Renal disease

Physiological changes in pregnancy
See Section 6.2.

Chronic renal insufficiency

Effect of pregnancy on renal function
The *prognosis* is influenced by:
- The type of renal disease
- The level of renal insufficiency at the time of conception, categorized as mild, moderate or severe

Hypertension:
- Worsening hypertension is a poor prognostic indicator

Proteinuria (≥500 mg/ 24 h):
- Generally, proteinuria in early pregnancy increases the risk of renal deterioration

Urinary tract infection (UTI):
- Triggers a decline in renal function

Mild renal insufficiency: serum creatinine ≤1.4 mg/dl (120 μmol/l):
- 16% have renal deterioration
- 6% progress to end-stage renal disease (ESRD)

Moderate: serum creatinine 1.5–2.0 mg/dl (124–168 μmol/l):
- 40% of patients have renal deterioration
- 20% have permanent deterioration
- 20% progress to ESRD

Severe: serum creatinine ≥2.0 mg/dl (177 μmol/l):
- 67% have renal deterioration which tends not to recover. 33% will progress to ESRD
- No guarantee that termination will reverse the decline

Effect of renal insufficiency on pregnancy
- Most common cause of perinatal mortality and morbidity in mothers with any renal disease is preterm birth
- Mild renal insufficiency: 96% perinatal survival
- Moderate renal insufficiency: 90% perinatal survival
- Severe renal insufficiency: 25% perinatal survival
- Perinatal mortality is increased in severe hypertension and nephrotic-range proteinuria
- Fetal growth restriction (FGR) and placental abruption
- Proteinuria ≥500 mg/day has 30% ↑ risk of pre-eclampsia
- Nephrotic syndrome ⇒ ↑ risk of thromboembolic disease

General management of pregnancy with chronic renal insufficiency

Prepregnancy management
Counsel that:
- Fertility diminishes as renal impairment progresses and conception occurs in only 1% of women with ESRD
- Serum creatinine ≥1.5 mg/dl (124 μmol/l) and hypertension are risk factors for permanent exacerbation of renal disease
- There is an increased risk of pre-eclampsia, placental abruption, FGR, preterm birth, perinatal mortality, and maternal mortality

Advise against pregnancy in women with:
- Severe renal insufficiency and those requiring dialysis
- Severe or uncontrolled hypertension
- Nephrotic syndrome
- Scleroderma
- Polyarteritis nodosa
- Active lupus nephritis (delay pregnancy until in remission for at least 6 months and normotensive)

- Diabetic nephropathy if serum creatinine is ≥1.5 mg/dl (124 μmol/l) because it is associated with a 40% risk of accelerated renal deterioration

Assess renal function: urinalysis, FBC, U&E, serum creatinine, 24-h urinary protein.

Control blood pressure:
- Maintain blood pressure ≤140/90 mmHg (see Section 7.4)
- In women with longstanding hypertension, assess cardiovascular status and consider echocardiography
- In women with diabetic nephropathy, prepregnancy treatment with ACE inhibitors combined with strict glycaemic control for ≥6 months has resulted in a high rate of successful pregnancies with few complications

Diabetic nephropathy: control diabetes (see Section 7.15). Caution: women with T1DM and diabetic nephropathy have an increased risk of severe hypoglycaemia.

Lupus nephritis:
- Screen for the presence of aPLs, anti-Ro/La, and check anti-ds DNA and complement levels
- Stop cytotoxic drugs for ≥3 months before pregnancy

Review medication:
- Substitute ACE inhibitors either preconceptually or as soon as pregnancy is confirmed, depending on the individual circumstances
- Discontinue statins preconceptually

General: folic acid supplement 5 mg/day, advise against smoking or alcohol intake, check for immunity against rubella.

Antenatal management
Multidisciplinary care: involve obstetricians, physicians, nutritionists, the general practitioner, and midwives.

Assess baseline renal function:
- Blood pressure
- Urinalysis and 24-h urinary protein
- FBC, U&E, serum creatinine, LFT, serum albumin
- Renal ultrasound scan for pelvicalyceal dimensions

Prophylactic treatment:
- Low-dose aspirin (LDA) 75–150 mg/day may reduce the risk of glomerular capillary thrombosis and pre-eclampsia
- Give thromboprophylaxis with LDA and LMWH if proteinuria ≥3 g/day, or if proteinuria ≥1 g/day with other risk factors

Increase antenatal surveillance:
- Checks every 2 weeks until 28 weeks' then weekly
- Check blood pressure and urinalysis at every visit
- 24-h urine protein
- Screen for urine infection 4-weekly, and treat promptly
- Screen for pre-eclampsia. Check serum urate and LFTs

Control hypertension (see Section 7.4):
- Maintain blood pressure ≤140/90 mmHg
- Avoid diuretics
- Admit patients with worsening hypertension
- Superimposed pre-eclampsia may be difficult to differentiate from worsening renal disease

Erythropoietin (EPO) and ferrous sulphate can be used for anaemia but use EPO with caution as it can worsen hypertension.

For women with diabetic nephropathy, refer to the management of diabetes in pregnancy (see Section 7.15 and also Section 7.20).

For women with lupus nephritis, refer to the management of SLE in pregnancy (see Section 7.24).

If haematuria, seek nephrologist's advice. Red cell casts suggest active renal parenchymal disease, thus consider early delivery.

Monitor fetal growth using serial ultrasonography.

Elective early delivery (34–36 weeks) depends on individiual severity and must be individualized.

Intrapartum management
- Withhold LMWH during labour and delivery
- Closely monitor blood pressure and fluid balance
- Maintain continuous electronic fetal monitoring

Postpartum management
- As before, closely monitor BP and fluid balance.

- If on LMWH, continue for 6 weeks
- Avoid NSAIDs as postpartum analgesia
- Reassess renal function
- Resume prepregnancy medication within 2 weeks; ACE inhibitors are safe in breastfeeding mothers

Further reading

Williams D. Renal disease. In: James DK, Steer PJ, Weiner CP, Gonik B (eds). *High Risk Pregnancy Management Options*. Elsevier Saunders: Philadelphia, 2005:1098–1124.

Diabetic nephropathy

A progressive disease characterized by proteinuria, hypertension, reduced glomerular filtration rate (GFR), and increasing renal failure.

Diagnosis

- Proteinuria ≥500 mg/day (urinary albumin excretion rate 300 mg/day) with no evidence of UTI
- Microalbuminuria is urinary albumin of 30–300 mg, also known as incipient diabetic nephropathy

Prevalence

- Found in 6% of patients with type 1 diabetes mellitus (T1DM) and 25% of all diabetics after 15 years' duration
- In the developed world, diabetic nephropathy is the cause of 40% of end-stage renal disease (ESRD)

Pathophysiology

- Hallmarks: glomerular basement membrane thickening and mesangial expansion ± nodule formation
- Prior to impairment, there is glomerular hyperfiltration and ↑ urinary albumin secretion resulting in microalbuminuria

Effect of pregnancy on diabetic nephropathy

Where serum creatinine is within the normal range, pregnancy does not accelerate the decline in renal function.
Women with moderate to severe renal insufficiency have a 40% risk of accelerated renal deterioration in pregnancy.

Effect of diabetic nephropathy on pregnancy

Fetal risks

- Perinatal survival is 95%
- Perinatal mortality is the same as women with T1DM without diabetic nephropathy
- Risk of congenital malformation in the baby is higher than in women with T1DM and normal renal function
- ↑ risk of small-for-gestational age babies
- Preterm delivery occurs in 45% of cases
- Children of mothers with diabetic nephropathy have an increased risk of neurodevelopmental problems

Maternal risks

The rate of pre-eclampsia is 50–60%. Women with T1DM and micro-albuminuria have a higher risk of pre-eclampsia than women with T1DM without microalbuminuria. The risk is highest in those with renal impairment and hypertension in early pregnancy and in women with severe proteinuria.

Lupus nephritis

Inflammation of the kidney associated with systemic lupus erythematosus (SLE).

Prevalence

Clinical lupus nephritis occurs in 50% of SLE patients.
Histological evidence is present in most SLE patients.
Usually arises within 5 years of diagnosis of SLE.

Pathophysiology

Occurs because of immune complex deposition, complement activation, and inflammatory damage.

Diagnosis

Presence of persistent proteinuria (75% cases) or haematuria or pyuria (40% cases) or urinary casts (30% cases) in a patient with SLE.

- Confirm by histology, via renal biopsy

Categories of glomerulonephritis

1. Diffuse proliferative (40% cases). Commonest and most severe, with hypertension, moderate to heavy proteinuria, nephrotic syndrome, haematuria, pyuria, and urinary casts. 10-year survival rate is 60%.
2. Focal proliferative
3. Membranous
4. Mesangial. Best prognosis. Usually no proteinuria

Effect of pregnancy on lupus nephritis

- Nephritis is unlikely to present for the first time in pregnancy without a past history of renal disease
- In general, 33% have renal flares in pregnancy
  - Between 7–10% chance of a renal flare if conceived after a 6-month period of remission
  - Between 50–60% chance of a renal flare if conception occurred at the time of active disease
- Increasing proteinuria is common owing to ↑GFR especially in the second trimester
- 21% have renal deterioration, 7% permanent

Effect of lupus nephritis on pregnancy

- Severe flares may cause acute renal failure, maternal mortality and perinatal mortality (up to 50% risk)
- An increased risk of pre-eclampsia. The two most common predisposing factors are chronic hypertension and presence of antiphospholipid antibodies (aPL)
- aPLs also ↑ the risk of perinatal mortality
- Risk of neonatal lupus (discoid rash, congenital heart block, thrombocytopenia)

Differentiating a renal flare from pre-eclampsia

Increasing proteinuria, thrombocytopenia and new onset seizures may occur in both worsening SLE and lupus nephritis, and in severe pre-eclampsia.

The following factors point towards a *renal flare*:

- Development of proteinuria before the third trimester
- Presence of haematuria and/or urinary casts
- Active disease within 6 months of conception
- Raised anti-ds DNA levels, reduced complement levels
- Occasionally, other SLE symptoms may be present (extreme fatigue, discoid rash, arthralgia)

The following factors point towards *pre-eclampsia*:

- A normal baseline 24-h urinary protein excretion
- Elevated serum urate and/or abnormal LFT
- Antithrombin deficiency

Confirmation via renal biopsy is not generally recommended

Pregnancy in women on dialysis

Incidence

Patients receiving dialysis usually have a marked decrease in fertility, but pregnancy occurs in about 1%.

Effect of dialysis on pregnancy

- Diagnosis of pregnancy is difficult as >50% of women on dialysis have irregular periods. HCG levels are normally elevated
- Obtain an ultrasound scan to confirm pregnancy
- Increased risk of polyhydramnios as high urea levels promote osmotic diuresis in the fetus

- Increased risk of second trimester miscarriage, premature rupture of membranes, and preterm birth
- Up to 60% of pregnancies result in a live birth, of which 85% are preterm and 28% are small-for-gestational age
- Maternal deaths have been reported

Effect of pregnancy on dialysis
- Hypertension worsens in more than 80% of patients

Management
Prepregnancy management
- Pregnancy is a contraindication whilst on dialysis
- Counsel that pregnancy outcomes are improved after a renal transplant when compared to women on dialysis
- Fertility is improved with haemodialysis (compared to peritoneal) and erythropoietin (EPO) for anaemia
- Give contraceptive advice

Antenatal management
- Ensure that the patient is on a transplant list
- Low-dose aspirin 75 mg/day and folic acid 5 mg/day
- Monitor serum haemoglobin, iron, K+, Ca2+ and phosphate level. Give EPO and iron. Aim Hb 10–11 g/dl
- Give potassium supplements if required
- Adjust calcium and phosphate binders as required

Haemodialysis is preferred to peritoneal dialysis. Regimen should mimic physiological changes in pregnancy.
- Avoid dialysis-induced hypotension
- After first trimester, increase dialysis to 20–24 h/week. Aim serum urea <17 mmol/l. This improves nutritional status as greater protein intake allowed, prevents polyhydramnios and worsening of hypertension
- Maintain good fluid balance. Potassium supplements may be required
- After 24 weeks, fetal monitoring during dialysis

Control blood pressure
- Maintain blood pressure <140/90 mmHg
- Increase in BP may be reversed by correcting fluid overload

Peritoneal dialysis. Complications include peritonitis—treat with intraperitoneal antibiotics as for the non-pregnant
- Monitor fetus with serial US for growth and liquor

Intrapartum management
- 50% of cases are delivered by CS
- Close monitoring of blood pressure and fluid balance
- Continuous electronic fetal monitoring

Postpartum management
- Post-CS, women on peritoneal dialysis will need temporary haemodialysis
- Close monitoring of blood pressure and fluid balance
- Avoid NSAIDs for postpartum analgesia
- Return to prepregnancy medication within 2 weeks

Pregnancy after a renal transplant

Incidence
Renal transplant patients usually have a return of fertility. Pregnancy occurs in up to 12% of patients.

Effect of pregnancy on renal transplant
- The effect on a transplanted kidney's function is unclear
- Pregnancy does not adversely affect the graft function if serum creatinine <1.4 mg/dl (120 μmol/l) and woman treated with prednisone and/or azathioprine
- Obstruction of the transplanted ureter by the pregnant uterus is rare but has been reported

Effect of renal transplant on pregnancy
- Fetal survival after the first trimester is >90%
- Prepregnancy renal function, worsening hypertension and worsening proteinuria affect pregnancy outcome
- Serum creatinine <1.4 mg/dl (120 μmol/l): 96% fetal survival rate
- Serum creatinine >1.4 mg/dl (120 μmol/l): 74% fetal survival rate and a higher risk of renal deterioration
- Main concern: safety of immunosuppressive drugs during pregnancy and breastfeeding, and opportunistic infections as a result of immunosuppression
- Prednisone is associated with maternal hypertension, pre-eclampsia, gestational diabetes, preterm birth
- Prednisone in doses ≥15 mg/day is rarely associated with neonatal adrenal insufficiency and thymic hypoplasia
- Azathioprine is associated with SGA babies and dose-related fetal myelosuppression
- Ciclosporin is not associated with an increase in congenital anomalies but is associated with SGA babies

Management
Prepregnancy management
- Delay pregnancy until renal function and immuno-suppression stable. Recommend wait 1 year after living relative donor transplant and 2 years after cadaveric
- Counsel about ↑ risk of pre-eclampsia, FGR and prematurity. Worse if hypertension, proteinuria, and UTI
- Assess renal function: serum creatinine levels should be <2.0 mg/dl (177 μmol/l)
- Quantify proteinuria
- Control blood pressure
- Immunocompromised patients are at risk of infections:
  - Check immunity to hepatitis B virus, herpes simplex virus, cytomegalovirus, *toxoplasma*, and rubella
  - Examine for genital warts
  - Live virus vaccine is contraindicated after transplant
- Review medication:
  - Substitute ACE inhibitors for other anti-hypertensives
  - Try to reduce prednisone to ≤15 mg/day, azathioprine to ≤2 mg/kg/day, ciclosporin to ≤5 mg/kg/day

Antenatal management
- Multidisciplinary care
- Give LDA 75 mg/day and folic acid 5 mg/day
- Continue immnunosuppressives at prepregnancy doses. Acute transplant rejection requires high-dose steroids
- Daily BP measurements by patient
- Twice weekly visits to the physician (less if graft is stable) for FBC, U&E, serum creatinine levels (and ciclosporin levels when indicated)
- Monthly urine cultures and renal scans. UTI is an indication for long-term low-dose antibiotic prophylaxis
- Determine IgM levels to CMV and toxoplasma for seronegative women every trimester
- In the last trimester, check levels of IgM for HSV
- Screen for pre-eclampsia
- Fetal growth scans every 2 weeks in the third trimester

Intrapartum management
- Aim for vaginal delivery
- Give prophylactic antibiotics
- Give hydrocortisone 100 mg IV 6-hourly to cover stress
- Continuous electronic fetal monitoring

Postpartum management
- Not to breastfeed whilst taking ciclosporin
- Avoid NSAIDs for postpartum analgesia
- Contraceptive advice

7.22 Transfusion-dependent anaemias and thalassaemia

Transfusion-dependent anaemias

Definition
Patients dependent on blood transfusions to survive include those with rare blood disorders and bone marrow failure, such as thalassemia, sickle cell disease, Fanconi's anaemia, aplastic anaemia, and myelodysplasia.

Prepregnancy: general
Review of previous blood transfusions, iron chelation, sickling crises and complications, obstetric history
- Blood tests:
  - FBC, reticulocyte count, ferritin and folate level
  - Hb electrophoresis
  - Blood group and red cell antibody screen
  - Screen for hepatitis A, B, C, HIV, rubella status
  - Screen for complications of iron overload: serum glucose, thyroid function, LFT, ECG, echocardiogram
  - Check renal function
- Vaccinate against hepatitis A and B
- All women should be given folic acid 5 mg/day
- Do not give iron. Stop iron chelation prepregnancy owing to potential risk of fetal skeletal anomaly
- Partner screening:
  - Women with β-thalassaemia major or HbEβ^0, risk is 50% if the partner is heterozygous
  - Women with HbSS, risk is 50% if partner has HbAS
- Counsel about maternal and fetal risks. Delay pregnancy until condition is stable
- Any contraceptive method is acceptable
- Sickling disorders:
  - Evaluate for pulmonary hypertension in patients with repeated acute chest syndrome
  - Assess risk by determining the level of HbS and HbF
  - If taking hydroxyurea: discontinue before pregnancy owing to teratogenic effects in animal studies
  - Advise avoiding crises by keeping warm and well hydrated
  - To prevent infection, give pneumococcal, meningococcal, and *Haemophilus influenzae* vaccinations
  - Prophylactic oral penicillin V 250 mg twice daily
  - Educate about symptoms and signs of infection
- Consider spinal X-ray in women with major thalassaemia and spinal abnormalities

Antenatal: general
- Follow prepregnancy management if not seen earlier
- If partner screening is positive: offer prenatal diagnosis and termination of affected pregnancy
- Continue folate 5 mg/day throughout pregnancy
- In women with β-thalassaemia major who had splenectomy:
  - Give prophylactic penicillin
  - Consider thromboprophylaxis
- Thalassaemia-dependent anaemia: regular visits for Hb check and blood transfusions to maintain Hb
- Sickling disorders (see Section 7.22)

Complications of regular blood transfusions
Alloimmunization—avoid by giving matched blood only; screen regularly for fetal anaemia if antibodies present.
Iron overload—prevent with iron chelation therapy

- *Endocrine failure*: hypothyroidism, diabetes mellitus, hypogonadotrophic hypogonadism
- *Cirrhosis*
- *Cardiomyopathy*
Bloodborne infections—avoid by hepatitis vaccination.
Transfusion reactions—avoid by giving leukoreduced blood.

Thalassaemia overview

Genetics
- Worldwide commonest inherited single gene disorders
- Result in defective globin chain synthesis
- Most cases are due to Mendelian recessive inheritance
- Heterozygous carrier state is called 'trait' and homozygous condition 'disease'

Types
1. Hereditary persistence of fetal haemoglobin, HPFH.
2. Structurally variant Hb due to single amino acid substitution that can cause sickling.
3. Thalassaemias: deficient globin chain synthesis:
   α$^+$ or β$^+$: notations used for ↓ globin chain synthesis
   α^0 or β^0 : notations used for no globin chain synthesis

Management of α- or β-thalassaemia trait
All women should be offered haemoglobinopathy screening:
- To identify early those at risk of affected baby
- To offer prenatal diagnosis and termination if affected
- To prevent ↑ infant morbidity and mortality from undiagnosed disease

Screening for thalassaemias by routine blood indices:
- Type of screening depends on local area prevalence
- In carriers: partner screening should be done prepregnancy or early in pregnancy to identify fetus at risk
- α-thal trait: fetal risk 25% if partner also has α-thal trait
- β-thal trait: fetal risk 25% if partner has β-thal trait, sickle-cell trait or HbE

Counsel about:
- Maternal and fetal risks
- Involve paediatricians if fetus may be affected
- Give folate 5 mg/day before and during pregnancy. Oral iron may be given in iron-deficiency anaemia
- No specific intrapartum or postpartum management

α-Thalassaemia (α-thal)

Prevalence
Commoner in South East Asia, China, Mediterranean, Middle East.

Pathophysiology
Mainly results from deletion of one or more of four α-genes.
One gene-deletion (α-/αα) or two gene-deletion (α-/α-), (--/αα) ⇒ α-thal trait.
- Those with (--/αα) are carriers of the α^0 mutation and often have a more severe blood picture than those with (α-/α-)
- At birth: Hb Barts (4 gamma chains, γ_4) is detected in 0.5–2% of (α-/α-) and up to 10% of (--/αα). These disappear by 6 months of age with no effect on development
- Hb synthesis in adults is normal
3-gene deletion (--/-α) ⇒ HbH disease.
   ↓ α-chain ⇒ some HbA + some HbH (β$_4$) in adults.

4-gene deletion (--/--)⇒ α-thal major. No α-chain ⇒ 80% Hb Barts and 20% Hb Portland, which is incompatible with life.
HbH and Hb Barts:

- Detected by Hb electrophoresis
- ↑ affinity for O_2 ⇒ poor oxygen delivery to tissues
- Precipitate within red cells ⇒ haemolysis in the spleen

Clinical features
α-thal trait: asymptomatic
α-thal major: incompatible with life
HbH disease:

- Childhood: mild to moderate haemolytic anaemia
- Adult: variable. Mild asymptomatic anaemia, to transfusion-dependent anaemia with jaundice, gallstones, bone abnormalities, hepatosplenomegaly, growth restriction
- Worsened by infection, fever, parvovirus B19, pregnancy

Effect of pregnancy on α-thal trait

- Normal outcome

Effect of α-thal trait on pregnancy

- If the fetus is unaffected - normal outcome
- If the fetus is affected - α-thal major

Fetal risks
Incompatible with life: severe anaemia, hydrops fetalis, hepatosplenomegaly, abnormal organogenesis, cardiac failure, polyhydramnios, placentomegaly, stillbirth.

Maternal risks
Are secondary to fetal and placental hydrops.

- Pregnancy-induced hypertension (50%)
- Pre-eclampsia (30%)
- Placental abruption
- Obstructed labour (large fetus)
- Antepartum (APH) and postpartum haemorrhage (PPH)
- Disseminated intravascular coagulation (DIC)

β-Thalassaemia (β-thal)

Prevalence
UK 1:10 000, South Asians 3:100, Cypriots 1:7.

Clinical features
One defective gene ⇒ β-thal trait: usually asymptomatic
Two defective genes ⇒ β-thal major:

- ↓β-chain ⇒ α-tetramers ($α_4$). Affects red cell maturation ⇒ haemolysis in the spleen and bone marrow
- Chronic dyserythropoietic anaemia ⇒ splenomegaly, infections, bone marrow expansion with deformity of long bones and skull
- Without adequate transfusion, death within a few years
- Regular blood transfusions may ⇒ iron overload
- Usually infertile owing to pituitary failure secondary to iron overload
- May have iron overload cardiomyopathy
- α-chains or ↑ HbF level improves the disease

Effect of pregnancy on β-thal

- β-thal trait: may develop mild anaemia in pregnancy
- β-thal major: may worsen disease ⇒ ↑ transfusion

Effect of β-thal on pregnancy
β-thal trait: normal outcome.
β-thal major:

- If Hb maintained ≥10 g/dl, well chelated and no bone abnormalities: normal outcome

- If maternal anaemia or inadequate transfusion ⇒ fetal hypoxia, FGR, preterm birth
- Maternal complication of iron overload
- If short stature with pelvic bone deformity ⇒ ↑ risk of cephalopelvic disproportion and CS

Diagnosis
α-thal trait and β-thal trait

- Red cell indices: ↓ mean cell volume (MCV <70 fl) and ↓ mean cell Hb (MCH <27 pg)
- Need to exclude iron deficiency anaemia
Hb electrophoresis
- α-thal trait: normal
- β-thal trait: ↑ HbA2 >3.5%, HbF may ↑ >1%
Prenatal diagnosis: confirm with DNA analysis using polymerase chain reaction (PCR) or Southern blot

HbH disease
Hb electrophoresis: some HbA and HbH

β-thal major

- Hb electrophoresis: no HbA
- For prenatal diagnosis, confirm with DNA analysis (PCR or Southern blot)

Hereditary persistence of fetal Hb (HPFH)
A complex group with persistent HbF synthesis in adult life.

Aetiology
Genetic heterogeneity. Generally, HPFH forms a continuum of β-thalassaemia.

Clinical features

- Homozygotes: 100% HbF, ↑ Hb, no clinical findings
- HPFH may decrease the severity of thalassaemias or structural Hb variants (such as sickle cell disease—see Section 7.22) by increasing the amount of HbF synthesis

---

◉ Box 7.14 Types of haemoglobin

Normal haemoglobin (Hb):

- Consists of haem and four globin chains.
- Four globin-chain-synthesis is normally 'balanced', one pair each by the α- and the β-globin genes
- Two α-globin genes are positioned on chromosome 16
- One β-globin gene is positioned on chromosome 11
- Normal person has four α-genes (one pair each derived from maternal and paternal chromosomes, i.e. genotype αα/αα) and two β-genes (one from each parent)

Types of globin chains:

Embryo:
Hb Gower1 ($ζ_2ε_2$), Hb Portland ($ζ_2γ_2$), Hb Gower2 ($α_2ε_2$)

Fetal:
Mainly HbF ($α_2γ_2$)

Adult:
≥96% HbA ($α_2β_2$), <3.5% HbA2 ($α_2δ_2$), <1% HbF

7.23 Sickle cell disease

Sickle cell disease (SCD) is an inherited autosomal recessive condition, characterized by sickle-shaped red blood cells (RBCs) and chronic anaemia caused by homozygous inheritance of HbS (HbSS).

Pathophysiology of sickle cell disorders

- Haemoglobin S (HbS) is caused by a point mutation in the β-globin gene where valine replaces glutamic acid at position 6
- Significant sickling results from a sickle cell gene (HbS) on one chromosome and another mutation on the other (i.e. HbS + another mutation)
- When deoxygenated, HbS aggregates leading to red cell rigidity
- The deoxygenated haemoglobin chain is less soluble, causing RBCs to form a characteristically sickle shape
- This results in abnormal adherence to vascular endothelium, leading to infarction and premature removal from the circulation of the sickled RBCs
- HbF protects from sickling crises (e.g. in early life, HPFH, or treatment with hydroxyurea)

Sickling disorders

- Homozygous sickle cell disease (HbSS)
- HbC mutation (HbSC)
- β-thalassaemia, sickle cell thalassaemia (HbSβ⁰)
- D-punjab mutation (HbSD-Punjab)
- HbE mutation (HbSE)
- O-Arab mutation (HbSO-Arab)

Prevalence

- HbSS: in London 1: 500.
- HbAS: West Africans 1:4, Afro-Caribbeans 1:10, Cypriots 1:100, Indians 1:100
- HbSC: Ghanaian 1: 6, Afro-Caribbeans 1:30
- HbSD: Indians 1:100

Clinical effects of sickle cell

HbSS

- HbF in the first 6 months of life protects from crises
- As HbF ↓, chronic haemolytic anaemia develops
- Patients are generally healthy except during periods of crises, which are often precipitated by infection
- Life expectancy is decreased by 25–30 years

Anaemia due to haemolysis (consequent ↑ gallstones and acute cholecystitis), red cell aplasia or splenic sequestration.

Vaso-occlusive disease ↑ blood viscosity, tissue hypoxia, infarction, severe pain and organ damage ⇒ stroke, renal papillary necrosis, retinopathy, leg ulcers, aseptic bone necrosis.

↑ risk of infections due to loss of splenic function.

Acute chest syndrome usually caused by fat emboli from bone infarction. Fever, tachypnoea, pleuritic chest pain, leukocytosis, worsening anaemia and pulmonary infiltrates, caused by pulmonary or intravascular infarction, or thrombosis.

Sudden death in sickle cell disease
Has been reported in HbSS and HbSC. Post mortem shows:
- Intravascular plugs of sickled red cells
- Extensive fibromuscular dysplasia
- Abnormal foci of fibrosis and degeneration throughout the myocardial conducting system

Effects of pregnancy on HbSS

- ↑ frequency of sickling
- ↑ frequency of painful crises
- ↑ susceptibility to infection, chest and urinary tract

- Beware: HbSC patients are not usually anaemic, but at risk of severe sickling in pregnancy and puerperium

Effect of HbSS on pregnancy

- Fetal risks: ↑ risk of miscarriage, fetal growth restriction (FGR), preterm birth, fetal distress and ↑ perinatal mortality by 4-6-fold
- Maternal risks: ↑ pre-eclampsia, placental abruption, thromboembolism, bone marrow embolism, CS, and ↑ mortality (rate of up to 2.5%)
- Patients with HbAS also have ↑ risk of pre-eclampsia, renal papillary necrosis and urinary tract infection

Diagnosis

HbSS Hb electrophoresis: HbS makes up 90–95% of total Hb. HbF and HbA2 are present but HbA is absent

- Blood film: sickled cells and hyposplenism (Howell–Jolly bodies, target cells, ↑ platelet and ↑ white cell count)

HbSC Electrophoresis show both HbS and HbC are present

- ↓ MCV suggests iron deficiency or thalassaemia

Early diagnosis allows:
- Prophylaxis with penicillin and vaccines
- Early identification of complications and treatment

Management

Antepartum management

- Partner screening to consider prenatal diagnosis
- Folic acid 5 mg/day thoughout pregnancy
- Prophylactic penicillin 250 mg BD
- Regular visits for Hb, urinalysis, and BP checks
- Regular fetal growth scan
- No evidence for routine thromboprophylaxis
- No evidence for prophylactic blood transfusions

Intrapartum management

- Operative delivery for obstetric indication only
- Keep warm, ensure adequate hydration and O₂
- Continue prophylactic penicillin
- Ensure adequate pain relief
- Avoid prolonged labour
- Continuous CTG
- Blood transfusion if Hb <8 g/dl

Postpartum management

- Maintain good hydration and oxygenation
- Early mobilization and chest physiotherapy if CS
- Encourage breastfeeding
- Contraceptive advice
- Thromboprophylaxis

Newborn screening for sickle-cell disease

- Part of neonatal dried blood spot to identify and decrease morbidity and deaths from sickle cell disease
- Babies are at risk of severe infections and splenic sequestration crises

Management of sickle cell crises

- Admission with early involvement of haematologists and anaesthetists. Patient may require intensive care
- Good analgesia with IV/SC opiates, morphine infusion
- Keep warm, well hydrated and well oxygenated. Regular blood gases and pulse oximetry required
- Continue prophylactic penicillin and prompt treatment of any suspected infections

- Blood transfusion for severe anaemia, splenic sequestration or acute chest syndrome
- In acute chest syndrome: consider differential diagnosis e.g. pulmonary embolism, amniotic fluid embolism, pulmonary oedema
- Thromboprophylaxis
- Blood transfusion and exchange transfusion

Further reading

Dauphin-McKenzie N, Gilles JM, Jacques E, Harrington T. Sickle cell anemia in the female patient. *Obstet Gynecol Surv* 2006; **61(5)**:343–52.

www.sickleandthal.org.uk NHS sickle cell and thalassaemia screening programme.

Clark P, Greer IA. Hereditary red cell disorders. In: *Practical Obstetric Hematology*. London: Taylor & Francis, 2006: 163–83.

Johnston TA. Haemoglobinopathies in pregnancy. *The Obstetrician and Gynaecologist* 2005; **7(3)**:149–57.

> **Box 7.15 Blood transfusion in sickling disorders**
>
> - Transfusion may precipitate a crisis if sudden ↑Hct
> - Anaemia may be precipitated by haemolysis, infection, aplasia, inflammation or folate deficiency
> - Blood transfusion is generally not required. Hb of 6–8 g/dl is typical for HbSS
> - HbSC or HbSβ^0 often have higher Hb levels
> - Blood transfusion to reduce sickling if:
>   - Acute anaemia evidenced by ↓ Hb accompanied by ↑ reticulocyte count, bilirubin, and lactate dehydrogenase levels, indicating ↑ haemolysis
>   - ↓ reticulocyte count indicating aplastic anaemia (usually associated with parvovirus B19 infection)
> - Consider transfusions in severe anaemia, multiple pregnancy, pre-eclampsia, acute chest syndrome, acute renal failure, septicaemia, cerebral ischaemia of arterial origin or increased painful crises
> - Target level: <30% of sickle cells in circulation
>   - Hb 8–10 g/dl: top up to 12–14 g/dl with sufficient dilution
>   - Hb <5 g/dl: partial exchange transfusion. Remove 500 ml whilst transfusing two red cell units

7.24 Bleeding disorders

Classification

Familial
Haemophilias A and B, von Willebrand disease.

Acquired
Liver disease, malabsorption, vitamin K deficiency, use of anticoagulants, disseminated intravascular coagulation (DIC).

Haemophilia

Haemophilia is an inherited blood clotting disorder where an essential clotting factor is deficient.
- Haemophilia A: factor (F) VIII deficiency
- Haemophilia B: factor (F) IX deficiency
- Haemophilia C: factor (F) XI deficiency

Pathophysiology
- X-linked recessive disorders
- Mainly affect males, females are usually carriers

Haemophilia A
- Severity of the disease remains constant in a family
- 40% of severe disease is caused by an inversion in intron 22 of the FVIII gene on the X chromosome
- Most mild disease is caused by point mutations
- 30% of cases have no family history

Haemophilia B
- Severe disease is less common than in haemophilia A
- More often associated with a positive family history

Prevalence
- Haemophilia A: 1/10 000 population
- Haemophilia B: 1/50 000 population

Female carrier types
Obligate:
- A haemophiliac father, or
- Family history of haemophilia and an affected son
- ≥one child with haemophilia

Potential:
- A maternal relative with haemophilia

Sporadic:
- One affected child but no family history

Von Willebrand disease (vWD)

Prevalence
One per cent of the population. Commonest inherited bleeding disorder.

Pathophysiology
- Inherited deficiency in von Willebrand factor (vWf) and factor VIII leads to a defect in primary haemostasis. Gene is on chromosome 12
- vWf enhances platelet adhesion to damaged subendothelium and stabilizes FVIIIc in plasma
- ↓ vWf ⇒ platelet dysfunction and FVIIIc deficiency

Lifelong tendency to bleeding. May be mild, moderate or severe and there are many subtypes:
- Type 1: mild vWf deficiency
- Type 2: qualitative defect, type 2b associated with thrombocytopenia
- Type 3: non-functional, severe vWf deficiency

Type 1 and 2 are autosomal dominant and type 3 vWD is autosomal recessive.

Haemophilia and vWD in pregnancy

Carriers of vWD and haemophilia
Haemophilia carriers: factor levels ~50% of normal (as random inactivation of an X-chromosome in all cells).

Diagnosis of haemophilia/von Willebrand disease
- Activated partial thromboplastin time (APTT) is prolonged in vWD and haemophilia
- Normal time does not exclude mild disease in haemophilia carriers

Diagnostic test: factor levels in APTT-based test.
- Haemophilia A: ↓ FVIIIc level but a normal level in pregnancy does not exclude carriership
- Haemophilia B: ↓ FIXc level
- Haemophilia C: ↓ FXIc level
- Functional vWf activity is measured by ristocetin cofactor activity (RiCOF)
- vWD: ↓ vWf:RiCOF ratio, ↓ vWf antigen (vWf:Ag), ↓ FVIIIc

Further tests are requried to classify the type of vWD.

Effect of pregnancy on haemophilia and von Willebrand disease
- FVIII and vWf levels ↑ with increasing gestation ⇒ improvement in haemophilia A and type 1 vWD by the second trimester
- FVIII and vWf levels ↓ rapidly after delivery
- There is no increase in FIX levels in pregnancy
- In type 2B vWD, thrombocytopenia oftens worsens in pregnancy
- In type 3 vWD, there is no increase in vWf activity with gestation

Effect of haemophilia and von Willebrand disease on pregnancy
Maternal risks
- ↑ risk of excessive bleeding with early pregnancy miscarriage, ectopic pregnancy or chorionic villus sampling (CVS) as factor levels are only increased substantially after the first trimester
- ↑ risk postpartum haemorrhage (PPH) (risk is 20% in vWD), mainly secondary

Risks in affected fetus
- Spontaneous bleeding is rare
- Traumatic delivery may cause intracranial haemorrhage (ICH) and cephalhaematoma

Severity of haemophilia and von Willebrand disease
Bleeding disorder correlates with factor levels.
- <10 iu/dl: severe spontaneous bleeding
- 10–40 iu/dl: moderate bleeding after minor trauma
- ≥50 iu/dl: mild bleeding after major trauma

Factor level
- Factor level ≥40 is safe for vaginal delivery
- If <40, treatment is required at the onset of labour to cover delivery and postpartum
- Factor level ≥50 is safe for invasive procedures (CS, CVS, amniocentesis, evacuation)
- If <50, treatment is required before the invasive procedure

Management of von Willebrand disease and haemophilia

Treatment with deamino-D-arginine vasopressin (DDAVP)

- ↑FVIII and vWf levels by 2–5 times within 1 h
- Suitable for patients with type 1 vWD and haemophilia A
- Contraindicated in patients with type 2b vWD and ineffective in type 3 vWD
- Infusions can be repeated 12–24-hourly but repeated use over 3 days ⇒ ↓ response, possibly due to tachyphylaxis
- Fluid restrict for 24 h; advise patient to drink only when thirsty
- Monitor fluid balance if using oxytocin
- Side effects: hypotension, flushing, tachycardia, headache, volume overload (ADH effect) and hyponatraemia

If DDAVP not suitable or ineffective:

- Recombinant factor concentrate may be used. Plasma-derived concentrate ↑ risk of transmission of infection
- Plasma-derived FVIII concentrate containing vWf that has undergone viral inactivation may be used for vWD as recombinant FVIII concentrates do not contain vWf
- Tranexamic acid may be used as adjunct. 1 g TDS orally, for 1 week following delivery to reduce the risk of secondary PPH

Prepregnancy management

Multidisciplinary care: close liaison with haemophilia centre. Ideally manage in a hospital with a haemophilia team.

Genetic counseling for all obligate and potential haemophilia carriers and women with vWD.

For haemophilia: confirm a true history and confirm carrier status with genetic studies:

- Direct method: establish mutation in affected family member. Screen potential carriers for same mutation
- Indirect method (linkage analysis of polymorphisms) is used if no affected male is available. Requires blood samples from as many family members as possible
- Preimplantation genetic diagnosis is possible with assisted conception but is only available in a few centres

For vWD: ascertain the subtype of vWD; avoid aspirin and NSAIDs in type 2b vWD.

- Discuss maternal and fetal risks
- Offer hepatitis A and B immunization to non-immune
- Coagulation studies identify those with ↓ factor levels
- Assess the effect of DDAVP in haemophilia A carriers with ↓ FVIII levels and in women with type 1 vWD

Antenatal management

- Measure factor levels in early pregnancy and before delivery. In vWD, measure FVIII, vWf:Ag and vWf:RiCOF levels
- Women with mild–moderate vWD or carriers of haemophilia A usually do not require treatment as FVIII and vWf often rise to safe levels by midtrimester
- Review by anaesthetist to discuss regional anaesthesia

Intrapartum management

- FBC and G&S should be taken
- Factor levels <50 iu/dl or ↓ vWf:RiCOF:
  - Treatment is required at onset of labour or after cord clamping
- Factor levels <40 iu/dl:
  - avoid intramuscular injections
- Risk of haematoma with epidural analgesia if factor levels are not within normal range. In type 2 and 3 vWD, epidural is not recommended
- In vWD and haemophilia carriers with high-risk fetus (affected fetus, male fetus with unknown haemophilia status or fetus of unknown sex):
  - Aim for atraumatic unassisted vaginal delivery
  - Avoid fetal scalp electrode and fetal blood sampling
  - Avoid ventouse extraction and difficult forceps
  - Low cavity forceps by an experienced operator is preferable to a difficult CS

Postpartum management

- Repair perineal trauma promptly
- Observe bleeding from wound sites
- Maintain vigilance for primary and secondary PPH
- Maintain factor levels ≥40 iu/dl for 3–4 days after vaginal delivery and for 4–5 days after CS
- Contraceptive advice
- Follow-up plan for mother and baby before discharge

Neonatal management

Obtain neonatal cord blood:

- Haemophilia carrier male baby for clotting factor assay
- If type 3 vWD or family history of severe vWD: testing for vWD is otherwise unnecessary unless there is bleeding or surgery is required
- Avoid neonatal intramuscular injections, heel stabs and circumcisions until haemophilia or vWD status are known. Give vitamin K orally
- Cranial scan if severe neonatal haemophilia
- Recombinant factor replacement if neonatal bleeding
- Debate regarding treatment with recombinant factor VIII to all affected males within 2 h of delivery

Prenatal diagnosis

Counsel haemophilia carriers and those at risk of type 3 vWD:

- Haemophilia carrier: 50% chance of a male fetus being affected, 50% chance of a female fetus being a carrier
- In haemophilia, maternal blood may be used to sex the fetus, by looking for free fetal DNA, after 9 weeks
- CVS at 11–13 weeks or amniocentesis >14 weeks for sexing or confirm diagnosis if the mutation is known
- Risk of miscarriage with invasive procedures
- If factor levels <50 iu/dl, use factor replacement or DDAVP to cover invasive procedures
- If no diagnosis, scan at 16–20 weeks for fetal sexing

7.25 Systemic lupus erythematosus

Relevant pregnancy physiology

There is a shift from cell-mediated immunity (Th1 response) to humoral immunity (Th2) which is reversed postpartum.

Systemic lupus erythematosus

Definition

Systemic lupus erythematosus (SLE) is an idiopathic, systemic connective tissue disease characterized by periods of disease activity and remissions.

Prevalence

- 1:1000 (10:1 female: male)
- Average age at diagnosis is 30 years
- Lifetime risk for developing SLE is 1:700 (white women)
- Commoner in Afro-Caribbean women

Pathophysiology

- Idiopathic
- There is a genetic predisposition:
  - 10% of patients have an affected relative
  - Concordance between twins is more than 50%
- Autoimmunity:
  - 6% of patients have other autoimmune disease
  - Circulating non-organ-specific autoantibodies
  - Polyclonal B cell activation, impaired T cell regulation of immunity and failure to remove immune complexes
- Environmental triggers: ultraviolet light, viral infection.

Diagnosis of systemic lupus erythematosus

Classification criteria for diagnosis

4 or more of the 11 criteria below must be present.

Those with <4 criteria have a lupus-like disease and may also benefit from treatment for SLE (American College of Rheumatology).

1) *Malar rash*: erythema over the malar eminences, sparing nasolabial folds

2) *Discoid rash:* thick, raised or flat red scarring with well-defined borders. Usually on sun-exposed areas and not itchy

3) *Photosensitivity*

4) *Oral ulcers*

5) *Arthritis:* non-erosive, ≥2 peripheral joints and characterized by tenderness, swelling or effusion. Occur in 90% of patients

6) *Serositis:* pleuritis or pericarditis

7) *Renal (lupus nephritis):* persistent proteinuria >0.5 g/24 h, haematuria, pyuria or urinary casts. Occurs in 50% of patients

8) *Neurological (lupus cerebritis):* new onset seizures, headaches, chorea, stroke, transverse myelitis, mood disorders or psychosis: in absence of drug use or metabolic derangements (electrolyte imbalance, uraemia, ketoacidosis). Occurs in 20% of patients

9) *Haematological:* haemolytic anaemia, leukopenia <4000/μl on ≥2 occasions, lymphopenia <1500/μl on ≥2 occasions, or thrombocytopenia <100 000/μl in absence of drugs

10) *Antinuclear antibody (ANA):* presence of ANA in absence of lupus-inducing drugs. Found in 96% of patients. ANA titres do not change with disease activity. Homogenous pattern of ANA binding is found in 65% of patients but its specificity is low. Peripheral pattern of ANA binding is most specific for SLE but its sensitivity is low

11) *Immunological*

- **Anti-DNA antibodies:** anti-double-stranded DNA (anti-ds DNA). Found in 80–90% of patients, elevated levels precede relapse in 80% of patients. Anti-single-stranded DNA is less specific for SLE

- **Anti-smooth (Sm) antibodies:** an antibody to extractable nuclear antigens (ENAs). Found in 40% of patients and is highly specific for SLE

- **Antiphospholipid antibodies (aPL):** positive test for anticardiolipin and/or lupus anticoagulant (see Section 7.26)

Other features of systemic lupus erythematosus

- Fever, fatigue, weight loss, myalgia, lymphadenopathy, Raynaud's phenomenon
- Antibodies to other ENAs such as Ro/SS-A and/or La/SS-B are found in 30% of patients, and are associated with neonatal lupus
- Reduced complement titres (C3 and C4)

Drugs which induce lupus erythematosis

- Mainly procainamide, quinidine, and hydralazine (but others e.g. methyldopa, valproate, carbamazepine, chlorpromazine, isoniazid, sulfasalazine, lovastatin, simvastatin, interleukins, interferon, griseofulvin, minocycline, penicillamine)
- Can take months or years to bring on lupus-like symptoms
- Diagnosis of exclusion—drug withdrawal leads to improvement in patient with previously normal immune system

Effect of pregnancy on systemic lupus erythematosus

- Flares in pregnancy are usually mild, occur at any stage, uncertain whether the frequency is increased or not
- Rate of SLE flare is lower when prior quiescent disease
- Lupus nephritis is unlikely to first manifest in pregnancy without a past history of renal involvement

In women with pre-existing lupus nephritis:

- In general, 33% have renal flares in pregnancy
- Between 7–10% have flares if conceive >6-month remission
- Between 50–60% have flares if conceive with active disease
- Increasing proteinuria is common in second trimester owing to increased glomerular filtration rate
- 21% experience renal deterioration
- 7% have permanent deterioration

Effect of systemic lupus erythematosus on pregnancy

- Normal outcome if remission for ≥6 months, no hypertension, lupus nephritis, thrombocytopenia or aPLs
- The risk of miscarriage, fetal death, pre-eclampsia, fetal growth restriction (FGR), and prematurity is increased in SLE with aPL, lupus nephritis (especially if hypertension or proteinuria), active disease at conception or first SLE presentation during pregnancy
- Presence of anti-Ro/La increases the risk of neonatal lupus

Detection of lupus flare in pregnancy

- There is symptom overlap between normal pregnancy and SLE flare and between lupus nephritis and pre-eclampsia.
- Increasing proteinuria, thrombocytopenia, and new onset seizures may occur in worsening SLE/lupus nephritis and in severe pre-eclampsia.

Presence of these factors point towards an SLE flare:

- Active disease within 6 months of conception
- Extreme fatigue (occurs in 80–100% of SLE patients), skin lesions (>90%), arthralgia (>80%), fever not due to infection, lymphadenopathy, pleuritic pain
- Leukopenia, raised anti-ds DNA levels, reduced complement levels (C3, C4)
- Presence of proteinuria before the third trimester, haematuria and/or urinary casts

Presence of the following points towards pre-eclampsia:
- A normal baseline 24-h protein excretion
- Elevated serum urate and/or abnormal LFT
- Antithrombin deficiency

Management of systemic lupus erythematosus
Prepregnancy management
- *History*: ask about current symptoms, recent SLE flares, any previous child affected by neonatal lupus
- *Examine:* for malar rash, discoid rash, and oral ulcers
- Assess *renal status*: check blood pressure, urinalysis, baseline 24-h protein, serum creatinine, urea and electrolytes (U&E). Arrange renal biopsy if lupus nephritis is suspected
- Assess *haematologic status*: FBC with white cell differentiation
- Assess *maternal and fetal risks*: anti-ds DNA, aPL, complement titres, anti-Ro/La
- *Counsel*: regarding maternal and fetal risks, and neonatal lupus:
  - Pregnancy outcome is best if the patient is in remission for at least 6 months with no history of renal disease, hypertension, thrombocytopenia, or aPL
  - Women with significant renal insufficiency (serum creatinine >2.0 mg/dl or 177 µmol/l) have a high risk of renal deterioration and poor fetal outcome, thus advise against pregnancy
- *Review medication*: avoid NSAIDs (may interfere with blastocyst implantation). Substitute ACE inhibitors for control of hypertension
- *Discontinue* cytotoxic drugs such as methotrexate and cyclophosphamide for ≥3 months before conception. In women taking high-dose methotrexate, pregnancy should be avoided for up to 2 years.
- *Avoid* mucophenalate in pregnancy.

Antenatal management
- Involve multidisciplinary team
- Prophylactic steroids do not prevent flares

Monitor disease activity: anti-ds DNA, complement titres and 24-h urinary protein should be done each trimester

For **control of hypertension**, see Section 7.4. Hydralazine and methyldopa have been associated with lupus-like syndrome but are not contraindicated in SLE.

Flares should be actively treated
- Lupus nephritis can only be confirmed with renal biopsy but this is generally not recommended in pregnancy
- Before fetal viability, confirmation with renal biopsy allows immunosuppressive treatment of SLE without delivery
- When the fetus is mature, consider delivery

CNS manifestations: consider electroencephalogram, brain imaging, followed by lumbar puncture to exclude infection.

Monitor the fetus:
- Fetal heart auscultation weekly from 16 weeks if Anti-Ro and/or Anti-La antibodies to screen for fetal complete heart block
- Anomaly scan should be performed at 18–22 weeks
- Fetal echocardiography if suspected complete heart block
- Serial ultrasound scans for fetal growth

Intrapartum management
- Aim for vaginal delivery
- Hydrocortisone 100 mg IM 6-hourly if women have taken >7.5 mg of prednisolone for >2 weeks

Postpartum management
- If mother anti-Ro/La-positive, baby should have an ECG
- No breastfeeding and use contraception if taking methotrexate or cyclophosphamide
- Azathioprine has theoretical immunosuppression but has been used in breastfeeding
- Hydroxychloroquine and NSAIDs can potentially displace bilirubin, so discontinue if baby jaundiced

Treatment of systemic lupus erythematosus in pregnancy
Hydroxychloroquine:
- Safe for use in malarial prophylactic doses
- Larger doses may cause fetal retinopathy
- If taken prepregnancy, should be continued to avoid increasing flares

Corticosteroids:
- Improve outcome in women with active SLE and/or raised anti-ds DNA levels
- Prednisolone or methylprednisolone are preferable because they are better metabolized by the placenta
- Doses are the same as prepregnancy but may be reduced if patient appears to be in remission
- Increase the risk of hypertension, pre-eclampsia, gestational diabetes, FGR, preterm birth, osteoporosis, and poor wound healing
- Monitor blood pressure, screen for gestational diabetes, and perform serial growth scans

Treatment of systemic lupus erythematosus flare in pregnancy
Mild to moderate flare without CNS or renal involvement:
- Initiate prednisolone or increase dose to 15–30 mg/day
Severe flare without CNS or renal involvement:
- Prednisolone 1.0–1.5 mg/kg/day should be used. Good response should be seen in 5–10 days, then taper dose
Severe flare with CNS or renal involvement:
- Intravenous methylprednisolone 10–30 mg/kg/day for 3–6 days
  - Then give prednisolone 1.0–1.5 mg/kg/day
- In postpartum women, azathioprine, methotrexate or cyclophosphamide may be used (avoid breastfeeding)
Lupus nephritis flare:
- Prednisolone 1.0–1.5 mg/kg/day should be used. If no response in 2 weeks, consider azathioprine or cyclophosphamide, and early termination, especially if there is deteriorating renal function
Plasmapheresis and intravenous immunoglobulin (IVIG) have been used to treat severe flare unresponsive to other treatment.

Further reading

Buyon JP. Management of SLE during pregnancy: A decision tree. *Rheumatologia* 2004; **20(4):**197–201.

Porter TF, Branch DW. Autoimmune diseases. In: James DK, Steer PJ, Weiner CP, Gonik B (eds.) *High Risk Pregnancy Management Options.* Elsevier Saunders: Philadelphia, 2005: 949–85.

7.26 Neonatal lupus erythematosus and rheumatoid arthritis

Neonatal lupus erythematosus

Incidence
One in 20 000 live births.

Pathophysiology
- Passively aquired autoimmunity from transplacental passage of anti-Ro and/or anti-La
- Of babies with neonatal lupus, 75–95% of mothers test positive for anti-Ro and 50–70% test positive for anti-La
- Anti-Ro is present in <1% of population, 30% of systemic lupus erythematosus (SLE) patients, and in those with Sjogren syndrome, subacute lupus erythematosus, Raynaud's phenomenon, and photosensitivity

The risk of delivering a baby with neonatal lupus
- Less than 5% in mothers with SLE
- In mothers with anti-Ro/La: risk of cutaneous neonatal lupus is 15%, risk of neonatal heart block is 2–5%
- Neonatal lupus is not related to severity of maternal disease
- Risk is increased if a previous child is affected: 16–18% if one and 50% if two previous children affected

Haematological neonatal lupus is rare. May manifest as autoimmune haemolytic anaemia, leukopenia, thrombocytopenia, and hepatosplenomegaly.

Cutaneous neonatal lupus: commonest manifestation of neonatal lupus. Erythematous, scaling plaques on the face and scalp usually appear in the first 2 weeks, and can last for 6 months. Avoid sunlight and phototherapy

Cardiac neonatal lupus: permanent congenital complete heart block (CCHB), endocardial fibroelastosis, myocarditis, dilated cardiomyopathy, pericardial effusion, and mitral insufficiency. Mortality rate of CCHB is 30%, mainly <90 days.

The pathogenesis of CCHB is dependent on a specific antiRo causing inflammation and fibrosis of the cardiac conducting system, especially the atrioventricular node.

Heart block may progress through first, second, and then third degree. In severe cases heart failure leads to hydrops fetalis and intrauterine death (IUD).

Diagnosis of congenital heart block
- Bradycardia detected during routine scan or check
- Fetal echo shows atrioventricular dissociation with a structurally normal heart
- Maternal autoantibodies confirm neonatal lupus
- Patients with a previous affected child and/or anti-Ro/La should have regular fetal auscultation

Management of congenital complete heart block
Antenatal management
CCHB is permanent but first and second degree heart block may be reversible with maternal dexamethasone therapy. However, this is controversial and increases maternal hypertension, pre-eclampsia, and gestational diabetes.

Permenant heart damage can occur within 1 week of a normal fetal echo or first degree heart block.

Close monitoring is required with frequent auscultation. If bradycardia is detected at or near term, deliver immediately.

After delivery
- Arrange for neonatal ECG, FBC and LFT
- Avoid sunlight and phototherapy
- 60% of survivors require pacemakers in early infancy, or by early teens to prevent sudden death
- Counsel the mother about recurrence (10–20%)

Rheumatoid arthritis
Rheumatoid arthritis (RA) is a chronic inflammatory disease mainly affecting synovial joints.

Incidence
- Peak incidence is at the age of 35 years
- Affects 1:1–2000 pregnancies

Pathophysiology
- 70% of cases are associated with HLA-D4
- Unknown endogenous or exogenous antigens activate CD4 T cells which stimulate monocytes, macrophages, and synovial fibroblasts to produce cytokines and B cells to produce antibodies and rheumatoid factor (RF)

Diagnosis
Classification criteria for the diagnosis of rheumatoid arthritis
At least 4 of the following must be present for >6 weeks (American College of Rheumatology):
- Morning stiffness in and around the joints for ≥1 h before maximal improvement
- Arthritis of ≥3 joint areas simultaneously with soft tissue swelling or fluid
- Arthritis of hand joints
- Symmetrical arthritis
- Rheumatoid nodules (subcutaneous, over bony prominences, extensor surfaces or in juxta-articular regions)
- Serum rheumatoid factor (RF): found in 5% of general population and 90% of RA patients
- Changes on posteroanterior hand and wrist radiographs, including erosions, unequivocal bony decalcification localised in or most marked adjacent to involved joints

Other features
- Deformities such as ulnar deviation of the metacarpophalangeal joints, Swan neck, and Boutonniere deformities of the fingers may be apparent in later stages
- Extra-articular features: fatigue, vasculitis, subcutaneous nodules, normocytic normochromic anaemia, pulmonary granulomas, effusions and fibrosis, pericarditis and amyloidosis
- Immune complexes are common in the synovial fluid and circulation
- Antinuclear antibodies are positive in about 30% cases.
- About 5–10% have antiphospholipid antibodies

Effect of pregnancy on rheumatoid arthritis
- Between 70–80% of patients improve during pregnancy, most of whom will relapse in the postpartum period
- About 16% of patients achieve remission
- Women who improved in a previous pregnancy are more likely to improve in subsequent pregnancies
- Postpartum flares may be related to resurgence of T cell-mediated immunity, and are exacerbated by breastfeeding
- There is a higher incidence of first presentation of RA postpartum, especially after the first child
- Age, duration and severity of RA, and presence of RF do not predict outcome in pregnancy

Effect of rheumatoid arthritis on pregnancy
- No adverse effect on pregnancy
- The main concerns relate to the safety of medical treatment
- Atlanto-axial subluxation rarely complicates general anaesthesia

Management
Prepregnancy management
- Avoid pregnancy during active RA
- Avoid NSAIDs: may affect blastocyst implantation and miscarriage (cause or association unclear)
- Use contraception when taking teratogenic drugs. Discontinue these drugs for >3 months before conception: methotrexate, cyclophosphamide, chlorambucil, cyclosporine, penicillamine, gold salts
- Leflunomide: the active metabolite takes up to 2 years to be undetectable in plasma and needs elimination with cholestyramine
- The following drugs lack safety data in pregnancy and should be avoided: mycophenolate mofetil, gold salts, penicillamine, tumour necrosis factor-α inhibitors (anakinra, etanercept, rituximab, infliximab)

Antenatal management and treatment of rheumatoid arthritis
Non-pharmacological control of arthralgia preferred:
- Paraffin baths, curtail physical activity, splinting, cold packs

Simple analgesics:
- Paracetamol

NSAIDs should be avoided in the last trimester:
- Effects on fetal kidney may cause oligohydramnios
- May cause premature closure of ductus arteriosus
- May increase the risk of neonatal haemorrhage via inhibition of platelet function
- Avoid COX-2 NSAIDs (associated with heart defects)

Corticosteroids:
- Preferable to NSAIDs, use lowest effective dose
- Increase risk of maternal hypertension, pre-eclampsia, gestational diabetes, preterm birth, and osteoporosis
- Monitor blood pressure and glucose levels regularly
- Calcium and vitamin D supplements recommended

Sulfasalazine:
- Safe for use in pregnancy and breastfeeding
- A dihydrofolate reductase inhibitor which increases neural tube defects, oral clefts, heart defects
- Give patients concomitant folate 5 mg/day

Hydroxychloroquine:
- Safe for use in malarial prophylactic doses
- Larger doses may cause fetal retinopathy
- Treatment may be stopped if RA improves

Azathioprine:
- For patients who require immunosuppression
- Safe in pregnancy, maybe because of fetal liver immaturity that converts it to active metabolites
- May be used as a steroid-sparing agent but its onset of action is ≥3 weeks
- Theoretical risk of immunosuppression in the neonate if breastfeeding but not a contraindication

Monitor patients:
- Check FBC for normocytic, normochromic anaemia
- Patients on sulfasalazine: check liver function
- ESR and RF levels are not useful

Assess the range of motion of hip and neck joints:
- Ensure that the patient is able to abduct and externally rotate her hips for vaginal delivery
- Neck X-ray and refer the patient to anaesthetists if neck or neurological symptoms—to identify those with ligamental instability of the atlantoaxial joint

Intrapartum management
- Aim for vaginal delivery
- Hydrocortisone 100 mg IM 6-hourly if taking >7.5 mg prednisolone for >2 weeks in pregnancy

Postpartum management
- Inform patients not to breastfeed and to use contraception when taking methotrexate, cyclophosphamide, chlorambucil or ciclosporin
- Hydroxychloroquine and NSAIDs can potentially displace bilirubin, so discontinue if baby jaundiced

7.27 Antiphospholipid antibodies and syndrome

Antiphospholipid antibodies are common and do not, alone constitute the disease antiphospholipid syndrome (APS).

Antiphospholipid antibodies (aPL)

A heterogenous group of antibodies directed against anionic phospholipids and/or phospholipid-binding proteins (which include β2-glycoprotein-1 (β2GP1), prothrombin, factor V, protein C, protein S, annexin-V).

The commonest detected aPLs are anticardiolipin antibody (aCL) and lupus anticoagulant (LA). LA causes agglutination of phospholipids important for coagulation ⇒ increased clotting time. It is associated with false positive tests for syphilis.

Prevalence

- Between 2–10% of normal population
- Between 10–20% of women with recurrent miscarriage. aPLs are less common in women with <3 miscarriages
- 30% of patients with thrombosis
- 30% of severe, early-onset pre-eclampsia
- Between 30–50% of systemic lupus erythematosus (SLE) patients
- Most APS patients do not fulfil the diagnostic criteria for SLE and most primary antiphospholipid syndromes (APS) do not progress to SLE
- Higher in women with abruption, fetal death, or fetal growth restriction (FGR) without hypertension
- Also found in infections e.g. HIV and B cell lymphoma

Antiphospholipid syndrome

Definition

APS is a disorder characterized by:

1. Thrombosis (venous, arterial, microcirculation) and/or
2. Pregnancy morbidity, i.e
   - ≥3 consecutive miscarriages <10 weeks' gestation, or
   - ≥1 fetal death >10 weeks or
   - ≥1 preterm birth <34 weeks with normal fetal morphology due to pre-eclampsia or placental insufficiency
3. Combined with the presence of aPL (either aCL +/or LA) on two separate occasions at least 6 weeks apart.

Types of antiphospholipid syndrome

1. Primary APS: occurs alone
2. Secondary APS: associated with other conditions, mainly SLE

Other clinical features

- Immune thrombocytopenia (ITP), haemolytic anaemia
- Cerebral involvement: epilepsy, cerebral infarction, chorea, migraine, transverse myelitis
- Heart valve disease (particularly mitral valve)
- Systemic and pulmonary hypertension
- Livedo reticularis
- Amaurosis fugax
- Leg ulcers

Pathophysiology

The *in vivo* mechanisms responsible for thrombosis and fetal loss are uncertain, but several pathways are suggested:

- aPL binding with phospholipids may interfere with the coagulation cascade ⇒ a procoagulant state
- aCL binding requires the presence β2GP1 and may interfere with its anticoagulant. Anti-β2GP1 antibodies are more specific for APS but there is poor lab standardization

- aPL affects *in vitro* trophoblast differentiation, proliferation and invasion ⇒ impaired implantation
- Annexin-V, an anticoagulant on normal placental villi, is ↓ with aPL. There is placental infarction and thrombosis, possibly owing to spiral artery vasculopathy
- In the mouse model, the mechanism of APS pregnancy loss is complement activation and not thrombosis

Effect of pregnancy on antiphospholipid syndrome

- Risk of thrombosis, including CVA, in APS is exacerbated by the hypercoagulable pregnant state
- Pre-existing ITP may worsen in pregnancy

Effect of antiphospholipid syndrome on pregnancy

- Increased risk of recurrent miscarriage, hypertension, pre-eclampsia, FGR, fetal death, preterm birth, abruption, and thrombosis
- Complications are less in women with previous recurrent miscarriages than previous thrombosis or late fetal death
- Risk is related to antibody titre, especially IgG aCL
- Thrombosis is more strongly associated with LA than with aCL
- Past obstetric history is the best predictor of outcome

Fetal death can follow FGR, oligohydramnios, pre-eclampsia.

- The risk of FGR is more than 30%
- ↑ risk of non-reassuring fetal heart rate pattern in labour

Pre-eclampsia is often severe. Risk is 10% in those with previous recurrent loss but 30–50% in those with previous thrombosis or late fetal death. It may develop as early as 15 weeks, especially if previous thrombosis or late fetal death.

Preterm birth risk is 10% with past recurrent loss but 30–40% in those with SLE, previous thrombosis or late fetal death.

Laboratory criteria for the identification of aPL

LA requires ≥2 phospholipid-dependent coagulation tests. Activated partial thromboplastin time (APTT) and dilute Russell viper venom time (dRVVT) are both prolonged. Addition of normal plasma fails to correct the prolonged time and addition of excess phospholipid corrects the prolonged time.

aCL are measured using commercially available enzyme-linked immunosorbent assay (ELISA) kits. Medium to high titres of IgG or IgM aCL are required.

Treatment

Immunosuppression with intravenous immunoglobulin (IVIG), prednisone, azathioprine or plasmapheresis is ineffective. Prednisone increases the risk of preterm birth, pre-eclampsia, hypertension, and gestational diabetes.

Currently the mainstay of therapy is anticoagulation, but prophylaxis against APS thrombosis with low-dose aspirin (LDA) 75 mg/day has not been proven to be effective.

In a non-pregnant APS patient with prior thrombosis:

- Recurrence risk of thrombosis is up to 70% and often occurs in the same vascular distribution as the first event

Venous thrombosis

- Occurs in 32% of APS patients
- Warfarin therapy with a target INR of 2.0–3.0 reduces recurrence by 80–90% and is as effective as an INR of 3.0–4.0
- Recurrence rate is highest in the first 6 months after stopping warfarin therapy, thus lifelong warfarin anticoagulation is warranted

Arterial thrombosis

- The commonest is stroke (13%)
- Next are transient ischaemic attacks (7%)

- Aspirin 300 mg/day alone is as effective as moderate-intensity warfarin (INR 1.4–2.8) in preventing recurrence

In women with aPL and ≥1 fetal loss but no thrombosis:
- LDA alone has no benefit over placebo in reducing pregnancy loss
- Heparin and LDA reduces pregnancy loss by 54%, when compared with LDA alone. The effects of high dose unfractionated heparin (UFH) do not differ from low dose UFH

Recommendations for treatment of APS in pregnancy

Where heparin is used, the current practice is to:
- Use LMWH. This has the advantage of once-daily dosing and carries less risk of heparin-induced thrombocytopenia and osteoporosis than UFH. However, there is currently insufficient evidence to compare efficacy between UFH and LMWH
- Interrupt heparin therapy during labour or on the day of delivery and recommence postnatally for 6 weeks, or until warfarin has been reintroduced and the target INR has been reached for at least 2 consecutive days

Where LDA is used, the current practice is to:
- Start 75 mg per day prepregnancy and continue during pregnancy until 4 weeks before delivery

Previous late fetal loss, neonatal death or adverse outcome due to pre-eclampsia, FGR or abruption:
- LDA prepregnancy and start prophylactic LMWH once pregnancy is confirmed

Prior thrombosis
- LDA prepregnancy
- If on maintenance warfarin before pregnancy:
  - Change warfarin to therapeutic dose of LMWH <6 weeks' gestation to avoid warfarin embryopathy. Recommence warfarin postpartum
  - It may be necessary to use warfarin in pregnant women with previous cerebral arterial thrombosis if heparin is inadequate to prevent transient ischaemic events
- If not on maintenance warfarin:
  - Commence LMWH once pregnancy is confirmed and for 6 weeks postpartum

No previous thrombosis
- Many advocate LDA alone, although this has not been proven to be effective in preventing fetal loss or thrombosis

Women with SLE (secondary APS)
- Hydroxychloroquine may provide some protection from thrombosis and should be continued in pregnancy

Prepregnancy
- Women with a history of recurrent miscarriages, thrombosis, severe early-onset pre-eclampsia or FGR, or fetal death should be screened for the presence of aCL or LA

- Check for anaemia, thrombocytopenia, renal compromise
- Discuss anticoagulation prophylaxis and risk of warfarin versus heparin therapy

Antenatal
- Multidisciplinary care involving obstetricians, rheumatologists and haematologists
- Start anticoagulant prophylaxis with LDA and LMWH
- Prenatal visits every 2–4 weeks initially, then 1–2 weekly in second half of pregnancy. BP checks and urinalysis should be performed to detect early-onset pre-eclampsia
- Fetal surveillance:
  - Ultrasound monitoring of fetal growth and uteroplacental blood flow is important
  - Uterine artery waveforms can be assessed at 20–24 weeks' gestation. Those with early diastolic notching should have 2–4-weekly growth scans and regular BP checks because of the high risk of FGR and pre-eclampsia
  - Those with low risk (e.g. aPLs only and no notches) can have midwifery care (add 4-weekly USS for growth and amniotic fluid volume if poor history or anxious)

Intrapartum
- Aim for vaginal delivery near term
- Unless low risk (e.g. aPLs only and no notches), induction should be considered by the estimated date of delivery
- Discontinue heparin during labour and delivery
- Consider sequential compression devices
- Continuous electronic fetal monitoring

Postpartum
- Resume anticoagulation
- Women on long-term warfarin therapy may recommence this on day 2–3 postpartum and LMWH is discontinued when the INR is >2.0 for 2 consecutive days
- Encourage breastfeeding
- Avoid the COCP

Further reading

Lim W, Crowther MA, Eikelboom JW. Management of antiphospholipid antibody syndrome: a systematic review. *JAMA* 2006; **295(9):**1050–7.

www.cochrane.org Empson M, Lassere M, Craig J, Scott J. Prevention of recurrent miscarriage for women with antiphospholipid antibody or lupus anticoagulant. *Cochrane Database of Systematic Reviews,* 2005.

Petri M, Qazi U. Management of antiphospholipid syndrome in pregnancy. *Rheum Dis Clin North Am* 2006; **32(3):**591–607.

Porter TF, Branch DW. Autoimmune diseases. In: James DK, Steer PJ, Weiner CP, Gonik B (eds.) *High Risk Pregnancy Management Options.* Elsevier Saunders: Philadelphia, 2005: 949–85.

Definitions

Crohn's disease

Crohn's disease (CD) is an idiopathic, relapsing, chronic granulomatous inflammatory disease affecting the full thickness of the bowel wall. It affects mainly the terminal ileum but can be anywhere in a discontinuous pattern.

Ulcerative colitis

Ulcerative colitis (UC) is an idiopathic, relapsing, chronic inflammatory disease of the rectum. It usually affects only the mucosa and submucosa. May extend proximally to involve the entire colon in continuity.

Prevalence

- CD: 50 in 100 000, M:F = 1:1
- UC: 80 in 100 000, affects F > M

Pathophysiology

A genetic predisposition exists in both CD and UC. Infection, autoimmunity, and environmental toxins may also be involved.

Bowel inflammation is caused by immune dysregulation in response to normal gut flora in the genetically susceptible. In CD, there is mutation in *NOD2*, a gene encoding an intracellular receptor for bacterial lipopolysaccharide.

The inflammatory response is caused by:
- Interleukin-12 and interferon-γ in CD
- Interleukin-13 in UC

Smoking is associated with ↑ risk of CD but ↓ risk of UC.

Clinical features

Crohn's disease

- Abdominal pain, diarrhoea, weight loss, rectal bleeding (fresh or malaena), fistulae, perinanal sepsis
- Affects terminal ileum and colon in 50% cases, terminal ileum alone in 30% cases, colon alone in 20% cases

Ulcerative colitis

- Lower abdominal pain, watery diarrhoea, faecal urgency, rectal passage of blood and mucus. May have fever and abdominal distension (toxic megacolon)
- Confined to the colon and rectum

Extraintestinal manifestations include:

- Arthritis (sacroileitis, ankylosing spondylitis)
- Aphthous ulcers (CD)
- Gallstones
- Ascending cholangitis, sclerosing cholangitis
- Conjunctivitis, iridocyclitis, episcleritis

Complications

CD: perforation, stricture formation, perianal problems, fistulae, and abscess formation.
UC: toxic megacolon and malignancy if longstanding

Diagnosis

Most women have been diagnosed before pregnancy. The diagnosis is based on imaging, colonoscopy, and biopsy.

Effect of pregnancy on inflammatory bowel disease

- Risk of relapse is similar during and outside pregnancy for both CD and UC (30–50% per year)
- Relapse more common in first trimester. More frequent postpartum relapse reported in CD but not UC

Most women with prior surgery and quiescent disease tolerate pregnancy well.

Complications include:
- Malabsorption of fat, fat-soluble vitamins, vitamin B12, electrolyte imbalance
- Obstruction of ileostomy as pregnancy progresses
- Peristomal cracking and bleeding may occur owing to abdominal wall stretching

Effect of inflammatory bowel disease on pregnancy

- Fertility may be ↓ in active CD
- Active disease at the time of conception is associated with ↑ risk of miscarriage and preterm birth

Management

Prepregnancy management

- Encourage conception during remission, avoid pregnancy during active disease
- Folate supplementation 5 mg/day
- Consider changing drug therapy to those with a good safety record in pregnancy

Antenatal management

- Continue folate supplementation
- Monitor fetal growth

Intrapartum management

- Operative delivery for obstetric indications only
- Prepare for surgical problems if previous abdominal surgery
- Avoid vaginal delivery or episiotomy in severe perianal CD, impaired anal continence with ileal pouch-anal anastomosis

Postpartum management

- ↑ frequency of relapse is reported in CD but not in UC
- Encourage breastfeeding. This is safe in women taking sulphasalazine, mesalazine, corticosteroids, metronidazole
- Limited date about safety of azathioprine and breastfeeding but the benefits of continuing therapy to maintain remission outweigh the risks of discontinuing therapy
- Advise regarding contraception

Management of acute inflammatory bowel disease relapse

- Multidisciplinary: obstetrician, gastroenterologist and surgeon
- Management of IBD in pregnancy is the same as outside, but abdominal pain may have obstetric causes, i.e. preterm labour
- Check blood for anaemia, electrolyte imbalance, serum albumin or impaired liver function
- Stool culture to exclude infection
- Check C-reactive protein (CRP). Erythrocyte sedimentation rate (ESR) is normally ↑ in pregnancy unlike CRP
- Plain abdominal X-ray: if toxic megacolon suspected
- Surgery for obstruction, toxic megacolon, haemorrhage or perforation should not be delayed due to pregnancy
- Treatment with 5-aminosalicylate derivatives (sulphasalazine, mesalazine, olsalazine, balsalazide), corticosteroids, azathioprine, metronidazole, loperamide is safe in pregnancy and breastfeeding
- 5-aminosalicylic acid (5-ASA) derivatives:
  - To induce and maintain remission of colonic CD and UC
  - Salazopyrin (sulfasalazine) used orally or rectally splits in the colon into sulphapyridine and 5-ASA
  - Sulfasalazine is a dihydrofolate reductase inhibitor that blocks the conversion of folate to its more active metabolites
  - Folate supplement 5 mg/day should be given before and during pregnancy

Chapter 8

Problems arising during pregnancy

Contents

Covered elsewhere

8.1 Antepartum haemorrhage

Definition
Antepartum haemorrhage (APH) is bleeding of >5ml from the genital tract after 24 weeks' gestation.

Incidence
- Between 2 and 5% of all pregnancies

Causes
- Placental abruption (10–15%)
- Placenta praevia (15–26%)
- Local
- Undetermined

Clinical relevance
In the last Confidential Enquiry into Maternal and Child Health 2003–2005, there were five deaths from antepartum haemorrhage (three from praevia and two from abruption).

Of the 3791 stillbirths in 2004, 10% were due to APH.

Clinical evaluation
History
- Gestational age
- Presence or absence of fetal movements
- Timing and amount of bleeding
- Fresh or old (brown) or mixed with mucus
- Association and nature of pain and contractions
- History of preceding coitus or trauma
- Site of bleed (from vagina, rectum, urethra)
- Placental site on scan
- Blood group

Examination
- Observations (BP, pulse, respiration rate)
- Evidence of shock (pallor, cool peripheries, slow capillary refill, nausea, vomiting, restlessness)
- Abdominal examination
- Assess fundal height: can be large-for-gestational age in massive abruption or small-for-gestational age (SGA) when associated with fetal growth restriction (FGR)
- Assess the lie, presentation, and viability of fetus(es)
- Uterus may be soft, tender, irritable or 'woody' hard
- External examination to assess amount of blood loss and whether it is continuing
- Speculum examination once placenta praevia excluded to look for lower genital tract bleeding
- Digital examination should not be performed unless placenta praevia definitely excluded owing to the risk of heavy bleeding

Investigations
- FBC, G&S, crossmatch if heavy bleeding
- Kleihauer in Rhesus-negative women
- Clotting and U & Es in abruption or heavy bleeding
- CTG to assess fetal wellbeing and uterine activity
- Ultrasound for placental site and presentation once maternal and fetal condition stable

Inform anaesthetic staff if bleeding is significant or continued.

Inform SCBU and neonatologists if preterm delivery is expected or there is evidence of fetal distress.

Initial management
Management of APH depends on the cause, maternal and fetal condition, gestation, and degree of bleeding. It is best to treat APHs of unknown origin as if they were small abruptions.

Large bore cannula (14–16G), or two if significant bleed (>500 ml) or continued bleeding.

Initial resuscitation in heavy bleeding should be with colloids (maximum 2 l, then red blood cell transfusion). Liaise with haematology early and order at least 4–6 units of blood. If in shock or massive haemorrhage anticipated, consider requesting 10 units initially. For example, a concealed bleed that has led to intrauterine death (IUD) is likely to be >1.5 l. Owing to the high risk of disseminated intravascular coagulation (DIC) with massive APH, order fresh frozen plasma (FFP) as well.

In massive haemorrhage, the differential diagnosis will only be placenta abruption or praevia (see Sections 8.2 and 8.3).

It is important to estimate blood loss as accurately as possible to guide replacement—weigh swabs and measure volume of blood in massive haemorrhage.

Postpartum haemorrhage (PPH) will nearly always complicate a significant (>500 ml) APH (see Section 11.1).

All Rh-negative women will need to receive anti-D according to the RCOG guidelines (**B**).

Consider corticosteroids if preterm delivery (<36 weeks) is expected as per RCOG guidelines (**A**).

Local and undetermined bleeding

Show
Bleeding when the mucous plug is shed from the cervix.

Cervical causes
Cervicitis, cervical polyps, and, rarely, cervical carcinoma. Hence the need to perform a speculum on anyone who presents with bleeding once placenta praevia has been excluded.

Cervical polyps should be assessed postnatally, and removed if still present.

If a cervical carcinoma is expected, then refer immediately to colposcopy.

Postcoital
This is a common presentation. Light painless bleeding from the cervix occurs secondary to sexual intercourse. It is usually noticed immediately after intercourse or when the woman next goes to the toilet.

On speculum, a bleeding point or ectropion may be seen. If confirmed postcoital bleed (i.e. painless spotting immediately after intercourse with bleeding point seen on cervix and placenta not low), then the woman can be discharged.

However, if the cause is in doubt then always consider abruption or placenta praevia and treat appropriately.

Genital infections
Bleeding can be secondary to vaginitis (thrush, bacterial vaginosis and *Trichomonas vaginalis*) and cervicitis (Neisseria, Gonoccocus, and *Chlamydia trachomatis*). Thrush is very common in pregnancy and can be diagnosed clinically on speculum. Take swabs (see also Sections 3.2 and 3.3).

Vasa praevia

A rare but dangerous cause of bleeding.

A velamentous cord insertion occurs when the cord inserts into the membranes and the umbilical vessels run through the membranes to the placenta. If this occurs in the lower segment, it is known as a vasa praevia. The vessels can be torn when the membranes rupture (spontaneously or artificially), causing sudden fetal distress and exsanguination if delivery is not immediate. This can also occur when there are vessels travelling through the membranes to a succenturiate lobe.

Undetermined

In a proportion of cases, the cause of bleeding is undetermined. These probably represent cases of minor placenta praevia or abruption and should be monitored as such.

Further reading

www.rcog.org.uk Use of anti-D immunoglobulin for Rh prophylaxis. Green top guideline no. 22, 2002.

www.nice.org.uk Pregnancy—routine anti-D prophylaxis for Rh-D negative women, 2002.

8.2 Placental abruption

Definition
Placental abruption is the premature separation of a normally sited placenta from the uterus and occurs in about 1% of pregnancies.

Risk factors
- Idiopathic (majority)
- Increasing age
- Increased parity
- Hypertension
- Smoking
- Trauma (traffic accident, seat belt injury, assault and domestic violence—see Section 1.9)
- Cocaine use
- External cephalic version (ECV)
- Sudden uterine decompression following membrane rupture in polyhydramnios and multiple pregnancy
- Raised second trimester alpha fetoprotein levels
- Bilateral notching on uterine artery Doppler

Clinical evaluation
Diagnosis of an abruption is clinical and women tend to present with vaginal bleeding and pain, premature labour or CTG abnormalities.

The supposedly typical features of pain (particularly if the placenta is posterior) and bleeding will not always be present. Probability of abruption depends on background risk.

Always consider the diagnosis even if the typical signs are not present.

Revealed abruption: blood tracks from the site of placental separation between the decidua and chorion to the cervix causing vaginal bleeding.

Concealed abruption: blood forms a retroplacental clot between the placenta and uterus with no vaginal bleeding. This can lead to a mismatch between the amount of blood seen and the degree of maternal shock.

Extravasation of blood into the myometrium (giving rise to the blue-coloured Couvelaire uterus) causes pain and uterine irritability.

With severe abruption the uterus becomes woody hard and extremely tender to touch.

In about 50% of cases the woman will be in labour. It may be difficult to distinguish the pain and uterine irritability of abruption from labour. Consider the diagnosis if there is bloodstained liquor and uterine hyperstimulation. The CTG may show signs of fetal distress and the 'saw tooth' effect of frequent uterine activity (see Figure 8.1).

The degree of fetal distress will depend on the extent of placental separation.

Management
Presence of maternal and/or fetal compromise
- Resuscitate mother
- In severe cases, delivery will be inevitable. If the fetus is alive, deliver by the most expedient route. If fully dilated then instrumental may be possible; if not, then by CS
- In the presence of disseminated intravascular coagulation (DIC), regional anaesthesia is contraindicated owing to the risk of haemorrhage in the dural and epidural spaces. Those women will need general anaesthetic

- If the fetus has died, then vaginal delivery is the preferable mode. Assume the blood loss to be >1.5 l and expect DIC and postpartum haemorrhage (PPH). In these cases it is essential to liaise with haematology early and crossmatch at least 6–10 units of blood immediately along with other blood products (fresh frozen plasma (FFP) and cryoprecipitate)
- It is essential to monitor the mother closely as blood loss is often underestimated (especially in concealed abruption) leading to hypovolaemic shock
- Blood should be replaced as needed and coagulopathy corrected (see below)
- Strict fluid balance (hourly urine output)
- Invasive monitoring (CVP lines, arterial lines) may be necessary

Absence of maternal and/or fetal compromise
Labouring women can be allowed to proceed. Continuous maternal and fetal monitoring is necessary so that immediate recourse to CS can occur if there is evidence of fetal distress.

Antenatally, expectant management of mild cases can continue to improve fetal maturity. Admission until 24–48 h after the bleeding has settled is usual as subsequent bleeds are more likely to occur in that period. Growth scans are needed as growth restriction can occur with recurrent bleeds.

In general, if a mild abruption occurs at term, induction of labour (IOL) is advised.

In women with recurrent bleeds, IOL at 37–38 weeks should be considered.

In those with just a single small bleed with no evidence of compromise (normal growth, liquor, and uterine artery Dopplers), then there is no indication for induction.

Correct anaemia with oral supplements.

Complications
Disseminated intravascular coagulation
Incidence
- DIC complicates up to 35% of severe cases.

Pathophysiology
Thromboplastins released from damaged placental tissue cause activation of the extrinsic coagulation pathway. Clots can form in small vessels, leading to end-organ damage. Consumption of clotting factors such as fibrinogen, factors V, VII, VIII, and platelets occur. The fibrinolytic system is subsequently activated to dissolve fibrin which produces fibrin degradation products (FDPs). As the DIC worsens, clotting factors are used up, leading to uncontrolled bleeding. This will not resolve until the cause is treated (i.e. delivery and removal of the placenta) and clotting factors replaced. The situation is made worse by the fact that FDPs are potent anticoagulants and interfere with myometrial function.

Investigations
- Clotting screen-activated partial thromboplastin time (APTT), prothrombin time (PT), thrombin time (TT): APTT and PT are often prolonged with a short TT
- Platelet count: low
- Fibrinogen: low
- FDPs: raised

Management
Early contact with a senior haematologist is essential in the management of this condition so that the appropriate products can be ordered.

FFP and cryoprecipitate are used to replace fibrinogen and clotting factors. Consider giving platelets when the count falls <50 ×10⁹/l.

Acute renal failure

Pathophysiology
Hypovolaemia gives rise to prerenal renal failure while DIC causes vascular blockage within the kidneys. This can lead to oliguria or anuria.

Investigations
- Hourly urine output
- Monitor blood urea, electrolytes, and creatinine

Management
- Fluid management using a central venous pressure line
- Correct high K⁺ levels
- Advice from renal physicians should be sought

Postpartum haemorrhage (see also Section 11.1)
Poor myometrial contraction following an abruption and DIC contribute to PPH.

Fetomaternal haemorrhage
Rhesus-negative women need a Kleihauer test so that an adequate amount of anti-D can be administered to prevent immunization.

Fetal risks
Perinatal mortality is related to gestational age and has improved with use of steroids and improving neonatal care. In a recent study, the rate was found to be 9.2%.

Causes
- Prematurity
- Underlying disease states such as pre-eclampsia and fetal growth restriction (FGR)
- Hypoxia and respiratory distress
- Anaemia and coagulopathies secondary to fetal bleeding

Recurrence
The risk of an abruption occurring in a future pregnancy is between 6 and 16%. With two previous abruptions, the risk increases further (>30%).

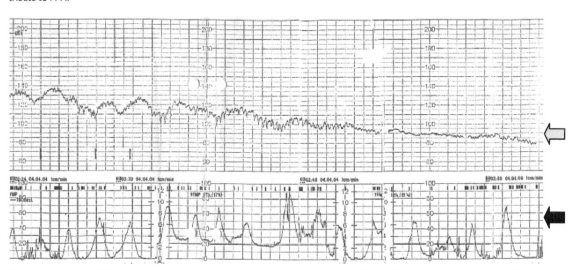

Fig. 8.1 Non-labour CTG during placental abruption showing uterine irritability and fetal demise (five or six contractions every 10 min ◀■) with a pathological (terminal ⇦) fetal heart rate.

8.3 Placenta praevia

Definition and incidence

One in five women will have an apparently low-lying placenta at 24 weeks' gestation. Placenta praevia occurs when the placenta is partially or wholly inserted into the lower segment of the uterus. As the lower segment of the uterus only forms later in pregnancy, placental 'migration' occurs, giving an overall incidence of 0.4–0.8%. Migration is less likely to occur with major degrees of placenta praevia, if the placenta is posterior or if there has previously been a CS (III).

Classification (see Figure 8.2)

Minor placenta praevia—the placenta is sited in the lower segment but does not cover the cervical os.
Major placenta praevia—the placenta covers the cervical os.

Risk factors

- Increasing age
- Increasing parity
- Previous CS (risk of 0.65% with one CS rising to 10% with four or more previous CSs)
- Previous placenta praevia
- Smoking
- Multiple pregnancy
- Previous dilatation and curettage

Clinical evaluation

- Classically, bleeding is painless (as opposed to abruption) and occurs with the development of the lower segment where shearing forces disturb placental vasculature
- Pain may be present as bleeding can be precipitated by uterine contractions and cervical dilatation. Conversely, bleeding from the low-lying placenta could cause lifting of the membranes and subsequent uterine contractions
- Some women will present for the first time with bleeding in labour
- Ten per cent of women with placenta praevia will also have a placental abruption
- In most cases, bleeding is unprovoked although it can be precipitated by sexual intercourse
- Bleeding can range from spotting with no maternal or fetal effect to torrential life-threatening bleeding and maternal shock
- The majority of women presenting with bleeding after 20 weeks will already have had an ultrasound determining placental site. However, a placenta praevia should still be excluded in a woman who presents with bleeding associated with a high presenting part or abnormal lie irrespective of previous ultrasound results

Management

Most low-lying placentae are diagnosed at the 20-week transabdominal anomaly scan and confirmed in the third trimester (see Section 6.8).

Hb levels should be optimized antenatally. Correct anaemia with iron sulphate, folate or B12 depending on the cause (see Section 6.5).

Antenatal—asymptomatic (no bleeding episodes)

Minor placenta praevia: should have a transvaginal scan (TVS) performed at 36 weeks to ascertain persistence of low position (C).

Major placenta praevia: should have a TVS performed at 32 weeks (C). Management plan for the third trimester must be made.

Traditionally, admission from 34 weeks until delivery has been advised owing to the risk of sudden and heavy bleeding. However, long admission to hospital in the absence of bleeding is not benign and can cause considerable distress, particularly with separation from family members (see Box 8.1).

Inpatient management remains the cautious, but not mandatory, option. A full discussion should take place with the mother, explaining the risks of haemorrhage. If she decides to remain at home:

- She should live close to hospital and have someone with her at all times
- She should know what to do in case of sudden heavy bleeding (call 999 immediately)
- She needs to attend hospital immediately if she has any bleeding, contractions or pain
- Keep up-to-date group and save in laboratory to reduce delays

Antenatal—symptomatic (bleeding episodes)

Any woman with a known placenta praevia who has an episode of bleeding should be admitted no matter how small the bleed.

DO NOT PERFORM A VAGINAL EXAMINATION.

The length of stay will depend on the amount of bleeding, gestation, and degree of praevia.

If bleeding is profuse with fetal or maternal compromise, resuscitation should start followed by delivery (see below). Crossmatch should be requested, and senior obstetric and anaesthetic staff informed immediately.

Traditionally, women with a major placenta praevia who have bled previously (episodes known as 'herald bleeds') should be admitted from 34 weeks' gestation in case of sudden heavy bleeding.

Expectant management until 39 weeks is preferable to reduce prematurity (with its associated morbidity and mortality). Many plan elective CS at 38 weeks to reduce the risk of maternal morbidity from emergency delivery in week 38–39. Gestational age and antepartum blood loss are directly related to perinatal mortality rate. In most cases, bleeding is self-limiting and does not cause significant morbidity, so delivery can be deferred until fetal maturation has occurred or there is a significant bleed requiring delivery. Blood can be transfused so that maternal haemoglobin remains above 10 g/dl.

An up-to-date group and save sample should always be present in the laboratory.

Clinical factors guide the need for transfusion.

Women with atypical antibodies form a high-risk group. Involve the local haematologist and blood bank early.

Fetal growth scans in those with repeated bleeds.

Encourage mobilization and use of prophylactic thromboembolic disease (TED) stockings when long inpatient stay is anticipated.

A full discussion regarding the risks of delivery should take place and be documented antenatally. This should include the risks of haemorrhage, blood transfusion, and hysterectomy. The risk of hysterectomy with a placenta praevia is about 2%. This rate increases to 10% in those with a previous lower segment CS (LSCS) and to 66% in those with a placenta accreta (see Section 8.4).

Delivery

Mode of delivery is decided on an individual basis. Blood should always be available during delivery, the amount depending on the clinical circumstance. As a minimum, 2 units should be available in cases of minor placenta praevia in labour with no bleeding. At least 4 units should be available for asymptomatic women with major placenta praevia undergoing a CS. In the presence of massive antepartum haemorrhage, it will be necessary to crossmatch 6–10 units initially and order fresh frozen plasma (FFP).

Women with a major placenta praevia at term should have an elective CS at 39 weeks. Delivery may occur at any point if bleeding is profuse.

Review of controlled clinical trials that assessed the impact of interventions on women with placenta praevia.

On hospital versus home care for women with symptomatic placenta praevia, the only significant difference was a reduction in hospital stay (**Ib**).

Conclusion: insufficient evidence to recommend a change in practice.

Recommended RCOG good practice points:

- Any woman going to theatre with a placenta praevia should be delivered by the most experienced obstetrician and anaesthetist on duty
- As a minimum, a consultant obstetrician and anaesthetist should be present within the delivery suite during a planned CS for placenta praevia

Vaginal delivery is more likely if the placenta is:

- Anterior (**B**).
- More than 2 cm from the cervical os and <1 cm thick (**B**)
- Fetal head is engaged and below the leading edge of the placenta (**IIb**)

With minor degrees of placenta praevia:

- If a woman presents in labour with no bleeding, labour can continue
- If there is heavy or continued bleedings, or bleeding causing maternal or fetal compromise at any point, then delivery should be by the most expedient way
- Examination under anaesthesia (EUA) ± amniotomy can be performed if there is ongoing but non-life-threatening bleeding. This can be under either general anaesthetic or epidural so that quick recourse to CS can occur if there is profuse bleeding. The vaginal fornices are examined with care for the presence of placenta tissue (feels boggy). If no placenta is felt then a finger can be passed through the cervical os and amniotomy can be performed. In the presence of placental tissue or heavy bleeding, CS should be performed

Risks and prognosis

Maternal risks

Postpartum haemorrhage See also Section 11.1.

When a placenta is in the upper segment of the uterus, bleeding from the placental bed is stopped when the myometrium contracts and retracts, causing occlusion of the sinuses. As the lower segment contains fewer muscle fibres, this process can be inadequate, leading to continued bleeding.

Uterotonics may be of some use by maintaining a contracted uterus.

If bleeding continues, surgical techniques include:

- Haemostatic sutures to the placental bed
- Hydrostatic balloon catheterization
- Uterine packing
- B-Lynch suture
- Internal iliac artery ligation
- Uterine artery embolization
- Hysterectomy

Coagulopathies should be corrected.

Fetal risks

- Prematurity
- Cord prolapse
- Fetal growth retardation (FGR)
- Anaemia and exsanguination (can occur if the placenta is incised during the delivery)
- Fetal mortality (42–81/1000)

Recurrence

The risk is 4–8%, increasing with the number of CSs.

Further reading

www.cochrane.co.uk Neilson JP. Interventions for suspected placenta praevia. *Cochrane Database System Reviews* 2003; **2**:CD001998.

www.rcog.org.uk RCOG. Greentop guideline no. 27. Placenta Praevia and Placenta Praevia Accreta: Diagnosis and Management, 2005.

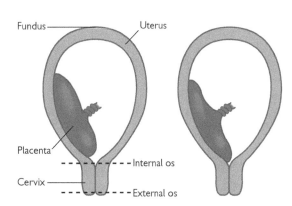

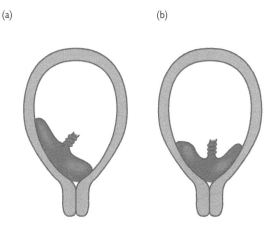

Fig. 8.2 Classification of placenta praevia. Minor: (a) placenta encroaching the lower segment; (b), placenta impinges but does not cover the cervix. Major: (c) placenta partially covering cervix; (d) placenta completely covering cervix. (Kindly produced by Miss A. Kumar.)

8.4 Placenta accreta, increta, and percreta

Definitions (see Figure 8.3)
Placenta accreta is an abnormal adherence of the placenta to the uterine wall (80%).
Placenta increta occurs when the placenta invades deeply into the myometrium (15%).
Placenta percreta is placental invasion through the uterus to the serosa (5%). Invasion of bladder and other pelvic structures can occur.

Incidence
The incidence is 1:2500. It is increasing because of rising CS rates.

Risk factors
- Placenta accreta is often associated with placenta praevia as the endometrium is deficient in the lower segment. It occurs in 3% of women with a placenta praevia
- Previous CS—incidence increases with the number of previous CS (accreta occurs in 10% of placenta praevia with one previous CS, rising to 40-60% with placenta praevia and two or more CS)
- Short CS-to-conception interval
- Increased maternal age

Investigations
- Colour flow Doppler ultrasonography in women who are at an increased risk of placenta accreta (anterior placenta praevia and previous low segment CS (LSCS)) (**C**)
- MRI has been used to diagnose placenta accreta but with poor sensitivity, therefore Doppler is the preferred option (**III**)

Risks and prognosis
- As for placenta praevia (see Section 8.3)
- However, the risk of haemorrhage, transfusion, and hysterectomy (66%) are greater

Management
- Counselling and consent regarding risks of blood transfusion and Caesarean hysterectomy
- Consultant obstetric and anaesthetic inputs are vital in planning and conducting delivery (**C**)
- Delivery should only be performed in a unit with facilities for high volume blood transfusion and availability of other blood products (**IV**)
- At least 4 units of crossmatched blood should be available
- Colleagues from other specialities (vascular, urology, radiology) may be needed. Alert them in advance of a planned procedure (**C**)
- An ultrasound scan can be performed at the time of CS to identify the exact location of the placenta. A uterine incision away from the placenta can then be performed
- If a morbidly adherent placenta is diagnosed at the time of CS, severe uncontrolled bleeding can occur if attempts are made to separate the placenta
- Haemostatic sutures in the placental bed may help
- Conservative management with the placenta left *in situ* ± uterine artery embolization, internal iliac artery ligation, and postpartum methotrexate have been used with varying success. The main risk is secondary postpartum haemorrhage

Further reading

www.cemach.org.uk Why Mothers Die (2004) Confidential Enquiry into Maternal Deaths in UK 2000–2002.

www.cemach.org.uk Saving mothers lives (2007) Confidential Enquiry into Maternal Deaths 2003–2005

www.rcog.org.uk RCOG Greentop guideline no. 27. Placenta praevia and placenta praevia accreta: diagnosis and management, 2005.

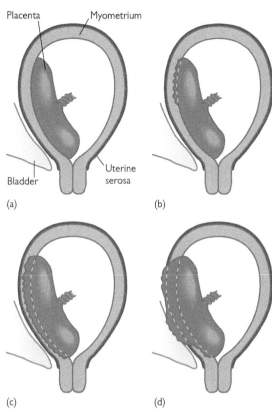

Fig. 8.3 (a) Normal placental adherence; (b) placenta accreta;
(c) increta; and (d) percreta. (Kindly produced by Miss A. Kumar.)

Abdominal pain is common in pregnancy. A thorough history and examination is essential to make a diagnosis and exclude any underlying serious pathology.

There is a long list of differential diagnoses (see Box 8.2).

Clinical evaluation

History
- Pain: type, site, duration, radiation
- Any exacerbating or relieving factors
- Use of analgesia required
- Associated urinary and bowel symptoms
- PV loss, i.e. discharge, bleeding or 'show'
- Rupture of membranes
- Uterine activity
- Presence or absence of fetal movements
- Past medical and surgical history

Examination
- Vital signs: look for tachycardia, pyrexia or hypotension
- Site of pain: localized or generalized
- Presence of rebound, guarding, and bowel sounds
- Uterine or abdominal tenderness
- Assess for uterine irritability (palpation and CTG)
- Speculum: cervical dilatation, liquor, blood or abnormal discharge
- Urinalysis
- Presence of fetal heart and CTG

Investigations and management are discussed for each cause (see below). Many women experience pain that spontaneously settles. It is important in abdominal pain to have a wide differential diagnosis and hone down using the detailed history and examination rather than inappropriate imaging. Although UTI is common, it is not the cause of all abdominal pain.

Useful tip: Remember that abruption can never be disproved and that premature labour can only be disproved in retrospect. When the cause is not clear, or there are recurrent admissions, it is better to say 'abdo pain ? cause' and keep an open mind than carry on with the wrong diagnosis.

Obstetric causes of abdominal pain

Abruption (see Section 8.2)

Labour (including preterm) (see Sections 9.1 and 8.18)

Uterine rupture (see Section 9.16)

Acute fatty liver of pregnancy (see Section 8.14)

Pre-eclampsia /haemolysis, elevated liver enzymes, low platelets syndrome (HELLP) (see Section 8.14)

Miscarriage and ectopic (see Sections 5.6 and 5.7)

Chorioamnionitis

Pathophysiology

Commonly an ascending infection from the vagina and cervix causing an inflammatory reaction in the decidua, followed by a chorionitis.

Other routes are transplacental, retrograde infection from the abdominal cavity via the Fallopian tubes, and inadvertent infection during invasive procedures (e.g. amniocentesis).

Infection of the amnion and amniotic cavity (amnionitis) can occur with subsequent infection of the cord (funisitis) and fetus.

Common isolates include *Ureaplasma urealyticum*, group B streptococcus, *Escherichia coli*, *Fusobacterium* spp., and *Bacteroides* spp.

Frequently, multiple microorganisms are involved.

History
- Preterm and/or prolonged rupture of membranes (but chorioamnionitis can occur with intact membranes)
- Generalized abdominal pain
- Contractions
- Abnormal, offensive vaginal discharge
- Fever and generally feeling unwell
- Nausea, vomiting, and diarrhoea
- Recent amniocentesis or chorionic villus sampling

Examination
- Flushed, tachycardia, and pyrexia
- Hypotension in severe infection
- Tender uterus
- Offensive discharge or liquor on speculum
- Cervical dilatation
- Fetal tachycardia

Investigations
- Raised WCC and CRP (but low WCC if septic)
- U&Es, LFTs and clotting (disseminated intravascular coagulation (DIC)) in severe infection
- Blood cultures if pyrexial
- High vaginal swab and endocervical swabs
- Amniocentesis

Management
- If good evidence of infection, delivery should be expedited whether fetus is viable or not
- Broad-spectrum antibiotics should be commenced in consultation with the microbiologist.
- Inform anaesthetic and neonatal colleagues.

Complications
- Maternal septic shock and death
- Fetal infection and inflammation (fetal inflammatory response syndrome), stillbirth, and intrauterine death
- Neonatal infection, bronchopulmonary dysplasia, neurological impairment (periventricular leukomalacia, cerebral palsy)

Symphysis pubic dysfunction

Incidence
The incidence of symphysis public dysfunction (SPD) is common at 1:36 to 1:300.

Pathophysiology
- Multifactorial
- The fibrocartilaginous symphysis pubic joint relaxes by 2–3 mm in normal pregnancy, widening the pelvis before delivery
- In SPD, this is increased, causing pelvic girdle instability and pain of varying degrees
- Relaxin and progesterone are thought to cause collagenolysis of the pelvic joint, leading to laxity and pain
- Altered pelvic load, poor posture, lack of exercise, and previous difficult deliveries are also implicated

History
- Pain over symphysis pubis and lower abdominal pain with radiation down legs
- Difficulty walking, standing, going down stairs, turning in bed
- In severe cases, immobility

Examination
- Tenderness (sometimes extreme) over symphysis pubis and sacroiliac joints
- Range of hip movements reduced, waddling gait

Investigations
- Imaging techniques can be used to assess width of symphysis pubis joint but not routine in clinical practice
- Important to exclude UTI and sciatica

Management
- Review by obstetric physiotherapist for advice on posture and gentle exercises
- Pelvic support may give some relief
- Paracetamol and codeine are safe to use in pregnancy
- In severe cases, crutches or a walking frame may be required along with hospital admission for stronger analgesics
- Consider venous thromboembolism prophylaxis if immobile
- Advise avoidance of heavy lifting and prolonged standing
- When turning in bed or getting in and out of a car, avoid hip abduction by keeping knees together
- Rarely, induction is justified for severe symptoms
- During labour, avoid leg separation and excessive hip abduction.
- Lithotomy position should be kept to a minimum

Symptoms usually resolve postpartum but high chance of recurrence in future pregnancies.

More information can be found at www.pelvicgirdlepain.com

Fibroids

During pregnancy, fibroids can grow and undergo haemorrhagic infarction, causing pain (red degeneration). Rarely, torsion of subserosal pedunculated fibroids occurs.

History
- Much commoner in black women
- May have been seen on US or known before
- Severe localized pain
- Fever

Examination
- Fibroids can often be palpated and will be tender

Investigations
- Raised WCC and CRP
- US if not previously performed and to exclude other causes of pain

Management
- Conservative management with analgesics

Round ligament pain
- Occurs in 10–30% of pregnancies
- Typically pain occurs during the second trimester
- Often sharp pain worse on sudden movement
- Pain and tenderness is lateral to the uterus and radiates to the groin. It can be on one or both sides
- Self-limiting, usually settles within 2–3 weeks

Braxton Hicks contractions
- Non-progressive uterine contractions in latter half of pregnancy (usually painless but sometimes painful)
- Tend to be irregular in frequency and intensity
- Preterm labour is the main differential diagnosis
- Speculum examination should be performed to assess the cervix. If there is any doubt about the diagnosis, repeat after 2–4 h to see if there is any cervical change (see also Sections 8.18 and 8.19).

⊙ Box 8.2 Differential diagnosis of abdominal pain in pregnancy

Obstetric causes	Non-obstetric causes
Abruption	Urinary tract infection (UTI)
Labour and preterm labour	Pyelonephritis
Braxton Hicks	Appendicitis
Chorioamnionitis	Pancreatitis
Uterine rupture	Cholecystitis
Miscarriage	Bowel obstruction
Pre-eclampsia /HELLP	Inflammatory bowel disease
Acute fatty liver	Ovarian cyst accident (rupture or torsion)
Symphysis pubis dysfunction	
Fibroid degeneration	Ulcer
Round ligament pain	Heartburn
Divarification of recti	Constipation
Fetal movements	Trauma, domestic violence, assault
Ectopic pregnancy	Psychogenic
	Renal colic
	Pneumonia
	Other rare medical, e.g. myocardial infarction, diabetic ketoacidosis, porphyria, diverticulitis

Also see Inflammatory bowel disease (see Section 7.27) and Domestic violence (see Section 1.9).

Heartburn

- Heartburn is a frequent problem in pregnancy, exacerbated by smooth muscle relaxation of the gastrointestinal tract (progesterone effect) and pressure from the gravid uterus
- Burning epigastric discomfort, particularly after eating
- Avoid bending and lying flat in bed
- Antacids and H_2 receptor antagonists can be used
- Dilute HCl can also be tried as some cases are caused by bile reflux

Constipation

- Frequent problem in pregnancy (up to 40%) exacerbated by smooth muscle relaxation of the gastrointestinal tract
- Colicky pain outside the uterus
- Increase water and fibre in diet
- Laxatives should be reserved for severe cases

Urinary tract infections

See also Section 13.12.

Incidence

Symptomatic lower UTI (cystitis) occurs in 1% of pregnant women. Asymptomatic bacteriuria occurs in 2–10% (similar to non-pregnant women). Upper UTI (pyelonephritis) occurs in 1–2%.

Pathophysiology

Anatomical and physiological changes in the urinary tract make UTI more likely during pregnancy

- Ureteric dilatation caused by muscle relaxant effect of progesterone and mechanical obstruction of ureters by uterus at the pelvic brim
- Ureteric dilatation results in urinary stasis in second and third trimesters
- Bladder hyperaemic and more capacious due to progesterone

Risk factors

- Recurrent UTIs
- Diabetes
- Catheterization
- Urinary tract calculi
- Obstruction to urinary tract
- Reconstructed urinary tract, e.g. clam cystoplasty
- Congenital abnormality of renal tract
- Neuropathic bladder
- Immunosuppression

Lower UTI—cystitis

History

- Frequency, urgency dysuria, haematuria, offensive urine
- Preterm labour

Examination

- Lower abdominal tenderness
- Urinalysis: if nitrites and leukocyte esterase are positive, then UTI is likely. If negative, this does not exclude UTI. Haematuria and proteinuria are unreliable indicators of UTI

Investigations

- MSU for microscopy and culture. Significant bacteriuria if colony count >10^5/ml
- Most common uropathogens during pregnancy are *Escherichia coli* (70–80%), *Klebsiella*, *Proteus*, *Enterobacter*, and *Staphylococcus saprophyticus*
- If non-significant culture or mixed growth, sample should be repeated

Management

- If high clinical suspicion of UTI (symptomatic and positive urinalysis), commence antibiotics for 5–7 days while awaiting MSU result.
- Amoxicillin and cephalosporins are safe in pregnancy and are effective against most possible urinary pathogens.
- Nitrofurantoin should be avoided in the third trimester (neonatal haemolytic anaemia) and trimethoprim avoided in the first trimester (folate antagonist).
- In women with recurrent UTIs, review of previous results may aid antibiotic choice.

Lower UTI—asymptomatic bacteriuria. (See also section 6.6)

- If asymptomatic but positive urinalysis, await result of MSU before starting treatment.
- Women with asymptomatic bacteriuria should receive treatment as it reduces the risk of developing pyelonephritis (by 75%), preterm delivery, and low birth weight babies.

Complications

Pyelonephritis

Upper UTI—pyelonephritis

Incidence

- The incidence of pyelonephritis in women with untreated asymptomatic bacteriuria is up to 29%.

History

- Loin pain, abdominal pain
- Fever, rigors
- Vomiting

Examination

- Pyrexia and tachycardia
- Renal angle and lower abdominal tenderness
- Urinalysis—nitrites, leukocyte esterase, blood and protein
- CTG—fetal tachycardia

Investigations

- MSU
- FBC, CRP, U&Es, and blood cultures
- Renal tract US (hydronephrosis, congenital abnormality).
- US can be inconclusive in diagnosing calculie
- If suspicion of an obstructed infected kidney, a plain abdominal X-ray (90% of stones) or one-shot intravenous urogram at 20–30 min can be performed with minimal radiation risk to the fetus
- Alternatively, MRI can give excellent anatomical detail without radiation

Management

- Commence IV antibiotics before result of MSU available. Cephalosporins will cover most microorganisms. Gentamicin can be added in severe cases (care with high-dose gentamicin and fetal ototoxicity)
- Change to oral antibiotics once apyrexial for 24 h and complete a 2-week course

- Maintain hydration with IV fluids if not tolerating oral fluids
- Thromboprophylaxis if reduced mobility and dehydration
- Urgent nephrostomy drainage will be required in those with an infected obstructed kidney, typically due to calculus. Advice from a urologist should be sought

Complications
- Prompt treatment reduces the risk of sepsis and preterm labour

Follow-up of upper and lower UTIs
- MSU result should be checked to make sure that correct antibiotic treatment has been given
- Repeat MSU 1 week after completion of antibiotics to ensure adequate treatment

- MSU should be sent monthly to screen for recurrent infections
- Consider antibiotic prophylaxis and renal tract imaging in those with two or more UTIs in pregnancy

Further reading

www.cochrane.org.uk Vazquez JC, Villar J. Treatments for symptomatic urinary tract infections during pregnancy. *Cochrane Database System Reviews* 2003; **4**:CD002256.

Smaill F. Antibiotics for asymptomatic bacteriuria in pregnancy. *Cochrane Database System Reviews* 2001; **2**:CD000490.

Appendicitis

Incidence
The incidence is 1:1000. Appendicitis is the most common non-obstetric surgical emergency and 'typically atypical'.

History
- Abdominal pain, anorexia, vomiting

Examination
- Pyrexia
- Guarding and rebound tenderness may not be present owing to muscle laxity
- Tenderness is not always in right lower quadrant as the appendix can be displaced upwards with the growing uterus

Investigations
- Raised WCC and CRP
- Blood cultures
- MSU to exclude UTI
- US—look for appendix mass, free fluid, and non-compressibility of the appendix

Management
- Keep nil by mouth (NBM) if diagnosis suspected
- Surgical review
- Appendicectomy
- Laparoscopic removal is possible before 20 weeks' gestation
- For open procedures in the first trimester, a McBurney incision can be used. After this, a right paramedian incision over area of maximal tenderness is needed

Complications
- The main risk is delay in diagnosis and subsequent increased risk of perforation, peritonitis, and preterm labour
- There is a 33% risk of miscarriage after first trimester appendicectomy, and 14% risk of preterm labour in the second trimester
- Postoperative tocolysis has been advocated but there are no reported trials

Pancreatitis

Incidence
Incidence is 1:4000.

Pathophysiology
Gallstones are the commonest cause of pancreatitis in pregnancy. Other causes should be considered, including alcohol, hypertrigyl-ceridaemia and hypercalcaemia (secondary to hyperparathyroidism).

History
- Epigastric pain radiating to back
- Nausea, vomiting, and fever

Examination
- Tachycardia and pyrexia
- Epigastic tenderness ± rebound, guarding, and reduced bowel sounds

Investigations
- FBC, CRP, U&Es, LFTs, Ca^{2+}, glucose, clotting, serum amylase, and lipid profile (hyperlipidaemia may mask rise in amylase)
- Arterial blood gases
- US upper abdomen
- Differential diagnosis includes cholecystitis, pre-eclampsia, haemolysis, elevated liver enzymes, low platelets syndrome (HELLP), and acute fatty liver of pregnancy

Management
- Surgical review
- Supportive treatment. IV fluids and analgesia as required, nasogastric tube
- NBM and gastric acid suppression
- Urinary catheter to monitor hourly urine output
- Antibiotics (cephalosporin and metronidazole)
- Close monitoring of bloods (as above)

Complications
Ten per cent have serious complications, including sepsis, cardiorespiratory failure, renal failure, pseudocyst formation, and maternal death.

Cholecystitis

Incidence
Incidence is 1:1000 pregnancies. There is an increased incidence of gallstones in pregnancy; most are asymptomatic.

History
- Colicky, right upper quadrant pain radiating to back
- Nausea, vomiting, and fever

Examination
- Pyrexia and tachycardia
- Right upper quadrant tenderness, rebound, and guarding
- Positive Murphy's sign (inspiratory arrest due to pain during deep palpation of right upper quadrant)

Investigations
- Raised WCC and CRP
- LFTs and amylase may be mildly abnormal
- US to visualize gallstones
- MRI cholangiography if suspect stone in common bile duct
- Differential diagnosis includes severe pre-eclampsia, HELLP, and acute fatty liver of pregnancy

Management
- Surgical review
- Conservative management. Keep NBM, nasogastric tube, IV fluids, and analgesia
- IV antibiotics (cephalosporin and metronidazole)

Complications
Surgery is indicated only if recurrent attacks, failure to respond to conservative treatment, perforation or empyema of the gallbladder. It is preferable to perform elective surgery in the second trimester as there is a lower risk of miscarriage and better access. Endoscopic retrograde cholangiopancreatography (ERCP) (with limited fluoroscopy) is an alternative.

Bowel obstruction

Incidence
The incidence is 1:1500–66 000. The main causes are adhesions (58%) and volvulus (24%).

History
- Colicky abdominal pain, vomiting, and constipation
- Previous history of abdominal surgery

Examination
- Dehydration, tachycardia
- Tender outside uterus

- Abdominal distension, tympanic on percussion, high pitched or absent bowel sounds
- Evidence of peritonitis

Investigations
- Raised WCC and CRP
- Erect abdominal X-ray to assess for dilated loops of bowel (low risk of radiation outweighs risk of delayed diagnosis)

Management
- Surgical review
- NBM
- If no evidence of strangulation or perforation, then short trial of conservative management with fluid resuscitation and nasogastric aspiration
- If perforation or strangulation is a possibility, then laparotomy is needed
- Tocolysis should be considered
- Antibiotics

Complications
High maternal (6%) and fetal mortality (26%) is reported. Increased risks with delayed diagnosis, strangulation or perforation of the bowel and electrolyte imbalance.

Ovarian cysts

See also Section 13.3.
- Small simple ovarian cysts (<5 cm) are frequently seen on first trimester scanning and are usually corpus luteal cysts which resolve spontaneously. If identified during US, then no further action is needed.
- Complex cysts and cysts >5 cm need to have a repeat scan after 4 weeks to exclude rapid growth. Most resolve spontaneously or remain unchanged. If there is no suspicion of malignancy, then an US can be performed 6 weeks' postpartum.
- Cysts which are >5 cm and persist into the second trimester are more likely to cause complications such as torsion (6%) and are most likely to be dermoid cysts (42%).

- Indications for surgery during pregnancy are suspicion of malignancy (complex cyst, solid components, multiseptate, papillary projections) and torsion.

Ovarian torsion

See also Sections 13.3 and 13.4.
History
- Pain, nausea, and vomiting
Examination
- Tachycardia and pyrexia
- Localized pain ± rebound and guarding. Pain may be higher than expected in the abdomen owing to the ovaries rising with the gravid uterus
Investigations
- WCC and CRP can be raised
- US to identify cyst
- Differential diagnosis includes appendicitis (if on right)
Management
- Keep NBM, IV fluids, and analgesia
- Laparoscopy or laparotomy for correction of torsion and cystectomy ± oophorectomy if non-viable ovarian tissue
- Tocolysis should be considered
Complications
Malignancy (rare), miscarriage, and preterm labour following surgery.

Further reading
www.sages.org Society of American Gastrointestinal and Endoscopic Surgeons. *Guidelines for Diagnosis, Treatment, and Use of Laparoscopy for Surgical Problems during Pregnancy*, 2007.

Carpal tunnel syndrome

Pathophysiology
- Median nerve (C6–T1) compression at the wrist
- May be caused by fluid retention and narrowing

Incidence
- The incidence is 2–3%
- Higher in pre-eclampsia and older primips

Clinical presentation
- Numbness, tingling and pain in the thumb, index finger, middle finger and radial side of the ring finger
- Symptoms worse at night. Nocturnal waking and shaking the wrist to relieve symptoms is a classic symptom
- Motor loss ⇒ wasting of thenar eminence, weakness, and loss of two-point discrimination
- Usually occurs in third trimester in one or both hands
- Symptoms usually resolve after delivery but may persist for 6 months in breastfeeding women
- Ulnar nerve may also be compressed ⇒ numbness in the fourth and fifth fingers (ulnar nerve syndrome)

Diagnosis
Often diagnosed clinically. Symptoms can be reproduced by:
- Tinel's sign: tapping of the carpal tunnel
- Phalen's sign: sustained flexion of wrist for ≥30s

Management
- Reassurance that condition improves after delivery
- Avoid flexion of the wrist using wrist splints
- Local steroid injections but complications include median nerve injury and tendon rupture
- Diuretics have been used, but efficacy is not proven and should be avoided in pregnancy
- Surgical division of the flexor retinaculum rarely indicated in pregnancy because of complications

Bell's palsy

Pathophysiology
- Unilateral lower motor neuron lesion of the facial nerve (seventh cranial nerve) ⇒ weakness of upper and lower facial muscles
- Accounts for 60–75% of all cases of unilateral facial weakness

Incidence
Affects 45:100 000 pregnant women, mainly peripartum (2 weeks either side of delivery).

Aetiology
- Outside pregnancy: mainly caused by reactivation of herpex simplex and zoster virus sequestered in the geniculate ganglion
- In pregnancy: possibly caused by swelling of the facial nerve within the petrous temporal bone
- In bilateral palsy (rare), consider myasthenia gravis, Guillain–Barre, and lesions at the base of the brain (lymphoma, sarcoidosis, and Lyme disease)

Clinical presentation
- Facial weakness, including ipsilateral loss of frontalis muscle (cannot wrinkle forehead)
- Cannot close the eye and attempts to do so result in the eyeball deviating upward and inward (Bell phenomenon)
- Absent corneal reflex and inability to produce tears on the affected side
- May be associated with ipsilateral retroauricular pain and loss of taste on the anterior two-thirds of the tongue
- Associated pre-eclampsia (22%) and hypertension (7%)
- Increased Caesarean, prematurity, and low birth weight

Diagnosis
The diagnosis is made on clinical grounds.
- Determine if peripheral seventh nerve lesion or central lesion (patients cannot wrinkle their foreheads with Bell's palsy but can with central lesion owing to bilateral innervation of the forehead).
- Main cause of central lesion is a stroke involving the pons, thus there would be additional cranial nerve deficit.

Management
- Reassure that 80–90% resolve, usually within 6 weeks
- Recovery is less likely in patients with complete paralysis, hypertension, and taste impairment
- Monitor for pre-eclampsia or pregnancy-induced hypertension

Treatment
- Artificial tears to lubricate the cornea
- May need to have the eye taped shut to prevent drying and infection
- If the diagnosis of Bell palsy is made <2 weeks of onset, oral prednisolone may be given for 7 days and stopped without a taper to increase the chance of recovery
- The addition of antiviral agents to prednisolone has been shown to be effective out of pregnancy, but the safety of this in pregnancy has not been established
- Surgical treatment is controversial
- Recurrence risk: 12%

Meralgia paraesthetica

Pathophysiology
- Compression of the lateral cutaneous nerve of the thigh (L2, L3) as it passes under the inguinal nerve just medial to the anterior superior iliac spine
- Causes numbness and pain in the anterolateral aspect of the thigh. Associated with pregnancy, prolonged labour, obesity, and exaggerated lumbar lordosis

Clinical presentation
- Symptoms usually begin in third trimester
- Aggravated by standing or walking and relieved by sitting

Management
- Resolves after delivery
- Treatment is usually not required
- In severe cases, carbamazepine, amitriptyline, local steroid injections or lidocaine injections may be used

Obturator nerve (L3, L4) injury
- Injury may be caused by pressure from the fetal head during a difficult labour
- Results in weak hip adduction

Sciatic nerve (L4–S3) injury

Incidence
- Rare

Pathophysiology
- May be injured by intramuscular injection
- Causes complete paralysis of the ankle and toes and weakness of leg flexion. The patient can stand but the leg is raised to correct for footdrop when walking

Sciatica is usually caused by ruptured intervertebral disc, resulting in pain in the lower back which radiates along the course of the nerve down the posterior leg

Common peroneal nerve injury

Incidence
- Most frequently injured nerve in the body owing to superficial position in the relation to the head of the fibula

Pathophysiology
- Contains nerve roots L4–S1
- May be injured by pressure on the nerve, e.g. in delivery stirrups, sustained knee flexion or prolonged squatting
- Injury results in footdrop, usually self-resolving

Management
Physiotherapy and use of a footbrace

Lumbosacral plexopathies (L4, L5, S1)

Incidence
- The incidence is 1:2000 deliveries

Pathophysiology
- Injury ocurs as nerve roots pass over the pelvic brim, possibly from pressure of the fetal head during rotation and descent, particularly if macrosomia, prolonged second stage, and cephalopelvic disproportion
- Commonest neurological deficit develops in sciatic nerve distribution, mainly common peroneal nerve, with walking difficulties, foot drop, weakness of ankle inversion, dorsiflexion, and eversion
- Recovery depends on the severity of the deficit

Further reading

Gilden DH. Bell's palsy. *New England Journal of Medicine* 2004; **351:**1323–31.

Mabie WC. Peripheral neuropathies during pregnancy. *Clin Obstet Gynecol* 2005;**48(1):**57–65.

Prevalence

Thirty-five per cent of pregnant women suffer from headaches. Most headaches in pregnancy are primary:

- 64% : tension headaches
- 26% : migraines without aura
- 10% : migraines with aura
- Cluster headaches are rare in pregnancy

Secondary headaches occur in 1–2% of the general population. In pregnancy, <1% of headaches are secondary.

Primary headaches in pregnancy

Tension headache

Prevalence

Lifetime: 88%. Commonest headache in pregnancy.

Aetiology

Related to stress, possibly caused by muscle contraction.

History

Bilateral, non-pulsating, mild to moderate intensity and not aggravated by activity. May be chronic, daily headache. About 50% improve during pregnancy. Difficult to differentiate from pathological causes of headaches. Normal neurological history.

Examination

Normal neurological examination.

Management

Reassurance, advice on relaxation techniques, and paracetamol for analgesia.

Migraine headache

Prevalence

Affects 25% of women over a lifetime.

Pathophysiology

Of female migraineurs, 50% have menstrual migraines. Attacks correlate with declining plasma oestradiol levels. Oestrogen levels increase in pregnancy and decline sharply postpartum. Possibly caused by cerebral vasodilatation, or platelet aggregation and serotonin release with stimulation of nociceptors.

Diagnosis

- ≥5 repeated attacks lasting 4–72 h
- At least two of: throbbing pain, unilateral pain, aggravation by activity, moderate or severe intensity
- One of: nausea/vomiting, photophobia/phonophobia
- Normal neurological examination
- No test to confirm the diagnosis of migraine
- No other reason for headache
- May have precipitating factors: chocolate, cheese, stress
- Often relieved by sleep

Migraine with aura (classical migraine):

- Visual changes (scotoma, fortification spectra), sensory changes (numbness, tingling) +/or dysphasia
- Lasts up to 1 h, followed by headache
- Usually resolve but may last many hours in hemiplegic migraine

Migraine without aura (common migraine)

- May be preceded by neck stiffness, fatigue, and nausea
- May be aggravated by overuse of migraine medications

Effect of pregnancy on migraine

- New-onset migraines are unusual in pregnancy
- In 50–80% of cases: migraine improves, particularly those with menstrual migraine and in the third trimester
- In 10% cases: migraine worsens during pregnancy
- In 34% cases: recurrence within 1 week of delivery
- In 50% cases: recurrence within 1 month of delivery

Effect of migraine on pregnancy

Associated with increased risk of pre-eclampsia, especially severe

Management of migraines in pregnancy

- Attention to avoidance of precipitating factors
- Rest, adequate sleep, avoid light

Treatment:

- Analgesia: paracetamol. NSAIDs may be used in first two trimesters. Opioids in severe cases (meperidine, morphine)
- Antiemetic: prochlorperazine, metoclopramide
- Prophylaxis: for frequent migraines. Low-dose amitriptyline or beta-blockers may be used
- Avoid ergot derivatives (FDA category D)
- Avoid triptans: safety in pregnancy is unproven (FDA category C)

Owing to difficulty excluding other causes of headache, women with first time focal migraine or worsening migraines in pregnancy should be investigated with CT or MRI.

Secondary headaches in pregnancy

Subarachnoid haemorrhage (SAH)

A type of haemorrhagic stroke caused by bleeding into the subarachnoid space around the brain.

Incidence

Eight per 100 000. Accounts for about 5% of strokes.

Pathophysiology

Ruptured arterial (berry) aneurysms: 70% of cases. 50% of patients with aneurysmal SAH will die or suffer serious disability. If untreated, 25% re-bleed within 4 weeks, with 70% mortality. Risk factors include smoking, hypertension, alcohol, and genetic tendancy.
Ruptured arteriovenous malformations (AVM): 10% of cases.
Idiopathic: 10%.
Out of pregnancy, the ratio of aneurysm to AVM is 7:1. The average age of aneurysmal SAH is 52 years. In pregnancy, relatively more cases are due to AVMs, with a ratio of 1:1.

History

- Sudden onset, severe, often occipital headache
- Nausea, vomiting, photophobia, neck stiffness
- Sudden collapse or impaired consciousness
- Impaired speech
- Hemiparesis and seizures

Examination

- Focal neurological signs may be present
- Papilloedema

Investigations

CT scan: for presence, amount, and source of bleeding. Sensitivity of 90% if performed within 24 h and 50% within 72 h.
Lumbar puncture: if CT scan normal, examine cerebrospinal fluid (CSF) for blood.
Cerebral angiography: to identify the presence and site of aneurysm or other vascular abnormality.

Effect of pregnancy on aneurysms or AVMs

- ↑ incidence of aneurysmal SAH (~5-fold), ↑ with gestation
- No evidence that labour increases the risk of SAH
- AVMs are oestrogen-sensitive and tend to dilate. Controversial whether AVM rupture is increased
- Risk of re-bleeding from AVM may be as high as 50%

Effect of SAH on pregnancy
- Mortality rate is about 40% in and out of pregnancy
- Subarachnoid haemorrhage is a common cause of 'indirect' maternal death (11 deaths in 2003–2005)

Management
Prepregnancy
Advise defer pregnancy until after treatment of AVM

Antenatal
- Investigate abnormal neurological symptoms and signs
- Multidisciplinary team care
- Management is the same as out of pregnancy but extra care with intraoperative hypotension and hypothermia
- Anticonvulsants, high-dose steroids, mannitol, and nimodipine are used depending on clinical problems

Surgical treatment
- Is associated with lower maternal and fetal mortality
- Consensus is to treat asymptomatic aneurysms >7 mm
- Clipping and endovascular coil embolization of aneurysms has been successful in all stages of pregnancy
- Embolization is a new development

Intrapartum
- Vaginal delivery preferable if AVM or aneurysm is successfully treated. CS is only indicated if acute bleeding near term or perimortem for fetal salvage
- Recommend epidural and shorten the second stage
- Regional anaesthesia is preferable. If GA used, β-adrenergic blockade will attenuate a hypertensive response to intubation
- Regional anaesthesia is contraindicated in recent SAH, as there is a risk of raised intracranial pressure (ICP)

Idiopathic intracranial hypertension
Incidence
Rare. Commonest in obese, young women. Recurrence 10%.

Clinical features
- Usually self-limiting, resolves postpartum
- Progressive, daily, bilateral, non-pulsating, mainly retro-orbital headaches, aggravated by coughing or straining
- Often associated with obesity +/or rapid weight gain
- Diplopia (15%) may become permanent if untreated
- Papilloedema and raised ICP. Headaches improve with removal of CSF to normalize pressures
- In severe cases, optic nerve infarction may cause blindness

Effect of pregnancy on idiopathic intracranial hypertension
- Tends to worsen, possibly related to weight gain
- May present in pregnancy, commonly in second trimester

Diagnosis
- Papilloedema, due to raised intracranial pressure
- Normal CSF composition
- CT/MRI show no hydrocephalus or space-occupying lesion

Management
Regular ophthalmology for visual fields and acuity.
Advise limitation of weight gain.
Treatment for pain relief and prevention of visual changes:
- Oral analgesia
- Thiazide diuretics and acetazolamide may diminish CSF and reduce intracranial pressure. Avoid acetazolamide in first trimester. Thiazides in third trimester may cause neonatal thrombocytopenia
- Corticosteroids may be used for rapid relief in a patient with severe papilloedema or visual changes

- Refractory cases: serial CSF drainage or shunt insertion
- In extreme cases where vision is threatened, surgery with optic nerve fenestration may be an option

Headaches with pre-eclampsia
- New-onset or change in character of headache
- Usually bilateral, throbbing, worsened by activity. Tend to worsen with increasing BP. May be associated flashing lights
- Linked to ↑ vascular reactivity, vasoconstriction, endothelial damage, and platelet hyperaggregation (also typical of migraine).

Postdural puncture
- Onset about 1 day after siting an epidural block
- Frontal headaches, relieved by lying down. May be associated with neck stiffness, tinnitus, visual symptoms, and rarely seizures
- Prompt review by anaesthetist for blood patch

Further reading
Goadsby PJ. Headache. In: Warrell D, Cox TM, Firth JD, Benz EJ (eds). *Oxford Textbook of Medicine*. Oxford: Oxford University Press, 2004.

Martin SR, Foley MR. Approach to the pregnant patient with headache. *Clin Obstet Gynecol* 2005; **48(1):**2–11.

⊙ Box 8.3 Investigation of headache in pregnancy

Neurological history and examination:
- New-onset, sudden onset or worsening headache
- Fever, neck stiffness
- Papilloedema
- Neurological disturbance (e.g. weakness)

Exclude pre-eclampsia if ≥24 weeks' gestation: check BP and urine. Consider U&E, uric acid, platelet count and LFTs
- CT or MRI if focal signs persists for more than 24 h
- Lumbar puncture is indicated once an intracranial mass effect has been ruled out by imaging studies

---

⊙ Box 8.4 International Headache Society Classification

Primary headaches:
- Tension-type headaches
- Migraine headaches
- Cluster headaches
- Exertional headaches

Secondary headaches:
- Head injury
- Vascular disorders (subarachnoid haemorrhage and cerebral vein thrombosis)
- Non-vascular intracranial disorders (idiopathic intracranial hypertension, neoplasm, and postdural puncture)
- Infections (meningitis)
- Homeostasis disorders (pre-eclampsia, hypoglycaemia)
- Disorders of cranial structures (sinusitis, temporomandibular joint pain)
- Psychiatric disorders (depression, anxiety)
- Neuralgias (trigeminal neuralgia)

8.10 Pregnancy-induced hypertension

Definitions

- Hypertension is defined as a BP of >140/90 mmHg on two occasions 4 h apart, or one reading of >170/110 mmHg
- Pregnancy-induced hypertension (PIH) is hypertension developing after 20 weeks' gestation in the absence of proteinuria and other features of pre-eclampsia (see Section 8.11) that resolves after pregnancy

Incidence

- Hypertension is a common complication of pregnancy (10%) with a spectrum of consequences.
- PIH affects 5–6% of pregnancies

Clinical evaluation

History

- Asymptomatic, raised BP identified during routine screening
- Previous history of PIH/pre-eclampsia
- Increasing age
- Obesity
- Pre-existing renal disease
- Vasculitic conditions, e.g. systemic lupus erythematosus (SLE)
- Absence of symptoms of pre-eclampsia

Examination

- BP (see Box 8.5 for correct measurement)
- Absence of proteinuria on urine dipstick (≤trace proteinuria)
- Absent signs of pre-eclampsia (see Section 8.11)

Investigations

- Blood should be taken for FBC, U&Es, LFTs, and urate
- A 24-h urine protein collection or protein:creatine ratio (see Box 8.6) is performed if proteinuria is detected on urine dipstick

Management

A rise in diastolic blood pressure which does not reach 90 mmHg is usually associated with an uncomplicated pregnancy. PIH is associated with far fewer complications than pre-eclampsia in terms of maternal morbidity and fetal mortality.

Monitoring is important in women with PIH owing to an increased risk of developing pre-eclampsia.

The overall risk of progressing to pre-eclampsia is 15–20% but depends on the gestation at which hypertension develops:

- <32 weeks' gestation—50% will progress
- 32–35 weeks—40% will develop pre-eclampsia
- At 38 weeks—<10% will progress to pre-eclampsia

New hypertension developing at 24–28 weeks' gestation is predictive of severe pre-eclampsia.

Inpatient assessment may be necessary initially to establish the diagnosis and exclude pre-eclampsia. Baseline bloods should be performed along with daily urinalysis. Once the diagnosis of PIH is confirmed, then women may be monitored as outpatients, ideally in Day Assessment Units.

Frequency of monitoring will depend on degree of hypertension and may range from weekly in those with mild PIH (140–150/90–95 mmHg) to three times weekly if BP is close to treatment levels. Both BP and urinalysis should be performed. Women with PIH should be aware of symptoms of pre-eclampsia and should attend if present.

Although bed rest may be associated with reduced risk of severe hypertension and preterm birth, there is insufficient evidence to provide clear guidance for clinical practice. Bed rest has no effect on the incidence of pre-eclampsia.

Treatment of hypertension reduces the risk of severe hypertension but does not improve neonatal outcomes or reduce the risk of pre-eclampsia.

It is unclear whether there is any benefit in treating mild to moderate hypertension with antihypertensives.

Consider treatment of hypertension when diastolic blood pressures are persistently above 105 mmHg (A). See Section 8.12 on pre-eclampsia for choice of antihypertensives.

Before 28 weeks, consider starting treatment when diastolic BP is greater than 90 mmHg (A). Aim for BP of ≤140/90. The main concern with treatment of hypertension is reduced placental perfusion and fetal growth restriction.

Monitor growth with serial US in women on antihypertensives.

With mild hypertension, induction of labour is indicated for the usual postmaturity criteria. In women requiring two agents to control blood pressure or where there are concerns with fetal growth, induction will need to be considered earlier.

Postnatally

- The BP usually settles within 6 weeks of delivery.
- If hypertension persists, consider essential hypertension.
- Women with PIH are at increased risk of recurrence of PIH in future pregnancies and of hypertension in later life.
- Therefore they should have regular BP monitoring by their GP.

Further reading

Scottish obstetric guidelines and audit project. The management of mild non-proteinuric hypertension in pregnancy. Guideline update, March 2002.

> **Box 8.5 Correct blood pressure measurement (A, Ib and IIb)**

- Automated machines tend to under estimate blood pressure in pregnancy and pre-eclampsia
- Therefore always check manually
- Woman should be rested and at a 45° angle
- Choose correct cuff; too small a cuff will overestimate blood pressure, and too large a cuff can underestimate it (although to a lesser extent)
- Cuff should be at the level of the heart
- Use Korotkoff phase V (disappearance of sound) for diastolic BP as it can be more accurately reproduced compared to phase IV sounds
- Always measure to within 2 mmHg

> **Box 8.6 Protein:creatinine ratio**

- Protein (mg):creatinine (mmol) ratio is more convenient than a 24-h collection as it can be performed on a one-off urine sample
- A level of ≥0.25 has been shown to have a sensitivity of 96.6% and specificity of 92.3% in detecting significant proteinuria (≥0.3 g/24 h)
- A result can be obtained on the same day and therefore reduces costs and inconvenience of admission if significant proteinuria is not present. In women with a raised protein: creatinine ratio, a 24-h urine collection can be performed to assess the degree of proteinuria

Definition

Pre-eclampsia(PET) is a multisystem disease of pregnancy of unknown origin and protean manitestation. It is defined clinically by pregnancy-induced hypertension (PIH; see Section 8.10) and proteinuria (>0.3 g/24 h) after 20 weeks' gestation.

Clinical relevance

While women with PIH (hypertension without proteinuria) are much less likely to have complications, those with pre-eclampsia (hypertension with proteinuria) and HELLP syndrome (haemolysis, elevated liver enzymes and low platelets) have a significant risk of maternal and fetal morbidity and mortality. (See Section 7.4 for more on chronic hypertension and Section 10.3 for eclampsia.)

Pre-eclampsia is the second largest cause of direct maternal deaths. In the 2003–2005 Confidential Enquiry, 18 women died from severe pre-eclampsia and its complications. The commonest cause of death (10) was intracranial haemorrhage, with 2 deaths from cerebral infarction, 2 deaths from multiorgan failure (including acute respiratory distress syndrome, ARDS), 1 from massive liver infarction, and 3 other causes. Failure of antihypertensive therapy was the commonest cause of substandard care.

Identification of at-risk women, antenatal screening, appropriate investigations, and treatment are essential in the management of hypertension in pregnancy.

All units should have protocols in place for the management of women with moderate and severe pre-eclampsia. It is vital that those looking after pregnant women know their local protocol.

Incidence

- Between 2 and 3% of pregnancies are affected, of which 2% develop eclampsia.
- 15% of women with chronic hypertension develop pre-eclampsia.

Risk factors

See Box 8.7.

Pathophysiology

The aetiology of pre-eclampsia is unknown. However, vasospasm (causing hypertension) and generalized endothelial damage (leading to leakage of protein and fluid from the intravascular space) are the final common pathways by which the maternal syndrome develops.

Normally in early pregnancy extravillous trophoblast invades uterine spiral arteries to transform them from thick-walled muscular vessels to high-flow, low-resistance, thin-walled vessels, thereby increasing blood flow to the placenta. The process involves the decidual segments initially, followed by the myometrial segments, being complete by 20–24 weeks. In women with pre-eclampsia, there is a failure of trophoblast invasion so that the myometrial spiral arteries retain their thick-walled high resistance features.

It is thought that this causes uteroplacental underperfusion and placental hypoxia, resulting in oxidative stress and the release of anti-angiogenic (e.g. s-VEGFR1) and other factors into the maternal circulation, causing widespread endothelial damage.

Reductions in levels of the vasodilator (and antiplatelet aggregator) prostacyclin and increases in the vasoconstrictor thromboxane A_2 are thought to bring changes in vascular tone, blood pressure, and platelet thrombosis. Increased vascular sensitivity to angiotensin II is also seen in pre-eclampsia, leading to increased vascular tone and hypertension.

The multisystem effects are shown in Box 8.8.

Clinical evaluation

History

Asymptomatic with raised BP and proteinuria found on routine antenatal screening or the woman may present with a combination of symptoms and signs, namely:

- Headache, visual disturbance, epigastric and/or right upper quadrant pain
- Worsening peripheral and periorbital oedema
- Nausea and vomiting
- Small-for-dates on routine clinical palpation
- Reduced fetal movements
- Abdominal pain and bleeding with abruption (see Section 8.2)
- Cerebrovascular accidents
- Seizures

Examination

- The BP should be rechecked
- Oedema is not necessary for the diagnosis of pre-eclampsia but facial oedema and oedema persisting after 12 h rest are significant
- Symphyseal fundal height to assess for fetal growth retardation (FGR)
- The fetal heart rate should be checked
- Tenderness over the liver is an ominous sign
- Clonus ≥3 beats is associated with cerebral irritation

Investigations

- **Urinalysis:** ≥+1 protein on urine dipstick is significant and quantitative measurement is necessary. Approximate equivalents for proteinuria are 1+ = 0.3 g/l, 2+ = 1 g/l, 3+ = 3g/l
- **FBC:** raised haemoglobin and haematocrit with haemoconcentration; low haemoglobin with haemolysis, low platelets
- **U&Es:** raised creatinine (mean levels first, second, and third trimesters are 60, 54 and 64 µmol/l) and urea
- **LFTs:** raised transaminases (ALT and AST). Normal pregnancy levels 20% lower than non-pregnant state
- **Urate:** levels equate to gestation (i.e. <320 µmol/l at 32 weeks, <360 µmol/l at 36 weeks) but are raised in pre-eclampsia
- **Clotting:** only needed if abnormal liver function, low platelets or severe pre-eclampsia. Look for evidence of disseminated intravascular coagulation (DIC)
- **MSU:** to rule out infection as cause of proteinuria
- **US:** asymmetrical growth retardation, reduced liquor volume, abnormal Doppler waveforms (reduced, absent or reversed umbilical end-diastolic flow, redistribution with low resistance in middle cerebral artery)
- **24-h urine collection:** for protein is the 'gold standard' quantitative measurement for proteinuria
- **PCR** (protein:creatinine ratio): can be performed on a one-off urine sample and has been found to be accurate in predicting significant proteinuria (see Box 8.6 Section 8.10)

Pre-eclampsia can range from mild to severe. Mild pre-eclampsia is the absence of symptoms and signs of severe pre-eclampsia (see Section 8.13).

Prediction

- Identify risk factors at booking (see Box 8.7)
- Uterine artery Dopplers at 20–24 weeks for at-risk women

- Elevated indices or bilateral notching of the diastolic waveform suggests increased peripheral vascular resistance and increased risk of pre-eclampsia, FGR and placental abruption

Prevention

Aspirin: a Cochrane review has shown that antenatal aspirin provided a small-to-moderate benefit when used for the prevention of pre-eclampsia, i.e. a 15% reduction in the risk of pre-eclampsia. There was a greater reduction in the risk of pre-eclampsia in those taking >75 mg aspirin/day, compared with <75 mg/day. However, the subgroup numbers were small and the current reassurance about safety of aspirin in pregnancy only applies to lower doses.

- 8% reduction in the risk of delivery <37 weeks
- 14% reduction in the risk of death (stillbirth, neonatal/infant death) in the antiplatelet group
- No overall difference in risk of placental abruption and small-for-gestational age
- No overall difference in the risk of PIH

Calcium supplements: halve the risk of pre-eclampsia and reduce serious morbidity and death in women at high risk and with low dietary intake. Calcium is safe and cheap with no adverse effects. Further research is needed to establish the optimal dose.

Vitamins C and E: a large randomized controlled trial (RCT) (*n* = 1877) investigating the effect of vitamin C and E supplements in nulliparous women found no reduction in the risk of pre-eclampsia, FGR, the risk of death or other serious outcomes in infants.

Recurrence

Between 10 and 20% of women with previous pre-eclampsia will develop it in subsequent pregnancies.

➕ Box 8.7 Risk factors for developing pre-eclampsia

- Extremes of age
- Genetic (increased incidence if mother and sisters affected)
- Ethnic origin (increased risk among Africans)
- Primigravida
- Previous history of pre-eclampsia
- Multigravida with new partner
- Obesity
- Essential hypertension
- Pre-existing renal disease
- Diabetes mellitus
- Antiphospholipid antibodies
- Inherited thrombophilia

➔ Box 8.8 Multisystem effects of pre-eclampsia

Cardiovascular

- Peripheral resistance ↑ in pre-eclampsia, as opposed to the ↓ in normal pregnancy
- ↑ sensitivity to angiotensin II increases BP further

Renal

- Glomerular endothelial swelling—'glomerular endotheliosis'—characteristic of pre-eclampsia
- Increased glomerular vascular permeability
- Enhanced tubular reabsorption and ↓ renal clearance of uric acid
- Reduced renal blood flow and glomerular filtration rate
- Renal artery spasm
- Acute tubular necrosis and cortical necrosis

Hepatic

- Liver oedema
- Periportal haemorrhagic necrosis
- Subcapsular haemorrhage

Haematological

- Endothelial damage, hypertension, and low plasma colloid oncotic pressure contribute to increased capillary leakage
- Microangiopathic haemolysis
- Activation of the coagulation system in severe PET with raised fibrinogen degradation products and prolonged thrombin time
- Increased capillary leakage in pulmonary vessels

CNS

- Vascular autoregulatory dysfunction causing cerebral oedema, poor cerebral perfusion, and haemorrhage
- Retinal oedema and detachment

Uteroplacental and fetal

- Failed trophoblast invasion of uterine spiral arteries
- Reduced uteroplacental perfusion
- Compensatory redistribution of blood flow to brain and ↓ blood flow to fetal kidneys ⇒ ↓ urinary output
- Severe hypertension causing placental separation
- Severe pre-eclampsia necessitating preterm delivery

Further reading

Hofmeyer GJ, Atallalh AN, Duley L. Calcium supplementation during pregnancy for preventing hypertensive disorders and related problems. *Cochrane Database of Systematic Reviews* 2006 **3**: CD001059

8.12 Management of mild pre-eclampsia

Women with new onset pre-eclampsia, those who are symptomatic, or have significant hypertension (≥140/90), ≥2+ protein on urinalysis or fetal effects (reduced movements, fetal growth retardation (FGR), oligohydramnios, abnormal fetal Doppler waveforms) must be admitted for further assessment.

Initial monitoring should include:

- 4-hourly BP, including mean arterial pressure;
  MAP = ([Systolic–diastolic]/3) + diastolic
- Twice daily fetal heart rate (FHR)
- 24-h urine collection for protein
- Thromboembolic disease (TED) stockings
- Daily urinalysis
- US for fetal size, liquor volume, and umbilical artery Doppler
- If fetal growth restriction (FGR), twice daily CTGs

Pre-eclampsia can progress rapidly and unpredictably from mild to severe life-threatening condition so close monitoring is essential. In most units, if pre-eclampsia is confirmed, it is managed as an inpatient unless mild and stable.

Mild pre-eclampsia

If pre-eclampsia is mild and stable, women may be managed as outpatients with regular (at least twice weekly) review.

Most units have a Day Assessment Unit whereby women can be seen regularly for BP checks, urinalysis, fetal monitoring, and blood tests.

If there is change in any of the variables or the woman is non-compliant, then admission is warranted.

Such women should be aware of the symptoms and signs of pre-eclampsia (headache, blurred vision, vomiting, epigastric discomfort, reduced fetal movements) and must attend if present.

Management

- The only treatment is delivery
- The outcome depends on clinical severity and gestation
- Antihypertensives control BP but do not stop the disease process
- In women with mild pre-eclampsia (asymptomatic, mildly raised BP not requiring treatment, and stable bloods with a normally grown fetus), expectant management is preferred
- Expectant management to gain fetal maturity is justified as long as complications are not present
- Close monitoring is essential, as fulminating life-threatening severe pre-eclampsia can develop over a short space of time
- Consider induction of labour at term, particularly if the cervix is favourable

Antihypertensives

- Consider starting antihypertensives when BP persistently ≥140/90
- All antihypertensives reduce the risk of severe hypertension in women with mild–moderate pre-eclampsia.
- There is insufficient evidence as to whether there is a reduction in serious outcomes and whether treatment is worthwhile in those with mild–moderate hypertension
- The main concern with antihypertensive therapy is of reduced placental perfusion and increased FGR
- Sudden drastic drops in BP should be avoided and the aim is to keep the BP >130/80 mmHg
- ACE inhibitors are contraindicated because of fetal effects (oligohydramnios, renal failure, and hypotension).
- Diuretics should only be used for treatment of pulmonary oedema as they further deplete the intravascular volume
- No difference in drug choice

First line—methyldopa

- Safe drug profile and many years of experience in pregnancy
- No evidence of long-term adverse effects in exposed infants
- Long half-life and slow onset of action
- The alpha-agonist effect inhibits vasoconstriction by a centrally mediated effect
- Main adverse effects are depression and drowsiness.
- Sedative effect usually resolves after a week
- Avoid if abnormal LFTs
- Treatment starts with a loading dose, 500–750 mg orally followed by a maintenance dose of between 250 mg BD and 1 g TDS

Second line—nifedipine

- No evidence of harm to fetus but limited safety data compared with more established treatments
- A Ca^{2+} channel blocker which inhibits influx of Ca^{2+} ions to vascular smooth muscle, resulting in arterial vasodilatation
- Side effects include headache and facial flushing
- Initial dosage of nifedipine slow release 10 mg BD swallowed- may be increased to 40 mg BD
- Slow-release preparations preferred as less likely to cause precipitous BP drop

Beta-blockers

- Act on heart, peripheral blood vessels, airway, pancreas, and liver receptors
- Labetalol is a combined alpha- and beta-blocker with arteriolar vasodilating action that lowers peripheral resistance
- Possibility of an increased risk of small-for-gestational age (SGA) baby in those treated with beta-blockers
- Side effects are few
- Avoid in asthmatics
- Start with labetalol 100 mg BD orally, increasing to 200 mg TDS

Thromboprophylaxis

- TED stockings should be worn by inpatients
- Women with significant proteinuria are at an increased risk so consider prophylactic low molecular weight heparin

Fetal monitoring

- Maternal monitoring of fetal movements (>10 in 12 h) is subjective but should be taken seriously
- FHR ± CTGs twice daily are advised as a minimum
- Fortnightly growth measurements by US. Pre-eclampsia <36 weeks is associated with a high risk of impaired fetal growth and neonatal mortality/morbidity
- Weekly liquor volume and umbilical artery Doppler assessments are arranged in the intervening week. If the pulsatility index is abnormal (>+2SDs), increase to twice weekly. If absent or reversed end-diastolic frequencies, arrange daily monitoring by fetal venous Doppler and/or fetal biophysical profile and/or computerized CTG

Steroids

If delivery is anticipated before 36 weeks, then consider steroids for fetal lung maturity.

Delivery

The decision to deliver is multifactorial and includes all aspects of maternal and fetal wellbeing, including past obstetric history and current gestation.

In women who are at or near term, the decision to deliver is easier.

However, in women who are <34 weeks, the risks of expectant management (eclampsia, HELLP syndrome, renal insufficiency, hepatic rupture, abruption, and intrauterine death) have to be weighed against the risks of prematurity and failed induction.

Delivery needs to be expedited in women with:

- Signs/symptoms of severe pre-eclampsia or HELLP syndrome (see Sections 8.13 and 8.14)
- More than 3 antihypertensives needed to control BP
- Static fetal growth, reduced fetal movements, oligohydramnios
- Abnormal ductus venosus Doppler flow (reversal of flow during atrial contraction wave) and/or abnormal fetal biophysical profile and/or computerized CTG
- End-organ damage (renal, hepatic, neurological, haematological and pulmonary)

Induction of labour is preferable. If there is evidence of fetal compromise, careful monitoring of the fetus during induction is essential. Continuous CTG is necessary when regular contractions start.

Further reading

Abalos E, Duley L, Steyn DW, et al. Antihypertensive drug therapy for mild to moderate hypertension during pregnancy. *Cochrane Database of Systematic Reviews* 2001; **2:**CD002252.

Duley L, Henderson-Smart DJ, Knight M, King JF. Antiplatelet agents for preventing pre-eclampsia and its complications. *Cochrane Database of Systematic Reviews* 2004; **1:**CD004659.

Magee LA, Duley L. Oral beta-blockers for mild to moderate hypertension during pregnancy. *Cochrane Database of Systematic Reviews* 2003; **3:**CD002863.

Meher S, Duley L. Rest during pregnancy for preventing pre-eclampsia and its complications in women with normal blood pressure. *Cochrane Database of Systematic Reviews* 2006; **19(2):**CD005939.

PRECOG. Evidence used to develop the PRECOG guideline. Action on pre-eclampsia, 2004. www.apec.org.uk

8.13 Management of severe pre-eclampsia

Definition

BP ≥170/110 on two occasions along with significant proteinuria (>5 g in 24 h). Clinical features of severe pre-eclampsia (which may be apparent at BP <170/110) are summarized in Box 8.9

Management

- Involvement of senior obstetric and anaesthetic staff is essential
- The single major failing in clinical care in the last triennial Confidential Enquiry was inadequate treatment of hypertension, with subsequent intracranial haemorrhage
- Diastolic BP is one of a number of useful indices of severity of pre-eclampsia
- The pressure during systole is more important in cases of intracerebral haemorrhage
- It is essential to commence antihypertensive treatment promptly in any woman with severe pre-eclampsia

Antihypertensives

- Antihypertensive treatment should be administered when BP >160/110 and/or mean arterial pressure (MAP) >125
- With MAPs >145 there is a loss of cerebral autoregulation with a risk of cerebral haemorrhage
- BP can drop suddenly with intravenous treatments and cause fetal bradycardia
- Preloading with colloid (<500 ml) and continuous fetal monitoring is therefore necessary with parenteral antihypertensives
- Hydralazine (IV bolus or infusion), labetolol (IV bolus or infusion) or nifedipine (orally) are used for the acute management of hypertension (**A**)
- Aim for BP 140–150/80–90 mmHg
- Hydralazine is a vasodilator with a direct relaxing effect on smooth muscle in the blood vessels, predominantly in the arterioles. Tachycardia is a side effect. Further doses should be avoided with a maternal heart rate >120 bpm
- BP should be checked every 15 min until stable, then every 30 min

Fluid balance

- Strict fluid balance is essential. Owing to the risks of fluid overload and pulmonary oedema, input should be restricted to 85 ml/h (**C**). Remember to include all infusions (syntocinon, antihypertensives, magnesium sulphate, $MgSO_4$)
- Output needs to be monitored and, in the acute situation, a catheter with hourly urometer should be used
- Oliguria is often seen with severe pre-eclampsia and is defined as <100 ml/ 4 h
- Renal failure rarely complicates pre-eclampsia and in most cases, a diuresis occurs postpartum
- An initial 500 ml bolus of colloid can be given if necessary. However, further fluid replacement should not be given without invasive monitoring (CVP line), particularly in the presence of acute blood loss
- Continuous O_2 saturation monitoring with pulse oximetry is necessary to detect early pulmonary oedema

Seizure prevention

- In women who are at risk of seizures, particularly with CNS symptoms (severe headache, agitation, clonus), magnesium sulphate $MgSO_4$ should be administered to prevent seizures
- In the MAGPIE study, women allocated to $MgSO_4$ had a 58% reduction in developing seizures

- See local guidelines. In general, 4 g of diluted $MgSO_4$ is given over 5–10 min as a loading dose followed by an infusion of 1 g/h
- $MgSO_4$ toxicity presents with somnolence, blurred vision, weakness, loss of patellar reflexes, respiratory and cardiac arrest.
- O_2 saturation, respiratory rate, urine output, and deep tendon reflexes should be monitored hourly
- Calcium gluconate 1 g (10 ml) over 10 min can be given if respiratory depression is present
- For the treatment of eclampsia see Section 10.3

Delivery

- Once BP is controlled in women with severe pre-eclampsia, delivery needs to be considered
- Individual circumstances will dictate whether delivery can be delayed for the administration of steroids in preterm gestations
- Conservative management at very early gestations may improve neonatal outcome, but this needs to be balanced against maternal wellbeing (**A**)
- Mode of delivery will depend on gestation, maternal and fetal wellbeing. If <32 weeks, vaginal delivery is less successful, but still worth considering. If >34 weeks, the chance of a vaginal delivery is up to 65%
- Syntocinon 5 iu IM should be given for the third stage. Products containing ergometrine should be avoided owing to the risk of further hypertension

Postpartum

- Strict fluid balance and BP control
- BP tends to fall initially. However, it tends to rise again >24 h and often additional anti-hypertensive treatment is needed
- Avoid methyldopa postnatally owing to the risk of postpartum depression. Labetolol, atenolol, nifedipine, and enalapril can be used with breastfeeding
- One-third of seizures occur postnatally. Therefore $MgSO_4$ should be continued for 24 h postpartum in those at risk
- The incidence of severe pre-eclampsia falls after day 4 postnatally
- Women with severe pre-eclampsia need to remain in hospital for 4 days owing to the risk of seizures
- On discharge, arrangements for regular BP checks should be made. Antihypertensives should be reduced as needed
- A postnatal review should be offered to discuss events surrounding the delivery as well as advice for future pregnancies
- BP and urine should be checked at the 6-week postnatal check to ensure that hypertension and proteinuria have resolved

Women who have hypertension during pregnancy are at increased long-term risk of cardiovascular disease and hypertension. The risk is greater in women with pre-eclampsia compared with PIH. This is associated with a higher risk of metabolic syndrome

Further reading

RCOG Greentop Guidelines. The management of severe pre-eclampsia/eclampsia. Guideline No. 10A. London, RCOG Press, 2006. www.rcog.org.uk

Altman D, Carroli G, Duley L, Farrell B, Moodley J, Neilson J, Smith D. Magpie Trial Collaboration Group. Do women with pre-eclampsia, and their babies, benefit from magnesium sulphate? The Magpie Trial: a randomised placebo-controlled trial. *Lancet* 2002; **359**:1877–90.

> **Box 8.9 Symptoms and signs of severe pre-eclampsia**

- Severe headache
- Visual disturbance
- Epigastric pain or vomiting
- ≥3 beats clonus
- Papilloedema
- Liver tenderness
- Platelet count <100x10^6/l
- ALT or AST >70 iu/l
- ≥5 g proteinuria/24 h
- Creatinine >120 µmol/l
- Pulmonary oedema
- HELLP syndrome

HELLP syndrome

HELLP syndrome is considered a complication of severe pre-eclampsia and is characterized by Haemolysis (microangiopathic haemolytic anaemia), Elevated Liver enzymes (secondary to parenchymal necrosis), and Low Platelets (consumption).

Maternal mortality is 1–10%. Serious complications include renal failure, abruption, disseminated intravascular coagulation (DIC), and pulmonary oedema. Fetal mortality rates range from 8% to 60% depending on gestation at birth.

Incidence
- Affects 20% of pregnancies complicated with severe pre-eclampsia
- Increases with increasing age and parity
- 15% present in the second trimester, 50% in the third trimester, and 35% postpartum

Clinical evaluation

History
Symptoms most commonly reported are:
- Epigastric pain and right upper quadrant tenderness (65%)

In addition, there may be:
- Nausea and vomiting
- Headache
- Generalized oedema and significant weight gain
- Feeling unwell with flu-like symptoms
- Haematuria

Examination
- Epigastric and right upper quadrant tenderness
- Jaundice
- Hypertension and proteinuria (although not always present)

Investigations
- FBC and film: haemolysis identified by abnormal blood film, fragmented red blood cells, and raised reticulocyte count. Thrombocytopenia (platelets <150x109/l)
- Lactate dehydrogenase (LDH): raised in haemolysis (>600 iu/l)
- LFTs: raised transaminases and bilirubin (secondary to haemolysis). Aspartate aminotransferase (AST) levels >2000 iu/l are associated with disordered mental state, jaundice, and extreme hypertension
- Clotting: DIC complicates HELLP in about 20% of cases
- Liver US: excludes haematoma
- Differential diagnoses include acute fatty liver of pregnancy and TTP-HUS (thrombotic thrombocytopenic purpura–haemolytic uraemic syndrome)

Management
The management of HELLP syndrome follows that of severe pre-eclampsia (see Section 8.13), focussing on BP control and the correction of coagulation disorders (fresh frozen plasma (FFP) and cryoprecipitate) and platelets.

Liaise with haematology early. Platelet transfusion is considered when platelet count is <20x10⁹/l or when platelets <50x10⁹/l, and procedures such as CS or CVP line insertion are needed.

If <36 weeks, administer steroids to improve fetal lung maturity. Severity of HELLP will dictate whether delivery can be delayed for 24 h until steroids have had optimal effect. A Cochrane review looked at the effect of corticosteroids in improving the maternal morbidity and mortality of HELLP syndrome. No improvement was seen in placental abruption, pulmonary oedema, liver haematoma or rupture in the treatment group. There was a tendency to an increased platelet count after 48 h in those treated with corticosteroids. This could potentially avoid the need for general anaesthetic for CS delivery in those with an initial platelet count <80x10⁹/l. This relates to steroid use over and above that given for fetal lung maturity.

Again, treatment is delivery. If >34 weeks and time allowing, vaginal delivery can be attempted. However, in severe cases, delivery by CS may be warranted independent of gestation.

Regional anaesthesia is contraindicated with abnormal clotting and platelet count <80x10⁹/l. IM analgesia should be avoided with platelet counts <80x10⁹/l.

Strict fluid balance is essential ± CVP line. Acute renal failure is a significant complication of HELLP syndrome secondary to acute tubular necrosis.

Eclampsia is more often seen with HELLP compared with severe pre-eclampsia therefore MgSO₄ should be administered (see Section 8.13)

Subcapsular haematoma can form in association with severe parenchymal necrosis, leading to stretching of the capsule which can eventually rupture. Inform surgical (liver) team urgently if suspected to decide on conservative or surgical management.

HELLP can deteriorate within the first 48 h of delivery, therefore close monitoring is essential. Red cell transfusion may be needed with continued haemolysis.

Recurrence
- Between 3% and 27% recurrence for HELLP syndrome
- There is a 42% risk of any type of pre-eclampsia or eclampsia

Acute fatty liver of pregnancy

Incidence
The incidence of acute fatty liver in pregnancy (AFLP) is between 1:9–13 000 pregnancies.

Pathophysiology
Unknown but thought to be a variant of pre-eclampsia.
In some cases there is an association with an autosomal recessive abnormality in fetal long-chain fatty acid ß oxidation. The affected fetus produces abnormal fatty acid metabolites which accumulate in the maternal liver

An association with obesity, male fetuses, multiple pregnancy, and primigravidae has been reported.

Clinical evaluation

History
The symptoms are non-specific:
- Nausea, anorexia, and malaise
- Vomiting and abdominal pain
- Jaundice
- Pruritis
- Altered consciousness secondary to hepatic encephalopathy

Examination
The same as for pre eclampsia (see Section 8.11)

Investigations
- LFTs: raised transaminases (3–10 times normal). Raised bilirubin
- Uric acid: raised (often out of proportion to degree of pre-eclampsia)

- U&Es: raised creatinine
- FBC: neutrophilia
- Clotting: prolonged prothrombin time
- Glucose: low (often marked hypoglycaemia)
- Liver US
- Liver biopsy: confirms diagnosis but often not necessary and will be contraindicated in the presence of ↑ coagulopathy

Management
- Inform senior anaesthetists, obstetricians, and hepatologists early. Delivery is advisable once the maternal condition is stabilized
- Intensive monitoring of blood glucose, clotting, and LFTs is needed with strict fluid input/output. Invasive monitoring is often required. Treat hypoglycaemia with 50% glucose intravenous infusion (IVI)
- Liaise with haematologists for FFP to correct coagulopathy
- If fulminant liver failure or encephalopathy, then transfer to a liver unit
- Plasmapheresis is sometimes needed

Risks
- Maternal mortality is 10–20% (three deaths in the last Confidential Enquiry)
- Fetal mortality is 20–30%

Thrombotic thrombocytopenic purpura (TTP), haemolytic uraemic syndrome (HUS), and TTP–HUS

Incidence
Rare: 4–6 per million adults per year. However, it may rise as high as 1:25 000 in pregnancy, hence recognition is important as it may be fatal.

Pathophysiology
Characterized by thrombocytopenia, microangiopathic haemolytic anaemia, and multi-organ failure secondary to ischaemia.

Damage to microvascular endothelial cells causes release of multimers of von Willebrand factor (vWF). There is a decrease in the vWF cleaving factor metalloproteinase which can be either hereditary or acquired. Accumulation of vWF leads to platelet aggregation and obstruction of arterioles and capillaries by microthrombi, causing organ damage. Platelets are consumed, leading to thrombocytopenia; microangiopathic haemolysis causes anaemia.

Factors that can precipitate TTP–HUS include pregnancy (10–25% of cases), malignancy, drugs, and infection (HIV, E. coli).

Clinical features
Crossover in the symptoms commonly occurs.

Thrombotic thrombocytopenic purpura (TTP)
- TTP is increasing, possibly related to drug exposure
- Chronic relapsing TTP may be congenital. Two-thirds are non-recurrent
- More extensive than HUS, with CNS involvement
- Classic pentad present in ~50% of cases.
- Pentad consists of thrombocytopenia, microangiopathic haemolytic anaemia, renal impairment, fever, and neurological features (headaches, drowsy, seizures, coma)
- 50% occur before 24 weeks' gestation
- Relapse is more common

Haemolytic uraemic syndrome (HUS)
- No metalloproteinase ADAMTS-13 deficiency
- Less extensive than TTP, mainly renal involvement
- Classic triad consists of thrombocytopenia, microangiopathic haemolytic anaemia, and renal impairment
- Typically a single episode
- Usually presents postnatally with acute renal failure
- HELLP syndrome may evolve into HUS

Risks
Untreated there is a high risk of fetal growth restriction (FGR), fetal and maternal mortality (as high as 90% or 20% with treatment).

Clinical features in pregnancy
History
- Fever and malaise
- Nausea, vomiting, and abdominal pain
- Headaches and seizures

Examination
- BP can be raised and urine output may fall

Investigations
- FBC: thrombocytopenia, haemolytic anaemia
- Blood film: ↑ reticulocytes, red cell fragmentation
- U&Es: creatinine is often raised
- LFTs: transaminases are often normal but unconjugated bilirubin is raised with haemolysis
- LDH: raised secondary to haemolysis
- Clotting: is normal in TTP (antithrombin level is ↓ in pre-eclampsia, HELLP and AFLP)
- Urine dipstick: proteinuria and haematuria can be present because of renal damage
- There is no definitive test and classic features are not always present

Management
- Involve ITU staff and haematologists at the start
- Platelet transfusions are contraindicated
- Plasma exchange is the treatment of choice for TTP–HUS. FFP and platelets are comparatively less effective
- Continue plasma exchange until ≥48 h after remission. Repeated cycles may be required until delivery
- Red cell transfusion as required for anaemia
- Give folate supplementation
- High-dose steroids may confer benefit
- Low-dose aspirin if platelet count >50 x 10^9/l
- Supportive therapy for renal and CNS impairment
- Consider delivery in refractory cases

TTP–HUS does not necessarily resolve postpartum (as opposed to HELLP and AFL)

Thrombocytopenia in pregnancy

Definition
Platelet count below non-pregnant range of 150–400 x 10^9/l.

Incidence
Between 5–10% of pregnant women have low platelets at term.

Aetiology
- Spurious (clumping of blood sample)
- Gestational or pregnancy-associated thrombocytopenia (PAT)
- Immune thrombocytopenic purpura (ITP)
- Pre-eclampsia, HELLP, acute fatty liver
- Thrombotic thrombocytopenic purpura (TTP)
- Haemolytic uraemic syndrome (HUS)
- Disseminated intravascular coagulation (DIC)
- Splenic sequestration: hypersplenism, liver disease, portal hypertension, hepatic vein thrombosis, infection (malaria), myeloproliferative and lymphoproliferative disorders
- Bone marrow suppression: aplastic anaemia, bone marrow infiltration, parvovirus B19

History
Review of medical and obstetric history. Enquire about:
- Drug and alcohol history, including use of heparin
- Recent infections or blood transfusion
- CNS symptoms: headaches, drowsiness, seizures
- Visual disturbances
- Abdominal symptoms: epigastric pain
- Arthralgia

Examination
- Look for petechiae, purpura, and mucosal bleeding
- Examine for splenomegaly or hepatomegaly
- Check reflexes and presence of clonus

Investigations
- Exclude spurious thrombocytopenia: repeat platelet count in citrate to prevent clumping
- Check BP and urinalysis
- FBC, film, reticulocyte count, lactate dehydrogenase
- U&E, uric acid, LFT, HIV
- Coagulation screen
- Consider autoantibody screen: antinuclear, anti-DNA, anti-Smith, antiphospholipid, and rheumatoid factor (see Section 7.26)

Diagnosis
- Severe hypertension points to pre-eclampsia/HELLP
- Fever, severe CNS or renal impairment suggest TTP/HUS
- Coagulation screen is normal in TTP/HUS
- Fibrinogen level is decreased in DIC

Blood film
- Platelet clumping: spurious result
- Red cell fragmentation: thrombotic microangiopathies
- Hypersegmented neutrophils and oval macrocytes: folate deficiency
- Other abnormal red and white cell: bone marrow disease
- Normal: PAT or ITP

Onset of disease
- If <24 weeks' gestation: consider ITP, TTP
- If >24 weeks' gestation: consider pre-eclampsia, HELLP
- If postnatal: consider pre-eclampsia, HELLP, HUS

Following delivery
- Normal platelet count: PAT
- Resolution of pre-eclampsia/HELLP (there may be transient deterioration before resolution)
- TTP, HUS and ITP are not resolved by delivery

General management
- Close liaison between obstetricians and haematologists
- Exclude pre-eclampsia, HELLP, SLE, TTP, HUS

Treatment
- Maternal treatment does not affect fetal platelet count
- >80: regional anaesthesia is generally safe
- <80: general safer than regional anaesthesia. Treat before regional anaesthesia
- <50: increased risk of bleeding. Treat before delivery
- <20: severe; treat as increased risk of spontaneous bleeding
- Treat if symptomatic at any stage of pregnancy

Gestational thrombocytopenia

Incidence
- Between 5 and 10% of pregnancies
- Responsible for 75% of thrombocytopenia cases, mainly in the third trimester

Effect on pregnancy
- Haemodilution, increased platelet activation and clearance leads to fall in platelet count during pregnancy
- Maternal risk relates to platelet count
- No adverse fetal effect. No need for fetal blood sampling

Diagnosis of exclusion
- Platelet count is often >80x10^9/l
- Diagnosis confirmed when maternal platelet count returns to normal after delivery

Management
Gestational thrombocytopenia is a benign condition with no adverse consequence for mother or baby even if the platelet count falls <100x10^9/l. Therefore no treatment is required.

However, it is difficult to distinguish from ITP. If ITP is not excluded, follow the management as for ITP.

Immune thombocytopenic purpura

Incidence
ITP usually affects young women more than men, with an estimated incidence of 1–2 in 10 000 pregnancies. Three per cent of cases occur in pregnancy.

Pathophysiology
Autoantibodies are directed against platelet surface glycoproteins IIb/IIIa or Ib/IX, resulting in platelet destruction by the reticuloendothelial system, mainly in the spleen.
Primary (idiopathic)
Secondary associations:
- *Helicobacter pylori*
- Infections: HIV, Epstein–Barr, cytomegalovirus, varicella
- Connective tissue disorders: SLE, rheumatoid arthritis
- Antiphospholipid syndrome (APS)
- Lymphoproliferative disorders
- Post-transfusion purpura

- Heparin-induced thrombocytopenia
- Drug-induced

Clinical features

It is a diagnosis of exclusion.

ITP should be considered if thrombocytopenia is detected in the first half of pregnancy. If detected in the third trimester, then consider gestational thrombocytopenia.

Eighty per cent of patients have chronic disease and may have:

- No symptoms (i.e. incidental finding)
- Easy bruising, worsened by aspirin or alcohol ingestion
- Acute onset of petechiae, purpura, mucous membrane bleed

Effect of pregnancy on immune thrombocytopenic purpura

- None

Effect of immune thrombocytopenic purpura on the mother

- Relates to platelet count

Effect of immune thrombocytopenic purpura on the fetus/neonate

Antiplatelet IgG may cross the placenta leading to:

- Thrombocytopenia in 10–30% of cases
- Platelet count of 20–50 x 10^9/l in 5–10% of cases

Predictors of fetal/neonatal thrombocytopenia include maternal symptoms, prepregnancy ITP, and an affected sibling.

The risk of bleeding in fetus/neonates is low:

- Risk of neonatal intracranial haemorrhage (ICH) is 2%

Intrauterine fetal blood sampling (FBS) is not justified:

- Risk of bleeding before labour is small (placental IgG transfer occurs late in pregnancy)
- The risk of cordocentesis is similar to risk of ICH

Clinically severe bleeding is associated with neonatal alloimmune thrombocytopenia (NAIT). In this situation intrauterine FBS for fetal platelet count is justified as fetal platelet transfusion may be required

Management

Prepregnancy

- Close liaison between obstetricians and haematologists
- Advise women with refractory ITP and severe thrombocytopenia to avoid pregnancy
- Optimize therapy and consider splenectomy
- Women who had a splenectomy require:
  - Prophylactic oral penicillin V 250 mg BD
  - Vaccination against pneumococcal, meningococcal, and *Haemophilus influenzae*
- Counsel about maternal and fetal risks

Antenatal

- Monitor platelet count every 2–4 weeks
- Aim for safe platelet count for delivery (>80x10^9/l)
- Treatment depends on platelet count and symptoms
- Anaesthetist review to discuss regional analgesia plan

Intrapartum

- Inform anaesthetists and paediatricians of delivery
- Aim for vaginal birth. No evidence that Caesarean decreases the risk of ICH when compared with vaginal birth
- Platelet count <80x10^9/l, avoid regional anaesthesia
- Platelet count <50x10^9/l, platelets should be available (use only if active bleeding)
- Avoid fetal scalp electrode, FBS, ventouse extraction, and difficult forceps delivery (simple lift-out only)

Postpartum

- Repair perineal trauma promptly
- Any wound sites should be observed closely
- Avoid NSAIDs. Thrombosis prophylaxis with LMWH is safe if platelet count is >50x10^9/l
- Obtain cord blood for neonatal platelet count. If low, monitor daily as nadir is only reached at 2–5 days in affected babies, when splenic circulation is established
- In neonates with severe thrombocytopenia or bleeding:
  - Perform ultrasonography of brain
  - Treat with intravenous immunoglobulins (IVIG)
  - Platelet transfusion if life-threatening bleeding

Treatment of thrombocytopenia in ITP

Prednisolone

- 1 mg/kg/day until response obtained, then gradually decrease to lowest dose that maintains platelet count >50x10^9/l
- Possible adverse effect: hypertension, gestational diabetes, osteoporosis, and psychiatric disorders

Intravenous immunoglobulin

- Use for women who are intolerant/resistant, or require prolonged therapy/high dose of prednisolone
- May be used as first line instead of prednisolone
- Possibly delays the clearance of IgG-coated platelets
- Peak response is usually 4–5 days after the infusion
- Response is temporary, usually lasting 2–4 weeks
- Possible adverse effect: small risk of infection transmission, allergic reactions, and aseptic meningitis
- IVIG can cross the placenta but no evidence that the fetal platelet count is affected

Bolus anti-D IgG

- May help increase platelet count in Rhesus-positive women
- Possibly competitively inhibit clearance of IgG-coated platelets

Splenectomy

- May be performed in pregnancy in refractory cases
- Ideally in second or third trimester at time of CS (if required for obstetric indication)

Azathioprine

- May be used when other measures fail
- Monitor fetal growth as FGR may occur

Platelet transfusion

- Prophylactic platelet transfusions are usually ineffective
- Give as a last resort for bleeding or prior to surgery
- Increases antibody titres and increased platelet count is not sustained

Further reading

www.bcshguidelines.com British Committee for Standards in Haematology. Guidelines on the diagnosis and management of the thrombotic microangiopathic haemolytic anaemias. *British Journal of Haematology* 2003; **120:**556–73.

Clark P, Greer IA. Thrombocytopenia in pregnancy. In: *Practical Obstetric Hematology*. London: Taylor & Francis, 2006: 140–62.

Horn EH, Kean L. Thrombocytopenia and bleeding disorders. In: James DK, Steer PJ, Weiner CP, Gonik B (eds). *High Risk Pregnancy Management Options*. Elsevier Saunders: Philadelphia, 2005: 901–24.

8.16 Thromboembolism

Clinical relevance

Deep vein thrombosis (DVT) and pulmonary embolus (PE) are life-threatening conditions, but clinical assessment of DVT and PE is unreliable. Women presenting with symptoms and signs of venous thromboembolism (VTE) need to have their diagnosis confirmed by objective testing and to start treatment without delay (**A**, **Ib**). Failure to appreciate the significance of symptoms and signs, delay in treatment, and inadequate anticoagulation are all factors associated with maternal death from VTE.

PE remains the leading direct cause of maternal deaths in the UK. In the last 2003–2005 Confidential Enquiry, there were 33 deaths from PE (1.56 per 100 000 maternities) and 8 from cerebral vein thrombosis, of which 13 occurred in the first trimester, 1 in the second, and 4 others were followed by perimortem or post mortem CS after collapse. Of the 17 postpartum deaths, 8 ocurred after vaginal delivery and 7 after CS.

Guidance for thromboprophylaxis during pregnancy and postpartum has been extrapolated from advice on how to manage thromboembolic disease in non-pregnant women.

Incidence

- 0.1% incidence of non-fatal DVT and PE
- Pregnancy increases the risk of VTE 6-fold
- Risk is greatest in the puerperium
- Mortality of untreated PE is 13%

Pathophysiology

Pregnancy is a hypercoagulable state. Factor VIII, IX, and X levels increase in pregnancy, along with fibrinogen. Fibrinolytic activity decreases and levels of endogenous anticoagulants (protein S and antithrombin) are lower. Venous stasis further raises the risk of thromboembolic disease (TED).

Risk factors

See Box 8.10.

Clinical evaluation

History

'Classical' symptoms are often absent.

DVT

- Unilateral pain, discomfort, and swelling of the leg
- Affects left leg in 90%

PE

- Dyspnoea, tachypnoea, pleuritic chest pain, haemoptysis, faintness, apprehension
- Symptoms and signs of DVT
- Collapse and central chest pain with massive PE

Examination

'Classical' signs are not often present, therefore it is important to have a high index of suspicion.

DVT

- Tenderness, oedema, asymmetry of the legs
- Increased calf diameter
- Pain in calf with dorsiflexion of the foot
- Increased temperature, pelvic pain

PE

- Raised respiratory rate, tachycardia, low O_2 saturations
- Raised jugular venous pressure (JVP), focal chest signs
- Signs of DVT
- Hypotension and respiratory distress with massive PE (difficulty breathing, cyanosis)

First line investigations

- **FBC** elevated WCC (neutrophilia)
- **CRP** elevated
- **D-dimer levels are not indicated**: These are increased in normal pregnancy owing to physiological changes in the coagulation system and in the presence of medical problems, especially with pre-eclampsia. Low level probably excludes VTE, but a raised level is not dignostic
- **Arterial blood gases:** May be normal with small PEs (15%). Hypoxia and respiratory alkalosis are signs of PE.
- **ECG:** Sinus tachycardia, right heart strain or (rarely) right bundle branch block.
  Classical triad of 'S1, Q3, T3' (deep S waves in lead I, Q waves and inverted T waves in lead III) is rarely seen.
- **Chext X-ray:** Excludes other causes of symptoms and aids interpretation of the V/Q scan. Normal in 50% with PE. Wedge infarct rarely seen. Non-specific changes in PE include segmental collapse, raised hemidiaphragm, consolidation, and unilateral pleural effusion (see Figure 8.4)

Objective tests for venous thromboembolism

Lower limb vascular studies (see Figure 8.5)

These comprise duplex scanning or power Doppler ultrasound. Accuracy is uncertain in pregnancy but these procedures are more practical than venography. Accuracy is greater for proximal DVT compared with calf DVT. They can be used in patients with suspected PE to detect DVT as a surrogate marker to avoid ionizing radiation.

Ventilation/perfusion scan (V/Q) (see Figure 8.6)

- If the CXR is normal, a V/Q scan is the first line test for PE
- A perfusion scan is performed first, followed by the ventilation scan if perfusion is abnormal (**IV**)
- The mother and fetus are exposed to a very low radiation dose. The increase in risk of fatal cancer up to the age of 15 is 1:280 000 (background risk 5 in 10 000)

CT pulmonary angiography (see Figure 8.7)

- CT pulmonary angiography (CTPA) is recommended as the first line investigation for PE in non-pregnant women (British Thoracic Society)
- Exposes the mother to higher levels of radiation than a V/Q scan
- Absorbed dose to breasts is 40 times that of a perfusion scan, which raises the lifetime risk of breast cancer by up to 13.6%
- However, the radiation dose to the fetus is lower compared with that of a V/Q scan (see above). CTPA should be considered when the CXR is abnormal or results of V/Q are equivocal
- Neonatal thyroid function should be tested in the first week of life to exclude hypothyroidism if iodinated contrast has been used

MRI

MRI techniques are being developed in the diagnosis of PE. The safety is not yet established but it is unlikely to cause harm.

Box 8.10 Risk factors for venous thromboembolism

- >35 years (if >40, risk increased 100-fold)
- Immobility (including paraplegia)
- Obesity (BMI >30 kg/m^2; >80 kg)
- Parity >4
- Operative delivery (CS increases risk 2–8-fold)
- Dehydration (hyperemesis; long haul flights)
- Haemoconcentration (pre-eclampsia; ovarian hyperstimulation syndrome)
- Surgical procedures in pregnancy or puerperium (e.g. postpartum sterilization)
- Previous TED
- Excessive blood loss
- Sickle cell disease
- Inflammatory disorders and infection (inflammatory bowel disease; UTI)
- Congenital thrombophilias:
  - Antithrombin deficiency
  - Protein C deficiency
  - Protein S deficiency
  - Factor V Leiden
  - Prothrombin gene variant
- Acquired thrombophilias:
  - Lupus anticoagulant
  - Anticardiolipin antibodies

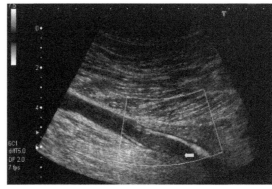

Fig. 8.5 Power Doppler US demonstrating a central thrombus (⇐) with surrounding blood flow in the distal left superficial femoral vein. (Kindly provided by Dr William Partridge and Dr Stephen Fenn.)

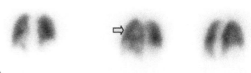
(a)

(b)
Fig. 8.6 V/Q scan. Row (a) is the perfusion part of the scan. Note the perfusion defects (⇒). Row (b) is the ventilation part. Note the mismatch.

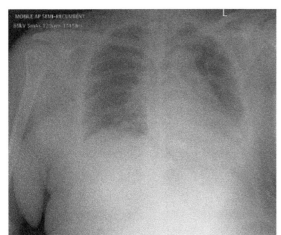

Fig. 8.4 CXR of patient with a left-sided PE. Notice non-specific changes (left lower lobe consolidation).

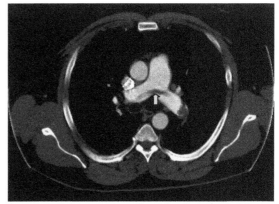

Fig. 8.7 CTPA demonstrating a filling defect ('saddle' embolus) at the main pulmonary artery bifurcation extending into both the right and the left main pulmonary arteries (⇑). (Kindly provided by Dr William Partridge and Dr Stephen Fenn.)

Overview

Always approach with care while awaiting results.

As clinical evaluation of venous thromboembolism (VTE) is unreliable and the risks when untreated are potentially fatal, always treat with unfractionated heparin (UH) or low molecular weight heparin (LMWH) without delay if VTE is suspected, until a diagnosis is excluded by objective testing, unless treatment is strongly contraindicated (**A**).

Objective testing should be performed quickly to avoid risks, inconvenience, and costs of inappropriate anticoagulation (**B, III**).

Before starting anticoagulant treatment, FBC, U&Es, thrombophilia screen, coagulation screen, and LFTs should be performed (to exclude renal and hepatic dysfunctions which are cautions to anticoagulant treatment). A thrombophilia screen will not affect current management but may influence duration and intensity of anticoagulant treatment. Results need to be interpreted with care, as pregnancy and the presence of a thrombus can affect values.

Treatment of VTE in pregnancy is with heparin as it does not cross the placenta so has no direct effect on the fetus. The interpretation of results and suggested action are shown in Box 8.11.

Fetal risks

- These arise secondary to hypoxia in acute VTE or the investigations required.
- Acquired and inherited thrombophilias can affect placental function and cause early and late fetal loss, growth retardation and pre-eclampsia (see Section 7.26).
- Warfarin is associated with embryopathy.

Initial treatment of venous thromboembolism

Low molecular weight heparin

LMWHs are as effective (PE) or more effective (DVT) than UH, with lower mortality and fewer haemorrhagic complications in non-pregnant subjects (**A, Ib, Ia**).

A systematic review of prophylaxis and treatment of VTE in pregnancy found LMWHs to be effective and safe. Risk of recurrence of VTE while on treatment was low (1.15%).

The greater bioavailability from subcutaneous tissue, longer plasma half-life (4 versus 1.5 h) and the ease of administration without the need for continuing laboratory monitoring have made LMWHs the choice of drug in the management of VTE.

LMWH increases the ratio of anti-Xa to anti-IIa activity, therefore resulting in less risk of bleeding compared with UH.

It also has a lower risk of thrombocytopenia and osteoporosis compared with UH.

Twice daily dosing of dalteparin and enoxaparin are recommended during pregnancy owing to changes in pharmacokinetics of these drugs in pregnancy (increased plasma volume and renal excretion). If the diagnosis of VTE is confirmed and treatment continued, peak anti-Xa activity (3 h post injection) should be measured to confirm appropriate dosing. The target level is 0.6–1.0 u/ml.

Intravenous unfractionated heparin

- Traditionally, given in acute VTE.
- The preferred treatment in massive VTE because of its rapid action and extensive experience (see below).
- Loading dose of 5000 iu, followed by continuous infusion of 1000–2000 iu/h
- Measure activated partial thromboplastin time (APTT) 6-hourly after loading dose then at least daily
- APTT should be 1.5–2.5 times the average laboratory control

Subcutaneous unfractionated heparin

Effective alternative to intravenous unfractionated heparin for initial management of DVT (**A, I and II**). Mid interval APTT should be 1.5–2.5 times the control.

Maintenance treatment for VTE

Oral anticoagulants

- Readily cross the placenta
- Associated with characteristic embryopathy in first trimester (6.4% risk of nasal hypoplasia and or stippled epiphyses), CNS abnormalities (any trimester), fetal haemorrhage, miscarriage, and stillbirth
- Avoided in pregnancy
- Can be used postpartum as safe with breastfeeding.

Heparins

- LMWH is the drug of choice (see above)
- Women should be taught injection technique and safe disposal of needles and syringes
- Outpatient monitoring of platelets starting 7–10 days after initiating treatment and then monthly to exclude thrombocytopenia
- Arrange antenatal anaesthetic review and prepare plan for labour (preferably spontaneous)

Fondaparinux

- This is a synthetic pentasaccharide with anti-Xa activity. The therapeutic effect is narrow. There is no placental transfer.
- Can be used as an alternative in cases of heparin-induced thrombocytopenia

Clopidogrel

This is a prodrug which selectively inhibits ADP-induced platelet aggregation. It increases the bleeding time by 1.5–2-fold. The effects are irreversible and it acts within 2 h. Note that this interacts with low-dose aspirin to prolong the bleeding time.
It must be stopped 7 days before delivery.

Vena cava filters

Vena cava filters prevent PEs and are indicated in pregnant women with a DVT when:

- Anticoagulants are contraindicated
- Diagnosis is made shortly before delivery
- DVT is extensive and the woman is preoperative requiring anticoagulation interruption

Duration of treatment

- Treatment of proximal VTE in pregnancy should continue for 6 months from initiation or 6 weeks postnatally, whichever is longer
- The duration is 3 months if distal DVT
- If VTE develops in early pregnancy, the dose can be reduced to prophylactic levels after completing treatment (e.g. enoxaparin 40 mg OD), in view of the high recurrence risk

Delivery

Labour

Once in labour, further doses of heparin should be withheld. Restart treatment dose postpartum.

Induction

Administer a thromboprophylactic dose on the day prior to induction and continue at this dose until labour has established. Restart treatment dose postdelivery.

If DVT confirmed on Doppler scan:
- Continue anticoagulant treatment (**IV**)
- Leg should be elevated and a graduated elastic compression stocking applied to reduce oedema initially followed by mobilization

If low level of suspicion of DVT and Doppler scan is negative
- Discontinue treatment (**IV**)

If high level of clinical suspicion for DVT and negative Doppler scan
- Continue treatment and repeat US in 1 week. If repeat testing is negative, then discontinue treatment (**IV**)

If medium or high probability of PE on V/Q scan
- Continue treatment (**IV**)

If low probability of PE on V/Q and Doppler US positive
- Continue treatment (**IV**)

If low probability of PE on V/Q, Doppler US negative but high degree of clinical suspicion
- Continue treatment for 1 week and repeat V/Q and Doppler. If still high clinical suspicion and tests are still negative, consider pulmonary angiography, CTPA or MRI (**IV**)

Regional analgesia
- To avoid epidural haematoma, no regional anaesthesia for 12 h after prophylactic heparin and 24 h after treatment dose
- LMWH should not be given for at least 4 h after epidural catheter inserted or removed and the cannula should not be removed within 10–12 h of most recent injection

Elective Caesarean section
Thromboprophylactic dose on the day prior to delivery and omit on morning of delivery. Thromboprophylactic dose given 3 h after delivery (or 4 h after epidural removed), then treatment dose that evening.

There is an increased risk of wound haematoma (2%), so consider intra-abdominal drains and interrupted sutures to allow drainage (RCOG good practice point).

Women who have a high risk of haemorrhage (e.g. significant APH), coagulopathy, progressive wound haematoma, suspected intra-abdominal bleeding and PPH) and who need anticoagulation can be given intravenous unfractionated heparin. It has a shorter half-life than LMWH and is more easily reversed with protamine sulphate in case of haemorrhage.

Postnatal anticoagulation
(See also duration of treatment.)
- Warfarin is safe in breastfeeding mothers
- Start on day 2 or 3 postpartum

- Check INR 2 days after starting
- Target INR should be 2.0–3.0
- Stop heparin when INR>2.0 on 2 successive days
- After treatment is complete, test for inherited and acquired thrombophilias
- Future thromboprophylaxis is advised for high-risk situations (i.e. subsequent pregnancies, periods of immobility, surgery)
- Avoid oestrogen-containing contraceptives

Massive DVT
If DVT threatens leg viability through venous gangrene, the leg should be elevated with consideration of surgical embolectomy or thrombolytic therapy.

Recurrent PE
- If recurrent PE occurs while on anticoagulant treatment, assess adequacy of anticoagulation (anti-Xa levels with LMWH or APTT with unfractionated heparin)
- A temporary caval filter may be required in women with recurrent PE despite satisfactory anticoagulation

Massive PE
- Presents with collapse, severe cardiorespiratory compromise or cardiac arrest
- Initial ABC management (see Section 10.1)
- Urgent senior obstetric, anaesthetic, and medical review
- IV heparin is the drug of choice in this situation owing to rapid onset of action
- Thrombolytic therapy, percutaneous catheter thrombus fragmentation or surgical embolectomy may be required

Post-thrombotic syndrome
- The features of pain, swelling, hyperpigmentation, and ulceration occur secondary to valve incompetence
- Graduated elastic compression stockings should be worn on the affected leg for 2 years after the acute event to reduce this risk (**A**)

Further reading
www.rcog.org.uk RCOG: Thromboembolic disease in pregnancy and the puerperium: Acute management. Guideline No. 28. London: RCOG Press, 2007.

www.rcog.org.uk RCOG: Thromboprophylaxis during pregnancy, labour and after vaginal delivery. RCOG Greentop Guideline No. 37. RCOG Press, 2004.

Definitions
- **Preterm birth (PTB):** birth before 37 completed weeks
- **Preterm labour (PTL):** the progressive effacement and dilatation of the cervix in the presence of regular painful contractions
- **Threatened PTL** is diagnosed in the event of uterine contractions without cervical change

Clinical relevance
- PTB is associated with significant perinatal morbidity and mortality, particularly before 30 weeks' gestation (very PTB)
- The financial and emotional costs associated with PTB are extremely high
- While improved neonatal intervention has increased the survival rate of very preterm infants (see Figure 8.8), morbidity remains high
- Improved techniques to identify, prevent, and treat women at risk of PTL and PTB are needed (see Section 6.8)

Incidence
- PTB occurs in 5–10% of pregnancies
- A third present in PTL with intact membranes, a third with preterm prelabour rupture of membranes (PPROM), and a third will be iatrogenic
- The incidence of PTB has increased with assisted reproduction due to increased multiple pregnancy

Causes
See Box 8.12. PTB happens either due to spontaneous causes of labour (e.g. associated with twins, APH, infection, polyhydramnios or trauma) or by iatrogenic causes (medical induction of labour (IOL) or surgical CS for maternal or fetal indications before term).

Clinical evaluation
History
- Accurate and detailed history to identify at-risk women (see Box 8.12)
- Abdominal or back pain, period cramps
- Vaginal bleeding, spotting or 'show'
- Dysuria, diarrhoea
- Asymptomatic or vague symptoms with cervical incompetence
- Short cervix or funnelling identified in high-risk women undergoing cervical length screening or during routine US (dating, anomaly)
- It is important to review LMP and early US dates and pick up any discrepancies

Examination
- Pyrexia and tachycardia in the presence of infection
- Hypotension in severe infection and APH
- Abdominal tenderness (see Section 8.5): may be localized, generalized, intermittent with contractions, constant with abruption
- Regular palpable contractions
- Assess presentation and degree of engagement
- Sterile speculum to assess cervical effacement and dilatation
- Look for bulging membranes, blood, offensive discharge, and pooling of liquor
- CTG: uterine activity. Fetal heart may be normal, tachycardic (infection) or fetal distress pattern (abruption, fetal growth retardation (FGR))

Investigations
- Urinalysis and MSU
- High vaginal swab (HVS)
- Swab for *Chlamydia trachomatis*
- Fetal fibronectin (FFN) test (see Section 6.8)
- US to assess presentation, liquor volume, placental position, cervical length, and estimated fetal weight
- FBC and CRP: raised WCC and CRP in the presence of infection

Infection is associated with oligohydramnios (though it is not clear whether this is related to PPROM, or whether it is because liquor has anti-infection properties).

Worse outcomes are associated with very low birth weight babies (<1500 g).

✚ Box 8.12 Risk factors for preterm labour and birth

Previous preterm labour

Strongest predictor for recurrence.
- 15% risk with 1 previous PTB
- 30% risk with 2 previous PTBs
- 45% risk with 3 previous PTBs

Intrauterine infections
- Commonest cause is ascending from the genital tract, e.g. bacterial vaginosis, *Ureaplasma urealyticum*, *Neisseria gonorrhoeae*, *Chlamydia trachomatis*, and *Trichomonas vaginalis*
- Transplacental from maternal blood
- Trans-Fallopian from the abdominal cavity
- Inadvertent infection following invasive procedures (e.g. amniocentesis)

Extrauterine infections
- Asymptomatic bacteruria
- Pyelonephritis
- Periodontal disease
- Malaria
- Typhoid

Cervical causes
- Previous terminations of pregnancy, particularly if recurrent, second trimester or cervical dilatation >10 mm
- Cervical surgery, e.g. knife cone or large loop excision of transformation zone for cervical intraepithelial neoplasia (volume of cervical tissue removed is important)
- Cervical trauma in previous deliveries

Fetal
- Congenital abnormality
- Chromosomal abnormality

Uterine causes
- Uterine abnormalities
- Overdistension, e.g. multiple pregnancy, polyhydramnios
- Trauma (accidents, falls)

Social
- Increasing age
- Low prepregnancy weight
- Short pregnancy interval
- Poverty
- Smoking
- Alcohol
- Drugs
- Stress
- Domestic violence

Other
- Antepartum haemorrhage (found in 20% of preterm births)
- Pre-eclampsia
- Uteroplacental insufficiency

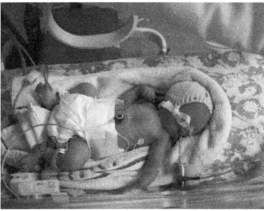

Fig. 8.8 Preterm infant—the lower the gestation and birthweight, the greater the complications. Image provided courtesy of Nicola, Chris, and Callum James Giddens.

Management

The diagnosis of premature labour is very difficult. Between 70 and 80% of women who present with threatened preterm labour will deliver at term. It is important not to expose women to the potential side effects of tocolytics if they have a low chance of delivering preterm. However, identifying women with a high risk of preterm birth (PTB) can allow timely administration of steroids and/or transfer to the appropriate neonatal unit. The results of tests, such as fetal fibronectin (FFN) and cervical length, can help decide who to treat.

There is no evidence to support or refute bed rest in hospital or at home. Thromboembolic disease (TED) stockings should be worn if there is reduced mobility.

Corticosteroids

- Between 40 and 50% of babies born before 32 weeks develop respiratory distress syndrome (RDS)
- Intramuscular betamethasone (two injections of 12 mg, 24 h apart) significantly reduces the incidence of RDS, intraventricular haemorrhage (IVH), necrotizing enterocolitis (NEC), and neonatal deaths in preterm babies (**A**)
- The optimal treatment-to-delivery interval is >24 h, but <7 days (**A**)
- Corticosteroids should be offered to women at risk of preterm delivery between 24 and 34 weeks' gestation (**A**)
- Between 35 and 36 weeks, treatment should be considered, although the NNT (number needed to treat) will be higher
- A single course does not appear to be associated with any significant maternal or fetal adverse effects (**A**)
- Specialized care from endocrinologists/obstetricians is needed for diabetic women owing to the risk of hyperglycaemia. (Good Practice Point)
- Systemic infections (such as tuberculosis) are a contraindication.
- In general, administration is advised for women with clinical chorioamnionitis. (Good Practice Point)
- The ACTORDS trial demonstrated that repeated courses of steroids reduced neonatal morbidity. However, concerns remain about long-term consequences

Tocolytics

10% of women in PTL will be suitable for tocolytic therapy. Those in advanced labour (>4 cm dilated), with evidence of intrauterine infection, antepartum haemorrhage (APH) and most with preterm prelabour rupture of membranes (PPROM) will not be candidates for tocolysis.

Tocolytics reduce the rate of PTB measured at 48 h and 7 days.

Symptomatic relief does not treat the cause, hence it is no surprise that tocolytics fail to delay delivery further or confer any long-term benefit. This, along with the side effects and poor efficacy, make the case against tocolysis. However, they are of benefit when delay of birth by 48 h is necessary to administer corticosteroids or for *in utero* transfer (**A**).

Longer use requires a strong justification.

β-mimetics

- Intravenous ritodrine and salbutamol
- Stimulate β2-adrenergic receptors and thus relax smooth muscle (e.g. uterus, arterioles, and bronchi)
- Reduce the odds of delivery within 24 h, 48 h, and 7 days, but do not significantly reduce births before 30, 32, and 37 weeks
- Not associated with any clear effects on the important measures of perinatal death or neonatal morbidity related to prematurity (e.g. RDS, IVH or necrotizing enterocolitis)

- High frequency of side effects, including palpitations, tremor, nausea, headache, chest pain, pulmonary oedema, hypokalaemia, and hyperglycaemia
- Ritodrine is no longer the drug of choice. Nifedipine and atosiban have comparable effectiveness with fewer side effects (**A**)

Calcium channel blockers

- Oral nifedipine blocks the influx of calcium through voltage-dependent channels, leading to a reduction in both intracellular calcium and subsequent myometrial contraction
- Reduce the number of women giving birth within 7 days and before 34 weeks and, as a consequence, reduce incidence of RDS, NEC, IVH, and jaundice
- Fewer adverse effects compared with β-mimetics
- Theoretical risk that nifedipine could reduce placental and fetal blood flow
- Inexpensive and comparatively easy to administer
- Not licensed for treatment of PTL, therefore responsibility lies with prescriber
- Side effects include headaches, hypotension, and flushing

Atosiban

- Intravenous competitive oxytocin–vasopressin receptor antagonist
- Reduces the odds of delivery within 24 h, 48 h, and 7 days, but no significant reduction in births before 30, 32, and 37 weeks
- Fewer adverse effects compared with β-mimetics
- Expensive but licensed for use in the UK (RCOG recommendation)

NSAIDs

- Indomethacin
- Reduction in the odds of delivery within 24 h, 48 h, and 7 days
- Main concern is its effect on the fetus (constriction of the ductus arteriosus, NEC, IVH, and renal effects)
- Long-term use mandates scanning for oligohydramnios

Infection and antibiotics

Intrauterine and extrauterine infections are associated with PTB (see Box 8.12 Section 8.18). Pathogens can cause infection of the decidua, chorion, fetal vessels, and amniotic fluid. Aspiration of infected amniotic fluid can lead to pneumonia, and fetal microbial infection can cause a systemic inflammatory response. This can lead to significant neonatal morbidity such as RDS, NEC, IVH, and periventricular leukomalacia (PVL).

Bacterial vaginosis

- Bacterial vaginosis (BV) is characterized by an imbalance of the normal vaginal flora, with a decrease in the number of protective H_2O_2-producing lactobacilli and an overgrowth of BV-associated organisms.
- These include *Gardnerella vaginalis* and anaerobes such as *Bacteroides*, *Peptostreptococcus*, *Mobiluncus*, and *Mycoplasma* species.
- BV is associated with PTL, PTB and PPROM. In one study, women with BV were 6.9 times more likely to have a PTB.
- Conflicting results regarding the benefits of screening and treating women who are high and low risk for PTB, and for those who are asymptomatic.
- A recent Cochrane review found that antimicrobial treatment effectively treated BV but there was no reduction in the incidence of PTB or PPROM.
- It may be that treatment at an earlier gestation (<20 weeks) would be more effective in reducing the incidence of PTB, but further studies are needed. In women who had previously had a PTB, treatment did reduce the risk of PPROM but not PTB.

Antibiotic prophylaxis

A Cochrane review found a reduction in the incidence of chorioamnionitis and endometritis in women treated with antibiotics who were in PTL with intact membranes. However, there was no reduction in PTB.

Antibiotics did not improve neonatal outcomes.

A trend was noted of an increase in neonatal death and cerebral palsy among those who received antibiotics.

ORACLE II was the largest study in the review and the results are summarised in Box 8.14.

Group B streptococcus

PTB and prolonged rupture of membranes are major risk factors for group B streptococcus (GBS). (See Section 6.6)

Involving the neonatal unit

- It is important to have good face-to-face relationships with neonatal doctors and nurses
- Visit your babies (well or sick)
- It is essential to know the minimum gestation your neonatal unit (NNU) will accept and the availability of cots
- An *in utero* transfer may be organized to another unit as long as maternal condition permits. Evidence suggests that *in utero* as opposed to *ex utero* transfer is better for fetal outcome. However, the health of a sick mother should not be compromised by a long ambulance transfer (e.g. in sepsis, significant active bleeding, severe pre-eclampsia).
- *Ex utero* transfers can cause significant anxiety to the mother, particularly if concomitant illness or CS delay the transfer of the mother to follow her baby.
- All obstetricians need to know survival chances by gestation and should counsel parents using same data as neonatologists.

Review by neonatologist

- In-depth discussion between the parents and a senior neonatologist is essential
- Outcomes need to be discussed in full along with treatment options

Labour and delivery

For very preterm infants there are risks of asphyxia and trauma during labour, and these have to be placed against the very real dangers of iatrogenic premature delivery with a false diagnosis of labour.

Mode of delivery needs to be discussed sensitively with the parents.

There are conflicting views regarding the optimal mode of delivery. CS at early gestations (particularly classical) is associated with significant maternal morbidity such as sepsis and increased blood loss, and has implications for future deliveries (repeat CS, rupture placenta accreta) without necessarily improving outcomes for the baby.

One review looked at elective CS versus expectant management for the delivery of the small baby. Those born after CS were less likely to have died or had neonatal seizures, although this was not statistically significant. Women undergoing CS were more likely to have serious morbidity.

The term breech trial did not look at preterm babies. However, the risks of cord prolapse and head entrapment can occur during preterm delivery (the latter also at CS). CS for preterm breech (<32 weeks) may confer benefit (see also Section 9.11).

Decisions regarding mode of delivery depend on the individual case along with the opinions of the parents.

CTG monitoring in labour of very preterm infants (limits of viability) should be discussed with the parents. If the decision has been made not to intervene in the presence of fetal distress, watching an abnormal fetal heart trace can be distressing for both parents and staff. However, knowing the condition of the baby during labour (maybe by intermittent monitoring) can help the neonatologist decide whether to continue with active resuscitation and support.

Labour should be managed as for a term pregnancy.

Instrumental delivery is not indicated routinely for preterm delivery. If needed for obstetric reasons, vacuum extraction should be avoided in gestations below 34 weeks owing to the risks of cephalohaematoma, intracranial haemorrhage, and neonatal jaundice. There is insufficient evidence to establish safety between 34 and 36 weeks (**IV**).

The interpretation of CTGs <28 weeks is more difficult as decelerations are common.

Preterm fetuses are more susceptible to progressive hypoxia and acidaemia.

8.20 Preterm labour and birth—outcomes

Maternal outcomes

- Maternal risks are associated with tocolytic use, underlying causes of preterm labour (PTL) (e.g abruption, sepsis) and with a CS (postpartum haemorrhage (PPH) and classical CS).
- Risk of postnatal depression, particularly if there has been a neonatal death. Appropriate support and counselling is important (see Section 11.6).
- A postnatal follow-up appointment should be offered so that events surrounding the preterm birth (PTB) are discussed in full and a plan formulated for future pregnancies.

Fetal outcomes

(See also Box 8.13.)

- Immaturity is the greatest cause of neonatal deaths and accounts for approximately 50%
- Risks of hypoxia and trauma during labour and delivery
- Respiratory distress syndrome (RDS), necrotizing enterocolitis (NEC), and intraventricular haemorrhage (IVH) contribute to a significant proportion of neonatal morbidity and mortality. Very preterm babies are more likely to develop these problems
- RDS can cause significant morbidity up until 34 weeks' gestation
- Hypoxaemia can lead to organ failure and IVH
- Intrauterine infection can cause IVH, damage to the white matter of the brain, and cystic change, leading to periventricular leukomalacia (PVL)
- Cerebral palsy is seen in 60–90% of babies with PVL
- Patent ductus arteriosus can lead to congestive cardiac failure
- Jaundice can develop secondary to liver immaturity. The fetal brain is more susceptible to the neurotoxic effects of unconjugated bilirubin (immature blood–brain barrier)
- Hypothermia
- Difficulty in feeding as the suck reflex is not established until 34 weeks' gestation. Very preterm babies require nasogastric feeding
- Chronic lung disease can develop in the long term
- Retinopathy of prematurity

In a study looking at the morbidity and mortality of preterm infants born in 1983 and 1993, the neonatal mortality rate decreased from 23.8% to 15.1% owing to improved neonatal care. However, the rate of IVH was the same, and the incidence of bronchopulmonary dysplasia increased. Therefore, the actual number of babies with disability had increased with the number of infants surviving.

It is good practice to visit babies in the neonatal unit/ special care baby unit to find out about their long-term follow-up and progress, and parents appreciate it.

Management in future pregnancies

- Minimize risk factors, e.g. stop smoking, reduce alcohol intake, normalize BMI, improve diet
- Treat any vaginal infections
- Transvaginal cervical length measurement to monitor for cervical shortening in high-risk women (usually 2-weekly from 2 to 4 weeks prior to earliest loss)
- Shortening and funnelling of the cervix (see Figure 8.9) is associated with preterm labour
- Women who have a cervical length measurement of ≤15 mm between 14 and 24 weeks' gestation, have nearly a 50% chance of delivery ≤32 weeks
- If cervical shortening is detected, a cervical cerclage can be considered (see below). There is contested evidence about the protective use of progesterone therapy

- Systematic reviews of cerclage in short cervix are not supportive and it should not presently be recommended

Cervical cerclage

A history of recurrent second trimester miscarriage or early preterm delivery where there is painless dilatation of the cervix suggests cervical incompetence (or 'premature cervical opening').

The aim of cervical cerclage is to provide cervical support and prevent dilatation in the incompetent cervix. It is also thought that it prevents exposure of the membranes to vaginal flora and pathogens, therefore reducing preterm prelabour rupture of membranes (PPROM) (see Figure 8.10).

It is often performed despite lack of evidence of efficacy. A Cochrane review found no evidence that a cervical suture reduces the risk of pregnancy loss, PTB or fetal morbidity associated with PTB. Therefore, women at a low or medium risk of PTB should not be considered for a cervical suture. They concluded, however, that there might be a place for cervical cerclage in high-risk women (>2 second trimester losses, shortening cervix on US). Among these women, an elective cervical cerclage at 12–14 weeks can be considered. At this stage, the risk of spontaneous miscarriage is lower (than in the first trimester) and nuchal translucency scan has been performed to screen for chromosomal abnormalities.

Routine cervical cerclage in multiple pregnancy does not improve outcome.

Vaginal sutures: purse-string non-absorbable suture around the cervix. Types include the Shirodkar suture (incision through anterior vaginal wall to reflect the bladder so that the suture is close to the internal os) and MacDonald suture (without bladder reflection). They are usually removed at 35–37 weeks' gestation.

Abdominal suture: considered only when vaginal sutures have failed. The bladder is reflected and the suture placed over the internal os. Can be inserted prepregnancy; delivery is by lower segment CS (LSCS).

Risks include bleeding, infection, spontaneous rupture of membranes (SROM), miscarriage, and trauma to the cervix.

Rescue cerclage can be inserted if a woman presents with painless effacement and early dilatation of the cervix or if there is cervical shortening or funnelling on US screening.

Rescue cerclage is contraindicated in the presence of contractions, bleeding, infection, and SROM. It is less likely to be of benefit with cervical dilatation.

Maintenance tocolytics

Oral β-mimetics do not reduce the risk of PTB when used as maintenance after PTL.

The role of calcium channel blockers in preventing preterm labour is not clear and randomized controlled trials (RCTs) are needed.

Progesterone

The current studies show benefit conferred with specific progesterones, 17-OHP (17-hydroxyprogesterone caproate) and medroxyprogesterone.

IM progesterone reduces the rate of preterm birth <37 weeks. Infants are less likely to weigh <2.5 kg and less likely to have an IVH. However, there is no reduction in perinatal death.

Vaginal progestogens reduce the risk of birth before 34 and 37 weeks, but there is insufficient information regarding clinically relevant maternal and neonatal outcomes.

In clinical practice, progesterone is used after discussion with the woman of its inconclusive evidence.

232

http://www.nottingham.ac.uk/obgyn/Epicure/epicurehome/

Study design

A series of prospective population-based observational studies established in 1995 to determine the outcome of survival and rates of disability of extremely premature infants in the UK.

Definition of disability

● 'Severe disability' refers to children who are likely to be highly dependent on care-givers, e.g. non-ambulant cerebral palsy, profound hearing loss or blindness

● 'Moderate disability' refers to children who are likely to be reasonably independent, e.g. ambulant cerebral palsy, some hearing loss, some visual impairment

● 'Mild disability' refers to children that have neurological signs with minimal functional consequences

Survival by gestation

Gestation (weeks)	Died in delivery room (%)	Survival to discharge (%)
22	84	1
23	60	11
24	41	26
25		44

Disability of surviving children by gestation

Gestation (weeks)	Severe disability (%)	Moderate disability (%)	Mild disability (%)	No disability (%)
22	50		50	
23	25	38	25	12
24	29	22	36	14
25	18	22	35	24

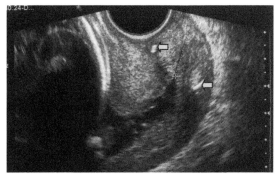

Fig. 8.10 Transvaginal USS at 21 weeks showing a short cervix (15 mm) with funnelling and a MacDonald cervical suture in situ (⇦). (Kindly provided by Dr Manju Chandiramani.)

Further reading

www.rcog.org.uk Guideline No. 7. RCOG Antenatal Corticosteroids to Prevent Respiratory Distress Syndrome, 2004.

www.rcog.org.uk RCOG Guideline No.1b Tocolytic Drugs for Women in Preterm Labour, 2002.

www.cochrane.org.uk Sosa C, Althabe F, Belizan J, Bergel E. Bed rest in singleton pregnancies for preventing preterm birth. *Cochrane Database of Systematic Reviews* 2004; **1**:CD003581.

Dodd JM, Flenady V, Cincotta R, Crowther CA. Prenatal administration of progesterone for preventing preterm birth. *Cochrane Database of Systematic Reviews* 2006; **1**:CD004947.

Drakeley AJ, Roberts D, Alfirevic Z. Cervical stitch (cerclage) for preventing pregnancy loss in women. *Cochrane Database of Systematic Reviews* 2003; **1**:CD003253.

King JF, Flenady VJ, Papatsonis DN, Dekker GA, Carbonne B. Calcium channel blockers for inhibiting preterm labour. *Cochrane Database of Systematic Reviews* 2003; **1**:CD002255.

McDonald H, Brocklehurst P, Gordon A. Antibiotics for treating bacterial vaginosis in pregnancy. *Cochrane Database of Systematic Reviews* 2007; **1**:CD000262.

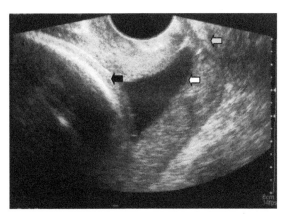

Fig. 8.9 Transvaginal USS at 30 weeks showing shortening (⬒) and funnelling (⬒) of the cervix. Fetal head (◀). (Kindly provided by Dr Manju Chandiramani.)

Incidence

Preterm prelabour rupture of membranes (PPROM) occurs in 2% of pregnancies, contributing to over a third of preterm births.

Risk factors

- Infection
- Placental abruption
- Uterine overdistension (e.g. polyhydramnios, multiple pregnancy)
- Smoking
- Drug use

Subclinical infection is a major cause of PPROM. Microorganisms are thought to cause weakness of the membranes with subsequent rupture. Bacterial vaginosis (BV) (7.3-fold increase risk of PPROM) and STIs (*Chlamydia trachomatis*, *Neisseria gonorrhoeae*, and *Trichomonas vaginalis*) are associated with PPROM.

Clinical evaluation

History

- Sudden gush of fluid, soaking clothes. Sometimes only dampness of underwear noted, can be mistaken for urinary incontinence
- Abdominal pain, contractions
- Mild pyrexia, generally feeling unwell, abnormal vaginal discharge
- PV bleeding
- Dysuria
- Cord prolapse

Examination

The diagnosis is made on speculum, not scan.

- **Vital signs**: raised temperature and tachycardia with infection, hypotension with severe infection
- **Abdominal**: tender abdomen in the presence of abruption or infection. Contractions palpated if threatened or actual preterm labour (PTL)
- **Sterile speculum**: to assess for liquor. If liquor not seen, ask the woman to cough as it may cause a trickle through the cervix. Do not perform vaginal examination (VE) as this increases the risk of intrauterine infection (**C**)
- If cord prolapse, call for immediate help (see Section 10.5)
- **CTG**: fetal heart may be normal, tachycardic (infection) or show signs of fetal distress (abruption, cord compression)

Investigations

- Urinalysis and MSU
- High vaginal swab (HVS)
- Swab for *Chlamydia trachomatis*
- FBC and CRP: raised WCC and CRP with infection
- US to assess presentation, liquor volume, and estimated fetal weight. Anhydramnios is associated with a poorer outcome than oligohydramnios

Management

Immediate

- Delivery occurs within 7 days in 80% of cases of PPROM
- Corticosteroids (see Section 8.19). There is no increased risk of infection to mother or baby
- 4-hourly observations (temperature, pulse, BP).
- CTG 8-hourly
- Bloods twice weekly to look for leukocytosis (corticosteroids can cause a temporary rise in WCC) and rising CRP
- Monitor for evidence of intrauterine infection (feeling unwell, flu-like symptoms, abdominal pain, fetal tachycardia, offensive or green liquor)

- If no contractions, prophylactic tocolysis is not recommended (**A, Ib**). In women with contractions who need corticosteroids or *in utero* transfer, tocolysis could be considered for <48 h as long as there is no evidence of infection or fetomaternal compromise. There is lack of evidence that tocolysis improves neonatal outcome and could potentially have adverse effects on the fetus if infection present
- A Cochrane review looking at the effect of antibiotics in women with PPROM found there was a reduction in the risk of chorioamnionitis and birth within 48 h and 7 days.
- ORACLE I was the largest study in the review. The results are summarized in Box 8.14. The recommended antibiotic regime is erythromycin 250 mg orally 6-hourly for 10 days
- See Section 6.6 Screening for infections for treatment of group B streptococcus (GBS)
- If there is doubt about diagnosis (e.g. good history of spontaneous rupture of membranes (SROM) but no liquor seen during speculum), pad checks and repeat speculum 1 h after lying down in the left lateral position (so that any liquor will accumulate in the vagina). Also, repeat US for amniotic fluid index may be helpful
- A 'hindwater' leak (membrane rupture occurring above the intact cervical membranes) should be treated as PPROM

If labour has not started after 48–72 h

Most women with PPROM will go into PTL. Those that do not can be managed as outpatients if there is no evidence of maternal or fetal infection or compromise. Amniotic fluid index (AFI) is useful here, as if the deepest pool >2 cm (after 72 h), then there is a lower risk of infection and imminent PTB.

- Outpatient monitoring should only be considered after rigorous individual selection by a consultant obstetrician (**B**)
- At home, the woman should check her temperature at least twice a day. She must be aware of the symptoms and signs of infection, labour, and cord prolapse, and should attend hospital immediately if these develop
- Maternal monitoring of fetal movements
- FBC and CRP should be checked twice weekly along with CTG monitoring
- 2-weekly growth scans, including liquor volume and umbilical artery Doppler
- Thromboembolic disease (TED) stockings if reduced mobility. Consider thromboprophylaxis if multiple risk factors and delivery not imminent
- Amnioinfusion: this can be performed diagnostically in a Fetal Medicine Unit where there is doubt about ROM (mainly <24 weeks), or therapeutically to prevent pulmonary hypoplasia. Although there is some evidence of benefit, there are no good trials
- It has also been used in labour to prevent or treat recurrent decelerations caused by presumed cord compression and to prevent meconium aspiration syndrome

Delivery

Immediate versus expectant

PPROM at very early gestations (<24 weeks): the outlook is poor—survival is low and babies that survive are at a high risk of severe morbidity. A balanced discussion between the parents and neonatologists is essential regarding the prognosis for the baby. Some may consider termination rather than expectant management owing to the poor prognosis.

PPROM between 24 and 34 weeks: expectant management with monitoring should be attempted, with delivery in the presence of infection, fetal compromise or cord prolapse.

If the pregnancy reaches 34 weeks or PPROM occurs after 34 weeks, delivery should be considered (**B**) as the risks of expectant management (infection, cord compression, cord prolapse, and stillbirth) are greater than the risks of immediate delivery (prematurity and failed induction). If the woman wishes to continue with expectant management, then she should be counselled regarding the increased risks of infection versus reduced risks of respiratory problems, admission to neonatal unit, and CS (**B**).

Mode of delivery and CTG monitoring in labour should be discussed with the parents. The same considerations regarding labour and delivery apply as per preterm labour (see Section 8.19).

Maternal outcomes

- Maternal systemic infection is rare but can be very serious. If not delivered, then deliver immediately and commence aggressive antimicrobial treatment. Liaise with microbiologist, senior obstetrician, and anaesthetist (see also Section 10.2).
- There may be psychological impact owing to prolonged hospital stay, uncertain outcome, and separation from baby on the neonatal unit (NNU)
- Risk of CS (including classical CS) in the presence of cord prolapse, failed induction or infection
- Increased risk of postpartum endometritis

Fetal outcomes

See also Section 8.20.

- Morbidity and mortality related to prematurity (RDS, death, cerebral palsy), infection (chorioamnionitis, cerebral damage, and neonatal infection) and oligohydramnios (pulmonary hypoplasia, limb deformities and poor fetal growth)
- The earlier the gestation at PPROM, the greater the chance of neonatal infection
- Fetal distress secondary to cord compression and cord prolapse
- Depending on the gestation of PPROM <24 weeks, even when pregnancy is prolonged, there is an associated significant risk of mortality from pulmonary hypoplasia

Management of future pregnancies

Treating BV in pregnancy in women who have had a previous PTB can reduce the risk of PPROM in future pregnancies (See also Section 8.19).

STIs should be treated.

Further reading

www.rcog.org.uk RCOG Guideline No. 44 Preterm prelabour rupture of membranes, 2006.

Kenyon S et al. Antibiotics for preterm rupture of membranes. *Cochrane Database of Systematic Reviews* 2003; **2:**CD001058.

→ **Box 8.14 Landmark research: the ORACLE Trials**

ORACLE I

Women <37 weeks admitted with PPROM where there was uncertainty regarding commencing antibiotics (i.e. no clinical evidence of infection) were randomized to co-amoxiclav plus erythromycin, co-amoxiclav plus placebo, erythromycin plus placebo or placebo only.

A total of 4826 women were randomized. Erythromycin was found to reduce the chance of delivery within 7 days after randomization, reduce the need for neonatal surfactant use, chronic lung disease, major cerebral damage on US, and death.

There was a significant increase in the risk of necrotizing enterocolitis (NEC) in babies of women treated with co-amoxiclav, therefore use should be avoided.

ORACLE II

Kenyon SL et al. ORACLE Collaborative Group. Broad-spectrum antibiotics for spontaneous preterm labour: the ORACLE II randomised trial. ORACLE Collaborative Group. *Lancet* 2001; **357:**989–94.

Women <37 weeks admitted with suspected or actual PTL where there was uncertainty regarding commencing antibiotics (i.e. no clinical evidence of infection) were randomized to co-amoxiclav plus erythromycin, co-amoxiclav plus placebo, erythromycin plus placebo or placebo only.

A total of 6295 women were randomized and neither β-lactam nor macrolide antibiotics prolonged pregnancy or improved neonatal health.

Antibiotics should therefore not be routinely prescribed to women presenting in PTL in the absence of infection.

Non-significant doubling in the rate of NEC in babies of women treated with co-amoxiclav suggests that this antibiotic should be avoided in labour.

ORACLE FOLLOW UP

Kenyon S, Pike, Jones DR. Childhood outcomes after prescription of antibiotics to pregnant woman with spontaneous preterm labour: 7 years follow up of the ORACLE II trial *Lancet* 2008; **372:** 1319–27.

Follow up at 7 years of the children has shown an increase in functional impairment if erythromycin was given. Cerebral palsy rates were also increased with administration of either erythromycin or co-amoxiclav. The number needed to harm was 64 (95% CI 37–209) and 79 (95% CI 42–591) respectively.

Kenyon SL et al. ORACLE Collaborative Group. Broad-spectrum antibiotics for preterm, prelabour rupture of fetal membranes: the ORACLE I randomised trial. ORACLE Collaborative Group. *Lancet* 2001; **357:**979–88. Erratum in: *Lancet* 2001; **358:**156.

8.22 Obstetric cholestasis

Obstetric cholestasis (OC) is a pregnancy-specific condition characterized by pruritus without a rash, abnormal liver function tests (LFTs), and resolution postpartum.

It is a diagnosis of exclusion (see Box 8.15). It is associated with an increased risk to the fetus, including prematurity and intrauterine death (IUD).

Incidence
- A total of 0.7% of pregnancies are affected
- OC occurs more commonly in the third trimester
- The incidence is doubled in the South-Asian population

Pathophysiology
OC is a multifactorial condition (genetic, endocrine, and environmental factors are involved). Women with OC may have an increased sensitivity to the cholestatic effect of oestrogens. It is more likely if there is a personal or family history of OC (mother, sisters).

Clinical evaluation
History
- Typically, there is generalized pruritus, including the palms and soles without a rash, but women can present with pruritus of the abdomen only. The itching is worse at night and disturbs sleep
- Dark urine, pale stools, and jaundice are uncommon
- Ask specifically about a previously affected pregnancy, rashes, symptoms of pre-eclampsia, recent foreign travel, viral illness, personal and family history of liver disorders and gallstones, drug history (including over-the-counter medicines), and alcohol use

Examination
No rash but excoriation and permanent scars can be present when pruritus is severe.

Investigations
LFTs
- Normal pregnancy values are 20% lower than non-pregnant
- Alanine aminotransferase (ALT), aspartate aminotransferase (AST), gamma-glutamyl transferase (GGT) and bilirubin. Transaminases are commonly raised in OC, typically 30–200 u/l
- Bilirubin is rarely raised.
- Alkaline phosphatase is normally raised in the third trimester owing to a placental isoenzyme

Bile acids
- The most useful test in the diagnosis of OC, though results can take up to 10 days. Normal levels do not exclude the diagnosis
- Levels are not predictive of fetal risk

In the event of abnormal LFTs or bile acids, a number of investigations are undertaken to exclude other diagnoses:
- BP and urinalysis to rule out pre-eclampsia
- Viral hepatitis screen (hepatitis A, B, C, cytomegalovirus (CMV) and Epstein–Barr virus (EBV))
- Autoimmune hepatitis screen (antimitochondrial antibodies for primary biliary cirrhosis, anti-smooth muscle antibodies for chronic active hepatitis)
- A liver US scan

If all normal, then OC should be considered.

If pruritus persists despite normal LFTs and bile acids, repeat tests every 1–2 weeks. Pruritus can precede abnormal biochemistry by several weeks.

Management
Antenatally
Once OC is diagnosed, LFTs should be checked weekly (**C**). If levels return to normal, then OC is unlikely. Check clotting if high levels of transaminases as there may be hepatic impairment.

There is no evidence that any specific treatment for OC improves symptoms or neonatal outcome.

Topical emollients
Examples are calamine lotion and aqueous cream with menthol. These are safe and may provide relief from pruritus.

Antihistamines
Chlorpheniramine may help with pruritus and provides night sedation.

Ursodeoxycholic acid
Ursodeoxycholic acid (UDCA) is most commonly prescribed for the relief of pruritus in OC, though unlicensed for this use. Not found to be unsafe.

There is insufficient data to support the widespread use of UDCA outside clinical trials. Women should be aware of the lack of robust data concerning improvement of OC, protection against stillbirth, and safety to the fetus (**A**).

Dexamethasone
Results of improvement of symptoms and biochemistry are conflicting. Not recommended outside of randomized controlled trials (**B**).
Concerns exist regarding safety of repeated doses of steroids (adverse fetal and neonatal effects).

Vitamin K
Women should be offered oral vitamin K (10 mg OD) from diagnosis to reduce risk of postpartum haemorrhage (PPH), and fetal or neonatal bleeding (**C**).

Reduced fat absorption with OC may lead to vitamin K deficiency and subsequently low levels of vitamin K-dependent clotting factors (II, VII, IX, and X), more likely in the presence of steatorrhoea.

Fetal monitoring
No specific fetal monitoring modality predicts fetal death (**C**). Some mothers may feel reassured by intermittent CTG monitoring during pregnancy, although unable to predict future fetal wellbeing.

US is not reliable in predicting intrauterine death (IUD) in OC (**B**) as there is usually no evidence of placental insufficiency.

The importance of maternal monitoring of fetal movements should be explained, and women advised to attend for fetal assessment if any concerns arise.

Decision to deliver
OC is associated with increased rates of spontaneous and iatrogenic prematurity, fetal distress, and IUD. There is no correlation between degree of biochemical abnormality and risk of IUD. Thus the decision to deliver should not be based on these values (**B**) unless there are maternal health concerns.

The decision to deliver is based on the diagnosis and gestation.

Delivery at 37–38 weeks is commonly advised owing to the risk of stillbirth. Death is usually sudden and thought to be due to acute anoxia. One study found a 7% risk of IUD in women with OC with a median gestation of 38 weeks amongst singleton pregnancies. With active management of 70 women with OC, no IUDs were reported (alternate day CTG, weekly US, and induction of labour (IOL) at 37–38 weeks).

The RCOG guideline states that there are insufficient data to support or refute the popular practice of IOL at 37 weeks to reduce the risk of late stillbirth (**B**).

The main concerns with IOL at 37–38 weeks are of fetal respiratory morbidity (respiratory distress syndrome, transient tachypnoea of the newborn and ventilation) and failed IOL leading to CS.

- Premature delivery rates are reported to be between 17 and 38% with 22–67% iatrogenic
- Admission rates to SCBU/NICU range between 14 and 41%
- In one study of the 14% admissions to SCBU, 40% (4) required ventilation

A full antenatal discussion regarding the benefits of induction at 37–38 weeks should take place, explaining the risks of early delivery. Many women may find these risks more acceptable than the risk of IUD if not delivered by 38 weeks' gestation.

Difficulty arises when pruritus and abnormal LFTs are found after 37 weeks' gestation and bile acid results are not available (can take 10 days to get a result). Every effort should be made to exclude other causes of raised LFTs. If it is felt that OC is the cause and bile acid results are not available, then the woman should be offered IOL after discussion of the risks and benefits.

Postpartum

- Active management of third stage as increased risk of PPH
- Diagnosis of OC is confirmed with resolution of pruritus and LFTs to normal postpartum. As LFTs can increase postpartum, they should be checked after 10 days (**C**)
- If not resolved within 3 months, then other causes for abnormal LFTs should be sought, including tests for autoimmune hepatitis
- Postnatal review of blood should take place and women should be advised:
  - OC causes no long-term sequelae for mother or fetus
  - Ninety per cent recurrence rate in future pregnancies

- Female family members may be at increased risk (including daughters)
- Avoid oestrogen-containing contraceptives owing to the risk of pruritus and abnormal LFTs

A patient information leaflet can be obtained from www.britishliver-trust.org.uk

References

www.rcog.org.uk Green top guidelines. Obstetric cholestasis. Guideline No. 43. London, 2006.

Burrows RF, Clavisi O, Burrows E. Interventions for treating cholestasis in pregnancy. *Cochrane Database of Systematic Reviews* 2001; **4:** CD000493.

> **Box 8.15 Differential diagnosis of pruritus (with or without abnormal LFTs) in pregnancy**
>
> Skin-related:
> (See also Section 8.23)
> - Atopic dermatitis or eczema
> - Psoriasis
> - Pruritic eruption of pregnancy (PEP)
> - Herpes (pemphigoid) gestationis
>
> Others:
> - Pre-eclampsia
> - Acute fatty liver
> - Viral hepatitis (hepatitis A, B, C, EBV, CMV)
> - Gallstones
> - Drugs (e.g. methyldopa, antibiotics)
> - Alcohol
> - Recent viral illness

Physiological skin changes

The placenta produces a melanocyte-stimulating hormone that increases skin pigmentation. Melasma (mask of pregnancy), also known as chloasma, is a blotchy, brownish benign hyperpigmentation of the sun-exposed skin of the face. This results in symmetrical patches which commonly occur over the forehead, cheek bones, and upper lip (see Figure 8.11).

Stretch marks occur in the presence of high oestrogen levels on the abdomen, breast, and thighs. Thin-walled, dilated capillaries (especially in the lower legs) also increase. There is no effective prevention or treatment.

Normal pregnancy increases the amount of hair in the growth phase.

Skin disorders of pregnancy

If the rash is associated with itching, then one of the four pregnancy-associated dermatoses should be considered:

- Polymorphic eruption of pregnancy (see Figure 8.12)
- Prurigo of pregnancy
- Pruritic folliculitis
- Pemphigoid gestationis (see Figures 8.13 and 8.14)

The first three of these conditions are benign, but pemphigoid gestationis (also known as herpes gestationis) has an increased association with fetal growth retardation and fetal abnormality. It also has a high risk (>90%) of recurrence in subsequent pregnancies. See Table 8.1 for details.

Further reading

Burns T, Breathnach S, Cox N, Griffiths C, Subepidermal immunobullous disease, *Rook's Textbook of Dermatology*, Vol. 2, 7th edn. Blackwell Publishing, Oxford, 2004, 40–1.

Burns T, Breathnach S, Cox N, Griffiths C, Pregnancy, childbirth and the puerperium, *Rook's Textbook of Dermatology*, Vol. 4, 7th edn. Blackwell Publishing, Oxford, 2004, 15–70.

238

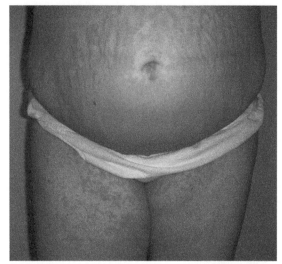

Fig. 8.12 Polymorphic eruption of pregnancy. Note the umbilical sparing.

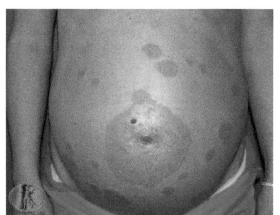

Fig. 8.13 Pemphigoid gestationis. (Courtesy of DermNetNZ.org.)

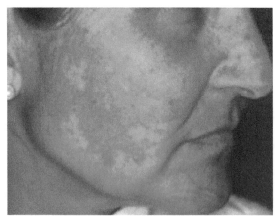

Fig. 8.11 Melasma. (Courtesy of DermNetNZ.org.)

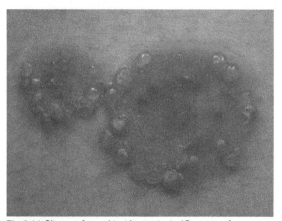

Fig. 8.14 Blisters of pemphigoid gestationis. (Courtesy of DermNetNZ.org.)

	Polymorphic eruption of pregnancy (PEP) or pruritic urticarial papules and plaques in pregnancy (PUPPP)	Pemphigoid gestationis (PG)	Prurigo of pregnancy	Pruritic folliculitis of pregnancy
Incidence	1:200 pregnancies	1 :10–50 000 pregnancies Commoner in whites than blacks	1:300 preguansies	1:3000 pregnancies
Pathophysiology	Unknown No hormonal abnormality Possibly occurs owing to stretching of the skin Associated with increased birth weight, greater maternal weight gain, primigravida, and multiple pregnancies	Pregnancy-specific autoimmune disease Associated with bullous pemphigoid, insulin-dependent diabetes, Graves', pernicious anaemia, vitiligo, rheumatoid arthritis Strong association HLA-DR3 and HLA-DR4	Associated with atopy	Unknown. Possibly hormone-induced acne
Onset	Third trimester	Abrupt onset anytime, usually second and third trimester	Second and third trimester	Second and third trimester
Eruption	Severe pruritis, urticarial papules and plaques, rarely vesicles (but not bullae) and target lesions	Intensely pruritic, urticarial erythematous papules and plaques; target lesions, annular wheals after 2 weeks vesicles and large tense bullae may form, secondary skin infection may occur	Pruritic groups of red or brown excoriated papules	Acneiform eruption consisting of multiple, pruritic, 2–4-mm follicular papules or pustules
Distribution	Abdomen (typically sparing the umbilical area), along striae, spreading to thighs, buttocks, under the breasts and upper arms	Periumbilical, spreading peripherally to limbs, palms, soles	Abdomen, extensor surface of limbs	Widespread, mainly on the shoulders, upper back, arms, chest, and abdomen
Resolution	Self-resolves after delivery	May improve at the end of pregnancy, but flares can occur postpartum Occasionally persists for several months postpartum. In a few it may develop into bullous pemphigoid May recur in subsequent pregnancies or use of combined oral contraception	Pruritis improves after delivery but papules may persist for several months postpartum May recur in subsequent pregnancies	Self-resolves within 2 weeks postpartum
Fetal effects	None	Low birth weight, preterm birth, stillbirth Similar transient bullous eruption in 10% of babies	None	None
Diagnosis	Usually clinical. A negative immunofluorescence test distinguishes PEP from PG	Skin biopsy and direct immunofluorescence test shows C3 deposition at the basement membrane zone	Clinical	Clinical
Management	Reassure Resolves by delivery Discuss risks versus benefits of treatment Cool soothing baths, emollients, 1% menthol in aqueous cream. Topical steroids 1% hydrocortisone, stronger Betnovate if required Sedative antihistamines Severe cases require systemic corticosteroids	Cool soothing baths, emollients. Potent topical corticosteroids 0.1% mometasone furoate or very potent 0.05% clobetasol propionate Most require systemic steroids prednisolone 40 mg/day Some require topical or systemic immunosuppression with azathioprine or ciclosporin Sedative antihistamine chlorpheniramine 4 mg TDS or QDS or promethazine 25 mg *nocte*	Topical steroids 1% hydrocortisone Antihistamines if required	Topical 10% benzoyl peroxide Topical steroids 1% hydrocortisone Antihistamines if required

Table 8.1 Pregnancy-specific dermatoses

8.24 Infections in pregnancy—varicella zoster and cytomegalovirus

Introduction

Acute viral infections in pregnancy tend to produce few symptoms in the mother. However, these viruses can cause severe congenital infections in the fetus with associated risks of miscarriage, fetal growth retardation (FGR), non-immune hydrops, intracranial calcifications, microcephaly, and intrauterine death (IUD). Treatment options for viral infections are limited and therefore minimizing the risk of transmission is essential. Bacterial and parasitic infections also cause significant perinatal morbidity and mortality, and it is important that prompt diagnosis is made so that the appropriate treatment can be started.

See Sections 6.6 and 6.7 for rubella, HIV, hepatitis B, syphilis and group B streptococcus infections in pregnancy. See Sections 3.2 and 3.3 for *Chlamydia trachomatis*, *Neisseria gonorrhoeae*, *Trichomonas vaginalis*, and *Candida* (thrush) in pregnancy.

Varicella zoster and chickenpox

Incidence

The incidence of varicella zoster (VZV) is 3:1000 pregnancies; 90% women are immune.

Transmission

Highly contagious DNA virus of the herpes family transmitted via respiratory droplets, direct contact of vesicle fluid, or airborne spread.

Incubation

Incubation is 10–21 days. Infectious from 48 h before rash appears until the vesicles crust over. VZV IgM increases 3 days after onset of symptoms and VZV IgG increases after a further 4 days.

Clinical evaluation

History
- Prodromal symptoms of fever, malaise, and myalgia
- Rash

Examination
Pruritic rash that becomes maculopapular, then vesicular, and finally crusts over

Investigations
Diagnosed clinically on the characteristic exanthema

Management of chickenpox
- The woman should attend her GP surgery and not labour ward or antenatal clinic owing to the risk of transmitting infection to other pregnant women
- Oral aciclovir reduces the duration of fever and symptoms of varicella when given within 24 h of the rash appearing (avoid first trimester) (C)
- Women with severe infection (pneumonia, neurological symptoms, haemorrhagic or dense rash, bleeding or significant immunosuppression) or risk factors for pneumonia (smokers, chronic lung disease, steroid use or in the latter half of pregnancy) should be assessed in hospital (C). IV aciclovir may be necessary

Contact with VZV
- After the contact with chickenpox, a detailed history of the significance of the contact and the susceptibility of the patient needs to take place (C)
- If unsure of previous VZV infection, check VZV IgG. If positive, no further action is needed
- If susceptible to VZV and significant contact with a person who is infectious (household, face-to-face for 5 min or indoors contact for 15 min), varicella zoster immunoglobulin (VZIG) can be given. VZIG is most effective when given within 72 h but may still have benefits up to 10 days (C). VZIG diminishes the severity of the disease but not the risk of fetal varicella syndrome (FVS; see below)

Maternal risks

Adults have an increased risk of pneumonia, hepatitis, and encephalitis compared with children. Disease is more severe in pregnancy, i.e. 10% risk of pneumonia among pregnant women, with higher mortality than non-pregnant subjects. With antiviral treatment, maternal mortality <1%.

Fetal risks

Before 20 weeks: 2% risk of FVS. FVS is characterized by skin scarring in a dermatomal distribution, eye defects (microphthalmia, chorioretinitis, and cataracts), hypoplasia of the limbs and neurological abnormalities (microcephaly, cortical atrophy, and mental retardation).

Offer a detailed US at 16–20 weeks or 5 weeks after infection to detect abnormalities. Presence of VZV in amniotic fluid is not predictive of FVS.

After 20 weeks: between 20 and 36 weeks, maternal VZV is not associated with adverse fetal outcome. Shingles may occur in first few years of life.

Varicella infection of the newborn occurs with maternal infection near delivery (within 4 weeks of delivery). Up to 48% of neonates will develop clinical varicella.

Major risk is for the fetus born between 2 days before, and 5 days after maternal chickenpox has developed. The neonate has no immunity and so has a greater risk of disseminated disease and death. VZIG should be given to the fetus in these circumstances as it reduces mortality (C).

Neonate
- If the baby has contact with VZV during first week of life and the mother is immune then no further action required
- If mother is non-immune, then administer VZIG
- If the baby develops varicella, treat with aciclovir

Shingles

Shingles is the reactivation of VZV which remains dormant in sensory nerve root ganglia. It causes a vesicular erythematous skin rash in a dermatomal distribution. If immunocompetent, then viraemia is uncommon with no risk to the fetus.

Shingles is unlikely to cause chickenpox in someone susceptible unless disseminated shingles or exposed lesions.

Cytomegalovirus

Incidence

Cytomegalovirus (CMV) is the most common cause of congenital infection and non-hereditary deafness. Between 1 and 2% primary infection in pregnancy; 50–80% of women are seropositive.

Transmission

DNA virus of herpes family transmitted in saliva, urine, and genital secretions as well as via blood products. Transmission to fetus is transplacental and via direct contact from birth canal.

Incubation

Thought to be between 3 and 12 weeks. IgM present 4–8 weeks after self-limiting primary infection. The virus then becomes latent, with subsequent reactivation during mild immunosuppression (e.g. pregnancy and infections).

Clinical evaluation

History
- Primary infection is mainly asymptomatic but there may be fever and malaise
- Reactivation is asymptomatic

Examination
- Lymphadenopathy

Investigations
- Atypical lymphocytosis on FBC
- Viral culture with direct immunofluorescence from urine or blood
- Individuals previously infected with CMV can excrete the virus intermittently in urine, saliva, tears, cervical secretions, and breast milk for months, therefore take care when interpreting culture results
- Anti-CMV IgM and IgG: IgM levels remain raised for 4–8 months after primary infection. IgG titres increase with recurrent infection.
- Request additional antibody screen on saved booking blood serum to compare the presence and type of antibodies

Management
- No treatment
- Immunocompromised women may have some improvement in symptoms with antivirals

Maternal risks
- Rarely pnemonitis, hepatitis, meningitis, encephalitis, thrombocytopenia, Guillain–Barré, and myocarditis
- Reinfection and reactivation common

Fetal risks
- After primary maternal infection 40% of fetuses will be infected
- CMV is found in 1% of all newborns
- Of babies born to women with CMV in pregnancy 85% will have no CMV-related problems (including 75% of infected infants)

Congenital infection is three times more likely to occur with primary infection, particularly with advanced gestation (increased viral shedding from cervix with increased gestation).

Between 10 and 15% of infected neonates will be symptomatic at birth and have one or more features of congenital infection (hepatosplenomegaly, microcephaly, hyperbilirubinaemia, petechiae, thrombocytopenia, and fetal growth retardation (FGR)). Between 20 and 30% of these babies will die.

Between 5 and 15% of asymptomatic infected neonates will develop long-term problems (sensorineural deafness, microcephaly, low IQ, and seizures).

Owing to intermittent viral shedding, a fetus may be affected despite maternal antibodies. However, complications with maternal recurrent CMV are much lower. In one study of children with congenital infection, 25% had sequelae following primary infection compared with 8% with recurrent infection.

Offer counselling to the mother regarding the risks of congenital CMV. Owing to the significant risks associated with congenital infection, some women will decide on termination. If the pregnancy proceeds, culture of the amniotic fluid (6 weeks after infection) for CMV can help guide management. Serial US scans should be performed to monitor growth, structural abnormalities, and the development of non-immune hydrops.

Women who need transfusion during the antenatal period should receive CMV-negative blood.

Further reading

Royal College of Obstetricians and Gynaecologists Greentop guidelines. Chickenpox in pregnancy. Guideline No.13. London: RCOG Press, 2007.

Herpes simplex virus

See also Section 3.5.

Incidence

- There is <1% seroconversion during pregnancy
- It may be difficult to distinguish primary and recurrence

Antenatal management

Women without a history of herpes simplex virus (HSV) should be advised to avoid sexual intercourse if their partner has active oral or genital herpes. Asymptomatic viral shedding can still occur, posing a risk of primary infection in the absence of lesions (**C, IV**). Consider condom use during asymptomatic intervals to reduce risk of infection, particularly in the third trimester. Antenatal serum screening is not indicated.

Women with a previous history of genital herpes can be reassured that if a recurrent attack develops, the risk of transmission to the fetus is low (0–3%). This should be weighed against the risks to the mother of a CS. Prophylaxis of HSV is sometimes considered at the end of pregnancy in women with very frequent attacks.

Women with primary HSV infection should be referred to a genitourinary physician. Aciclovir is well tolerated in late pregnancy and there is no evidence of maternal or fetal toxicity. A 5-day oral course should be given to those with a first episode to reduce the duration, severity, and decrease the duration of viral shedding (RCOG: Good Practice Point).

- In more severe infections, IV aciclovir may be required
- In case of difficulty in voiding due to pain, passing urine in the bath and the use of topical local anaesthetic gel may help
- If in urinary retention, then catheterize
- Daily suppressive aciclovir in the last 4 weeks of pregnancy may prevent recurrences at term
- Culture and diagnostic tests to predict viral shedding in late pregnancy are not indicated

Delivery

Neonatal infection is caused by contact with infected maternal secretions at delivery or from close contact with an infected individual. Risk of neonatal herpes (see below) with primary HSV genital infection at the time of delivery is about 40% with a vaginal birth.

Any woman who presents in labour with first-episode genital herpes lesions should be offered lower segment CS (LSCS) (**B**). If the woman presents with ruptured membranes <4 h with a first episode of genital HSV, CS has been shown to reduce the neonatal infection rate.

If the duration is longer, there may be no added benefit as the risk of infection increases once membranes have been ruptured for >4 h.

The risks are greatest with primary infection late in the pregnancy as the baby is delivered before development of protective maternal antibodies. Viral shedding can continue for 6 weeks following a primary episode.

Therefore, elective CS should be considered for women who present with first-episode genital herpes within 6 weeks of estimated date of delivery (EDD) or premature rupture of membranes (ROM) or labour. It is not indicated if the first episode was in the first or second trimester.

For women who opt for vaginal birth who have had a first episode of genital herpes within the last 6 weeks, IV aciclovir intrapartum to the mother and postnatally to the neonate may reduce the risk of neonatal herpes. Invasive procedures should be avoided (fetal blood sampling, fetal scalp electrode and instrumental delivery) (**C**).

For women presenting with recurrent genital herpes at the onset of labour, the risk of transmission to the neonate is very low (<3%) and should be set against the risks of CS (**B**). However, some women may feel that the small (but significant) risk of having a baby with neonatal herpes outweighs the risk of CS.

Recurrent genital herpes at any other time in pregnancy is not an indication for CS (**B**).

Postnatal management

- The paediatric team should be informed
- Close observation of the neonate
- Avoid direct contact between orolabial lesions and the neonate

Maternal risks

- Urinary retention
- Aseptic meningitis, encephalitis, and hepatitis if severe infection or immunocompromised
- Miscarriage and preterm labour with systemic disease

Neonatal risks

Not all infants exposed to HSV at birth become infected. In most cases, neonatal infection occurs from direct contact with infected maternal secretions. The incidence in the UK is 1.65 per 100 000 live births. Both HSV-1 and -2 can cause neonatal infection. It can affect the neonate in localized or disseminated forms.

Local infection can be:

- Meningoencephalitis
- Conjunctivitis, chorioretinitis, and keratitis
- Skin—vesicular lesions
- Lesions in the oral cavity, gingivostomatitis and involving the larynx

These can progress to disseminated infection.

Disseminated neonatal herpes is rare but is associated with a high morbidity (seizures, mental retardation) and mortality (70–80%). It can develop at birth or as late as 21 days afterwards. Organs affected include brain, trachea, lungs, oesophagus, stomach, kidneys, spleen, pancreas, heart, and bone marrow. It has a high morbidity and mortality.

Parvovirus B19

Incidence

- Also know as Fifth disease, erythema infectiosum or 'slapped cheek' syndrome
- About 1:400 pregnancies
- Infection peaks in late spring and early summer with periods of increased activity every 3–4 years.
- Between 50-60% women are immune to parvovirus B19

Transmission

DNA virus transmitted via respiratory droplets. Transplacental transmission to fetus.

Incubation

Incubation is 4–14 days. Parvovirus B19 viraemia occurs 6–8 days after exposure and lasts a week. The rash develops by day 16, after which the host is no longer infectious. IgM is raised within 10 days of exposure and remains high for >3 months. IgG is detected several days after IgM, and can be raised for life.

Clinical evaluation

History

- Fever, malaise, and arthralgia
- Rash

- Mild anaemia
- Twenty per cent of infections in adults are asymptomatic

Examination
- Lymphadenopathy
- Facial rash (slapped cheek) and reticulate lace-like rash on trunk and extremities in Fifth disease (common in children)

Investigations
- Serum IgM and IgG

Management
- If IgM-negative and IgG-positive, then reassure
- If IgM-positive, then acute infection

Maternal risks
- Aplastic crisis in women with sickle cell disease and other hereditary anaemias
- Chronic anaemia in severely immuno-compromised individuals
- Reversible pre-eclampsia owing to hydropic placenta (or 'mirror syndrome', where maternal water retention reflects fetal hydrops)

Fetal risks
- Parvovirus B19 is not teratogenic
- Of women infected with parvovirus B19 during pregnancy, 86% will have a normal outcome
- Parvovirus B19 is transmitted to the fetus in a third of cases
- The overall fetal loss from acute parvovirus B19 infection has been reported to be 6–12%
- The excess rate of fetal loss occurs in women infected in the first 20 weeks and is 9–11%
- Risk of fetal loss from acute infection >20 weeks' gestation is <1%
- Parvovirus B19 preferentially infects rapidly dividing cells, causing haemolytic anaemia and haemopoietic arrest
- This leads to high output cardiac failure and non-immune hydrops (ascites, pericardial and pleural effusions; see Figure 8.15)
- Risk of hydrops is 0.3–3%
- Hydrops usually develops 7–14 days after acute infection although it can develop after 8 weeks

- Serial US should be performed to assess for hydrops with subsequent referral to a tertiary fetal medicine centre if identified
- No evidence of long-term effects or congenital syndrome postnatally.

Conservative management can be considered as hydrops can resolve spontaneously. However, there is no way to predict which cases will resolve. Other options include delivery and transfusion if fetus is at an appropriate gestational age or fetal blood sampling to confirm anaemia with subsequent intrauterine blood transfusion. A large proportion (84%) of fetuses with severe hydrops will survive with intrauterine blood transfusions.

Further reading
www.rcog.org.uk RCOG Greentop guideline No. 30. Management of genital herpes in pregnancy. London: RCOG Press, 2007.

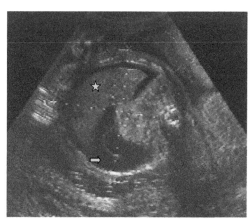

Fig. 8.15 Hydrops fetalis manifested as ascites (⇨). Liver (☆).

8.26 Infections in pregnancy—toxoplasma and listeria

Toxoplasma

Primary infection can cause severe neonatal problems. However, treatment options are available.

Incidence
- The incidence is thought to be 2:1000 pregnancies

Transmission
The parasite *Toxoplasma gondii* can be transmitted to humans from uncooked meat (especially pork, mutton, and wild game) and inadvertent ingestion of oocytes that are present in cat faeces (cat litter, soil, unwashed fruit, and vegetables). Transplacental transmission occurs during primary infection.

Incubation
- Up to 23 days
- IgM and IgG antibodies appear within 1–2 weeks of infection

Clinical evaluation
History
- 90% asymptomatic
- Glandular fever-like illness

Examination
Lymphadenopathy

Investigations
- IgM and IgG antibodies
- IgG antibodies peak within 1–2 months of infection, then decline but usually persist for life. IgM antibodies decline more rapidly
- Request additional antibody screen on saved serum from booking bloods to compare presence of antibodies

Infection if IgM-positive, IgG-negative then positive or a greater than 4-fold rise in IgG in two samples more than 3 weeks apart.

False-positive IgM with rheumatoid factor or antinuclear antibodies.

Management
- If a woman is found to have an acute infection with toxoplasmosis, then treatment should commence (spiramycin) to reduce the risk of transmission to her baby
- If acute infection is confirmed, amniocentesis can be performed to assess for fetal infection (PCR)
- If positive, perform US to look for structural abnormalities, namely microcephaly or hydrocephaly, intracerebral calcification, and hydrops fetalis
- Discussions with the mother should take place regarding the high risk of infection in the presence of structural abnormalities
- Termination can be offered if appropriate
- Alternatively, treatment with pyrimethamine, sulfadiazine and folinic acid alternating with spiramycin can be started, although there is a potential risk of teratogenicity and bone marrow toxicity to mother and fetus
- Serial US scans should be performed to monitor for fetal growth retardation (FGR), ventricular dilatation, and microcephaly
- Prevention is better than treatment
- Women should be advised to avoid undercooked or raw meat, unpasteurized milk, wash fruit and vegetables, wear gloves when gardening, and avoid contact with cat faeces.

Maternal risks
- Severe disseminated disease, chorioretinitis, and encephalitis in immunocompromised individuals

Fetal risks
- Toxoplasmosis prior to pregnancy makes congenital infection very unlikely

- Congenital infection can cause chorioretinitis, microcephaly, hydrocephaly, intracerebral calcification, and mental retardation
- Risk of transmission is highest in the third trimester (65%)
- The disease is more severe if transmission is in the first trimester (17% transmission). Spontaneous miscarriage often ocurrs with first trimester infection
- Seventy per cent of babies are born with no problems and 10% with chorioretinitis
- Perinatal death or disseminated disease in 1–2%

Toxoplasmosis is not routinely screened for in the UK (as opposed to France where there is a higher incidence of toxoplasmosis infection).

A Cochrane review on the effectiveness and safety of treatment in reducing congenital toxoplasmosis in acute infection failed to find any randomized controlled trials. Screening programmes should not be introduced until further evidence is available.

Listeria

Incidence
- Listeriosis affects 1:10 000 pregnant women

Transmission
Listeria monocytogenes is a Gram-positive bacillus transmitted in contaminated foods (soft cheese, milk products, and processed meats). Transmission to the fetus is thought to be transplacental and via ascending infection.

Incubation
- Incubation is 11–70 days

Clinical evaluation
History
- Flu-like illness, fever, and general malaise
- One-third are asymptomatic

Investigations
- Blood, vaginal, and cervical cultures
- Placental culture postpartum

Management
- Listeriosis responds to antibiotics, including ampicillin
- Treament should continue for 10–14 days

Maternal risks
- Cell-mediated immunity is primary host defence against Listeria, therefore increased risk of infection in pregnancy
- Rarely septicaemia, meningitis, and encephalitis

Fetal risks
- Early pregnancy infection often results in miscarriage
- Fetal infection can cause amnionitis with brown staining of liquor (often thought to be meconium), preterm labour, and early and late onset listeriosis
- In one study of women with listeriosis, the risk of intrauterine death was 19%. Fifty-four per cent of neonates developed early onset infection (<2 days) and 23% developed infection after 2 days
- The overall mortality rate from listeriosis was 50%
- Early onset infection occurs because of transplacental spread and results in congenital pneumonia. Late-onset infection tends to present with meningitis

8.27 Malpresentation

The presenting part of the fetus is the part which is lowest in the uterus. In most cases this is the head (cephalic presentation). Breech presentation, transverse, oblique, and unstable lie can all occur at term and are associated with specific risks (see also Sections 9.10 and 9.11 for labour management).

Breech presentation

Definition
A breech presentation is the *in utero* fetal position that leads to the feet or buttocks being delivered first.

Incidence
The incidence decreases with increasing gestational age.

Before 28 weeks, 20–30% of fetuses present as breech but most undergo spontaneous version so the incidence falls to 3% at term (>37 weeks). Four per cent of all deliveries (including preterm) are breech and up to 40% are undiagnosed before labour.

The breech position confers at least a 2-fold increase in perinatal mortality compared to a normal (cephalic) presentation. It is unclear whether this is due to the mode of delivery or confounding factors such as an underlying fetal abnormality. In the 7th Confidential Enquiry into Sudden Unexpected Deaths in Infancy (CESDI), 75% of deaths with breech presentation occurred after late recognition or delay in management of hypoxia.

Classification
There are three types of breech (see Figure 8.16).
- Frank (extended) 65%. Both legs flexed at hip and extended at the knee. Lowest risk of feto-pelvis disproportion and cord prolapse
- Complete (flexed) 10%. Both legs flexed at hip and knee
- Incomplete (footling) 25%. One or both legs extended at the hip

Risk factors See Box 8.16.

Prevention
- Postural management: adopting different positions such as the knee–chest, or supine with the pelvis elevated, has not been shown to change outcome
- Women may use moxibustion (burning herbs close to skin acupuncture point). Needs to be evaluated with a trial

Clinical evaluation

History
- Exaggerated subcostal discomfort or 'lump' under the ribs
- Fetal movements felt predominantly in lower part of uterus

Examination
- Ballotable round head at fundus and soft presenting part in the lower uterine pole
- Fetal heart sounds auscultated more commonly above umbilicus
- Often mistaken as 'deeply engaged head' at term
- Meconium seen in labour
- If in labour and cervix dilated, fetal sacrum and ischial tuberosities are aligned (versus face presentation where mentum and molar eminences form a triangle)

Investigations
- US: confirms fetal position and type of breech. Can detect fetal anomalies, fetal growth retardation (FGR) or liquor abnormalities

Fifteen per cent of breech presentations are not detected until 38 weeks' gestation and a further 21% are first detected in labour.

Antenatal management
- External cephalic version (ECV)
- Discuss vaginal breech delivery (VB) (see Section 9.11)
- Discuss CS (see Sections 9.11 and 9.14)
- There is no role for pelvimetry

246

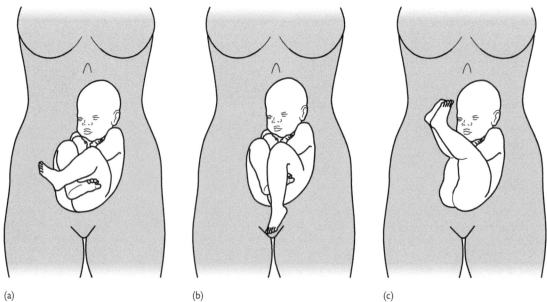

(a)   (b)   (c)

Fig. 8.16 Types of breech. (a) Complete (flexed); (b) incomplete (footling); (c) frank (extended). (Kindly provided by Miss Angel Kumar.)

Breech delivery
See Section 9.11

Transverse, oblique, and unstable lie

Definitions
- *Transverse lie:* the body lies transversely in the uterus
- *Oblique lie:* the head or breech is in one iliac fossa
- *Unstable lie:* the fetal lie and presentation continually change (longitudinal, transverse, oblique) >37 weeks' gestation

Risk factors
See Box 8.16.

Clinical evaluation
History
- Constantly feeling the baby turn
- Non-longitudinal lie diagnosed on routine antenatal examination or incidentally on US

Examination
- Transverse lie: the uterus may look wider than expected. Fetal poles felt laterally, and nothing palpated above or in the pelvis
- Oblique lie: fetal pole felt in the left or right iliac fossa with nothing above or in the pelvis. If a full bladder is suspected, voiding will often resolve the situation
- Unstable lie: different recorded positions in the last weeks of pregnancy

Investigations
- US to confirm the lie and identify cause (e.g. placenta praevia, ovarian cyst, polyhydramnios, fetal abnormality)

Antenatal management
- Most abnormal lies will stabilize in a longitudinal position
- Expectant management is reasonable
- Identify any causes of abnormal lie (e.g. placenta praevia) as this will influence management and delivery
- With abnormal presentations, limbs, cord, shoulder or back can be presenting, increasing the risk of cord presentation, cord prolapse, and compound presentation
- Some advocate inpatient management after 37–38 weeks while awaiting labour, particularly if the woman lives far from the hospital. If at any point a cord prolapse occurs, appropriate management is available immediately

- Risk of cord prolapse is probably higher for multiparous women as the internal os can be dilated 2–3 cm prior to labour
- Separation from family can have a huge psychological impact. The risks and benefits of inpatient management should be discussed before a decision is made
- If the baby spontaneously settles in a cephalic presentation for 48 h and maintains this, the woman can be discharged
- If spontaneous version does not occur, ECV can be tried. If successful and maintained, the woman can be discharged

Delivery
See shoulder presentation in Section 9.10.

Further reading

www.rcog.org.uk Guideline No. 20b. The management of breech presentation, 2006.

➕ Box 8.16 Risk factors for breech presentation

Decreased uterine polarity
- Grand multiparity
- Malformations (bicornuate, septate uterus)

Altered fetal mobility
- Prematurity
- FGR
- Macrosomia
- Polyhydramnios, oligohydramnios
- Multiple gestation
- Fetal abnormality (e.g. hydro- or anencephaly, cystic hygromas)
- Myotonic dystrophy, trisomies, Prader–Willi syndrome
- Very short umbilical cord

Pelvic block
- Pelvic shape
- Pelvic tumours
- Fibroids
- Placenta praevia

External cephalic version (ECV)

ECV involves applying gentle pressure to the maternal abdomen to turn the fetus in either a forward or a backward somersault to achieve a vertex presentation (see Figure 8.17).

This increases the chance of a non-breech presentation at delivery and reduces both the risks of VB and the chance of CS (**A**).

With a trained operator, the success rate is 35–50% in nulliparous and 50–80% in parous women (**B**). Tocolysis is effective (e.g. β_2-agonists such as terbutaline 250 μg SC or nifedipine 10–20 mg PO) and can increase the success rate. Regional anaesthesia may be helpful but needs further evaluation (**A**).

ECV should be offered from 36 weeks in nulliparous women and from 37 weeks in multiparous women (**B**).

Prerequisites are CTG monitoring (reassuring), a US machine (to check the presentation), and facilities for emergency CS in the rare case of bradycardia with cord entanglement (<1:200).

After successful ECV, spontaneous reversion to breech can occur, so confirm presentation when women present in labour.

Success rates for ECV are higher if:

- Multiparous
- Unengaged breech
- Extended or footling breech

Risks of ECV

- Low complication rate (**B**)
- Cord accident (especially if membranes ruptured), abruption (<1%), prolonged fetal bradycardia and emergency CS (0.4–4%)
- The most common side effect (20–35%) is transient tachycardia that spontaneously resolves
- Pain—stop procedure if not tolerated
- Feto-maternal haemorrhage. All Rh-negative women require prophylactic anti-D

Contraindications to ECV

See Box 8.17.

Further reading

www.rcog.org.uk RCOG Guideline No. 20a. External cephalic version and reducing the incidence of breech presentation, 2006.

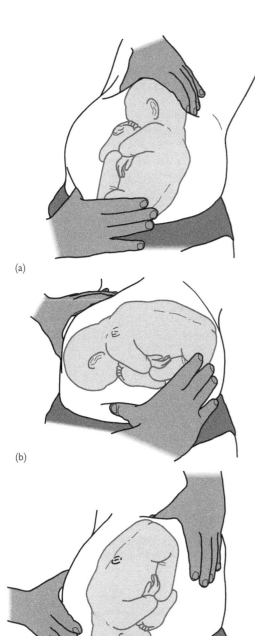

(a)

(b)

(c)

Fig. 8.17 External cephalic version. (Drawing kindly provided by Miss Mimi Kumar.)

8.29 Multiple pregnancy—maternal and pregnancy complications

See also Sections 6.11 and 9.17.

All adverse fetal and maternal pregnancy complications (except postmaturity) are significantly increased in multiple pregnancies versus singleton, and add a significant antenatal and neonatal workload.

Despite the increased rate of problems, the majority of twin pregnancies have a good outcome.

Maternal complications

Hyperemesis gravidarum
- High levels of hormones increase nausea and vomiting
- Women with hyperemesis should have an US to exclude a multiple pregnancy

Anaemia
- This is caused by greater haemodilution
- Iron supplements are recommended to reduce the risk of anaemia
- Folic acid 5 mg is also recommended owing to increased fetal demands of folate

Gestational diabetes
- Screening should be routinely performed because of the increased predisposition

First trimester miscarriage
- Increased risk of first trimester miscarriage (4%)
- Vanishing twin syndrome whereby one fetus dies *in utero* and is absorbed. The prognosis for the remaining twin is good
- Fetus papyraceous occurs when one twin dies at an early gestation and becomes shrunken and compressed

Pregnancy complications

Preterm rupture of membranes and labour
See Sections 8.21 and 8.18.
- Preterm delivery is the greatest cause of morbidity and mortality for multiple pregnancies
- There is an increased risk of preterm rupture of membranes (ROM) and preterm labour. The chance of spontaneous delivery at 24–32 weeks is about 1% in singletons, 5% in dichorionic (DC) and 10% in monochorionic (MC) twin pregnancies
- Mean gestation of delivery for DC twins is 37 weeks and for MC twins 36 weeks
- Cochrane reviews on bed rest and beta-mimetics do not show a reduction in the rate of preterm births

Cord prolapse (see also Section 10.5)
- Increased risk of malpresentation, polyhydramnios, and preterm ROM increases the chance of cord prolapse

Antepartum haemorrhage (see also Section 8.1)
- Owing to the larger placental surface there is an increased risk of placenta praevia and placental abruption
- Increased risk of velamentous cord insertion and vasa praevia

Polyhydramnios
- Increased liquor is seen in twin-to-twin transfusion (TTTS) and in monochorionic monoamniotic (MCMA) pregnancies (see Section 8.29)

- Increased discomfort, preterm rupture of membranes, cord prolapse, and malpresentation

Pre-eclampsia
- Pre-eclampsia is four times more prevalent in multiple pregnancies than in singleton but is comparable between MC and DC pregnancies
- There is an increased risk of pregnancy-induced hypertension and eclampsia as well
- Regular BP and urine checks are essential

Intrauterine death (IUD)
- The rate of miscarriage (death before 24 weeks) in a singleton pregnancy is 1%. The rate of fetal loss in DC twins is 2% and in MC twins is 10%
- There is an increase in antepartum stillbirth rate in multiple pregnancies. It is unclear why this occurs except in cases of TTTS (see Section 8.29)
- In twin pregnancies, the stillbirth rate is 3.5-fold and neonatal mortality 7-fold that for singleton pregnancies
- The greatest risks are for MC twins

Dichorionic twins
- Single IUD is commoner than double IUD
- Death of one fetus is associated with death or disability in the other fetus in about 5–10%, mainly due to prematurity
- Preterm labour is the main risk associated with death of one twin
- Monitor fetal growth and umbilical artery Doppler 3–4-weekly
- If there is a maternal cause for the IUD (such as severe pre-eclampsia), delivery may be required independent of the gestation
- Maternal disseminated intravascular coagulation (DIC) is rare in multiple pregnancies where one fetus dies. However, monitoring of clotting for DIC with one dead fetus is still necessary
- The risks of prematurity in the surviving twin need to be considered when planning delivery, along with the concerns and anxieties of the parents

Monochorionic twins
- Double IUD is commoner than single IUD
- The fetal loss rate is highest <24 weeks' gestation but ≥24 weeks' gestation, the perinatal loss is similar between MC and DC pregnancies (2.8% and 1.6%, respectively)
- If one fetus dies, the risk of death in the second fetus is 10–25%, with the risk of ischaemic cerebral lesions 25–45%
- Damage to the surviving twin in MC pregnancies is thought to be secondary to hypotension and exsanguination of the surviving twin into the hypotensive dead twin's fetoplacental circulation owing to the placental anastomoses. Iatrogenic preterm delivery to avoid a double IUD also contributes
- Death and cerebral damage occur soon after the death of one fetus
- A longer death-to-delivery time has been associated with better outcomes in the surviving twin, therefore this approach may be beneficial in very preterm pregnancies
- Regular US to identify cystic changes associated with fetal brain injury are needed. However, these changes can take a while before they become apparent. Fetal cerebral MRI imaging is likely to be more sensitive in detecting early brain injury.
- If severe cystic changes develop, then the parents may wish to consider termination
- The surviving twin will need close postnatal follow-up

In-depth counselling and psychological support is needed for parents when one twin dies *in utero*. Having become used to expecting two babies, it may be difficult to come to terms with now having only one. Mixed emotions of grief for the dead twin while looking forward to the birth of a surviving twin are often present. Anxiety near term can be significant and this should not be ignored when making a decision to deliver.

Cerebral palsy
- There is an 8-fold increased risk of cerebral palsy. This is associated with IUD of one fetus and intrapartum hypoxia

Delivery
See Section 9.17

Postpartum haemorrhage
(see Section 11.1)
- Increased risk of postpartum haemorrhage (PPH) due to:
  - Larger surface area of placental bed
  - Uterine overdistension prevents good uterine tone postpartum
- Ensure anaemia is corrected antenatally to reduce the risk of requiring a blood transfusion
- Encourage active management of the third stage

Postnatal depression
(see Section 11.6)
- Two babies can be very demanding, increasing the risk of postnatal depression

Maternal mortality
- Maternal mortality is twofold greater in twin pregnancies

Risks of higher order pregnancies
Risks are higher than for twin pregnancies:
- Preterm delivery–80%
- Triplets are 47 times more likely to have cerebral palsy than singleton pregnancies
- Fetal reduction, to twins, has been associated with a reduced preterm birth rate but higher miscarriage rate

Further reading
Crowther CA. Hospitalisation and bed rest for multiple pregnancy. *Cochrane Database of Systematic Reviews* 2001; **1**:CD000110.

Yamasmit W, Chaithongwongwatthana S, Tolosa JE, Limpongsanurak S, Pereira L, Lumbiganon P. Prophylactic oral betamimetics for reducing preterm birth in women with a twin pregnancy. *Cochrane Database of Systematic Reviews* 2005; **3**:CD004733.

RCOG. Multiple pregnancy study group. In: Kilby M et al. *Multiple Pregnancy*. London: RCOG press, 2006.

8.30 Multiple pregnancy—fetal risks

Fetal abnormalities

Chromosomal

Dizygotic twins

- The age-related risk of Down's syndrome for each dizygotic (DZ) twin is the same as singleton pregnancies
- The overall risk of having a pregnancy with one Down's syndrome baby is double that of a singleton

Monozygotic twins

- The age-related risk for Down's syndrome is the same as singletons, but both fetuses will be affected
- Biochemical serum screening has a low detection rate of chromosomal abnormalities in twins. Nuchal translucency (NT) is the investigation of choice
- If the NT is increased, invasive testing such as chorionic villus sampling (CVS) or amniocentesis can be offered
- Both are technically more difficult in twin pregnancies and there is an increased risk of sample contamination, especially with CVS.
- Miscarriage has been reported as higher with invasive testing of twins compared to singletons
- In a monozygotic (MZ) pregnancy without structural abnormalities, only one sac needs to be sampled at amniocentesis

Structural abnormalities

- **DZ:** the rate of structural abnormalities in each DZ twin is the same as for a singleton pregnancy. Therefore, the overall risk per pregnancy is double that of a singleton
- **MZ:** the risk of structural abnormalities is 2–3 times higher for MZ twins. These include cardiac abnormalities, bowel atresia, and neural tube defects. Detailed anomaly and cardiac scans are essential. The increased risk of structural abnormalities is thought to be due to uneven distribution of the inner cell mass during splitting. Vascular events may play a role

Use of selective feticide

- **Dichorionic (DC) twins:** selective feticide with potassium chloride can be offered to terminate the affected fetus. The risk of fetal loss in the healthy twin after feticide is 7%, with an average gestational age at delivery of 35.7 weeks
- **Monochorionic (MC) twins:** selective feticide is not possible owing to the vascular anastomoses present in the placenta. Alternative options include cord occlusion by bipolar coagulation. This is associated with a risk of death in the healthy fetus of 13% (41% fetal death in gestations <18 weeks and 3% in those ≥18 weeks) and rupture of membranes before 34 weeks in 23% of cases. The overall intact survival rate is 70%. The risks of cord occlusion have to be balanced against those of sudden fetal death in the affected fetus, which in turn is associated with a high risk of disability or death in the surviving twin (see Section 8.28)

Twin-to-twin transfusion syndrome

This is a problem unique to monochorionic pregnancies

Incidence

- 15% of MC twin pregnancies
- It can occur as early as 11–13 weeks' gestation and often develops in the second trimester

Pathophysiology

Twin-to-twin transfusion syndrome (TTTS) develops because of vascular anastomoses in the placenta which join the fetuses' circulation, enabling transfusion of blood from one fetus to the other.

Although 96% of MC placentas have vascular anastomoses, the type of anastomoses influences the development of TTTS.
Arterioarterial anastomoses (AAA) and venovenous anastomoses (VVA) are superficial and allow flow in both directions.

Arteriovenous anastomoses (AVA) are deep anastomoses and are present in 90% of cases of TTTS. Arterial blood from one twin drains into the venous system in the other twin, causing unidirectional flow.

Bidirectional AAAs are protective to the development of TTTS by balancing out the unidirectional flow caused by AVAs. In the absence of AAAs, there is a greater net flow of blood from one fetus (donor) to the other fetus (recipient), causing TTTS.

The donor fetus becomes hypovolaemic and develops oligohydramnios due to oliguria. The bladder can be small or absent. When oligohydramnios is severe, the appearance of a 'stuck twin' develops, with the fetus fixed at the edge of the placenta or uterine wall unable to move as it is held by the collapsed membrane of the oligohydramniotic sac.

Fetal growth retardation (FGR), anaemia, and hydrops can develop.

The recipient twin becomes fluid-overloaded, with a large bladder and evidence of polyhydramnios secondary to polyuria. Cardiomegaly and eventually hydrops can develop. The baby can be macrosomic and plethoric.

History

- Acute abdominal distension.

Examination

- Rapidly increasing symphyseal–fundal height
- Clinical polyhydramnios

Investigations

- MC twins require 2-weekly US scans for growth and liquor from 16 weeks to identify those developing TTTS
- The presence of oligohydramnios (deepest pool of liquor is ≤2 cm) in the donor and polyhydramnios in the recipient (deepest pool of liquor ≥8 cm) with discordant bladder sizes is diagnostic of TTTS
- Abnormal umbilical artery Dopplers (absent or reversed end-diastolic flow) are seen in the donor twin with abnormal venous Dopplers (reverse flow in the ductus venosus, pulsitile flow in the umbilical vein) in the recipient
- Severe TTTS occurs in about half of those affected, and ultrasonographic features may be present from as early as 11–13 weeks' gestation manifesting as increased nuchal thickness in one or both of the fetuses

Risks

- If untreated, the perinatal mortality of TTTS is 80%
- Increased risk of severe neurological impairment (20%)
- In severe TTTS with the presence of either abnormal umbilical artery Dopplers or abnormal venous Dopplers, the chance of one fetus surviving is 33% and 37%, respectively
- Cardiomyopathy can develop in the recipient, with a 10% chance of chronic cardiac problems, such as right ventricular outflow obstruction
- Increased risk of preterm rupture of membranes and cord accident with polyhydramnios
- Increased morbidity and mortality is associated with preterm birth and iatrogenic early delivery
- Risk of hypoplastic lungs in the donor twin

Management

Management of TTTS is specific to Fetal Medicine Units. Treatment options include serial amnioreduction, septostomy, and endoscopic laser coagulation of the communicating placental vessels (see Table 8.2). Alternatively, cord occlusion can be considered (see below).

Fetal growth retardation

About 25% of twin pregnancies are complicated by a birth weight below the 10th centile. The risks of FGR include fetal death and neurological damage caused by chronic hypoxia. If considering premature delivery, corticosteroids for lung maturity should be given.

DC twins

- FGR risk is 80%
- Four-weekly growth scans
- If FGR develops, increase surveillance with 2-weekly growth scans and at least weekly umbilical artery Doppler and liquor assessments
- Discordant growth (birth weight difference ≥25%) between dichorionic diamniotic (DCDA) twins tends to occur later in pregnancy and can be caused by different growth potential for each twin (dizygotic twins), poor placentation of one placenta, aneuploidy or congenital abnormalities
- Timing of delivery will depend on gestation, degree of FGR, and whether both fetuses are affected
- The risk of iatrogenic prematurity in the healthy fetus has to be weighed against the risk of neurological abnormality and death in the FGR fetus if the conservative approach is taken

MC twins

The risks of FGR are greater in MC than DC pregnancies:

- FGR risk is 16%
- Two-weekly US to detect FGR. If present, perform umbilical artery Doppler and liquor volume at least weekly
- Discordant growth can often happen early. Occurs when there is uneven distribution of the placenta between the twins and is influenced by the degree and type of vascular anastomoses
- Exclude congenital abnormalities, aneuploidy (in the very rare event that one fetus is affected) and infection
- TTTS is excluded if there is no evidence of polyhydramnios in the larger twin
- Discordant MC twins are at a higher risk of adverse outcome compared with DC twins
- This risk is greatest before 24 weeks' gestation, owing to TTTS, where the fetal loss rate is 12% compared with 1.8% in DC pregnancies

- Risks of prematurity need to be weighed against the risk of sudden death in the FGR fetus. This is associated with a high risk of death and cerebral damage in the surviving twin
- Should be managed in a tertiary centre

Problems unique to monoamniotic twins

All monochorionic monoamniotic (MCMA) twins will have their umbilical cords intertwined. If one cord becomes taut/entangled and cuts off the blood supply to the other twin, then death or hypoxia can ensue. This can happen both antenatally and in labour.

Table 8.2 Treatment options for TTTS		
Method	Survival outcomes	Other outcomes
Amnioreduction: amniotic fluid is drained to reduce polyhydramnios	Improves polyhydramnios and reduces preterm labour due to polyhydramnios. Reduces intrauterine pressure and increases placental blood flow. In one study, at least one fetus survived in 71% of cases and both survived in 48% of cases	Preterm labour, preterm ROM and chorioamnionitis. 25% of survivors developed cerebral abnormalities. Does not treat underlying cause therefore recurrent procedures needed
Septostomy: needle or laser septostomy allows amniotic fluid to cross the amniotic membrane	In a study looking at amnioreduction versus septostomy, survival rate for at least one twin was similar (78% versus 80%)	Those undergoing septostomy were more likely to need a single procedure compared to amnioreduction (64% versus 48%). Does not treat underlying cause
Laser ablation: selective ablation (placental anastomoses are selectively ablated) and non-selective ablation (placenta is divided to make a dichorionic placenta)	In a study comparing selective laser treatment and amnioreduction, the survival rate of at least one twin at 6 months was higher for laser (76% and 51%, respectively)	Of those treated with laser, 52% were free of major neurological problems at 6 months compared with 31% who underwent amnioreduction. Treats underlying cause

8.31 Intrauterine death

Death of a baby before birth can cause considerable upset and grief to parents and their families. It can also be a distressing time for healthcare professionals. It is essential that we manage these women and their families in an appropriate and sensitive manner (see Section 1.8).

Definitions

Late fetal loss: *in utero* death delivered between 22^{+0} and 23^{+6} weeks gestation.

Stillbirth babies: born dead after 24 completed weeks.

Stillbirth rate: number of stillbirths per 1000 live births + stillbirths.

Neonatal death: death of a live born baby within 28 days of birth.

Early neonatal death: death occurs less than 7 completed days after birth.

Late neonatal death: death after 7 days, but before 28 completed days after birth.

Perinatal mortality rate: number of stillborn and early neonatal deaths per 1000 live births + stillbirths.

Incidence

- In 2005, the stillbirth rate was 5.5/1000 (3676 stillbirths) for England, Wales and Northern Ireland

Risk factors and causes

Box 8.18 summarizes the risk factors and causes of intrauterine deaths (IUDs). Most, however, are unexplained. The Confidential Enquiry into Maternal and Child Health (CEMACH) classifies stillbirths using the extended Wigglesworth classification (based on a pathophysiological approach) supplemented by the obstetric (Aberdeen) classification (which emphasizes maternal causes), and the fetal and neonatal classification.

In 2005, the majority of stillbirths (>50%) were unexplained. This was followed by severe or lethal congenital anomalies (16%), antepartum haemorrhage (8%), and intrapartum causes (8%). More recent classifications (ReCODE) attribute many of the previously unexplained stillbirths to fetal growth retardation (FGR).

Clinical evaluation

History
- No fetal movements
- Term or preterm labour
- Symptoms associated with cause (e.g. vaginal bleeding and abdominal pain with abruption, itching with obstetric cholestasis)

Examination
- No fetal heart heard with sonicaid or CTG. Always record maternal heart rate as maternal tachycardia can be mistaken for the fetal heart
- Loss of fetal heart during labour with intrapartum deaths
- Examination findings associated with cause (e.g. hard uterus with abruption, hypertension with pre-eclampsia)

Investigations
- US: no fetal heart movements, Spalding's sign of overlapping of the skull bones in the dead fetus. May give a clue to the cause e.g. FGR, malformation
- Women who retain their fetus for ≥4 weeks can develop disseminated intravascular coagulation (DIC). Thus FBC, clotting profile, fibrin, fibrinogen and fibrin degradation products (FDP) levels are required
- Group and save
- Box 8.19 summarizes the investigations of causes of IUD
- If there is an obvious cause for the IUD, such as cord prolapse, further investigations may still be of value as post mortem not uncommonly identifies previously unrecognized anomalies or findings

Further reading

Cole SK, Hey EN, Thomson AM. Classifying perinatal death: an obstetric approach. *British Journal of Obstetrics and Gynaecology* 1986: **93(12):**1204–12.

Confidential Enquiry into Maternal and Child Health. Perinatal mortality 2005: England, Wales and Northern Ireland. CEMACH: London, 2007.

Hey EN, Lloyd DJ, Wigglesworth JS. Classifying perinatal death: fetal and neonatal factors. *British Journal of Obstetrics and Gynaecology* 1986; **93(12):**1213–23.

Wigglesworth JS. Monitoring perinatal mortality. A pathophysiological approach. *Lancet* 1980; **(8196):**684–6.

Box 8.18 Risk factors and causes of intrauterine death

Maternal
- Maternal age <20 (stillbirth rate 6.6/1000)
- Maternal age >40 (stillbirth rate 7.5/1000)
- Obesity (BMI >30)
- Social deprivation
- Drug use (cocaine), smoking
- Black and Asian ethnicity
- Pre-eclampsia, pregnancy-induced hypertension, essential hypertension
- Diabetes mellitus
- Obstetric cholestasis
- Systemic lupus erythematosus
- Thrombophilia (e.g. primary antiphospholipid syndrome, inherited thrombophilias)
- Hypoperfusion (e.g. maternal septicaemia, aggressive treatment of hypertension)
- Maternal thyrotoxicosis (rare)

Fetal
- Birth weight <1500 g (stillbirth rate 261/1000 for babies weighing <1000 g)
- Prematurity (this encompasses above): need to make distinction between prematurity and FGR which is probably most important cause of IUD
- Congenital anomalies
- Intrapartum causes (e.g. hypoxia, trauma)
- Postmaturity
- Fetal haemolytic disease (including Rhesus)
- Chromosomal abnormalities
- Fetal growth restriction
- Infection (e.g. group B streptococcus, rubella, parvovirus, syphilis, cytomegalovirus, toxoplasmosis)
- Multiple pregnancy, twin-to-twin transfusion syndrome

Placental
- Placental abruption
- Placenta praevia
- Cord prolapse
- Cord entanglement (including true knots, see Figure 8.18)

Box 8.19 Investigations into intrauterine death

Condition	Investigations
Maternal	
Pre-eclampsia	BP, urinalysis, PET bloods (see Section 8.11)
Diabetes	HbA1c, random blood glucose (see Section 7.15)
Obstetric cholestasis	LFTs and bile acids (see Section 8.22)
Thrombophilia	Anticardiolipin antibodies, lupus anticoagulant, antinuclear antibodies, inherited thrombophilia screen (see Section 7.26)
Infection	Check temperature. Bloods for toxoplasmosis, parvovirus, CMV, rubella, syphilis, listeria and CRP. Vaginal swab for group B streptococcus. (see Sections 8.24, 8.25, 8.26, 6.6 and 6.7)
Thyrotoxicosis	Thyroid function tests (see Section 7.16)
Feto-maternal haemorrhage	Kleihauer
Fetal	
Abnormal fetal karyotype	Skin sample if not macerated. If macerated, muscle and cartilage can be used. If unable to get sample and dysmorphic or structural features present, obtain parental blood for karyotyping
Infection	Swabs from baby (e.g. ear)
Congenital abnormalities	X-rays or MRI if post mortem declined
Placental	
Infection	Swabs from placenta
Karyotype	Wedge of placenta, including amniotic surface
Pathology	Histopathological examination of the placenta is very important (even if post mortem declined)

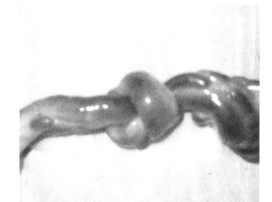

Fig. 8.18 True cord knot causing stillbirth.

8.32 Management of intrauterine death

Initial management and delivery

- If intrauterine death (IUD) is associated with maternal disease (e.g. placental abruption, eclampsia), the priority is to resuscitate, stabilize, and treat the mother. If the woman presents with contractions, labour should be allowed to proceed
- The woman and her partner should be informed about the death of the fetus immediately. It is important to relay any information in a clear, sensitive manner, avoiding the use of medical jargon
- Emotions can range from shock, disbelief, anger, blame, despair, fear, and anxiety
- Ask the parents if they would like to see the US. Seeing a static heart on scan may make the situation more believable. They may ask for more than one scan and it is important that requests are accommodated
- They may want time alone to grieve. Move to a side room away from the noises of labour ward (see also Section 1.8)
- A discussion regarding delivery should take place once the patient and family have had a chance to take in what has happened. Aim for a vaginal delivery, explaining the benefits of shorter hospital stay, less pain after delivery, and the risks of CS, including the implications for a subsequent pregnancy
- In some women (e.g. transverse lie, multiple previous CS), CS may be indicated
- Each unit will have their own protocol for IOL which should be followed in consultation with a senior obstetrician
- Some protocols will advise mifepristone followed 24–48 h later by either vaginal or oral misoprostol (side effects include nausea, vomiting, fever, tachycardia, and diarrhoea) which works well, particularly for earlier gestations. Other protocols use vaginal prostaglandin E_2
- Unless there are potential life-threatening conditions (e.g. infection, pre-eclampsia), the woman can go home if she wishes before commencing IOL
- IOL should not be delayed for too long owing to the increased risk of disseminated intravascular coagulation (DIC)
- As the fetus becomes increasingly macerated, it may be more distressing for the parents to see the baby and more difficult to identify a cause of death by post mortem
- Avoid amniotomy owing to the risk of ascending infection
- Review by anaesthetist to discuss analgesia options. These include entonox, pethidine, patient-controlled analgesia (PCA) and epidural (as long as there are no clotting abnormalities)

Postnatal management

- Ask the parents whether they would like to see, hold or name the baby
- Some may prefer time alone with their baby or would like the baby to be in a cot overnight by the bedside
- Photos, footprints, and a lock of hair can be kept. Even if the parents do not want to see a photo, with permission photos can be kept in the notes as some may change their mind later
- Ask whether they would like a chaplain or other religious representative. Some may wish for their baby to be blessed
- It can be difficult for siblings to understand what has happened. Parents can consider allowing them to see and hold their brother or sister. They may be worried that this will be upsetting, but children may be comforted to know that their sibling was real and did not look frightening
- Discussion regarding post mortem needs to take place. This can be distressing for the parents and needs to be approached sensitively. A post mortem may reveal a cause which can aid

management in future pregnancies. A negative post mortem is reassuring as the chances of recurrent IUD are low

- Discuss the process of a post mortem. Explain that their baby's face will not be cut and that afterwards, when clothed, there should be no evidence of the post mortem. All parts removed will be returned to the body
- If agreed, a consent form will need to be signed which includes options of a full or limited post mortem (i.e. exclusion of certain organs to be examined). If declined, X-rays or MRI should be discussed
- A Medical Certificate of Stillbirth needs to be issued to the parents and taken to the nearest office of the Registrar for Births, Marriages and Deaths within 6 weeks. Once registered, a certificate for burial or cremation will be given to the parents
- By law, babies born after 24 weeks' gestation must be buried or cremated. Discuss whether the parents would prefer for this to be arranged by them or by the hospital
- Administer anti-D if Rhesus negative
- 1 g oral cabergoline should be offered to suppress lactation
- Discuss counselling and refer appropriately
- Inform the GP, consultant, and midwifery team. Cancel antenatal appointments
- Most units will have protocols and checklists so that all investigations are performed and appropriate people informed

Follow-up

- Many maternity units provide separate bereavement support with approaches at approximately 2 weeks post IUD
- The purpose is to support and explain bereavement
- An appointment in an unhurried environment (preferably away from pregnant women) is essential to discuss the events surrounding the death of the baby and results of any investigations
- It is important not only to ask how the woman is but also how her partner is coping. Feelings of the partner can be overlooked after an IUD as care is concentrated on the mother
- Discuss future pregnancies and how to reduce the risks of another IUD occurring
- Most find serial US in future pregnancies reassuring
- Some disorders may need specific treatment (e.g. antiphospholipid syndrome) and this should be discussed
- A letter detailing the circumstances of the IUD and any results should be sent to the GP and patient. If she decides to book elsewhere in a future pregnancy, she has all the information to take with her
- If a couple is not planning a pregnancy in the near future, discuss contraception

Further reading

Further information for parents and healthcare professionals can be obtained from the Stillbirth and Neonatal Death Charity (SANDS, www.uk-sands.org) and the Child Bereavement Trust (www.childbereavement.org.uk)

Chapter 9

Care in labour

Contents

Covered elsewhere

9.1 Normal labour

Introduction

The human pelvis represents a compromise between the need to allow the passage of an offspring and the adoption of an upright stature. Human babies are born relatively premature compared to other mammalian species.

Intrapartum care has become an essential aspect of human labour and delivery. It serves always to support, frequently to supplement, and occasionally to replace the normal processes. This chapter will discuss the most important aspects of care in normal and abnormal labour.

Definitions

Labour is defined as the presence of contractions of sufficient frequency, strength, and duration to cause cervical effacement and dilatation

Lie is the relation of the fetal axis to that of the mother. It can be longitudinal, oblique, transverse, or unstable

Presentation is determined by the part of the body of the fetus that is foremost within or close to the birth canal. It can be cephalic, breech, cord or shoulder

Attitude is the posture assumed by the fetus. It can be flexion or extension. Extension (or 'deflexed' head) is associated with larger presenting diameters and malpositions (see Section 9.10)

Position refers to the relation of an arbitrarily chosen portion of the presenting part to the maternal pelvis. For cephalic presentations, the denominator is the occiput and the most common position is occipitoanterior (OA)

Caput is the swelling of the most dependent portion of the fetal head. It is normally only a few millimetres thick, but may be extensive in prolonged or obstructed labour

Moulding is the change in the shape of the fetal head from external compression. Severe moulding may indicate cephalopelvic disproportion (see Section 9.4)

Contractions of the uterine musculature occur from every 10 min in the early stages of labour to as frequently as every minute in the second stage. They last 30–90 seconds each. In the active phases of labour, their frequency is 3–4 every 10 min, but it may be less in parous women

Station (see Table 9.1) is the relation in centimetres of the bones of the presenting part to the level of the ischial spines. It is –5 at the pelvic inlet (presenting part just tipped), 0 at the spines (at vaginal examination two phalanges inserted to reach the presenting part), and +2 to +3 at the perineal floor (one phalanx inserted)

Engagement is the descent of the largest diameter of the presenting part (biparietal, or bi-ischial in breech) below the pelvic inlet. It usually occurs when station is zero. In nulliparas, it may happen before labour. The fetal head usually engages left occipitoanterior or occipitotransverse (LOA/LOT) owing to the presence of the maternal sigmoid colon in the posterior left aspect of the pelvis

Effacement is the shortening of the cervical canal from 3 cm to a mere circular orifice as a result of active or latent (painless) myometrial activity. It results in a release of a bloody mucousy plug, or 'show'

Dilatation. With contractions, the upper uterus progressively shortens to push forward the fetus, while the lower segment distends under pressure from the amniotic sac or the presenting part. Full dilatation is arbitrarily considered as 10 cm

Asynclitism refers to lateral deflection of the head anteriorly or posteriorly so that the sagittal suture lies closer to the sacrum (or, very rarely, closer to the symphysis pubis), rather than mid-way between the two. There is almost always some degree of asynclitism with occipitotransverse (OT) positions. Extreme asynclitism results in ear presentation.

Pelvimetry

- The female pelvis can be divided into three planes:
  - Inlet: bordered by the symphysis pubis (upper margin), the sacral promontory, and the linea terminalis
  - Midplane: bordered by the posterior surface of the symphysis, the ischial spines, and the sacrum at the level of S4–S5
  - Outlet: bordered by the lower margin of the symphysis, the ischial tuberosities, and the tip of the sacrum (not the coccyx, as it extends posteriorly during birth)
- The relevant diameters are important in determining the mechanism of labour. The longest are the transverse at the inlet and the anteroposterior at the outlet (see Table 9.2 and Figure 9.1)
- It is not possible to predict outcome of labour by pelvic assessment. X-ray pelvimetry, used in the past, does not improve perinatal outcome and may increase the CS rate. (Ib)

Physiology (stages) of labour

The *latent phase* ('early labour') begins with the onset of labour and ends when the cervix is 3–4 cm dilated and fully effaced.

The (active) *first stage* begins when the cervix is fully effaced and 3–4 cm dilated and ends when it is fully dilated.

Commonly there is an accelerative phase with gradual progress. This may be followed by a deceleration phase towards the end of the first stage (or 'transition') when the rate may slow somewhat before full dilatation.

The *second stage* is the interval between full dilatation and delivery of the fetus.

During the first and second stage, the following occur:

- Engagement in oblique or transverse position, if unengaged
- Descent to below the level of the ischial spines
- Flexion as a result of pressure of the presenting part against the pelvic floor
- Rotation to OA so that the largest occipitofrontal diameter occupies the longest anteroposterior diameter of the pelvic outlet. At the same time, the largest fetal diameter at the shoulders, the bisacromial, occupies the longest diameter of the inlet, the transverse
- Extension and delivery of the fetal head underneath the symphysis pubis
- Restitution with rotation of the fetus so that the bisacromial diameter now occupies the longest anteroposterior diameter of the pelvic outlet
- Delivery of the shoulders and the rest of the body

The *third stage* is the interval between the delivery of the baby and the delivery of the placenta, cord, and membranes, and usually lasts up to 30 min.

Management of normal labour

- Formal assessment programmes to diagnose active labour reduce hospital stay, use of oxytocics, and need for pain relief (A). There is, however, insufficient evidence yet to support the antenatal education of women to self-diagnose active labour to the same effect
- One-to-one trained support during labour should be pursued. Continuous support increases the spontaneous vaginal delivery rate and decreases the need for analgesia (A)
- A rapid evaluation of the maternal condition and a risk assessment should be performed if labour is diagnosed. Monitoring should be initiated according to the risk level assigned

- Regular bladder emptying should be encouraged
- Perineal shaving or enemas are not recommended; they do not decrease infectious morbidity (**A**). Perineal shaving may increase colonization with Gram-negative bacteria (**Ia**)
- Analgesia should be provided as requested
- A vaginal examination should be performed with consent every 2–4 h to assess progress. Dilatation, station, and amniotic fluid colour should be recorded. An abdominal examination to assess descent and contractions should also be performed. Use of a partogram is encouraged (see Section 9.4)
- Maternal observations should be regularly assessed (every 1–2 h) and recorded
- Women should be encouraged to push once the cervix is fully dilated, in the position they find comfortable. Upright or lateral positions are associated with a reduction in pain and assisted deliveries, but with an increase in tears and blood loss more than 500 ml (**Ia**)
- Restrictive use of episiotomy (only when thought to be clinically useful) decreases posterior perineal trauma and the need for suturing, but increases anterior trauma (periurethral, labial, periclitoral) (**Ia**)
- As the head delivers, the woman should be asked to give only small pushes or to pant. The shoulders should be delivered one at a time. The baby should then be placed on the maternal abdomen
- Active management of the third stage (oxytocic administration, early cord clamping, and controlled cord traction (see Figure 9.2) reduces blood loss but increases the risk of vomiting. Cord drainage (releasing the clamps) may reduce the length of the third stage (**Ia**)
- Combined ergometrine–oxytocin for the third stage reduces blood loss compared to syntocinon alone, but not the incidence of postpartum haemorrhage (PPH) of more than 1l. It increases the risk of vomiting and hypertension. Prostaglandins are less effective (**Ia**)

Tips

- Arbitrary limits on the duration of the latent or active stage only increase maternal dissatisfaction and have little evidence to support them
- Continuous support, as long as maternal and fetal wellbeing are ensured, and involving women in decisions is more important than adhering to stringent definitions

Table 9.1 Relation between engagement and station (assuming no massive moulding)

Fifths palpable abdominally	Description	Station
5/5	Fetal head free	−4/−5
4/5	Tip just below symphysis	−3
3/5	Occipitofrontal diameter palpable	−2
2/5	Sinciput and occiput palpable	−1
1/5	Only sinciput palpable	0/at spines
0/5	Nil palpable	Below spines

Table 9.2 Average pelvic diameters (see Figure 9.1)

Diameter→ Plane ↓	Antero-posterior (cm)	Oblique (cm)	Transverse (cm)
Inlet	11	12	13
Midplane	12	12	12
Outlet	13	12	11

- There is emerging evidence on the usefulness of an oxytocin infusion in the third stage in reducing the incidence of PPH. Even though its routine administration to all women cannot be recommended yet, it is good practice to have it ready for use, particularly in women at risk for PPH (see Section 11.1)
- A common mistake of juniors is to palpate the ischial tuberosity and mistake it for the ischial spine. The ischial spine is far more posterior. A good obstetrician will know whether you are performing it correctly by noticing whether the operators' fingers are inserted by at least two phalanges past the introitus

Further reading

WHO. *Normal labour. Managing Complications in Pregnancy and Childbirth: A guide for midwives and doctors* 2003. www.who.int/reproductive-health

NICE. Intrapartum care. Clinical Guideline. National Collaborating Centre for Women's and Children's Health. Commissioned by the National Institute for Clinical Excellence. London: RCOG Press, 2007. www.nice.org

The Cochrane Collaboration. *The Cochrane Database of Systematic Reviews*, No. 4. John Wiley and Sons Ltd, 2007. www.cochrane.org

These references have been used throughout this chapter and are strongly recommended for further reading.

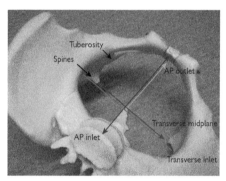

Fig. 9.1 Pelvic diameters (AP, anteroposterior).

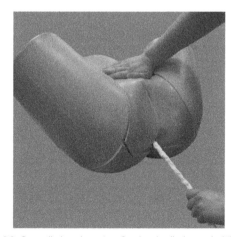

Fig. 9.2 Controlled cord traction. One hand pulls the cord while the other stabilizes the uterus by suprapubic pressure. Signs of separation should first be seen (cord elongation, fresh short gush of blood, uterus becomes smaller and rounded).

9.2 Risk assessment, home delivery, and water birth

Risk assessment

Definition
- Risk is the probability that an adverse outcome may occur
- There is no risk-free pregnancy with a guaranteed good outcome for mother and baby. The objectives are to reduce the maternal and perinatal mortality and morbidity
- Most pregnancies are low risk. The purpose of antenatal care is to provide an effective screening programme, to support pregnant women, and manage simple symptoms
- A few pregnancies can be regarded as high risk. The aim is to identify risk factors for adverse outcomes and instigate a plan for the prevention or treatment of complications

Approach

1. Risk scoring
Several risk scoring systems have been developed. They tend to be inflexible and their use has not been associated with reduction of adverse pregnancy outcomes.

2. Risk identification
The most common approach depends on the identification of risk factors from the history or examination at booking or subsequent visits or admissions. Management is then individualized and largely dependent on the preferences of the care provider (see Box 9.1).

3. Care plans
Care plans consist of a schematic approach to risk management. A predetermined management plan of common complications (e.g. gestational diabetes) is applied to every single pregnancy with such a complication (see Box 9.2).

This approach ensures consistency of care and facilitates audit. It is also more scientific, particularly if evidence-based recommendations are followed.

High risk factors
- Risk assessment should not only be part of the booking appointment, but a continuous dynamic process throughout pregnancy and should be repeated at the onset of labour
- Women should be reassigned to a high-risk group should any new factors present

Home delivery (see Box 9.3)

Incidence
- One in five women is interested in giving birth at home. The most recent recorded rate in the UK was just >2%. This is rising and rates of 4–5% are anticipated in the near future. There is large geographical variation (1–13.9%)
- A small number (<0.5%) of home deliveries are unplanned, usually in parous women
- Midwives have a professional duty to provide care to women, including home birth
- All competent low-risk women should be offered a home birth if there is adequate infrastructure and support

Good practice points
- Only low-risk women should be offered home birth. Local protocols should define the relevant criteria
- Multidisciplinary teams (MDTs) should draw up action plans for women who intend to give home birth against medical and midwifery advice
- Availability of a telephone (e.g. mobile) is advised

- Clear documentation is essential. Use of a partogram is encouraged
- A fetal Doppler should be available to establish the presence of a fetal heart rate when there is any problem identifying it or fetal distress is suspected
- Attendants need to be skilled in neonatal resuscitation, shoulder dystocia, and other emergency procedures
- There should be provisions in place for safe transfer to hospital if there are unexpected occurrences

Useful tips
You will frequently encounter women who request a home delivery despite multiple risk factors (e.g. twins, previous CS).
- Elicit the reasons for such a request. Often women are misinformed and afraid of medicalization of their care
- Provide balanced evidence-based information
- This may change their mind or help to prepare for the worst if unable to take standard advice
- Involve seniors (medical and midwifery) if women persist
- Protect the continuing and trusting relationship
- Do not be confrontational or make threats
- It is best to keep the lines of communication open so there is no delay or hesitation if the situation changes later

Water birth (see Box 9.4)
Immersion in water has become a popular choice in the last two decades. In the UK, it has been recommended that maternity services provide all women, regardless of ethnicity or educational status, the opportunity to labour and/or give birth underwater.
- Immersion in water has been used:
  - Antenatally
  - In early labour and for pain relief in the first stage of labour
  - For actual birth of the baby underwater
  - For the third stage
- There is no evidence to suggest any benefit or risk from immersion antenatally or in the early, latent phase of labour
- There are potential benefits from the use of water immersion for the active phase of labour in low-risk women
- There is a lack of good quality data on the safety of actual birth under water or of immersion for the third stage
- Water immersion should be offered only to uncomplicated pregnancies at term
- Spontaneous rupture of membranes is not a contraindication

Practical issues
- Attending midwives must be suitably trained
- In the absence of evidence for the latent phase, immersion should only take place in the active phase of labour, when the cervix is at least 4–5 cm dilated
- The temperature of the water should be 37°C. Alternatively, women can be encouraged to regulate it themselves
- The fetal heart should be monitored with underwater Doppler. If there are any concerns, the woman should be advised to leave the birthing pool for further management
- Strict infection control policies must be applied
- If the woman raises herself out of the water and exposes the fetal head to air in the second stage, she should be advised to remain out of water to prevent premature fetal gasping under water and freshwater drowning

- The baby needs to be brought to the surface face up for the same reason

Useful tips
- Suturing a perineal tear can be challenging, as tissues may be waterlogged, oedematous, and friable
- Allow 1 h before starting the repair
- Estimated blood loss can be inaccurate

Further reading

Cluett E R et al. Immersion in water in pregnancy, labour and birth (Cochrane review), 2002. www.cochrane.org

NICE. Antenatal care: routine care for the healthy pregnant woman. Evidence-based Clinical Guideline. National Collaborating Centre for Women's and Children's Health. London: RCOG Press, 2004. www.rcog.org.

Organisation of prenatal care and identification of risk. In: James DK, Steer PJ, Weiner CP and Gonik B (eds). *High risk pregnancy. Management options*, 2nd edn. London: Saunders, 2002.

Royal College of Midwives. Home birth. Position paper 25. London, 2005. www.rcm.org.uk

RCOG/RCM. Immersion in water during labour and birth. Joint Statement No.1, London, 2006. www.rcog.org

---

Box 9.1 High-risk factors at booking or evolving later

1. General history:
   BMI <18 or >35 kg/m^2
   Age <16 years or >40 old
   Smoking
   Cardiac disease, hypertension
   Renal disease
   Endocrine disease, diabetes
   Severe asthma
   Illicit drug use
   Haematological disorders
   Epilepsy on anticonvulsant drugs
   Psychiatric disease
   Malignant disease
   Autoimmune disorders
   HIV, hepatitis B or C infection

2. Previous obstetric history:
   Uterine surgery, including CS
   Stillbirth, neonatal death, second trimester loss
   Rhesus isoimmunization, other haemolytic diseases
   Previous postpartum haemorrhage
   Puerperal psychosis or depression
   Small or large for gestational age fetus
   Pre-eclampsia, HELLP (haemolysis, elevated liver enzymes, low platelets syndrome) or eclampsia

3. Index pregnancy:
   Any of the above (in 2)
   Amniotic fluid disorders
   Prematurity <37 or post-term pregnancy >42 weeks
   Multiple pregnancy
   Breech presentation
   Epidural
   Prolonged membrane rupture
   Induced or augmented labour
   Meconium staining
   Maternal infection
   Antepartum or intrapartum bleeding

Box 9.2 Simple care plan example—asthma

Booking visit
- Reassure regarding the safe use of asthma medication
- Refer to respiratory physicians if there is history of recent asthma exacerbation or hospital admission within last year

34 weeks
- Assess for symptoms and peak flow rates if appropriate
- Refer to respiratory physicians if exacerbations
- Growth scan if severe asthma or exacerbations antenatally
- Document plan for labour, third stage, and postnatal period

---

Box 9.3 Advantages and disadvantages of home birth

Advantages of home birth
- Psychological advantage—privacy, empowerment
- Continuity of carer
- A familiar environment
- Less medical intervention
- For selected low-risk women there is no strong evidence to support hospital birth

Disadvantages of home birth
- Less options for pain relief (though less pain experienced)
- Between 16–40% need to be transferred to another location during labour if a problem arises
- Increased perinatal mortality (1–2/1000, more than double the background) in the following situations:
  1. Evolving high-risk situations
  2. When there is a lack of skilled attendants
  3. When there is a need for transfer to hospital

Box 9.4 Water immersion—summary of benefits and risks

- Less pain leading to less need for epidural or pharmacological analgesia (Ia)
- No adverse effect on labour duration, operative delivery rates or neonatal outcome (Ia)
- Reduced obstetric intervention in prolonged labour (Ia)
- Mobility encouraged

Potential risks—for which little evidence exists
- Prolonged labour if immersion happens too early
- Maternal and neonatal infections
- Fetal hypoxia
- Neonatal hypothermia
- Cord rupture and haemorrhage
- Neonatal unit admission (only when associated with prolonged labour)

9.3 Analgesia and anaesthesia

Definition
Analgesia is the relief of pain without the loss of motor function or consciousness. Anaesthesia is the loss of feeling or sensation and can involve the loss of consciousness, of motor power, or of autonomic reflexes.

Physiology
Pain in labour is caused by contractions, cervical dilatation, and perineal distension. Sensory fibres from the uterus are carried to the T10–L1 spinal cord segments, from the perineum to S2–S4, primarily via the pudendal nerve.

Nearly all anaesthetic drugs cross the placenta by passive diffusion, even more so if they are lipid-soluble, less ionized, with low molecular weight and minimal protein binding.

Incidence
The incidence is partly dependent on availability. An anaesthetist is involved in up to 60% of labours in the UK.

Deaths
- There were 6 direct anaesthetic deaths in the 2003–2005 Confidential Enquiry, mostly associated with general anaesthesia (GA)
- Poor perioperative management may have contributed to a further 31 deaths
- The 7th Confidential Enquiry into Stillbirths and Deaths in Infancy (CESDI) investigated 25 UK cases with anaesthetic involvement, of which 19 were related to the use of GA

Techniques
Complementary therapies
Acupuncture and hypnosis may be effective in labour, but more research is needed on these and other therapies (aromatherapy, reflexology, massage, music). Even if the effects are placebo, this in itself can be valuable to help women cope with pain.

TENS
Transcutaneous electrical nerve stimulation (or TENS) provides relief for the first stage of labour (25–60% effective). It is also good for backache.

Entonox
- A 1:1 mixture of O_2/N_2O
- Most effective when used before pain starts

Side effects include nausea (reduced if use is intermittent), dehydration, hypoxia, alkalosis, and a long-term detrimental effect on vitamin B12 metabolism (an occupational health risk for midwives if exposed to leaking devices).

Local infiltration
- Perineal analgesia (see Figure 9.3) can be provided with 5–10 ml of lignocaine 1%, either before a low instrumental delivery, or when crowning of the fetal head is uncomfortable to the mother
- Pudendal block (see Figure 9.4) is an easy, rapid technique for providing analgesia for instrumental deliveries. Injecting 5 ml of lignocaine 1% each side is usually adequate. The rare risks include haematoma, sciatic nerve block, and rectal puncture

Systemic opiates
- Pethidine 100 mg IM 4-hourly is commonly used, together with sedatives to reduce narcotic demand
- Opiates are easy to administer, although pain relief may be inadequate

Risks include orthostatic hypotension, delayed gastric emptying, maternal and neonatal respiratory depression, less chance of successful breastfeeding. Their use must be avoided just before delivery to avoid neonatal respiratory depression.

Patient (woman)-controlled analgesia
Patient-controlled analgesia (PCA) has rapid onset and offset, and results in better pain scores and satisfaction compared to pethidine. Ideal for mid-trimester terminations and some cardiac patients.

Epidurals
Epidurals are performed with a 16–20-gauge needle in the epidural space at a level of L2–L5. Isobaric bupivacaine, 10–20 mls of a 0.25–0.5% solution or of 0.1% with fentanyl is used.

They offer better pain relief than other therapies for almost any obstetric situation without increasing the risk of CS or the incidence of lower Apgar scores at 5 min. Despite this, many clinicians still feel that epidurals slow down labour and increase interference. Others consider that social support, confidence, continuity of care, and early home assessment enable women to cope with the latent phase and thus avoid epidural and improve normal birth rates. There are ongoing studies to evaluate whether early initiation before the active stage increases the risk of CS.

Epidurals pose less maternal and fetal risks compared to systemic analgesia or GA. They are ideal for women with a ↑ difficult airway or symptomatic chest disease. They reduce the BP, which is beneficial to some cardiac conditions.

Their use is associated with an increased risk of instrumental delivery (Ia).

Discontinuation of the epidural before the second stage may allow women to feel the urge to push but there is no evidence to suggest it improves outcome or prevents instrumental births. In fact, it is only associated with inadequate pain relief (Ia).

Risks include side effects of the drugs, missed segment (10%), neurological damage, motor block and paralysis, dural tap (1%) (see Box 9.5), and accidental intravascular injection resulting in metallic taste, tinnitus, convulsions, or arrest.

There is a lower risk of hypotension with the recent low-dose local agents than in the past (Ia) and therefore preloading with IV fluids is not necessary.

Contraindications to epidural analgesia are shown in Box 9.6.

Spinal analgesia
Spinal analgesia is performed with a 24–27 gauge needle at L2–L5. A hyperbaric or isobaric local anaesthetic is used. Bupivacaine or lignocaine, with or without narcotics, is injected.

It is easy and fast compared to epidural and does not miss segments.

Disadvantages:
- Limited time span (2 h), unpredictable height of block, motor block necessary
- Unsuitable if woman has spina bifida cystica or abnormal neurological symptoms or findings (use epidural above lesion)
- Similar risks to epidural, but hypotension and fetal distress are more common

Combined spinal and epidural
This is performed with a needle-through-needle technique.

It provides faster relief than epidural and maintains the ability to prolong analgesia. It also increases maternal satisfaction. Besides an increase in incidence of itch, there is no difference in any other outcomes (Ia).

General anaesthesia
GA involves antacid prophylaxis, preoxygenation, induction with inhalational or intravenous agents, muscle relaxation, maintenance, and reversal of relaxation.

It is used when other techniques are rejected by the woman, contraindicated or have failed. It is very useful for when women are hypovolaemic or when a delivery must be undertaken with the minimum delay (e.g. category 1 CS).

It is fast and causes less hypotension than regional anaesthesia.

Experience, however, is necessary and all pregnant women are high risk for complications: aspiration, deep vein thrombosis (DVT), ileus, uterine relaxation and haemorrhage, anaphylaxis, and death.

The partner cannot be present, but this reduces psychological pressure on staff.

Good practice points
- Women with significant risk factors should be assessed by an anaesthetist prior to, or at the onset of, labour
- Women must be involved in decisions about analgesia in labour
- There should be clear verbal communication between professionals regarding the degree of emergency
- Have a low threshold for calling senior or expert help
- In emergencies, epidurals can be topped-up in the room but never initiated. Repeated attempts for a spinal anaesthetic should be avoided
- Meticulous record-keeping is essential

Useful tips
- Most operative deliveries can be performed without GA
- Asphyxia increases the placental transfer of drugs. If a CS category 1 under GA is performed, rapid-sequence induction should be started only after the Foley's catheter has been inserted and the surgeon is ready for knife-to-skin, to minimize the fetal exposure to anaesthetic drugs
- Adrenaline can and should be used for anaphylaxis and shock in pregnancy
- Women with an epidural should have continuous monitoring. It is a common mistake to discontinue the monitoring whilst the epidural is being sited. Fetal distress can go undetected during this period
- In severe fetal distress, use *in utero* resuscitation (IV fluids, stop oxytocin, left lateral position, terbutaline 0.25 mg SC) to buy time for a regional anaesthetic

Further reading

Guidelines for Obstetric Anaesthesia Services, 1998. London: Association of Anaesthetists of Great Britain and Ireland and Obstetric Anaesthetists' Association. www.aagbi.org.uk

Confidential Enquiry into Stillbirths and Deaths in Infancy. 7th Annual Report. London: CESDI, 1999. www.cemach.org.uk

Confidential Enquiry into Maternal Death. Saving women's lives, 2003–2005. London:CEMACH, 2007. www.cemach.org.uk

> **Box 9.5 Dural tap**
> - Incidence 1–3%
> - Accidental dural puncture with a large needle
> - Manifests with severe 'spinal' headache, worse on standing, thought to be caused by lower volume of cerebrospinal fluid (CSF)
> - Treatment consists of analgesics, fluids, and caffeine
> - If the symptoms do not resolve within 3–5 days, an autologous blood patch should be used
> - Up to 20 ml venesected maternal blood is injected into the epidural space at the original site
> - Works like a plug to prevent CSF leakage, relieve the headache, and allow the dural hole to heal
> - Success rate 75–90%

> **Box 9.6 Contraindications to the use of epidural analgesia**
> - Maternal refusal or inability to cooperate
> - Lack of trained staff to monitor woman
> - Local site sepsis—in pyrexia give antibiotics first
> - Proven or suspected bacteraemia
> - Bleeding disorders:
>   - Thrombocytopenia—platelet count below 80–100 × 10^6/dl
>   - Anticoagulated women are suitable if low molecular weight heparin was given more than 12 h before
> - Cardiovascular instability owing to haemorrhage or hypovolaemia
> - Fixed cardiac output (e.g. hypertrophic cardiomyopathy, aortic stenosis)
> - Intracranial hypertension
>
> Cautions:
> - The use of aspirin is not a contraindication
> - Women with HIV—epidural is safe, use standard precautions
> - Back pain—can be used with proper positioning but may become a medicolegal issue if the pain deteriorates after the epidural
> - Back surgery—avoid the scar; the block may be patchy
> - Spina bifida—an epidural can be inserted above the lesion

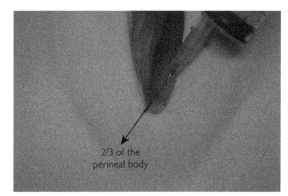

Fig. 9.3 Mediolateral perineal infiltration.

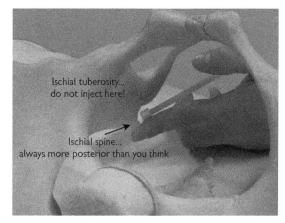

Fig. 9.4 Pudendal block. The anaesthetic is injected anteriorly to the ischial spine, in the area where the pudendal nerve re-enters the pelvis through the lesser sciatic foramen.

9.4 Poor labour progress

Incidence

In the National Sentinel Caesarean Section Audit, failure to progress (FTP) was the primary indication for CS in 35% of women with term cephalic pregnancy and no uterine scar. For 17% of these, dilatation at the time of CS was <4 cm whereas 25% of women were fully dilated.

In 1 in 4 women, augmentation was not attempted before reverting to a CS. These cases contributed 3.2% to the overall CS rate.

The management of labour progress is an essential component of intrapartum care and carries significant implications for women's satisfaction and cost.

Types of delay in progress

Latent phase delay is difficult to define. Diagnosing labour using pre-defined criteria can help to reduce the perceived incidence of such delays.

If the criteria are not met, the woman can be reassured that very early labour can last 2–3 days or stop, and be sent home.

If the criteria are met, and the cervix is not fully effaced and 3–4 cm dilated after 8 h, action must be taken.

Adequate sedation or pain relief are paramount in keeping women in either category satisfied.

Delay in the first stage consists of dilatation of <0.5–1 cm/h or crossing the 4-h partogram line.

Delay in the second stage—even though traditional approaches advocated limiting the duration of the second stage to <1 h, current practice is to allow up to 2 h for parous women or even 3 h for nulliparas, particularly when an epidural has been used.

Obstruction is suspected when there is arrest of cervical dilatation and descent of the presenting part. It is frequently combined with a large caput, excessive moulding, oedematous cervix and vulva, ballooning of lower uterine segment, formation of a retraction ring, and maternal or fetal distress.

Partogram

On a partogram, cervical dilatation and descent of the presenting part are plotted against time (see Figure 9.5).

The partogram should include an alert and action line:
- Alert line is set at a rate of 1 cm/h
- Action line is drawn 4 h right of the alert line

It is derived from a curve (Friedman's) that describes normal labour, using observational data from 100 primigravid women at term in spontaneous labour (98 singleton cephalic, one breech and one multiple pregnancy).

Graphs of dilatation versus time, or progress of labour, were produced, and resulted in a sigmoid curve with average progress during the active phase of 1.1 cm/h.

The average length of labour was 12 h for nulliparas and 6 h for parous women.

A 1999 study by Albers measured the length of labour in women who had not received oxytocin or epidurals, and reported that the active first stage was 7.7 h for nulliparas and 5.6 h for parous (upper statistical limits of two standard deviations (SD) from the mean = 17.5 and 13.8 h, respectively).

The mean length of the second stage was 54 min for nulliparas and 18 min for parous (upper statistical limits of two SDs from the mean = 146 and 64 min, respectively).

Variables associated with longer labours were electronic fetal monitoring (perhaps as a result of decreased mobility), maternal age >30 years, and narcotic analgesia.

Morbidity was not increased in longer labours.

Other studies have shown the fifth centile for cervical dilatation is 0.5 cm/h in both nulliparas and parous women.

Contributing factors

- **Age, obesity and first labour** are associated with less efficient contractions
- **Analgesia**—the use of epidurals may be responsible for delays if used in the latent phase, potentially by abolishing the Ferguson reflex (uterine activity in response to head descent). It can also prolong the second stage by affecting the tone of the pelvic musculature and the maternal urge to push. It is controversial whether it affects the active first stage; it can enhance uterine activity by reducing stress and therefore the release of maternal adrenaline (uterine musculature possesses beta-adrenergic receptors that inhibit contractions)
- **Maternal infection** is associated with slow labours, though it is difficult to establish cause and effect
- **Hypotonic contractions** may be the result of inherent defects (deficient oxytocin receptors), or more commonly, the result of stress or malposition
- **Malpositions or malpresentations** (see Section 9.10)
- **Cephalopelvic disproportion** (CPD) exists when the maternal pelvis is not of a sufficient size or shape to accommodate passage of the fetus. It can be absolute (rare), in which case a CS is necessary, or more frequently, relative when there is a malposition. It can result in obstruction. Since clinical and X-ray pelvimetry are not predictive, CPD is a diagnosis of exclusion
- **Fetal developmental abnormalities**—a large abdomen (hernias, ascites, organomegaly, megacystis) or hydrocephalus can lead to dystocia

Prevention

Interventions that decrease the risk of poor progress include:
- Education of all healthcare professionals about managing labour progress according to the available evidence
- Restrictive induction policy according to strict predetermined criteria
- Diagnosing labour using predefined criteria
- Avoiding arbitrary limits on the duration of either the latent or the active stage
- Water and home birth for low-risk women
- Encouraging the presence and support by a non-professional birthing partner ('doula')
- Selective oxytocin augmentation—may decrease the CS rates for 'failure to progress'
- Correction of malpositions (see Section 9.10)
- Acupuncture—may be beneficial but further research is necessary

Controversial strategies include:
- Routine active management of labour (see Box 9.7)—may shorten labour but does not decrease CS rates
- Routine amniotomy—may shorten labour by 30–120 min but can lead to intervention for fetal distress

Management of poor progress
(see Box 9.8)

Transfer to obstetric-led care
- **Treat any precipitating or causative factors**—give antibiotics if there are signs of infection. Treat any hypertony, empty the bladder
- **Expectant management** is still an option for cases where progress is slow but there is neither fetal distress nor evidence of CPD or obstruction, and uterine activity is of sufficient strength and regularity (3–4 contractions/10 min that last for more than 30–40 s)
- **Amniotomy** (selective) has a labour-promoting effect by releasing endogenous prostaglandins and encouraging application of the presenting part to the cervix. It has the additional benefits

of facilitating fetal monitoring by fetal scalp electrode application and assessing the amniotic fluid for quantity and colour. It carries the risk of cord compression, prolapse, and ascending infection

- **Augmentation** of labour with locally agreed oxytocin regimes should take place when the action line is crossed. In parous women, augmentation should only be decided by senior obstetricians and after obstruction has been excluded
- **CS** should be offered for FTP, but only after adequate uterine activity has been achieved for at least 2–4h. Ideally, the same observer should perform the vaginal examination before such a decision
- **Instrumental delivery** should be offered for delays in the second stage (see Section 9.12)
- Women should be involved in the decision-making process and their desires taken into account

Formal recommendations

Formal assessment programmes can be used to diagnose active labour (**A**).

Routine active management or early amniotomy should not be offered outside research studies (**A**).

The routine use of oxytocin infusion to shorten labour needs to be further researched. When such infusions are used for induction or augmentation, administration should be by trained personnel using electronic infusion pumps.

A partogram with a 4-h action line should be used as it decreases the need for vaginal examinations, oxytocin infusions, and CS rate without compromising the maternal or neonatal outcome (**A**).

Useful tips

- When used in the first stage, allow oxytocin time to have an effect. It usually takes 1–2 h for regular contractions to establish. Another 2 h are needed to assess progress. This means that vaginal examination should be planned for 3–4 h later after oxytocin use
- Contractions are best assessed by palpation, not by looking at the CTG (external transducers)
- Do spend a few minutes with the woman before making decisions that will affect her for the rest of her life
- Progress in labour is not only cervical dilatation. If there is clear evidence of descent and rotation in a single observation period, it is difficult to justify a CS for FTP even if the cervix has not dilated further. An expectant approach with reassessment in 2 h is usually better
- Intervention does not always mean, 'Get ready with your oxytocin, forceps or knife'. It means assessing and treating the causative factors in a stepwise manner while eliciting the desires of the parents
- Oxytocin infusions can be advanced much more quickly in the second stage
- A partogram of >1 page may well become a medicolegal case

Further reading

Albers LL. The duration of labor in healthy women. *Journal of Perinatology* 1999; **19**:114–19.

Friedman EA. The graphic analysis of labour. American Journal of Obstetrics and Gynecology 1954; **68**:1568–75.

O'Driscoll K, Jackson RJ, Gallagher JT. Prevention of prolonged labour. *British Medical Journal* 1969; **4**:477–80.

Thomas J, Paranjothy S. Clinical Effectiveness Support Unit. National Sentinel Caesarean Section Audit Report. RCOG, 2001. www.rcog.org.uk

www.who.int/reproductive-health Unsatisfactory progress in labour.

Assisted vaginal delivery. In: *ALSO provider manual*. ALSO (UK), 2000.

National Collaborative Centre for Women's and Children's Health. Intrapartum care: care of healthy women and their babies during childbirth NICE guideline, London, NCC-WC; 2007

> **Box 9.8 Time-keeping**
>
> Consider intervention when:
> - The latent phase is >8 h despite augmentation
> - Cervical dilatation proceeds at a rate of <0.5–1 cm/h
> - The partogram's 4-h action line is crossed
> - There has been no change in cervical dilatation or fetal descent despite 2 h of adequate uterine activity
> - Second stage has lasted for more than 2 h in parous or 3 h in nulliparas
> - Active labour has lasted for more than 12 h

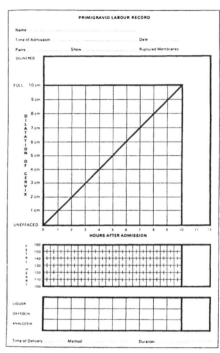

Fig. 9.5 This graph shows the simple Dublin partogram ('simple' because it does not show 'latent' phase of labour). It has a steep *x:y* gradient of ratio 1:1. Less steep ratios (e.g. 2:1) may prevent premature intervention, as does inclusion of the 'latent' phase on the partogram. Reproduced from Collier J, Longmore M, Brinsden M. *Oxford Handbook of Clinical Specialties*, published by Oxford University Press, 2006.

> **Box 9.7 Active management of labour (O'Driscoll)**
>
> This includes:
> - Accurate diagnosis of labour
> - One-to-one care
> - Frequent examinations to assess progress
> - Action for slow progress
>
> Active management may shorten labour but does not decrease the risk of CS for failure to progress.

9.5 Induction of labour

Definition
Induction of labour (IOL) is the artificial initiation of uterine contractions before their spontaneous onset, at a gestational age associated with a viable fetus >23–24 weeks (see recent Nuffield guidance). The expected outcome is cervical effacement and dilatation and eventually delivery of the fetus.

Indications for induction of labour
Any condition needing early delivery for maternal or fetal benefit where the vaginal route is deemed appropriate. Decisions are made on an individual basis. Reasons include the following:

Deteriorating maternal health
- Cardiac, renal, malignant, or autoimmune diseases

Obstetric conditions
- Pre-eclampsia
- Fetal growth restriction (FGR)
- Obstetric cholestasis (still debatable)
- Red cell isoimmunization
- Prelabour rupture of membranes at term
- Prolonged preterm ruptured membranes
- Suspected chorioamnionitis
- Marginal bleeding at term
- Unstable lie, after external cephalic version (ECV) and stabilization
- Prolonged pregnancy

Fetal conditions
- Anomaly requiring immediate treatment, e.g. cardiac
- In utero demise (IUD)
- Planned neonatal surgery, e.g. diaphragmatic hernia

For further indications for IOL see Box 9.9.

Special circumstances
Breech
There is little evidence and the risks cannot be quantified from the available trial literature. Successful ECV avoids dilemmas.

Previous uterine scar (e.g. Caesarean section)
The risk of uterine rupture in women with a previous scar is increased, and is as high as 1–2% when prostaglandins are used.

Women need to be informed of the potential risks and should participate in the decision-making. IOL is not contraindicated but a careful senior assessment should be made.

High parity
Potential risks in women of high parity include a higher rate of CS and a potentially increased risk of uterine rupture.

Methods for induction of labour
Membrane 'stretch and sweep'
Involves a digital vaginal examination (VE) and stretching of the cervix to reach the internal os and perform a cyclical 'sweeping' 360° motion. It acts by releasing local prostaglandins.

It does not increase the risk of maternal or neonatal infection but may cause discomfort and bleeding (A).

Membrane sweeping is not beneficial when routinely used before term but it can decrease the need for more formal methods when used beyond term (>40 weeks) (A).

Vaginal prostaglandin (PGE₂, Prostin)
Prostaglandins should be used in preference to oxytocin when induction of labour is undertaken in either nulliparous or parous women with intact membranes, regardless of their cervical favourability (A).

Vaginal tablets should be considered in preference to gel as they are cheaper and clinically equally effective (A).

Other routes (intravenous, oral, extra-amniotic, intracervical) are associated with an increased risk of side effects without any benefit in effectiveness.

Regimens for vaginal prostanglandins
Tablets—3 mg 6–8-hourly up to two (and occasionally three) doses.

Gel—2 mg in nulliparas with an unfavourable cervix (Bishop's score <4). For all other women, 1 mg. In both, a second dose of 1–2 mg can be administered 6 h later.

Artificial rupture of membranes (ARM)
Alone, it has no proven value for IOL. It is a prerequisite for the use of oxytocin. It will sometimes induce labour, especially in a parous woman with a favourable cervix.

Oxytocin (Syntocinon®)
In women who have rupture of membranes (ROM), either prostaglandins or oxytocin may be used for induction of labour, regardless of cervical status, as they are equally effective (A).

As women with ROM have a risk of chorioamnionitis, it is usual to administer one PGE₂ tablet only if the cervix is unfavourable, and then to proceed with oxytocin infusion.

Oxytocin should not be started for 6 h following administration of vaginal prostaglandins.

Oxytocin regimens are described in Table 9.3. It is best practice to use low-volume regimens (3 iu in 50 ml of normal saline) through an electrical pump, to avoid accidental overdose. The minimum dose possible of oxytocin should be used and titrated against uterine contractions, aiming for a maximum of 3 or 4 contractions every 10 min.

Other methods
- **Mechanical methods**—(laminaria tents, balloon catheters) are used to stretch the cervix and the membranes, and may prevent a CS when the other methods fail. Catheters can be passed through the cervix, blown up, and left for 24 h, and are particularly helpful when prostaglandins are avoided but there is an unripe cervix (e.g. vaginal birth after CS (VBAC))
- **Misoprostol**—can be given orally, sublingually, or vaginally, usually in doses of 25–50 μg. It is very effective, cheap, and stable but has a risk of uterine hyperstimulation and potentially rupture. Though widely used in the developing world, its use in developed countries cannot be recommended yet
- **Mifepristone**—potentially effective but not enough evidence yet
- **Acupuncture, homeopathy**—rigorous evaluation is lacking
- **Castor oil** causes nausea without any clear benefit
- **Baths, enemas**—there is no evidence to support use
- **Sexual intercourse**—the evidence is conflicting
- **Breast stimulation** may decrease the need for IOL and risk of postpartum haemorrhage (PPH). Not recommended for high-risk women as it has been associated with perinatal death
- **Intracervical hyaluronidase** is effective but invasive, and women's views have not been adequately explored yet
- **Relaxin, corticosteroids, and oestrogens**—not enough evidence yet to support their use

Box 9.9 Established indications for IOL

- Prelabour ROM at term—should be offered a choice of immediate IOL or after a maximum 96 h (**A**)
- Diabetes in pregnancy, at 38–39 weeks (**C**)
- Prolonged pregnancy >41 weeks' gestation as determined by an early pregnancy dating scan (**A**)
- Other conditions needing early delivery (e.g. pre-eclampsia)

Controversial indications for IOL

- Maternal request <41 weeks—where resources allow, IOL should be considered with compelling psychological or social reasons and a favourable cervix
- Multiple pregnancy—no definite conclusions can be drawn from the evidence. Perinatal mortality in twins is increased at term so IOL <40 weeks is reasonable
- Macrosomia without diabetes—there may be a potential decrease in shoulder dystocia and associated injuries with IOL <40 weeks. The evidence is inconclusive
- History of precipitate labour—in theory, IOL may avoid an out-of-hospital delivery. However, there is no evidence of any benefit in maternal or neonatal morbidity

The induction process

Decision and setting

- The woman needs to be involved in the decision and her wishes respected. Every effort should be made to ensure she is aware of the process, risks, and benefits involved
- For low-risk women, IOL can be conducted in outpatient or antenatal settings until active labour
- Where risk factors exist, IOL should occur in labour ward, e.g. suspected growth restriction, previous CS

Fetal monitoring

Fetal wellbeing should be established:

- Before induction (admission CTG for 30 min)
- After every intervention
- Intermittently thereafter
- Continuously once contractions start or with oxytocin

Induction protocol

- A VE is performed to assess the modified Bishop's score (see Table 9.4) as an indication of cervical favourability. A score of >8 is associated with ability to proceed to ARM
- In most cases, one dose of PGE$_2$ tablet or gel is given and a CTG performed again
- A further one dose of PGE$_2$ is given if necessary
- When it is possible to proceed to ARM, the woman is transferred to labour ward, if not already there
- Oxytocin infusion is started immediately after the ARM or 2–4 h later (in parous women) unless effective spontaneous contractions are present
- Continuous fetal monitoring thereafter

Risks

Failure of IOL—i.e. the cervix may not demonstrate changes sufficient for an ARM ('failed induction'). Later in labour, failure to progress (FTP) may occur. The earlier an IOL is performed, the higher the risk of CS for 'failed induction' or 'failure to progress'.

Uterine hyperstimulation—in such cases, oxytocin infusions should be stopped and no further induction agents should be given. A tocolytic (e.g. terbutaline 0.25 mg SC, one or two doses 15 min apart) should be given if there is any suspected fetal distress (see Section 9.9).

Fluid retention and hyponatraemia may occur with prolonged high-dose oxytocin infusions. Use of a syringe pump with a low-volume regimen (e.g. 3 iu in 50 ml of saline) is strongly advocated as it minimizes this risk.

Abruption and cord prolapse are associated with ARM, particularly where there is polyhydramnios.

Uterine rupture, especially high-order parity or uterine scar.

Atonic uterus and PPH are more common.

Useful tips

- Always explain the process of IOL in advance. Delivery may not occur for a couple of days. This avoids a common complaint, that labour was perceived as protracted and terrifying without warning
- Always re-check presentation in prolonged IOL with unengaged presenting part as it may be undiagnosed breech

Further reading

Bishop EH. Pelvic scoring for elective induction. *Obstetrics and Gynecology* 1964; **2(24):** 266–8.

Calder AA, Embrey MP, Hillier K. Extra-amniotic prostaglandin E2 for the induction of labour at term. *Journal of Obstetrics and Gynaecology of the British Commonwealth* 1974; **81:**39–46.

NICE. Induction of Labour. Evidence-based Clinical Guideline No. 9. Clinical Effectiveness Support Unit. Commissioned by the Department of Health and the National Institute for Clinical Excellence. London: RCOG Press, 2001 and 2008. www.rcog.org or www.nice.org

Nuffield Council on Bioethics. *Critical care decisions in fetal and neonatal medicine: ethical issues.* Latimer Trend and Company Ltd, Plymouth, 2006. www.nuffieldbioethics.org

Table 9.3 Oxytocin regimens

Time from start (min)	Oxytocin dose (mu/min)	Volume infused(ml/h)		
		3 iu in 50 ml	30 iu in 500 ml	10 iu in 500 ml
0	1	1	1	3
30	2	2	2	6
60	4	4	4	12
90	8	8	8	24
120	12	12	12	36
150	16	16	16	48
180	20	20	20	60
210	24	24	24	72
240	28	28	28	84
270	32	32	32	96

Doses highlighted with grey (>20 mu/min) are above those referred to in the summary of product characteristics and can be used only after senior decision.

Table 9.4 Modified Bishop's (Calder) score

Cervical Feature	Score			
	0	1	2	3
Dilatation	0	1–2	3–4	>4
Length	>4	3–4	1–2	<1
Station	–3	–2	–1/0	+1/+2
Consistency	Firm	Medium/Average	Soft	–
Position	Posterior	Central/Anterior	–	–

9.6 Fetal monitoring

Introduction

Monitoring of the fetal heart rate (FHR) has been introduced as a way of preventing cerebral palsy and perinatal mortality, which together account for the bulk of obstetric litigation.

Fetal monitoring and problems associated with it relate to the majority of comments on substandard care in most CESDI (Confidential Enquiry into Stillbirths and Deaths in Infancy) reports.

Fetal monitoring is usually performed in two ways:
- Using structured intermittent auscultation (IA)
- By continuous cardiotocography (CTG)

Intermittent auscultation

- Intermittent auscultation (IA) consists of auscultating the FHR after a contraction for a minimum of 60 s, and at least every 15 min in the first stage or every 5 min in the second stage (**A**)
- It is performed using either a Pinard stethoscope or a portable Doppler. Waterproof devices exist. IA cannot assess baseline variability

Cardiotocography

This is a method whereupon the FHR and the intensity and frequency of contractions are recorded using external (abdominal) or internal transducers (fetal scalp electrode and intrauterine pressure catheter, the latter rarely used). Internal transducers are more accurate. Recordings are standardized: paper speed is set to 1 cm/min, sensitivity displays are 20 bpm/cm, FHR range displays should be 50–210 bpm.

In a 1999–2000 survey (8th CESDI), the average percentage of women monitored either selectively or routinely, in units employing electronic fetal monitoring (EFM), was 93%. A guideline for interpretation of the EFM trace was available in only 74%.

The main criticism of EFM is that the various methods have been introduced into clinical practice before proper evaluation. This has led to increased obstetric intervention without a concurrent improvement in the target neonatal outcomes, either proxy (Apgar) scores, cord blood gases) or absolute (perinatal mortality, cerebral palsy).

The CTG is a sensitive method of detecting intrapartum hypoxia but its specificity is suboptimal: only 50% of abnormal traces are associated with fetal acidosis. Changes in FHR occur in response to altered O_2, CO_2, $[H^+]$, and arterial pressure; the fetal heart rate is an indirect measure of fetal oxygenation and pH.

Since the absolute target outcomes have a very low prevalence (altogether <1%, with only 10% of those actually related to intrapartum events), the number of false positives is high, leading to unnecessary interventions (see Box 9.10).

Admission CTG

A CTG performed at the onset of labour or on admission.

Even though a normal admission CTG is reassuring, it is poor at predicting later fetal compromise and cannot be recommended in low-risk women on the basis of the existing evidence (**B**).

Continuous CTG

See boxes 9.10 and 9.11

Practical points to consider

It is important:
- To perform a risk assessment analysis for every woman who presents in labour, if not already done
- To limit continuous CTG to high-risk cases where the expected prevalence of adverse outcomes (perinatal mortality, cerebral palsy) is higher and the number of false positives (and unnecessary intervention) will be low (**A**)
- To monitor low-risk women only with IA conducted appropriately, but then initiate continuous CTG if FHR abnormalities or intrapartum risk factors present (**A**)
- To interpret CTG traces using evidence-based guidelines

Important indications for CTG are described in Box 9.11

EFM is only as good as the people who use it

Radiotelemetric monitoring

A radiotelemetric system for monitoring FHR and uterine contractions during labour is available. A receiver system obtains the original signals and feeds them to a conventional fetal monitor.

It is used for women who desire increased mobility in labour and can have a positive effect on the maternal response to fetal monitoring.

Future directions

ST waveform analysis

This entails using an internal scalp electrode to record and interpret fetal ECG waveform changes.

When used as an adjunct to continuous CTG, compared to CTG alone, it is associated with: (**Ia**)
- Fewer babies with severe metabolic acidosis at birth or neonatal encephalopathy
- Fewer fetal scalp samples
- No difference in CS rates, Apgar scores <7 at 5 min, admissions to special care unit

Fetal lactate scalp sampling

This technique is currently under evaluation. It has the advantage of using a smaller sample volume. Levels of 2.90–3.08 mmol/l are considered suspicious and >3.08 abnormal.

Vibroacoustic stimulation

This has been proposed as a simple, non-invasive tool for assessment of fetal wellbeing but there is not enough evidence.

Near-infrared spectroscopy

Not enough evidence.

Fetal pulse oximetry

This technique measures the O_2 saturation of fetal haemoglobin by analysing the absorption patterns of infrared light, from 2 cm dilatation onwards. An SaO_2<30% for more than 10 min signifies hypoxia. A trial demonstrated that it decreased the CS rate for fetal distress but the overall CS rate remained constant owing to an increased CS rate for failure to progress (FTP). No difference was seen for any other maternal or neonatal outcome. It has similar limitations to CTG—good sensitivity but poor specificity.

> **Box 9.10 Continuous CTG—the evidence**

Continuous CTG during labour is associated with: (Ia)
- A reduction in neonatal seizures
- No significant differences in cerebral palsy, infant mortality or other standard measures of neonatal wellbeing
- An increase in operative deliveries (CS and instrumental) by about 30% unless supplemented by the use of fetal blood sampling (FBS)

> **Box 9.11 Continuous CTG—indications**

Antenatal
- Maternal—hypertension/pre-eclampsia, diabetes, antepartum haemorrhage (APH), other medical disease
- Fetal—small fetus, prematurity, oligohydramnios, abnormal umbilical artery Doppler velocimetry, isoimmunization, multiple pregnancy

Intrapartum
- Maternal—vaginal bleeding in labour, intrauterine infection, epidural analgesia, previous CS
- Labour—prolonged membrane rupture, induction, augmentation, hypertonic uterus
- Fetal—breech presentation, meconium staining of the amniotic fluid (especially fresh or with scanty liquor), suspicious FHR on auscultation or admission CTG if performed
- Post-term pregnancy—currently debated. Some units do not routinely continuously monitor post-term pregnancies

Box 9.12 Features of fetal heart rate (FHR) traces

Term	Definition
Baseline FHR (see Figure 9.6)	The mean level of the FHR in beats per minute (bpm) when it is stable over 5–10 min
Moderate bradycardia	100–109 bpm
Moderate tachycardia	160–179 bpm
Abnormal bradycardia	<100 bpm
Abnormal tachycardia	>180 bpm
Baseline variability (see Figures 9.6 and 9.7)	The difference in bpm between the highest peak and the lowest trough of fluctuation (occurring at 3–5 cycles per min) in a 1-min segment
Accelerations (see Figure 9.6)	Transient increases in FHR of 15 bpm or more for 15 s or more
Decelerations	Transient decreases in FHR of 15 bpm or more for 15 s or more
Early (see Figure 9.8)	Uniform, repetitive, with onset and recovery that coincide with the beginning and end of a contraction
Late (see Figure 9.9)	Uniform, repetitive, with onset mid to end of the contraction, nadir more than 20 s after the peak of the contraction, and ending after the contraction. Shallow (<15 bpm) late decelerations are still significant within the context of baseline tachycardia or persistent reduced variability (<5 bpm for >40 min) and may signify chronic hypoxia. Shallow brief decelerations may also occur in normal preterm fetuses of <32 weeks
Typical variable (see Figure 9.10)	Intermittent with variable shape and/or time relationships with contractions and a rapid onset and recovery
Atypical variable (see Figure 9.10)	Variable decelerations with loss of primary or secondary rise in baseline rate, slow recovery or prolonged secondary rise in baseline, continuation of baseline at a lower level, biphasic deceleration or loss of variability
Sinusoidal pattern (see Figure 9.11)	A regular oscillation of the FHR resembling a sine wave that is smooth, lasts for at least 10 min, and has a relatively fixed period of 3–5 cycles per min, amplitude of 5–15 bpm, and absent variability. If normal variability is present, the pattern is 'pseudo-sinusoidal'

Box 9.13 Categorization of FHR features

	Baseline (bpm)	Variability bpm	Decelerations	Accelerations
R	110–160	≥5 or <5 for ≤40 min (fetal sleep)	None present	Present (2 in 20 min)
NR	100–109 161–180	<5 for ≥40 but ≤90 min	Early decelerations Typical variable decelerations with over 50% of the contractions lasting for over 90 min. Single prolonged deceleration ≤3 min	Absence of accelerations is of uncertain significance in otherwise normal CTG
A	<100 >180 Sinusoidal pattern ≥10 min	<5 for ≥90 min	Late decelerations for over 30 min Atypical variable decelerations with over 50% of contractions for over 30 min Single prolonged deceleration >3 min	

R, reassuring; NR, non-reassuring; A, abnormal.

Box 9.14 Variable (typical) decelerations—physiology

These usually represent umbilical cord compression (see Figure 9.10):

- Once the cord is compressed, the first vessel to become occluded is the vein. Venous return is decreased, hypotension ensues, and reflex tachycardia is the outcome—the first shoulder
- As compression continues, the more elastic arteries are compressed as well. Peripheral resistance increases, fetal hypertension ensues, and reflex bradycardia is the outcome—the deceleration phase
- As compression eases off, the elastic arteries are released first and the rapid outflow of blood results in hypotension and reflex tachycardia—the second shoulder
- Further decompression releases the vein, and fetal blood pressure is restored—return to baseline
- The variable shape and onset is a reflection of variable compression owing to different intensity and duration of contractions, the cause and location of compression, the length and mobility of the cord
- A compromised fetus will be less able to elicit reflex responses of the FHR to BP changes: loss of shoulders or prolonged recovery to baseline. This is why atypical features are more sinister

Variable decelerations may also represent head compression and vasovagal reflex, and are sometimes associated with occipitoposterior positions.

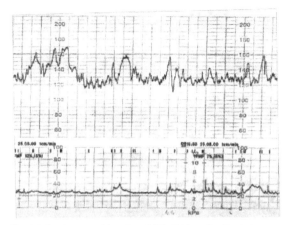

Fig. 9.6 Baseline rate. A baseline of 120–130 bpm for 10 min in a normal CTG. Variability is 10–15 bpm, and there are at several accelerations.

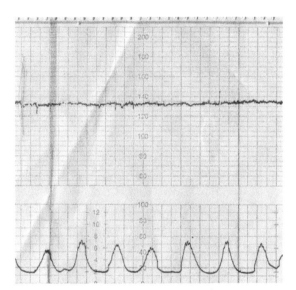

Fig. 9.7 Reduced variability. Compare with Figure 9.6.

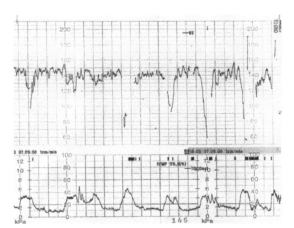

Fig. 9.8 Early decelerations. Note the peak and onset. The loss of contact indicates a need for a fetal scalp electrode to be applied.

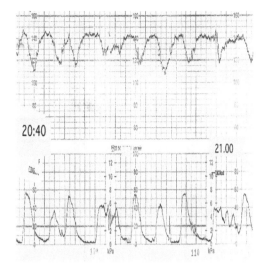

Fig. 9.9 Tachycardia and late decelerations.

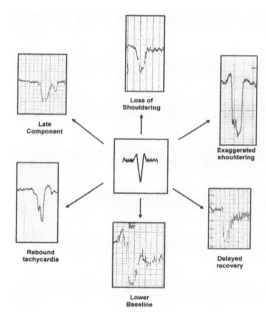

Loss of Shouldering

Late Component

Exaggerated shouldering

Rebound tachycardia

Delayed recovery

Lower Baseline

Fig. 9.10 Variable decelerations. A typical 'M'-shaped variable in the centre, with atypical features demonstrated with arrows. (Kindly provided by Ms Cathy Winter.)

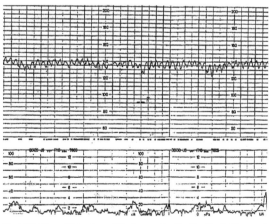

Fig. 9.11 Sinusoidal pattern. (Kindly provided by Mrs Sarah Gregson.)

9.8 Cardiotocograph interpretation

Categorization of CTG traces

- **Normal**—a CTG trace where all four features fall into the reassuring category
- **Suspicious**—when one feature falls into the non-reassuring category
- **Pathological**—when two or more features fall into the non-reassuring category or one or more falls into the abnormal category (see Figure 9.12)

Management of fetal heart rate trace categories
(See Section 9.9)
For suspicious traces, conservative measures should be used

- For pathological traces, conservative measures should be used in conjunction with fetal blood sampling (FBS) where appropriate and feasible (see Box 9.15). If FBS is not possible or appropriate, then delivery should be expedited (CS or assisted vaginal)

Further notes on interpretation

The presence of fetal heart rate (FHR) accelerations is associated with *good outcome.*

Most FHR features in isolation, with the exception of late or atypical variable decelerations, are *not good at predicting* adverse neonatal outcome:

- Uncomplicated moderate baseline tachycardia or bradycardia do not appear to be associated with poor neonatal outcome
- The predictive value of reduced baseline variability alone is unclear
- The absence of accelerations is of uncertain significance

Poor neonatal outcome is associated with:

- Repeated late, atypical variable, or prolonged decelerations
- Reduced baseline variability, if together with late or variable decelerations

Other situations

- During the second stage, a number of FHR abnormalities become more common, particularly early decelerations, but they are not associated with poor neonatal outcome unless there are other FHR features in the abnormal category
- The incidence and size of accelerations may be less at <30 weeks (i.e. <15 bpm), but then steadily increases to term
- Non-reassuring or abnormal FHR features are not only a result of hypoxia (see Box 9.14)

Documentation and risk management

The time and date need to be correctly set on electronic fetal monitoring (EFM) machines. The trace should be labelled with these and the mother's personal details.

Any event should be accompanied by an entry on the trace and the maternity notes.

CTG traces should be stored securely with the notes.

Labour wards should run regular (e.g. weekly) meetings to discuss important cases

Useful tips

- Look at the full picture and whether risk factors have been accumulating with time (progress, pyrexia, meconium)
- Fetal telemetry may be particularly useful for women with risk factors (e.g. previous CS) who are reluctant to accept continuous CTG for fear of immobilization

- Never 'eyeball' CTG traces. Unfold the whole strip. A systematic approach to interpretation is necessary
- Whether variability is normal or reduced during a deceleration is a useful sign
- It is good practice to have stickers that assist interpretation of the CTG traces. Use one every time a suspicious or pathological trace is encountered. It is common for these to follow the NICE guideline (see Figure 9.13)
- An alternative approach to CTG interpretation, particularly in units where the NICE algorithm or stickers are not available, is the ALSO mnemonic 'DR C BRAVADO' (see Box 9.17)
- It is a common mistake of junior doctors to assess a CTG without making a plan of action. The mnemonic (or the sticker) helps to remind of the importance of a plan. Sometimes the plan may just be to observe for further changes

Further reading

American Academy of Family Physicians. Advanced Life Support in Obstetrics Provider Manual, 4th edn. ALSO UK, 2000.

NICE. The Use of Electronic Fetal Monitoring. Evidence-based Clinical Guideline No. 8. Clinical Effectiveness Support Unit. Commissioned by the Department of Health and the National Institute for Clinical Excellence. London: RCOG Press, 2001. www.rcog.org.uk

The Maternal and Child Health Research Consortium. 8th Annual Report. Confidential Enquiry into Stillbirths and Deaths in Infancy. London: CESDI, 2001. www.cemach.org

Box 9.15 CTG features—differential

Bradycardia
- Post-term pregnancy
- Fetal cardiac malformations/heart block (SLE)

Prolonged deceleration
- Fetal head compression because of rapid fetal descent/cervical dilatation, vaginal examination
- Maternal hypotension, e.g. after epidural top-up or spinal

Tachycardia
- Increased fetal activity
- Prematurity
- Fetal anaemia
- Fetal cardiac disease/heart block (SLE)
- Maternal pyrexia, infection, dehydration, tachycardia
- Hyperthermia as a result of epidural

Reduced variability
- Fetal sleep (up to 40 min)
- Prematurity <32 weeks
- Drugs—opiates, ß-blockers, magnesium
- Incorrect recording sensitivity

Sinusoidal pattern
- Pseudosinusoidal—normal variability, lower frequency (1–2 cycles/min), 'saw-tooth' pattern rather than smooth wave, usually a result of fetal rhythmic movements (e.g. mouth)
- Fetal anaemia—any cause

Box 9.16 Fetal blood sampling

- Explain the procedure to the woman
- Obtain verbal consent
- Position her in left lateral position. The right leg is abducted (either by placing on a stirrup or being held by an assistant)
- Lithotomy is an alternative but may cause supine hypotension and iatrogenic fetal hypoxia
- The vulva and perineum are cleaned with antiseptic solution
- Aseptic technique is followed
- The amnioscope is inserted as posteriorly as possible and then angled anteriorly once the presenting part is encountered. Firm pressure is applied at the same time. This ensures the anterior cervix is displaced from view
- The fetal skin is dried with a swab. Ethyl chloride is sprayed on to it with the bottle held upright
- A thin uniform layer of paraffin or silicone is applied to facilitate formation of a blood droplet and help in displacing hair away from the chosen site
- A 2-mm blade is pushed against the presenting part in a firm quick motion perpendicular to the skin, avoiding areas of excessive caput
- Once a droplet has formed, a pre-heparinized capillary tube is touched on to the surface of the droplet (not the skin) and held. Avoid contact with hair or maternal fluids until at least two-thirds full
- Press on scalp at end if profuse bleeding
- Once the sample has been processed, remove the amnioscope and replace the woman's leg onto the bed

Box 9.17 DR C BRAVADO mnemonic (ALSO UK)

Determine **R**isk—maternal, pregnancy history, etc.
Contractions—frequency, intensity, regularity
Baseline **R**ate—normal, tachycardia, bradycardia
Variability—normal, reduced; for how long
Accelerations—present, absent
Decelerations—early, late, variable, atypical
Overall assessment—normal, suspicious, pathological
...and action plan: conservative, review time, FBS, delivery

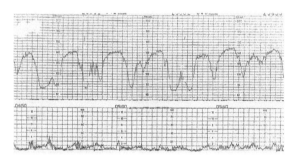

Fig. 9.12 Pathological CTG. Reduced variability and prolonged late decelerations.

CTG Sticker

	Reassuring	Non-reassuring	Abnormal	
Baseline rate (bpm)	110–160	100–109 161-180	<100 >180	Comments:-
Variability (bpm)	5 bpm or more	<5 for 40 mins or more but <90 min	<5 for 90 mins or more	Comments:-
Accelerations	Present	None	Comments:-	
Decelerations	None	Early Variable Single prolonged deceleration up to 3 mins	Atypical variable Late Single prolonged deceleration >3 mins	Comments:-
Opinion	**Normal CTG** (All four features reassuring)	**Suspicious CTG** (One non-reassuring feature)	**Pathological CTG** (two or more non-reassuring or one or more abnormal features)	
Dilatation		Cont's	:10	Liquor colour	Mat pulse	
Action						

| Date.................. | Time................. | Signature... | Status........................ |

Fig. 9.13 CTG sticker. It should contain an overall assessment and plan.

9.9 Fetal distress in labour

Introduction

Fetal distress in labour is an important contributor to perinatal morbidity and mortality. Hypoxia may develop as a result of reduced placental intervillous perfusion, oxygen transfer, or umbilical blood flow. Events leading to hypoxia cannot always be anticipated and vigilance for relevant signs is necessary.

Fetal hypoxia can lead to cerebral palsy or other neurodevelopmental disability, which account for the bulk (38%) of obstetric litigation.

The main problem is that clinical signs and CTG traces are poor predictors of a compromised fetus, and may lead to unnecessary intervention.

Presumed fetal distress is one of the most important contributors to CS rates, accounting for 40% of primary CS in the UK National Sentinel CS Audit. This equates to 15% of the overall CS rate.

Within trying to balance the identification of fetal distress and unnecessary intervention lies the importance of the diagnostic and therapeutic measures detailed here.

Outcome measures

Absolute

- **Death** from intrapartum 'asphyxia', 'anoxia' or 'trauma'. This definition covers any baby who would have survived but for some catastrophe occurring during labour. These babies will tend to be normally formed, stillborn or with poor Apgar scores, possible meconium aspiration or evidence of acidosis. Very premature infants (those <24 weeks' gestation) may be asphyxiated at birth, but are excluded
- **Cerebral palsy** (CP) is defined as non-progressive abnormal control of movement or posture of the spastic quadriplegia or dyskinetic type. The main causative factors are low birth weight and congenital malformations. Only 10% of CP cases are thought to be a result of intrapartum events and these are usually associated with abnormal CTG findings (**Ia**). The criteria for attributing CP to an acute intrapartum hypoxic event are detailed in Box 9.18
- **Neurodevelopmental disability**—any restriction of ability to perform an activity in the manner or within the range considered normal, with particular reference to difficulty in walking, sitting, hand use or head control

Intermediate (proxy)

- **Umbilical cord acid–base status**—predictive of short-term but not long-term complications
- **Apgar scores <3 at 5 min**—sensitive and predictive of long-term complications (see Section 11.8)
- **Neonatal encephalopathy**—is a syndrome of disturbed neurological function of the term infant in the first week after birth. If moderate or severe it is the most robust intermediate measure of potential long-term complications

Other

- Need for neonatal resuscitation or need for admission to special care unit—not predictive per se
- Neonatal convulsions—poor marker
- Meconium staining—poor marker
- Placental pathology—merits further investigation with rigorous studies to determine its usefulness as a predictive marker of neonatal outcome

Diagnosis of distress

Fetal monitoring

Electronic fetal monitoring (EFM) traces should be interpreted and categorized as detailed in Sections 9.7 and 9.8. The use of stickers is advised (see Figure 9.13). For pathological traces (see Figure 9.12), conservative measures (left lateral position, tocolysis) should be used in conjunction with fetal blood sampling (FBS) where appropriate or feasible.

Fetal blood sampling

FBS is a direct way of assessing the fetal pH and base excess as measures of hypoxia. It is possible to perform in at least half the cases of fetal distress. It is, however, invasive, uncomfortable for the mother, requires ruptured membranes, and a sufficiently dilated cervix (see Box 9.15).

The suggested actions are detailed in Table 9.5.

Situations where an FBS would be considered inappropriate or contraindicated are detailed in Box 9.19. In these cases, delivery should be expedited if there is suspicion of fetal distress.

Management

In utero resuscitation

- **Left lateral maternal position**—if there is a suspicion of fetal distress, the mother should be encouraged and assisted to adopt this position (**B**)
- **Stop oxytocin**—if there is a suspicion of fetal distress in the context of oxytocin use or hypercontractility, this should be managed by reducing or stopping the oxytocin infusion
- **Hydration (oral or IV)**—may alleviate changes, particularly to the FHR baseline, associated with maternal hypotension, dehydration or ketosis. Fluids containing dextrose are best avoided as they may increase lactic acidosis
- **Tocolysis**—betamimetics appear to reduce the number of FHR abnormalities and perhaps reduce uterine activity when there is fetal distress, especially with uterine hypercontractility (contractions >5 in 10 min (see Figure 9.14)

  A suggested regimen is SC terbutaline 0.25 mg, which can abolish more than 90% of fetal bradycardias (**A**)

  Prophylactic use of betamimetics during the second stage of labour increases forceps deliveries with no benefits in outcome
- **Oxygen therapy**—there is not enough evidence to support the use of prophylactic O_2 therapy for women in labour. There is a possibility that it may even be harmful (**C**)
- **Amnioinfusion**—is associated with a reduction in heavy meconium staining of the liquor, variable FHR decelerations, and reduced CS overall

  Under limited perinatal surveillance, amnioinfusion is further associated with a reduction in neonatal hypoxic ischaemic encephalopathy (HIE) and neonatal ventilation or intensive care unit admission. There is also a trend towards reduced perinatal mortality

Delivery

- In cases of suspected or confirmed acute fetal compromise that fail to respond to conservative measures, delivery should be expedited as soon as possible. The severity of the FHR abnormality and relevant maternal factors should be taken into account
- The accepted standard is that delivery should occur within 30 min, even though the evidence supporting it is weak
- Paired cord samples should be taken from the umbilical artery and vein after such deliveries. It must be noted, however, that they correlate poorly with FBS results
- If a CS is performed, women should be offered a vaginal delivery in their next pregnancy

Useful tips

- FBS in the early phase of the first stage (2–4 cm dilatation) may be difficult, but is always worth attempting
- pH can be assumed to be >7.20 if accelerations are provoked
- Positioning of the woman for FBS is important. The bed should be high and the woman as close to the right edge of the bed as possible, with her right leg lifted to provide adequate access and facilitate the procedure while minimizing the strain on the obstetrician's back
- Ethyl chloride spray both provides fetal analgesia and facilitates the sample by causing reactive skin vasodilatation after an initial vasoconstriction. Give it a few seconds to work so the vasoconstriction phase finishes
- It is good practice to perform an FBS while the oxytocin infusion is running, unless labour is expected to progress without it. If oxytocin has stopped, the FBS result may demonstrate the condition of the baby without contractions, but acute distress may ensue on restarting. If the EFM trace strongly suggests fetal compromise (e.g. prolonged deceleration), the necessary action is not an FBS with the infusion stopped but immediate delivery
- Obtaining an adequate sample can be easier if the puncture is performed during a contraction with or without fundal pressure or stabilization of the presenting part. Firm pressure on the amnioscope ensures the presenting part does not ballot away and that the sample is not contaminated with liquor, meconium or maternal blood
- Realistically, no more than three or four FBSs should be necessary throughout labour. If more, a CS should be considered
- It is important to discuss and respect the maternal preferences. Many will prefer a CS to an FBS when there is history of a previous compromised fetus or child

Further reading

MacLennan A. A template for defining a causal relation between acute intrapartum events and cerebral palsy: international consensus statement. *British Medical Journal* 1999; **319**:1054–9.

Thomas J, Paranjothy S. Royal College of Obstetricians and Gynaecologists. Clinical Effectiveness Support Unit. National Sentinel Caesarean Section Audit Report. London: RCOG Press, 2001.

Wigglesworth JS. Monitoring perinatal mortality—a pathophysiological approach. *Lancet* 1980; **ii**:684–6.

Table 9.5 FBS interpretation	
pH result	Action
≥7.25	Observe and repeat (e.g. after 60 min) if FHR abnormality persists
7.21–7.24	Repeat in 30 min *or* consider delivery if rapid fall since last sample
≤7.20	Delivery indicated

Box 9.18 Consensus criteria for defining an acute intrapartum hypoxic event

Essential
- Evidence of metabolic acidosis (pH<7.0 and base excess ≥12mmol/l) in fetal, cord or very early neonatal samples
- Early onset of moderate or severe encephalopathy in neonates of ≥34 weeks' gestation
- Cerebral palsy (spastic quadriplegic or dyskinetic)

Non-specific
- A sentinel hypoxic event occurring immediately before or during labour
- A sudden, rapid, and sustained deterioration in FHR pattern
- Apgar scores of ≤6 for >5 min (see Section 11.8)
- Early multisystem involvement
- Early imaging evidence of acute cerebral abnormality

Box 9.19 FBS is contraindicated or inappropriate

Clear evidence of acute fetal compromise
Prolonged bradycardia, cord prolapse, uterine rupture, abruption

Chorioamnionitis
The fetus may be distressed from sepsis despite a normal FBS result. Hypoxia is only a late event with chorioamnionitis, and occurs as a result of placental vasculitis

Maternal hepatitis B, C, HIV or active primary herpes
FBS should be avoided and, if performed, the risks should be discussed with the mother in advance

Fetal coagulopathy
Alloimmune thrombocytopenia, haemophilia, etc.

Prematurity <34 weeks
FBS results are difficult to interpret and the procedure carries additional risks to the fetus

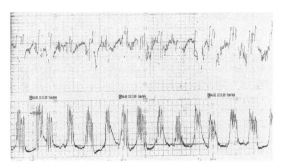

Fig. 9.14 Hypercontraction. Six or seven contractions every 10 min.

Vertex presentation (part of the head between the two fontanelles and parietal eminences) with the occiput positioned anteriorly in the pelvis (occipitoanterior—OA) is associated with the best labour outcomes.

Any other position of the occiput is termed a malposition: occipitoposterior (OP), occipitotransverse (OT). OT positions are commonly found at the initial stages of normal labour and will not be considered separately in this section. They pose problems when the fetal head is deflexed, in which case the implications and management are similar to the OP.

When any other fetal part or part of the head is presenting to the birth canal, there is a malpresentation: breech, shoulder (transverse), oblique, face, brow, compound (see also Section 8.27).

Risk factors
See Box 8.16 in Section 8.27

Incidence
The incidence at term is:
- OP—at least 5–10% by clinical diagnosis
- Breech—3%
- Shoulder (transverse lie) —0.3%
- Face—0.2%
- Compound—0.14%
- Brow—0.02%

Occipitoposterior and occipitotransverse malpositions

Malposition refers to cases where the fetal head is deflexed and the occiput positioned either transversely (OT) or posteriorly (OP) in the pelvis. The implications are similar for both situations.

OT positions occur normally at high transitory stations. The reason is that the transverse or oblique diameters are longer than the anteroposterior at the pelvic inlet (brim) (see Section 9.1). The fetal head usually engages transversely (or obliquely) and then rotates to the longer anteroposterior diameter of the pelvic outlet. Failure to do so, particularly at lower stations, comprises 'transverse arrest'.

Direct or oblique OP positions occur in one in three pregnancies at the onset of labour as determined by ultrasound studies. The majority then rotate, resulting in the clinical diagnosis of persistent OP later in labour in 5–10% of cases.

The significance is that labour may be prolonged by 1–2 h, and there is a higher risk of complicated perineal tears.

The risk of CS for failure to progress (FTP) or fetal distress is also significantly increased (variable decelerations and meconium are common).

Perinatal mortality is unaffected.

Risk factors include certain pelvic shapes (wider posteriorly) and the use of epidural at higher stations or in the latent phase.

Assuming the hands and knees or all fours posture either antenatally or in labour may decrease the incidence of malposition but needs to be further evaluated with a trial.

Diagnosis
Examination—scaphoid shape (central abdominal 'dip'), difficult to auscultate fetal heart (FH), impression of 0/5 palpable abdominally even though high vaginally, intense back pain with contractions ('back labour').

Vaginal examination (VE)—free presacral space owing to deflexion, persistent cervical lip, ears pointing downwards (towards occiput),

rotation of the examining finger by 360° encounters four suture lines (anterior fontanelle presenting).

Ultrasound—can be used to confirm the findings if there is any uncertainty and a rotational delivery is planned.

Delivery
1. **Spontaneous**—45% will deliver with expectant management but the use of oxytocin infusions, especially in nulliparas, is strongly recommended. Cephalopelvic disproportion (CPD) must be excluded first, but it must be remembered that it is usually relative rather than absolute: a result rather than cause of the malposition.

2. **Manual rotation**—the whole hand should be inserted and rotation to OA attempted using the thumb. The aim is to flex first then rotate.

   It can be tried either during contraction and pushing, or in between with slight upwards displacement of the head. The risks are minimal, but cord prolapse may follow excessive displacement.

3. **Ventouse**—both application and traction should be far more posterior (see Section 9.13).

4. **Direct traction forceps**—Neville–Barnes or similar can be used (see Section 9.13). Without an axis traction piece, Pajot's manoeuvre is essential (traction on the handle is made by the right hand while the left pulls or pushes downward on the shank). There is a high risk of complicated perineal tears.

5. **Kiellands**—can be used to rotate to OA first. This is only to be undertaken by experienced operators in carefully selected cases. The force applied is minimal (see Section 9.13)

6. **CS**—necessary if the vertex is not engaged or all other fails

Similar delivery options apply to OT positions.

Shoulder presentation

- This is usually a result of a transverse or unstable lie antenatally (see Section 8.27)
- It poses the risk of cord or hand prolapse. If neglected (developing countries), a retraction ring may form and maternal and fetal death may ensue as a result of uterine rupture

Diagnosis
- Abdominal examination and VE
- Ultrasound

Management

External cephalic version See Section 8.28.
- External cephalic version (ECV) is possible if the membranes are intact, not in active labour, and with tocolysis

Caesarean section
- A lower segment transverse incision with intraoperative version is usually performed. There is a high (25%) risk of uterine incision extension
- A vertical incision may be necessary if the fetus is back down or a poorly developed lower segment. In most cases it can be avoided

Stabilization and induction of labour
- ECV then artificial rupture of membranes (ARM) and oxytocin infusion if the cervix is favourable and >39 weeks' gestation (this gestation represents a balance between risks of labour starting with unstable lie versus risk of neonatal respiratory morbidity)

Face presentation

- Facial structures present to the birth canal as a result of hyper-extension of the neck
- It can be difficult to differentiate from breech presentation
- The denominator is the jaw ('mentum') and the relevant positions are mentoanterior or mentoposterior

Management

- Vaginal delivery can occur only if mentoanterior (see Figure 9.15) or if mentoposterior rotates early in labour
- Oxytocin infusion can be used to increase flexion
- Forceps can be used but with extra care to ensure that the head is engaged with abdominal examination
- Ventouse, fetal scalp electrode (FSE), or fetal blood sampling (FBS) are contraindicated as they may result in facial injury
- A large episiotomy may be beneficial
- A CS is necessary if persistent mentoposterior, not engaged, or all else fails
- After birth, there is considerable facial oedema and bruising

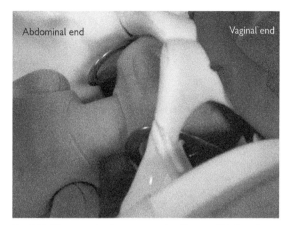

Fig. 9.15 Mentoanterior face presentation. The mandible is underneath the symphysis pubis. Here, forceps are used.

Brow presentation

- This describes a very deflexed head, where the presenting part is the area between the orbital ridges and the anterior fontanelle (see Figure 9.16)
- It is an unstable presentation and frequently only a transitory phase converting to vertex or face

Delivery

- The principles are similar to face presentation
- Usually needs CS if still brow at the level of the spines
- May deliver vaginally if small/premature fetus, particularly in parous women with an adequate pelvis

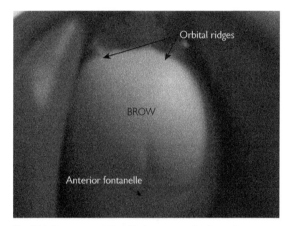

Fig. 9.16 Brow presentation. Oedema may make diagnosis difficult, as in face.

Compound presentation

- The term describes the occurrence of a prolapsed arm alongside the presenting part, usually the head
- The arm can be left alone or gently pushed back
- Care should be taken with delivery to avoid extensive perineal tears
- CS should be performed for obstetric reasons only

Breech presentation

See Sections 8.27 and 9.11.

Further reading

Akmal S, Kametas N, Tsoi E, Howard R, Nicolaides KH. Ultrasonographic occiput position in early labour in the prediction of caesarean section. *British Journal of Obstetrics and Gynaecology* 2004; **111(6):**532–6.

Lieberman E, Davidson K, Lee-Parritz A, Shearer E. Changes in fetal position during labor and their association with epidural analgesia. *Obstetrics and Gynecology* 2005; **105(5 Pt 1):**974–82.

See also Section 8.27.

Delivery options

Vaginal breech delivery

- Full consultation with the mother should occur
- Induction of labour and judicious use of oxytocics are not contraindicated, but extreme caution is advisable
- Epidural analgesia is often recommended, but is not essential and may adversely interfere with maternal effort and pushing
- An episiotomy is best performed when the posterior buttock is delivering
- A paediatrician should be present at delivery and the neonate's hips need to be checked postnatally

Criteria for selection:

- Normal fetal growth >2 kg, and estimated fetal weight <4kg
- Frank or complete breech
- Clinically adequate pelvis (on vaginal examination)
- Presence of experienced attendant

Spontaneous breech delivery

This occurs predominantly in very preterm deliveries. Pushing is avoided until the breech has reached the pelvic floor. No traction or manipulation is used and the baby is only held if necessary to keep the back upright and avoid falling.

Assisted breech delivery or partial extraction

The fetus delivers spontaneously up to the umbilicus and manoeuvres are then taken to assist delivery of the rest of the body:

- Maintain the sacrum anteriorly with hands grasping bony prominences only (the sacroiliac joints and the anterior iliac spines; see Figure 9.17), avoiding the soft abdomen (risk of organ rupture)
- If the legs do not deliver spontaneously, hook them anteriorly with the index finger to flex and deliver effortlessly
- Rotate the body 90–180° to deliver the shoulders once the scapula is visible (Lovsett's manoeuvre). The arms can be delivered in a similar manner to the legs
- Mauriceau–Smellie–Veit (MSV) manoeuvre (see Figure 9.18)—once the occiput is visible, place two fingers of the non-dominant hand on the malar prominences only, the other hand hooks neck and shoulders while the middle finger flexes the occiput. Suprapubic pressure can be used to increase flexion. The fetal body rests on the palm and forearm, and gentle downward traction and elevation is applied
- Forceps can be used for the aftercoming head (see Figure 9.19), especially if undelivered after 2–3 min. Kiellands or long forceps (e.g. Neville–Barnes) are best used, with the handles inserted from below before downwards traction is applied
- Lifting the ankles and the body against the maternal abdomen may effect delivery of the head, and several manoeuvres are described (Prague, Bracht, etc.). The risk is neck hyperextension and injury, but the manoeuvre may be used when the spine is posterior

Total breech extraction

- The feet are grasped and the entire infant is extracted
- Only indicated for delivery of a second twin (may decrease the risk of acidosis)

Risks of vaginal breech delivery

- Incompletely dilated cervix and/or head not moulded, resulting in head entrapment (up to 8%)—the cervix should be incised by 3 cm at 2, 6, and 10 o'clock
- Cord prolapse—7% overall, up to 20% with footling

- Nuchal arm—trapped behind the head. Rotate by 180° towards the side where the trapped arm points (e.g. with the spine anterior, a left nuchal arm will point to the right, therefore rotation should be clockwise to the right)
- Traumatic injuries—intracranial haemorrhage, spinal cord injury, limb fractures, nerve palsies, scrotal bruising

Elective Caesarean section

The Term Breech Trial (2000) profoundly altered practice, advocating delivery of all term breech infants by CS (A; see Box 9.19).

The aim is to reduce mortality to the infant but the technique does not reduce mortality and morbidity to the mother. Head entrapment can occur at CS and experience in breech extraction is still necessary. It is performed around 39 weeks' gestation, which represents the optimal balance between fetal maturity (mainly lungs) and the risk of spontaneous labour.

The evidence-based management of preterm breech delivery cannot be extrapolated from the Term Breech Trial. There is insufficient evidence to justify CS for preterm singleton infants or term second twin (C). The rate of head entrapment in premature breech delivery is the same at vaginal and CS deliveries. However, there is a significantly better survival for preterm breech after CS (III; CESDI Project 27/28 Report), but this evidence may suffer from bias.

The 2003 National Sentinel Caesarean Section Audit (NSCSA) showed an overall 88% CS rate for breech (56% elective and 44% emergency). Disappointingly, it also showed that only one in three women having a CS for breech presentation had been offered external cephalic version (ECV) despite this being a longstanding RCOG audit standard.

Delivery counselling

Offer ECV even in labour if intact membranes . If declined or unsuccessful then:

- Inform that babies delivered by planned CS have a lower mortality and early neonatal morbidity than those delivered by planned vaginal birth (A). The number needed to treat is 100
- There is no evidence that the long-term health of the baby is influenced by the mode of delivery (A)
- Planned CS has a 30% increase in risk of serious immediate maternal complications (see Section 9.14) compared with planned vaginal birth. However, CS does not carry any additional long-term risks outside pregnancy (A)
- The long-term effects of planned CS for breech delivery on future pregnancy outcomes for mother and baby is uncertain (C)

Useful tips

- At vaginal delivery, the rule of '5' has been traditionally used—5 min for each of the three delivery stages: to umbilicus, rest of the body and shoulders, head
- An episiotomy just before delivery of the head in a breech is extremely difficult but not impossible
- At CS, extreme care should be taken to avoid fetal laceration, as the risk is high with breech. A blunt final entry (finger puncture) to the uterine cavity is advocated
- CSs are a good opportunity for obstetricians to practise and teach the manoeuvres used for breech delivery. A common problem is difficulty delivering the head because of the face becoming entrapped with maternal soft tissues (peritoneum, sheath, bladder). Gently displacing the soft tissues with two fingers, rather than attempting heroic manoeuvres, will effect delivery
- In the MSV manoeuvre, the most important action is using the middle finger of the dominant hand to increase and maintain flexion. This by itself may be all that is needed to effect delivery

Further reading

RCOG. The management of breech presentation. Clinical Green Top Guideline No.20. London: RCOG, 2001. www.rcog.org

Whyte H et al. Term Breech Trial Collaborative Group. Outcomes of children at 2 years after planned cesarean birth versus planned vaginal birth for breech presentation at term: the International Randomized Term Breech Trial. *American Journal of Obstetrics and Gynecology* 2004; **191**:864–71.

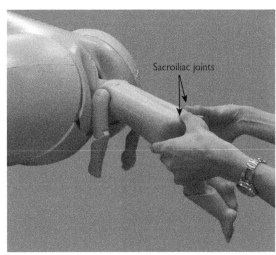

Fig. 9.17 Assisted breech delivery. The thumbs are on the sacroiliac joints, the index and middle fingers on the anterior superior iliac spines.

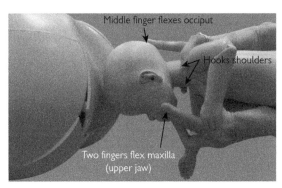

Fig. 9.18 MSV manoeuvre. This is the modified version which avoids mouth injuries.

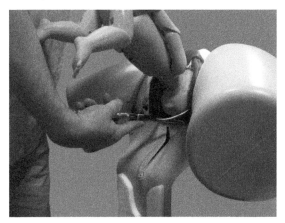

Fig. 9.19 Forceps for breech. The blades are inserted from below the head. Long forceps are essential and Kiellands are ideal. Here, application is complete and extraction is taking place.

➔ Box 9.20 Landmark research: The Term Breech Trial

Hannah ME et al. Planned caesarean section versus planned vaginal birth for breech presentation at term: a randomised multi-centre trial. Term Breech Trial Collaborative Group. *Lancet* 2000; **356**:1375–83.

Study design

2088 women with singleton frank or complete breech fetuses, at 121 centres in 26 countries were randomized to planned vaginal birth (VB) or planned Caesarean section (CS) from 38+ weeks' gestation. Both groups contained nulliparous and parous women. Randomization was stratified for parity.

Outcomes

Total breech extraction was not permitted. The trial stopped early in 2000 because interim trial analysis results showed:

- The overall risk of combined perinatal mortality or serious morbidity with planned CS was 1.6% versus 5.0% for planned VB (RR 0.33; CI 0.19–0.56, P<0.0001)
- Perinatal mortality was 0.3% (CS) versus 1.3% (VB)
- Serious neonatal morbidity was 1.4% (CS) versus 3.8% (VB)
- In countries with low perinatal mortality rate (PMR), such as the UK, neonatal morbidity for CS was even lower (0.4% versus 5.1% for VB)
- No significant difference in maternal mortality or serious morbidity was shown between the two groups

Study criticism

- The authors cite the NNT (number needed to treat), using the 'combined outcome measure', as 14 CS to one perinatal death or serious morbidity. This is misleading. Breakdown reveals that, excluding morbidity, 100 CS are necessary to prevent one perinatal death
- Insufficiently powered for maternal outcomes
- Interinstitutional variation of standard of care and varied levels of expertise of the birth attendants
- Most of the difference in perinatal outcomes is a result of the higher serious morbidity with VB in countries of low PMR (5.1% versus 0.4% with CS), with other outcomes being similar between the two groups. The difference in overall perinatal mortality is marginally statistically significant at P<0.01, and the difference in morbidity in countries with high PMR is similar in both groups (2.3% CS versus 2.5% VB)
- The emergency CS rate in the planned VB group was much higher in countries with low PMR (55.3% versus 31.7% in high PMR countries). This suggests that the difference in morbidity, likely to be linked to delivery technique, is probably not because of better expertise in low PMR countries, but due to a lower threshold for operative intervention
- Thus lost expertise may be the only factor responsible for the difference in outcomes, but the population and clinicians under study are too heterogenous for a meaningful conclusion to be reached
- Longer term follow-up (2 years) shows no difference in infant outcomes between those delivered by CS than for the VB group—the risk of death or neurodevelopmental delay was similar between the two groups (3.1% versus 2.8%)
- Overall, it is evident that vaginal delivery may not necessarily be the best current option to deliver a breech. However, if poor technique accounts for the poor outcomes, training should be the answer
- Very high rates of emergency CS and poor outcomes suggest that expertise is already lost (Working Party Report, RCOG)

Instrumental delivery rates in the UK are constant at about 10–15% (range 4–26%). The rates are a result of a variety of factors, such as current attitudes, the offer of epidural analgesia, the use of electronic fetal monitoring (EFM), and increasing litigation.

Several factors reduce the need for instrumental delivery:

- Antenatal perineal massage
- The presence of a support person (doula)
- Upright or lateral positions versus supine, or lithotomy
- Use of a 4-h partogram
- Epidural use after 3–4 cm dilatation, with reduced motor block
- Vaginal examination (VE) that establishes position early before caput or moulding
- Correction of malposition and inadequate contractions in nulliparas with oxytocin infusion
- Manual rotation of malposition at the end of first stage
- Amnioinfusion for variable decelerations
- Passive descent for 1 h if there is an epidural. Regard time to reach pelvic floor as an extension of first stage
- No time limit for second stage
- Selective use of fetal blood sampling (FBS) at the second stage
- Start pushing after 1–2 h or when there is the urge to push if the woman is a nullipara with an epidural

Box 9.20 shows the common indications for instrumental delivery.

Choice of instruments

Instrumental deliveries can be classified as:

- Midcavity—engaged at spines to +2 cm, 1/5 palpable abdominally
- Low—+2 cm or lower, visible with pushing only
- Outlet—at the pelvic floor, visible without spreading labia, <45° from midline

The choice of instruments is:

- Soft cups for uncomplicated deliveries of <45° rotation
- Metal anterior (e.g. Malstrom)—the handle is perpendicular to the cup, for difficult or oblique occipitoanterior (OA)
- Metal posterior (e.g. Bird, see Figure 9.20)—the suction tube is attached laterally to the cup to assist posterior placement, used for occipitoposterior (OP) or deflexed occipitotransverse (OT)
- Kiwi Omnicup® (see Figure 9.21)—comes in both anterior and posterior designs, the posterior can be used for any delivery
- Forceps—particularly useful for:
  - prematurity <34–36 weeks
  - specific malpresentations—face, aftercoming head in breech
  - when maternal effort is impossible or contraindicated, e.g. cardiac disease
  - excessive caput, large moulded heads and incoordinate maternal effort (but still ventouse may be safer)
  - when there has been ventouse failure but the head is crowning

The types of forceps are described in Box 9.21.

The most important factor, however, in making a choice, is the experience of the operator with the available instruments.

Assessment

History

- Previous obstetric history
- Current pregnancy—risk factors for maternal or fetal wellbeing
- Current labour—gestational age, estimated fetal weight, spontaneous/induced/augmented, progress, CTG

Vaginal examination

To assess presentation, engagement, dilatation, position, caput, and moulding.

Trial of instrumental

Performed when potential failure is anticipated, in a place where immediate recourse to CS can be undertaken, as delay to CS may be responsible for fetal injury.

Possible failure factors:

- Maternal BMI >30
- Estimated fetal weight >4 kg or clinically suspected big baby
- OP position
- Midcavity delivery

There is little evidence that CS after trial is worse than immediate CS, whereas the benefits of a vaginal delivery are significant.

Postpartum care

- Delaying cord clamping in preterm infants by 30–120 s reduces the need for transfusion and is associated with less intraventricular haemorrhage. There are no clear differences in other outcomes
- Paired cord samples
- Review for third or fourth degree tears
- Analgesia—regular paracetamol and diclofenac
- Thromboprophylaxis—reassess risk: prolonged labour, immobility, midcavity delivery are added risk factors
- Bladder care—encourage micturition every 2–3 h. Foley's catheter for at least 12 h if spinal or epidural. Postvoid residual if retention suspected. Risk factors are prolonged labour, epidural, birth weight >4 kg
- Physiotherapy—pelvic floor and abdominal exercises
- Information prior to discharge by obstetrician. Issues include indication, complications, future prognosis. Worth counselling soon after delivery and decision regarding future birth should be made early on. Vast majority should aim for SVD next time and >80% achieve it
- Midwifery-led debriefing may increase depression
- Further research required regarding timing and setting and avoidance of 'tokophobia' (morbid fear of childbirth). After operative delivery 50% of women avoid future pregnancy
- Critical incident reporting any adverse outcome—failure, SCBU admission, Apgar <7 at 5 min, pH<7.1, birth trauma

Fetal—Presumed fetal compromise

Maternal—Valsalva contraindicated

- Cardiac disease NYHA class III/IV
- Hypertensive crises
- Cerebrovascular disease
- Uncorrected vascular malformations
- Myasthenia gravis
- Spinal cord injury
- Dural tap only if headache worsens with pushing

Labour—Prolonged 2nd stage:

- Nulliparas 2 h or 3 h with epidural
- Parous 1 h or 2 h with epidural
- Maternal exhaustion / fatigue

➔ **Box 9.22 Types of forceps (see Figure 9.22)**

- **Direct traction**—Neville–Barnes, Simpson, Rhodes, Anderson: have a blade, shank, lock, and handle. Each blade has an inner cephalic curve to conform to the head and an upper pelvic one to fit to the pelvis
- **Rotational**—Kielland's do not have a pelvic curve, have a sliding lock to facilitate insertion and correction of asynclitism, and knobs that should point towards the occiput when correctly placed
- **Short**—Piper, Wrigley's are used for outlet deliveries, CS, and premature babies

◎ **Box 9.23 Prerequisites for instrumental delivery**

General

Analgesia:	Regional for midpelvis
	Pudendal for low
	Perineal for outlet
Asepsis:	Necessary
Bladder:	Empty
	Foley's removed or balloon deflated
Consent:	Explicit
Contraction:	Adequate
	Low threshold for syntocinon in nulliparas
	Rarely required in parous
Dilatation:	Fully (see exceptions in section 9.13)
Engaged:	0–1/5 palpable abdominally
Equipment and staff:	Back-up plan, neonatal resuscitation facilities, presence of paediatrician
Membranes:	Ruptured
Mother:	Informed, willing and not exhausted
Operator:	Skills, willingness to abandon, anticipation of complications
Pelvis:	Deemed adequate

Ventouse

Gestational age:	>36 weeks (insufficient evidence of safety at 34–36 weeks)
Presentation:	Vertex

Forceps

Presentation:	Vertex, face, breech

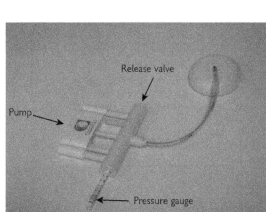

Fig. 9.20 Metal ventouse cup. The posterior cup (depicted here) is slightly smaller to facilitate manipulation.

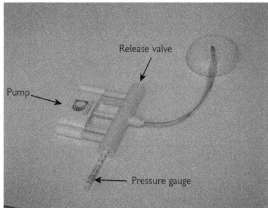

Fig. 9.21 Kiwi Omnicup®. Can be used either as a posterior cup (suction tube at the edge) or as anterior (tube perpendicular to the cup). The pressure should be at the upper limit of the green area. A check for tissue entrapment should be performed when pressure reaches the yellow line.

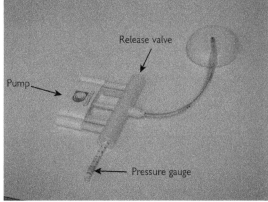
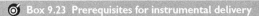

Fig. 9.22 Kiellands and Rhodes forceps. Neville–Barnes, Anderson, and Piper forceps are similar to Rhodes.

Comparison of instruments

Advantages

Ventouse

- Self-directing—need less traction and autorotation possible
- Less trauma—episiotomy, lacerations, third degree tears
- Less analgesia and less severe perineal pain at 24 h

Soft cups

- Less scalp trauma compared to rigid/metal

Forceps

- Specific indications—preterm, face, breech
- Less maternal morbidity than CS, even when rotational

Risks

Soft cups

- Higher failure rates

Ventouse

- More failure, needs proper angles and cooperation
- Minor scalp injury in 10%
- Caput, disappears in 2–3 days
- Cephalhaematoma in 10%—does not cross suture lines
- Subgaleal haemorrhage in 1–4%—weeks to disappear
- Retinal hemorrhage in 50%—transient only
- Jaundice, clinically only—no difference in phototherapy
- Maternal worries about baby's appearance—warn
- No difference:
  - CS rates
  - Apgar at 5 min, intubation
  - SCBU admissions
  - Need for phototherapy
  - Follow-up of mother and children

Forceps

- Tears—up to 75% occult third degree
- Short-term neonatal morbidity with rotational

Sequential use of both instruments

- Avoid when possible
- Risk of neonatal trauma—ICH, SCBU admissions
- Less risk than CS at full dilatation though—major postpartum haemorrhage (PPH), maternal hospital stay, SCBU admissions

Contraindications

- Not fully dilated—exceptions are second twin and severe fetal distress, e.g. cord prolapse at 8+ cms in parous woman
- Malpresentations—transverse lie, brow (may attempt ventouse with correct application)
- Fetal risks—hepatitis C (only relative), HIV, fetal coagulopathy, fetal predisposition to fracture (e.g. osteogenesis imperfecta)

Forceps technique

The forceps is held with the contralateral hand in a pencil grip, with the handle elevated towards the contralateral groin. The free hand protects the vaginal wall, and the forceps is pushed in place with only the thumb (see Figure 9.23). Once both blades are inserted, locking should be easy but does not have to be maintained throughout, only when pulling.

When correctly placed, the posterior fontanelle should not be more than one finger's distance from the level of the shanks, and the blades should be equidistant from the sagittal suture. The fenestrations should not admit more than one fingertip (see Figure 9.24). This applies similarly to malpositions, e.g. in occipitoposterior (OP), the posterior fontanelle should not be more than one finger's distance from the level of the shanks, and that is why Kiellands are always applied and held very posteriorly (almost in touch with the perineum) until rotation takes place. Otherwise, insertion should be reattempted or the delivery abandoned for a CS.

Ideally (but not necessarily, compare to ventouse), pulls should be performed with contractions. The force (Pajot's manoeuvre, see Figure 9.25) should be applied mostly perpendicular to the handle and downwards to maintain and increase flexion, whereas the actual straight pulling force should be much more controlled and subtle. The sum of these vectors will give the correct axis of traction, which is along the axis of the pelvis.

Once the posterior fontanelle is below the symphysis pubis, the handles are elevated in a 'J'. They are removed in reverse order, by sliding them along the fetal head, once the jaw has delivered.

Ventouse technique

Position

Modified lithotomy, 150° lateral tilt and wedge, top angled forward, buttocks at end of bed, woman pulling her legs, partner supporting head.

Cup insertion

Retract perineum and or labia, apply at flexion point 3 cm in front of posterior fontanelle, overlying the sagittal suture, leaving two-finger distance from anterior fontanelle.

- Outlet—apply to the most accessible portion
- Low—may need to manoeuvre laterally
- Occipitotransverse (OT)—apply posteriorly as always asynclitism and easier to manipulate at presacral space; flexion point will be more medial to the posterior fontanelle so slight lateral displacement only needed
- Occipitoposterior (OP)—apply as posteriorly as possible (11–12 cm = metacarpophalangeal joint)

Pressure

- -0.2 bar then check to ensure maternal tissue not trapped
- Then increase pressure in one step to –0.8 bar
- Gentle traction and wait 2 min, enough for chignon to form

Traction

- With contraction and maternal effort only
- Just after pushing has started, tuck elbow into your side to help prevent excessive force
- First pull always posteriorly
- Episiotomy if perineum does not allow
- Change angle when fontanelle or caput below symphysis
- Upwards when sagittal suture in AP diameter and visible
- Overall always perpendicular to the cup
- Thumb on cup, index on scalp not caput (see Figure 9.26)

Pulls

- One to train mother, especially if epidural
- Up to three for descent
- One (rarely two, especially if episiotomy not used) for the perineal phase
- Overall, usually three pulls are enough but occasionally up to five or six can be used, but only if there is progress with each one

Episiotomy

Episiotomy is performed when there is:
- Arrest at outlet
- Detachment at outlet
- Paramedian application
- Tear occurring
- Delivery requiring force

Avoid rocking motion or traction between contractions

Stop and proceed to CS
- If three detachments
- One or two pulls with no progress
- Delivery not imminent after three pulls
- 20 min from application
- 30 min from decision

Useful tips
- Be wary with head palpable in the abdomen (more reliably assessed with a bimanual in lithotomy)
- Always check your equipment before application (ventouse pump, forceps blades, resuscitation equipment)
- When the forceps do not lock, do not apply extra force but proceed to a different mode of delivery, usually CS
- The forceps do not have to be locked in between contractions. Avoiding this will reduce the risk of bruising or bradycardia during delivery

- Equally, traction is unnecessary in between contractions. Even if the head retracts, any position already gained is re-established as soon as the next contraction starts
- With proper technique, an episiotomy is not always necessary, even with forceps. The same principles should be applied as in normal deliveries
- It is good practice for the operator to take the cord blood samples for many reasons:
1. Earlier is easier as blood will not have clotted
2. Results are more accurate if taken early
3. It allows for subsequent clamp release or cord emptying as a method to expedite the third stage
4. It prevents premature traction applied to an unseparated cord—important for impatient carers
5. The arterial sample is the more difficult to obtain. It is also the one that more accurately reflects acute intrapartum events, while the venous reflects more chronic or subacute conditions
6. To assess your intrapartum care and your decision-making reliably

Further reading

RCOG. *Operative Vaginal delivery.* Clinical Greentop Guideline No. 26. Operative vaginal delivery. London: RCOG, 2005. www.rcog.org

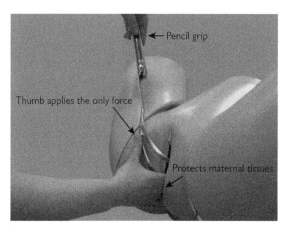

Fig. 9.23 Forceps insertion. **Left** blade with **Left** hand for **left** maternal side (and then similarly for the right side).

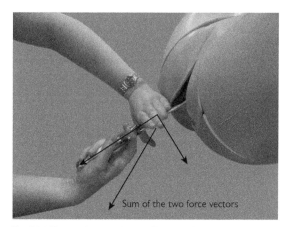

Fig. 9.25 Forceps force application. Downwards pressure is especially important with direct OP pulls or with higher OA stations.

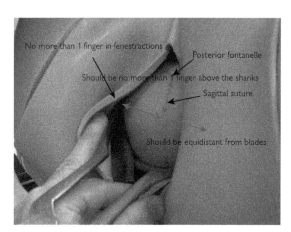

Fig. 9.24 Safe position for forceps.

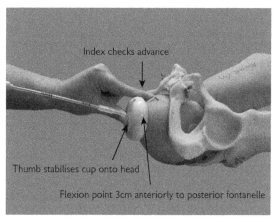

Fig. 9.26 Ventouse delivery. The index finger is used to ensure progress of the bony structures rather than just the caput.

9.14 Caesarean section

Current incidence of CS is 20–25%, whereas in the 1970s it was 10%. WHO defines a minimum acceptable rate of 2%, and an acceptable rate for a developed country as 10–15%, but this is not based on hard science. The impact on health systems is significant in terms of deskilling (e.g. breech vaginal delivery), complications, costs, and implications on fertility.

Indications and rates
Indications are shown in Box 9.23.

Factors responsible for rising CS rates
- Rising maternal age and obesity
- Rising multiple pregnancy rates (spontaneous and IVF)
- Neonatal survival at earlier gestation
- IVF—lower thresholds and higher intervention
- More women with serious medical problems (e.g. cardiac)
- Current management of breech presentation
- Increase of the previous CS rate; self-perpetuating effect
- Deskilled junior staff
- Litigation and obstetrician anxiety
- Safer CS makes it more attractive than it used to be (though vaginal delivery is also safer)
- CS on 'demand'—woman's choice, risks of instrumental delivery becoming less acceptable, media influence

No influence on likelihood of CS
- Active management of labour
- Early amniotomy
- Walking in labour
- Non-supine position during the second stage of labour
- Immersion in water during labour
- Epidural analgesia during labour
- The use of raspberry leaf

The effects of complementary therapies used during labour on CS rates (such as acupuncture, aromatherapy, hypnosis, herbal products, nutritional supplements, homeopathic remedies, and Chinese medicines) have not been properly evaluated. Further research is needed before they can be recommended.

Measures useful in reducing rates
- Educate patients, obstetricians, and midwives
- Address local intrinsic factors—wide variations
- National audits
- Home delivery, support in labour, doulas, one-to-one midwifery
- Increasing the uptake of external cephalic version (ECV)
- Increasing vaginal birth after CS (VBAC) rates
- Reliable dating
- Consultant level decisions
- Fetal blood sampling (FBS) for fetal distress
- 4-h action line partogram

Antenatal counselling and assessment
- Common indications for CS, e.g. failure to progress (FTP) or failed induction of labour (IOL)
- What the procedure involves
- Associated risks and benefits (see Box 9.24)
- Implications for future pregnancies and birth after CS

Haemoglobin assessment and correction of anaemia preoperatively is essential. Even though healthy women who have otherwise uncomplicated pregnancies should not routinely be offered a group and save (NICE), it has remained common practice.

Antacids and antiemetics should be given to reduce the risks of aspiration.

Consent for CS should be requested after providing evidence-based information in a manner that respects the woman's dignity, privacy, views, and culture whilst taking into consideration the clinical situation. Normally, consent must be written. However, in emergencies, verbal consent may be sufficient.

A competent pregnant woman is entitled to refuse a treatment such as CS, even when the treatment would clearly benefit her or her baby's health. Such a refusal and the relevant risks associated with it must be clearly documented.

Risks of CS See Box 9.24.

Timing categories
Elective (grade 4)
The risk of respiratory morbidity is increased in babies born by CS before labour, but this risk decreases significantly after 39 weeks. Therefore, planned CS should not routinely be carried out before 39 completed weeks.

Non-elective (grades 1–3)
Delivery at emergency CS for maternal or fetal compromise should be accomplished as quickly as possible, taking into account that too rapid delivery has the potential to do harm, especially psychological trauma.

Delivery within 30 min is the gold standard in cases of confirmed fetal compromise. The achievability is uncertain.

Evidence suggests that neonatal outcome is worse for very rapid deliveries (probably because the fetus is already compromised) or for CS deliveries accomplished >75 min from decision.

An urgency classification system has been devised and is now widely used (see Box 9.23) as the use of category names ('emergency', 'urgency' etc.) results in confusion.

Useful tip
To avoid confusion, the team should work to an exact time (e.g. "knife-to-skin by 11.20")

Robson classification
The need to improve information collection and to categorize women requiring CS led to the development of this classification system. It can be used to examine different indications and to compare units.

The rationale is that overall CS rates should not simply be considered too high or too low, but whether they are appropriate or not, after taking into consideration all the relevant information.

The ten ('Robson') groups are:
1. Nulliparous, >37 weeks, single, cephalic, spontaneous labour
2. Nulliparous, >37 weeks, single, cephalic, IOL or CS prelabour
3. Parous, no previous CS, >37 weeks, single, cephalic, spontaneous labour
4. Parous, no previous CS, >37 weeks, single, cephalic, IOL or CS
5. Parous, previous CS, >37 weeks, single, cephalic
6. Nulliparous, single breech
7. Parous, single breech
8. Multiple gestation, any
9. Singleton in oblique, unstable or transverse lie
10. Preterm <37 weeks single cephalic.

Further reading

Lucas DN et al. Urgency of caesarean section—a new classification. *Journal of the Royal Society of Medicine* 2000; **93**:346–350.

Robson M. Classification of caesarean sections. *Fetal and Maternal Medicine Review* 2001; **12**:23–39. Cambridge University Press.

Thomas J et al. National cross sectional survey to determine whether the decision to delivery interval is critical in emergency caesarean section. *British Medical Journal* 2004; **328**:665–7.

Box 9.24 Indications and grades of urgency

Grade	Criterion	Decision to delivery interval	Examples of indications
1	Immediate threat to life of mother or fetus	Aim to deliver within 30 min	FBS pH<7.2 and CTG remains pathological Severe fetal bradycardia of at least 3 min Cord prolapse with pathological CTG Abruption Uterine rupture Actively bleeding placenta previa
2	Distress not immediately life-threatening to mother or fetus	Aim to deliver within 30–75 min	FBS pH between 7.2 and 7.25 Suspicion of fetal distress and FBS impossible or failed
3	Needs early delivery but no maternal or fetal distress	The earliest possible at a time to suit the maternity team	Booked for CS but in labour or with spontaneous rupture of membranes Failure to progress with no fetal distress
4	Elective CS	At a time to suit the woman and the maternity team	Breech presentation at term Twins with first non-cephalic Placenta previa major Infections: 1. HIV+ve 2. Active primary genital herpes

Box 9.25 Risks of Caesarean section

Index pregnancy

- Haemorrhage and blood transfusion
- Abdominal pain
- Deep vein thrombosis
- Infection
- Bladder and ureter injury
- Hysterectomy
- Longer stay
- Reoperation, ICU admission, readmission
- Maternal mortality 3–4:10 000
  - Electives 5 times risk of vaginal delivery
  - Emergency 18 times risk of vaginal delivery
- Fetal lacerations 1–2%
- Neonatal respiratory morbidity

Risks in future pregnancies

- Delay in getting pregnant
- Future CS
- Placenta praevia (risk trebles)
- Placenta accreta (0.4%)
- Uterine rupture
- Adhesions, difficult surgery
- Possible adverse antepartum fetal effects, including stillbirth

9.15 Caesarean section—technical aspects and care

Anaesthesia for Caesarean section

In emergencies, the anaesthetist must be explicitly informed of the degree of urgency (knife-to-skin time).

Women are encouraged to have CS under regional anaesthesia because it is safer and results in less maternal and neonatal morbidity. This includes women who have a diagnosis of placenta praevia. Spinal is faster than epidural but carries a higher risk of hypotension.

Some women may still prefer a general anaesthetic (GA). This should be taken into account after counselling on the risks and benefits.

An indwelling bladder catheter is necessary.

Induction of regional anaesthesia for CS should take place in theatre because this does not increase anxiety. The partner is encouraged to attend when regional anaesthesia is used.

CS of urgency grade 1 (immediate risk to life of mother or fetus) may be under GA, but this must be justified. If a satisfactory epidural block is already established, appropriate topping-up by the anaesthetist may allow immediate operation.

GA for emergency CS should include preoxygenation, cricoid pressure, and rapid-sequence induction to reduce the risk of aspiration. The surgeon must be ready to start immediately.

Specific situations

Extreme prematurity (<28 weeks)
- A generous incision is necessary ('small baby large incision, large baby large incision, normal baby normal incision')
- A classical or vertical incision may be necessary
- Gentle technique and senior support is mandatory

Classical
- Consists of a vertical incision involving the upper segment. The DeLee modification starts from the lower segment
- It is associated with 5% prelabour rupture in subsequent pregnancies and increased postoperative pyrexia compared to transverse uterine incisions
- It may be necessary for cases involving:
  - Multiple previous CS
  - Extreme prematurity, especially breech or perimortem
  - Back down transverse lie
  - Anterior placenta praevia
  - Cervical cancer
  - Perimortem CS in premature pregnancy
  - Massive fibroids in lower segment

Occipitoposterior second stage
The uterine incision should be made higher and final entry should be digital to avoid fetal facial laceration.

Disimpaction may be necessary, either with vaginal assistance (an assistant flexing and pushing upwards) or by rotating the hand below the fetal head in a waving motion to release the vacuum before flexing and lifting it.

Breech
Digital entry to prevent fetal laceration (more common with breech), forceps or Mauriceau–Smellie–Veit (MSV) manoeuvre to flex the head; tocolysis should be ready.

Future directions
Carbetocin is a synthetic analogue of oxytocin with prolonged action, better distribution, and intensified effect that may reduce the incidence of postpartum haemorrhage (PPH) after CS.

Use of tocolysis for difficult CS needs further research.

Perimortem Caesarean section

In cases of antenatal maternal cardiac arrest, a perimortem CS should be performed. The aim is to aid maternal resuscitation by improving venous return rather than to save the baby.

Ideally, it should be performed within 5 min from the arrest. However, there is no maximum limit and there may be legitimate reasons for delay (e.g. instigating appropriate resuscitation). Babies have survived arrest for 20 min.

The availability of skilled personnel and equipment to care for mother and baby postoperatively is a prerequisite, but it does not have to be performed in an operating theatre.

The technique is 'splash and slash' and only an antiseptic, a knife, and a swab to pack the uterus is necessary. A Joel–Cohen or midline incision should be used. ALS should continue throughout.

The left lateral tilt, which is necessary for resuscitation, can be removed once the CS is performed.

Women who refuse blood
Specific precautions need to be in place for women who refuse blood transfusion, e.g. Jehovah's witnesses (see Box 9.27).

Postoperative care

Paediatric presence is not required at elective CS when all the following criteria are met:
- CS planned before onset of labour (urgency grade 4)
- Regional anaesthesia
- Term gestation (37–42 weeks)
- Within normal working hours
- No fetal disease or distress
- No severe maternal medical problems

Early skin-to-skin contact between the woman and her baby should be encouraged. Women who have had a CS should be offered additional support for breastfeeding.

After CS, women should be observed on a one-to-one basis by a properly trained member of staff until stable.

Regular analgesia for postoperative pain should be given. Providing there is no contraindication, non-steroidal anti-inflammatory drugs should be offered because they reduce the need for opioids.

Women who are recovering well can eat and drink as soon as they feel hungry or thirsty. The urinary bladder catheter should be removed once a woman is mobile.

Women who recover well should be offered early discharge after 24 h. It is not associated with readmission.

The best time to counsel women on the benefits (and risks) of vaginal birth after CS (VBAC) is immediately after a CS rather than at the next pregnancy. The indication for the CS and any other implications should be discussed.

Useful tips
- It is a common mistake to arrange CS for 38 weeks. This is associated with neonatal respiratory morbidity, and routine elective CS should be booked for 39 completed weeks
- Women should always have a plan for the event of labour in case of prematurity, even if elective CS is arranged

Box 9.26 Caesarean section—technique

- Check breech presentation with ultrasound before CS
- An indwelling bladder catheter should be sited immediately before the CS, if GA, or once regional anaesthesia is effective
- Assess thromboprophylaxis risk and instigate prophylaxis
- Accommodate woman's preferences where possible, e.g. lowering the screen to see baby born
- Follow infection control precautions. Double glove for HIV+ve
- The skin incision of choice should be transverse as it results in less postoperative pain and an improved cosmetic effect, but there is more bleeding compared to vertical incisions. A 15-cm length is usually enough (see Figure 8.27)
- Use Joel–Cohen technique if possible (straight skin incision, blunt dissection of deeper layers) as it results in shorter operating times and reduced postoperative febrile morbidity
- A lower segment incision should be used in most cases, as the risk of rupture is 0.5% (versus 2.2% with vertical)
- Blunt rather than sharp extension of the uterine incision results in less blood loss
- Forceps should only be used if there is difficulty delivering the baby's head
- Oxytocin 5 iu by slow IV injection should be administered with the anterior shoulder. The placenta should be removed using controlled cord traction and not manual removal to reduce the risk of endometritis. Spontaneous expulsion reduces blood loss
- Antibiotics (single dose) significantly reduce febrile morbidity. Both ampicillin and first generation cephalosporins have similar efficacy, with no added benefit using a broader spectrum agent (co-amoxiclav) or a multiple dose regimen
- Do not routinely exteriorize the uterus as it may increase the length of hospital stay
- The uterine incision should be sutured in two layers. The potential advantage of single-layer closure is a shorter operating time and lower incidence of infections, with similar scar strength, but further supporting evidence is necessary before routine use
- Neither the visceral nor the parietal peritoneum should be routinely sutured. Leaving the peritoneum open reduces operating time and the need for postoperative analgesia
- Close the subcutaneous tissue space ('fat stitch') if >2 cm depth of fat as it reduces the incidence of haematoma and seroma. Extremely thin patients may also benefit
- Superficial wound drains should not routinely be used because they do not decrease the incidence of wound infection or haematoma. However, most trials do not answer the question of whether wound drainage is of benefit when haemostasis is not felt to be adequate
- Subcuticular skin closure has higher patient satisfaction
- Umbilical artery gases should be performed after deliveries for suspected fetal compromise

Box 9.27 Caesarean section in women refusing blood transfusion

- Document refusal—be satisfied there is no pressure from others
- IV access, FBC, crystalloid fluids
- Consultant obstetrician to do CS
- Consultant anaesthetist, haematologist, and other senior staff aware
- Adequate incision
- Await spontaneous placental separation
- Use oxytocics sparingly
- Haemostasis should be secure
- Consider cell saver
- Rapid decision-making—lower threshold for intervention
- Early recourse to hysterectomy if there is major haemorrhage

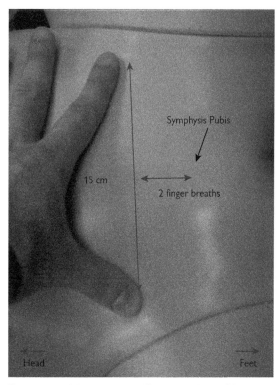

Fig. 9.27 Joel–Cohen skin incision. This is a straight line. Pfannenstiel is curved like a smile.

Further reading

Attilakos G, Psarovdakis D, Ash J et al. The haemodynamic effects of oxytocin and carbetocin following caesarean controlled trial. BJOG 2008; **115** (Suppl1): 140–1

National Collaborating Centre for Women's and Children's Health. *Caesarean section.* Commissioned by the National Institute for Clinical Excellence. London: RCOG Press, 2004. www.rcog.org.uk

Thomas J, Paranjothy S. Royal College of Obstetricians and Gynaecologists. Clinical Effectiveness Support Unit (2001). National Sentinel Caesarean Section. Audit Report. London: RCOG Press, 2001. www.rcog.org.uk

9.16 Vaginal birth after Caesarean section

Nine per cent of women in the UK have had a previous CS. There are two options in a subsequent pregnancy: planned elective repeat CS or planned vaginal birth (VBAC). They are both associated with benefits and risks. The available evidence for these is from non-randomized cohort studies only and therefore prone to bias.

In the UK, one in two women with previous CS attempts, and one in three overall achieves, a vaginal delivery. There is very wide unit variation, probably secondary to clinician preference. So long as VBAC is attempted, the rate of successful vaginal birth is about 75%. It is highest (90%) in women with only one CS and a previous vaginal delivery.

Repeat elective CS contributes to the overall CS rate by 14%. Increasing the VBAC rate is an important aspect of an effort to reduce CS rates and the self-perpetuating effect of the procedure. The USA has set a target of increasing the VBAC rate to at least 40%.

The 2003 National Sentinel Caesarean Section Audit (NSCSA) showed that 95% of women were recommended VBAC after CS for breech.

A number of complications increase with increasing number of previous CS: placenta accreta, perioperative injury to other structures, intensive care unit admission, hysterectomy, blood transfusion, and hospital stay.

Any decision should take into consideration:
- Maternal preferences and priorities
- A comprehensive and balanced discussion of the overall health risks and benefits of CS and VBAC
- Risk of uterine rupture
- Risk of perinatal mortality and morbidity

Women who choose an elective CS frequently do so because they are afraid of vaginal birth and the perceived lack of control. It is important that such fears are elicited and addressed by counselling with appropriate professionals (e.g. specialist midwives).

If the choice of planned VBAC is made, electronic fetal monitoring (EFM) during labour is necessary in the form of continuous CTG. Ambulatory EFM is an acceptable alternative that can be offered to women who desire increased mobility in labour.

Labour should be in a unit where there is ability to perform EFM, immediate access to CS, and on-site blood transfusion services.

Risks of vaginal birth after Caesarean

Compared to planned repeat elective CS, with planned VBAC some risks may be higher:
- Uterine rupture 1/150–500 versus virtually zero. The risk of maternal death is estimated <1/100 000
- Intrapartum perinatal death 1/1000–5000 (a risk comparable to the one for women in their first labour) versus 1/10 000
- Up to 1000 elective CS may be necessary to prevent one perinatal death (versus a possible downstream risk of stillbirth in future pregnancies)
- Risk of hypoxic ischaemic encephalopathy of about 1/1000. The impact on cerebral palsy risk is uncertain
- Risk of emergency CS is 20–30% but <10% if there has been a vaginal delivery after CS
- Potential need for GA, with its associated risks, with an emergency CS
- Maternal haemorrhage and infection rates are higher
- Hysterectomy, but evidence is conflicting

On the other hand, the risk of neonatal respiratory problems is decreased (2–3% versus 3–4%).

Contraindications to vaginal birth after Caesarean
- Congenital uterine abnormalities
- Prior classical J or T incision
- Prior transfundal uterine surgery
- Contracted pelvis
- Inability to perform EFM or revert to emergency CS
- Contraindications to vaginal delivery (e.g. major praevia)

Induction and vaginal birth after Caesarean
IOL can be offered but elective CS may be preferable.

Mechanical methods of cervical ripening (such as Foley's or balloon catheter) may avoid the use of prostaglandins.

In parous women it may be worth considering an artificial rupture of membranes (ARM) and waiting 24 h, e.g. in postdates pregnancy, but the possibility of using oxytocin, and the relevant risks involved, should be anticipated and discussed in advance.

The likelihood of uterine rupture is increased to:
- Between 0.8–1% with oxytocin
- Between 1–3% with prostaglandins

Macrosomia and vaginal birth after Caesarean
Successful vaginal delivery after one CS has been reported to be decreased in pregnancies complicated by macrosomia.

The success may be further decreased with:
- Previous CS for suspected cephalopelvic disproportion (CPD)
- Induction or augmentation in the current pregnancy

The risk of uterine rupture has been reported to increase.

However, the evidence is limited and there is uncertainty about the success rate and risks of VBAC in such context.

Vaginal birth after two previous Caesarean sections
Until recently, it had been common practice to advise women to have an elective CS after two previous CSs.

A rising number of women desire to try for a VBAC. It is important to elicit the woman's reasons for such a request before discussing the relevant risks and benefits, and to ask for a second opinion when the woman may be keen but the clinician not.

There is no solid evidence to support elective CS as routine practice and there is data to support VBAC. The chance of a successful vaginal delivery is in the region of 65–75%.

The usual contraindications to VBAC apply.

In the absence of reliable data, it would be unsafe to offer induction with either oxytocin or prostaglandins to women with two previous CS.

The risks are those of a VBAC in general, but major maternal morbidity is doubled versus women with one previous CS.

Tips
- Women should always have a plan for labour in case of prematurity. It is good practice if labour supervenes to discuss again the relevant risks and benefits of elective CS versus VBAC (if no contraindications). A significant proportion of women find they can cope and may alter their choice
- Elective CS should be planned for >39 weeks
- For women who are keen on VBAC, a clinic appointment should be given for 41 weeks to discuss the risks and benefits of membrane sweep and IOL. For those not keen on IOL, a CS may be arranged between 41 and 42 weeks

Further reading

Emmett C et al. On behalf of DiAMOND study group. Women's experience of decision making about mode of delivery after a previous caesarean section: the role of health professionals and information about health risks. *British Journal of Obstetrics and Gynaecology* 2006; **113:**1438–45.

RCOG. *Birth after previous caesarean birth.* Clinical Greentop Guideline No. 45. London: RCOG, 2007. www.rcog.org

9.17 Multiple pregnancy—labour and delivery

See also Sections 6.11, 8.28, and 8.29.

Increased risks of intrapartum hypoxia, fetal growth restriction (FGR), cord accidents, and malpresentations make twin deliveries higher risk than singleton deliveries. Mode of delivery depends on chorionicity, gestation, estimated fetal weight, and presentation of the leading twin.

Timing of delivery

For dichorionic diamniotic (DCDA) twins, there is an increased risk of intrauterine death with advancing gestation from 1:333 at 28 weeks to 1:69 after 39 weeks' gestation. Delivery of DCDA twins is recommended by 38 weeks to reduce the risk of intrauterine death.

For monochorionic diamniotic (MCDA) twins, the risk of death in uncomplicated pregnancies has been reported as 1:23 after 32 weeks' gestation. Some advocate delivery by 34 weeks, after steroids, to reduce the risk of intrauterine death (IUD) in one twin and subsequent neurological damage and IUD in the remaining twin. However, taking into account the small but significant risks of prematurity, delivery at 36 weeks may be more appropriate.

Mode of delivery

Dichorionic diamniotic twins

The most common presentation is cephalic/cephalic and vaginal delivery is recommended. If twin 1 is cephalic and twin 2 non-cephalic, vaginal delivery is still advocated. If the second twin is <1500 g, then delivery by CS to reduce the risk of trauma and hypoxia is advised. If twin 1 is non-cephalic, a CS is planned, based on research for term singletons. The main concern for vaginal delivery is 'locking' of the fetal heads when the first twin is breech and the second twin is cephalic. As the breech of the first twin delivers, delivery of the head may be prevented if the head of the second twin enters the pelvis first.

Women with a previous CS are often delivered by repeat CS because of a presumed greater risk of scar dehiscence, but a trial of vaginal delivery is perfectly reasonable if the mother wishes. It is important to have a plan for labour as it commonly starts before the recommended date for elective CS.

Monochorionic diamniotic twins

Many advocate that all MCDA twins should be delivered by CS owing to the risks of cord accidents, acute twin-to-twin transfusion syndrome (TTTS) in labour, and premature placental separation causing hypoxia.

One recent study has looked at the risks associated with MCDA delivery. Vaginal delivery of MCDA twins was significantly associated with a 5-min Apgar score of <7 compared with DCDA twins. However, the number with umbilical artery pH<7.2, admission to neonatal intensive care, and mortality were similar between the two groups. They concluded that vaginal delivery of MCDA twins was a reasonable management option.

Monochorionic monoamniotic twins

Delivery should be by CS by 34 weeks' gestation owing to the increased risk of IUD associated with cord entanglement.

🕐 Box 9.28 Vaginal delivery of twins

- There is an overall increased risk of instrumental and operative delivery
- Intrapartum IV access, FBC, and group and save should be performed
- Continuous CTG monitoring in labour aims to identify fetal distress. A fetal scalp electrode should be used to monitor twin 1 once the cervix has started to dilate
- Epidural anaesthesia is useful in the event of instrumental or operative delivery and if manoeuvres such as assisted breech delivery or internal podalic version are needed
- A paediatric or neonatal nurse team needs to be present for delivery and must be informed early of planned induction/delivery or spontaneous labour
- The place of delivery will depend on the clinical situation. Delivery in theatre enables quick recourse to CS if needed
- As the first twin is delivered, the position of the second twin should be stabilized, keeping it cephalic. Having an US machine available is essential
- If the second twin is not cephalic and does not rotate spontaneously, then external cephalic version can be attempted. Internal podalic version and subsequent breech extraction should only be attempted by those with appropriate experience
- After delivery of the first twin, the contractions often reduce in frequency and strength, therefore once the lie is stabilized it is usually necessary to augment contractions using a syntocinon infusion
- Hold off artificial rupture of membranes (ARM) until the presenting part is engaged in the pelvis to avoid the possibility of malpresentation and cord prolapse
- Delivery of the second twin should ideally be within 30 min of the first delivery. After this, there is an increased risk of hypoxia. Continuous CTG monitoring is essential
- There is a 5% risk of CS for the second twin after vaginal delivery of the first
- A 40 iu syntocinon IV infusion should be ready to commence once the second twin is delivered to reduce the risk of atonic postpartum haemorrhage (PPH)

Chapter 10

Obstetric emergencies

Contents

Covered elsewhere

- Antepartum haemorrhage (see Section 8.1)
- Postpartum haemorrhage (see Section 11.1)
- Fetal distress (see Section 9.9)
- Neonatal resuscitation (see Sections 11.8 and 11.9)
- When things go wrong (see Section 1.10)

10.1 Maternal collapse—obstetric causes

Peripartum emergencies

Structured approach

A structured approach to any emergency consists of:

- Assessing the maternal status and dealing with life-threatening problems (e.g. haemorrhage)
- Resuscitate the mother if necessary (see ABCDE boxes)
- If, and when, the mother is stable, assess fetal wellbeing and viability, and consider whether delivery is appropriate, when and how
- Deal with specific problems using protocols or algorithms to ensure a systematic approach
- Definitive care should follow (e.g. anticoagulation for pulmonary embolism)
- Teamwork cannot be overemphasized
- Equally crucial is leadership
- The person responsible for leading and coordinating the team should maintain a 'helicopter' attitude, rising above the situation to assess all the parameters in the round

Institutional requirements

Local protocols should exist in the labour ward to guide the management of the common or important complications.

The Clinical Negligence Scheme for Trusts (CNST) mandate a number of emergencies for which guidelines should exist. National guidelines (e.g. RCOG in the UK) may serve as a template or a substitute for local guidance.

Regular training and drills of all professionals involved should be run in labour wards.

Communication

- An important and often neglected part of an emergency for patients, their companions, and for staff
- Even one or two brief sentences to explain what is happening, and why, can make a great difference to women and their relatives during an emergency
- More details can follow later
- Clear communication is also vital between different health professionals (e.g. the anaesthetist)
- Accurate documentation is important from a clinical and medicolegal perspective. One person (e.g. a junior midwife) should be specifically assigned to keep a record of events. Structured proformas are valuable aids in documentation
- Remember clinical incident reporting (see Section 1.6)
- Root cause analysis can provide useful insights in retrospect
- There is not enough evidence to tell whether and how debriefing may be helpful or harmful
- Complaints come with the territory, and should be regarded as precious gems: most people want an explanation; only a small proportion of upset or damaged patients actually make them; they are a valuable source of learning, feedback, and improvement; they throw an important light on the people and systems who deliver care
- Do not be frightened of the aftermath
- Talk to someone senior

Collapse—first principles

- Resuscitate and then establish the cause
- Initial assessment as for all emergencies (see ABCDE boxes)
- Call for help—know the crash call number (usually 2222) and where the cardiac arrest trolley is kept

- Place the woman in a 15° left lateral tilt. This will increase cardiac output by preventing aortocaval compression from the gravid uterus
- Call for immediate senior obstetric and anaesthetic review if there is any maternal or fetal compromise
- All medical staff should be trained in immediate resuscitation to a nationally recognized level such as Advanced Life Support (ALS)
- Specialist courses provide additional training for obstetric and midwifery staff (e.g. Advanced Life Support in Obstetrics and Managing Obstetric Emergencies and Trauma; ALSO and MOET)
- Elicit a history from the woman or a witness and review antenatal care and concurrent medical problems
- Full examination should be performed including neurological
- Subsequent investigations and management depend on the presentation, clinical findings, and fetal wellbeing
- All obstetric and non-obstetric causes should be considered (see Table 10.1 Section 10.2)

Eclampsia

See Section 10.3

Haemorrhage

Antepartum (see Section 8.1) and postpartum (see Section 11.1).

Amniotic fluid embolus

Incidence

- Rare occurrence—1:80 000
- In the 2003–2005 Confidential Enquiry, there were 19 maternal deaths, which was a large increase and makes this the second largest cause of direct deaths

Pathophysiology

Amniotic fluid embolus (AFE) occurs when amniotic fluid and associated debris enters the maternal circulation, causing a devastating anaphylactic type reaction. Seventy per cent occur during labour, 19% during CS, and 11% are postpartum. Thirteen per cent occur within 3 min of amniotomy or insertion of an intrauterine pressure catheter.

History

Initial symptoms include breathlessness, chest pain, feeling cold, light-headedness, restlessness, distress, panic, a feeling of pins and needles in the fingers, nausea and vomiting, cyanosis, and abnormal behaviour.

The presentation may be:

- Sudden and catastrophic hypotension, hypoxia, and respiratory distress
- Cardiopulmonary arrest (87%)
- Disseminated intravascular coagulation (DIC) and haemorrhage (83%)
- Pulmonary oedema
- Seizures
- Fetal distress (if not delivered)

Investigations

Diagnosis is clinical: acute hypoxia (dyspnoea, cyanosis, respiratory arrest), acute hypotension or cardiac arrest, coagulopathy, and no other clinical condition or explanation for signs and symptoms.

- Accurate identification of fetal squames in the maternal circulation is difficult

- Urgent blood for FBC, clotting, fibrinogen, and fibrinogen degradation products to assess degree of coagulopathy
- CXR to look for pulmonary oedema and acute respiratory distress syndrome
- ECG

Management
- Supportive
- Immediate resuscitation with oxygen and fluids
- Involve obstetric, anaesthetic, haematological, and neonatal teams
- Deliver baby by quickest mode
- Liaise with haematology immediately and correct coagulopathy with fresh frozen plasma (FFP), cryoprecipitate and platelet transfusion (see DIC, Section 8.2)
- Treat haemorrhage (see Section 11.1). Crossmatch 6–10 units of blood
- Circulatory support with inotropes may be needed
- Early transfer to ITU is recommended by Confidential Enquiry into Maternal and Child Health (CEMACH) to improve survival rates

Prognosis
- High mortality rate of up to 61%. Most die within 1 h
- Of those who survive, 15% are neurologically intact
- AFE is one of the conditions being studied through the UK Obstetric Surveillance System (UKOSS; see Box 10.1). The aim is to identify the incidence, risk factors, management strategies and outcomes of this rare condition

Useful tips
- It is paramount to call for senior help early, especially if you need to use unfamiliar procedures or techniques
- For most emergencies, the bed will have to be flat
- In emergencies, the obstetrician must appear calm and composed
- Use the techniques you are most familiar with first

➜ Box 10.1 UKOSS (www.npeu.ox.ac.uk/UKOSS/)

The UK Obstetric Surveillance System was launched in 2005. It is a national reporting system to study rare disorders in pregnancy which are under-researched, with little evidence-based knowledge available to help guide prevention and management. This reporting system allows descriptive, case-control, and cohort studies to be conducted prospectively.

Each month UKOSS sends out reporting cards to identify conditions currently under surveillance and controls. A data collection sheet is then sent so that detailed information can be obtained. Surveillance is complete for eclampsia, peripartum hysterectomy, TB, pulmonary embolism, and acute fatty liver.

Data collection is in process for AFE, myocardial infarction, stroke, pulmonary vascular disease, gastroschisis, and fetomaternal alloimmune thrombocytopenia.

✚ Box A. Airway (with cervical spine protection if needed)

Obstructed airway: difficulty talking, cyanosis, use of accessory respiratory muscles of respiration, and abnormal breathing sounds
- Chin lift and jaw thrust if airway is compromised
- Supplementary O_2 via a face mask with reservoir bag at a flow of 15 l/min
- Urgent anaesthetic review if airway compromised. Consider oropharyngeal airway or tracheal intubation
- Tracheal intubation should only be attempted by those competent in inserting airways in pregnant women

---

✚ Box B. Breathing and ventilation

To ensure oxygenated blood to the brain
- Check respiratory rate

If not breathing, ventilate by:
- Mouth via a pocket mask, or
- A self-inflating bag and mask + O_2, or
- Self-inflating bag and tracheal intubation + O_2

Check O_2 saturation

✚ Box C. Circulation

To maintain cerebral perfusion
- If no pulse, call the cardiac arrest team and commence CPR according to Resuscitation Council guidelines
- If pulse present, check BP, pulse rate, capillary refill
- Two wide bore IV cannulae, 16G or more
- Blood tests—will depend on the clinical scenario. FBC, U&Es, LFTs, urate, glucose, G&S, and clotting should be taken after inserting cannula
- Crossmatch blood
- Commence colloids if hypotension, tachycardia or hypovolaemia is suspected
- Caution with fluids if severe pre-eclampsia or eclampsia
- Fluid balance and indwelling catheter
- ECG
- Fetal heart rate

✚ Box D. Disability or neurological status

Assess level of consciousness using AVPU:
- Alert
- Voice responsive
- Pain responsive
- Unresponsive

✚ Box E. Exposure and Environmental control
- Full exposure for initial assessment
- Keep warm (blankets, bear hugger)

10.2 Maternal collapse—non-obstetric causes

Pulmonary embolism

See Sections 8.16 and 8.17.

Septic shock

Septic shock occurs when there is evidence of systemic inflammatory response syndrome (SIRS) with evidence of infection. SIRS is defined as the presence of two or more of:

- Temperature >38°C or <36°C
- Tachycardia
- Tachypnoea
- White cell count >11 $\times 10^3$/ml or <4 $\times 10^3$/ml

Septic shock is the presence of sepsis with hypotension (systolic <90 mmHg or 40 mmHg below baseline). It is imperative to get early advice from microbiology. Vomiting, abdominal pain, and diarrhoea are features of pelvic sepsis, not necessarily simply gastroenteritis.

History

Antenatal causes of sepsis include:

- **Chorioamnionitis:** spontaneous rupture of membranes (SROM), prolonged labour, offensive discharge, abdominal pain, preterm labour, and recent amniocentesis
- **Pyelonephritis:** dysuria, frequency, haematuria, loin pain, recurrent UTIs, urinary tract abnormalities, stone disease, catheterization (see Section 8.6)
- **Chest infection:** cough, sputum, chest pain, shortness of breath, pre-existing respiratory disease, and smoking
- **Meningitis:** headache, neck stiffness, photophobia, vomiting, confusion, seizures, and rash (macular, petechiae, purpura)
- **Appendicitis:** abdominal pain (not necessarily McBurney's point), nausea, vomiting, and anorexia (see Section 8.7)
- **Cholecystitis:** right upper quadrant pain, vomiting, known gallstones (see Section 8.7)
- **Pancreatitis:** upper abdominal pain radiating to back, vomiting, known gallstones, alcohol abuse (see Section 8.7)

Examination

SIRS—hypotension, cyanosis, and peripheral shutdown (cold extremities, reduced capillary refill, mottled skin).

- Abdominal—loin, uterine or abdominal tenderness, peritonism (guarding, rebound), bowel sounds
- Speculum—offensive discharge or liquor
- Chest—air entry, crepitations, bronchial breathing
- Neurological—focal neurology, confusion

Investigations

Depend on suspected cause.

- Bloods as in Box C, Section 10.1, plus C-reactive protein (CRP) and blood cultures
- High vaginal and endocervical swabs if appropriate
- Urine dipstick and MSU
- Sputum culture
- Arterial blood gas (acidosis, hypoxaemia)
- Lumbar puncture for suspected meningitis

Management

The mainstays are circulatory support and antimicrobials. Intravascular release of vasodilator substances (nitric oxide) causes hypotension, reduced cardiac output, and tissue hypoperfusion. Multiorgan failure is an end result (respiratory, renal and liver failure, DIC).

Fluid resuscitation with colloids or crystalloids should be commenced immediately. If hypotension does not respond, then invasive monitoring should be considered (central venous pressure (CVP) line). Inotrope support may be needed and coagulopathy corrected.

Consult with microbiology and start broad spectrum antibiotics; the choice will depend on the clinical presentation. Empirical treatment should cover Gram-negative and anaerobic organisms. If chorioamnionitis is the cause, the fetus (whether viable or not) should be delivered. Puerperal pyrexia is considered in Section 11.5.

Intra-abdominal catastrophe

Although rare (9 deaths from dissecting aortic aneurysm in the 2003–2005 Confidential Enquiry), consider ruptured abdominal viscera or vessel in a woman presenting with abdominal pain, gastrointestinal symptoms and hypovolaemia out of proportion to external signs. Look for evidence of peritonism, increasing abdominal distension or free fluid on ultrasound. Fetal distress may also be present.

Differential diagnoses include:

- Ruptured peptic ulcer
- Ruptured liver or spleen
- Ruptured aneurysm (aortic, splenic, hepatic)

Resuscitation with colloids, blood products, and urgent review by surgical or vascular teams is necessary. Treatment will be laparotomy and repair.

Cardiac causes

See Sections 7.7, 7.8, and 7.9.

Arrhythmias

History

May predate pregnancy or be first presentation. Palpitations, shortness of breath, fainting, and dizzy episodes.

Examination

- Tachycardia
- Regular or irregular pulse (check apical and peripheral)
- BP and O_2 saturation

Investigations

- ECG, echo and 24-h tape
- Bloods—FBC, U&Es, Mg^{2+}, TFTs, and cardiac enzymes
- Cardiac monitoring
- Fetal monitoring

Management

- Arrange cardiology and anaesthetic reviews
- Sinus tachycardia, atrial and ventricular premature beats are common in pregnancy and need no treatment
- Try vagal manoeuvres for supraventricular tachycardias (SVT) before adenosine for persistent or symptomatic SVT (with cardiac and fetal monitoring).
- Correct low K^+ and Mg^{2+}

Dissection of thoracic aorta

Rare in pregnancy. It presents with severe chest pain.

- Associated with Marfan's syndrome, Ehlers–Danlos syndrome, and coarctation of the aorta
- CXR may show widening of the mediastinum
- Urgent cardiology and cardiothoracic review needed

Myocardial infarction

Extremely rare but consider if a strong family history, essential hypertension, obesity, diabetes mellitus or smoking.

There were 4 deaths from ischaemic heart disease in the 2003–2005 Confidential Enquiry, and 16 from myocardial infarction.

- Presentation is as for the non-pregnant (chest pain, shortness of breath, sweaty, distress)
- ECG and bloods, including troponin I, should be performed
- Initial treatment with oxygen, morphine, 300 mg aspirin PO and glyceryl trinitrate (GTN) can be commenced
- Arrange cardiology review

Cardiomyopathy

See Section 7.9.

Cardiac arrest

- Sudden loss of consciousness with no vital signs
- Resuscitate by beginning CPR within 3–4 min of onset, stabilize her condition, diagnose, and treat underlying cause

Neurological causes

Epilepsy

See also Section 7.14.

History

- Usually predates pregnancy but can be first presentation
- If post-ictal, obtain history from a witness if possible
- Ask about the frequency of fits, type and dose of antiepileptic medication, whether doses have been missed and why
- History of pre-eclampsia, diabetes, hyperemesis, drug or alcohol withdrawal

Examination

- Full neurological examination
- Look for trauma to the mouth or tongue
- Evidence of abruption (see Section 8.2)
- Blood pressure and urinalysis for protein

Investigations

- Drug levels
- Blood glucose, serum calcium, and sodium
- Blood and urine toxicology screen if indicated
- If first presentation, consider CT or MRI to exclude intracranial mass and EEG

Management

- Supportive treatment and treat any underlying cause
- If taking medication as prescribed, may need to increase dose if levels are low—liaise with neurology
- If first presentation, arrange neurological review
- In status epilepticus, urgent anaesthetic and neurological review are needed. Sub-buccal midazolam, IV lorazepam, PR diazepam, and IV phenytoin can be used to treat recurrent or single prolonged tonic–clonic seizures

Stroke

Stroke is rare, with a tendency to occur postpartum. It can be ischaemic or haemorrhagic. In the 2003–2005 Confidential Enquiry, 2 women died from cerebral infarct and 11 from intracerebral haemorrhage.

Causes of ischaemic stroke include atherosclerosis, vasculitis, antiphospholipid syndrome, protein C and S deficiency, antithrombin III deficiency, atrial fibrillation, mitral valve prolapse, subacute bacterial endocarditis, cardiomyopathy, sickle cell disease, thrombotic thrombocytopenic purpura, and paradoxical embolus.

Causes of a haemorrhagic stroke include eclampsia and arteriovenous malformations (AVM).

- An MRI or CT scan differentiates between ischaemic and haemorrhagic strokes

- Arrange investigations to establish cause, e.g. echocardiogram, ECG, thrombophilia screen
- Treat cause

Subarachnoid haemorrhage (SAH)

- Rare: 1–5/10 000 pregnancies
- Eleven deaths in the 2003–2005 Confidential Enquiry
- Caused by ruptured arterial aneurysm or arteriovenous malformation (AVM)
- Most occur postpartum
- No increased risk with Valsalva manoeuvres in labour
- Diagnose with CT or MRI
- MR angiography can identify the bleed
- Early neurosurgical review and treatment

Cerebral vein thrombosis

Cerebral vein thrombosis is rare. It usually occurs postpartum.

Substance abuse

Substance abuse (alcohol or drugs) and withdrawal should be a differential diagnosis for collapse, particularly if known drug or alcohol user.

Send blood and urine for toxicology (consent if conscious).

Commence supportive treatment with input from local Drug Dependency Unit.

See Sections 7.2 and 7.3.

Anaphylaxis

Laryngeal oedema, bronchospasm, and hypotension are features of anaphylaxis. Urgently involve anaesthetist.

After initial 'ABC' resuscitation, IM adrenaline is first line treatment (500 μg, 0.5 ml of adrenaline 1:1000) followed by 200 mg IV hydrocortisone and 10 mg IV chlorpheniramine (www.bnf.org).

Adrenaline can be administered every 5 min if required.

Fainting and vasovagal attack

Related to vasodilatation (progesterone effect).

Can be caused by lying supine and resulting aorto-caval compression.

Table 10.1 Causes of maternal collapse	
Obstetric causes	Non-obstetric causes
Eclampsia	Septic shock
Thromboembolism	Ruptured aneurysm
Amniotic fluid embolism	Rupture of liver or spleen
Uterine inversion	Cardiac arrhythmia
Uterine rupture	Myocardial infarction
Intra-abdominal bleeding	Cerebrovascular accident
Genital tract haematoma	Subarachnoid haemorrhage
	Anaphylactic shock
	Metabolic or endocrine cause
	Medication or substance abuse

Further reading

www.cemach.org.uk Why Mothers Die: Confidential Enquiry 2000–2002. London, 2004 and Saving mothers' lives. Confidential Enquiry 2003–2005. London, 2007.

www.library.nhs.uk emergency ID=79009.

www.nhsla.com Clinical Negligence Scheme for Trusts: Maternity Clinical Risk Management Standards. NHS Litigation Authority, 2006.

www.resus.org.uk for resuscitation guidelines.

10.3 Eclampsia

See also Sections 8.11, 8.12, and 8.13.

Introduction
Eclampsia is defined as the occurrence of convulsions superimposed on pre-eclampsia. Any convulsion in pregnancy should be treated as eclampsia unless proven otherwise.

The condition complicates ~1:2000 pregnancies, 1% of pre-eclampsia cases.

Twenty per cent of women are normotensive at presentation.

One-third occur postpartum, the highest risk being the first 24–48 h.

Complications
- Death—~1%
- Acute renal failure (reversible)—4%
- HELLP (haemolysis, elevated liver enzymes, low platelets syndrome)—3%
- DIC (disseminated intravascular coagulation)—3%
- Aspiration/RDS (respiratory distress syndrome)—3%
- Intracranial haemorrhage or transient blindness
- Fetal bradycardia

The single major failing in clinical care resulting in death is inadequate treatment of BP with subsequent intracranial haemorrhage.

Second, but equally important, is iatrogenic fluid overload and pulmonary oedema.

Diagnosis
History
- Headache, visual disturbances ('flashing lights'), abdominal pain, general malaise
- Post-ictal confusion

Observations and examination
- Grand mal generalized clonic convulsion
- Chest examination for signs of pulmonary oedema
- Brisk reflexes—the predictive value is uncertain
- 3+ beats of clonus
- BP and other vital observations
- Pulse oximetry—to detect pulmonary oedema
- Fetal heart rate (FHR) monitoring is one of the last (not first) priorities in an unstable patient—will only serve to increase distress

Investigations
- FBC, clotting, U&Es, LFTs, glucose, Ca^{2+}, Mg^{2+}
- Uric acid—may assist diagnosis but not useful for monitoring or clinical decision-making
- CXR—if low O_2 saturation check for aspiration after fit
- CT or MRI head (± venous angiography) if focal symptoms
- EEG
- Thrombophilia screen
- Toxicology screen

Management details
- The early involvement of consultant obstetricians and anaesthetists or ITU specialists in the management is essential

- BP values from automated machines should be compared with those from conventional sphygmomanometers. MAP (mean arterial pressure) = diastolic + (systolic–diastolic)/3
- $MgSO_4$ (see Box 10.3) is the anticonvulsant of choice in eclampsia and pre-eclampsia. It reduces the risk of recurrent seizures, maternal mortality, pneumonia, admission to ITU, baby death or admission to special care baby unit. It is more effective and safe than phenytoin, diazepam or lytic cocktail (usually a mixture of chlorpromazine, promethazine, and pethidine)
- The choice of antihypertensive depends on local protocols, availability, and the clinicians' experience. Labetalol orally or IV or nifedipine orally are first line treatments. Hydralazine IV can be used but has more side effects. Each unit should have an 'eclampsia box' with the necessary medications
- Fluid restriction (1 ml/kg/h or 85 ml/h) and central monitoring is essential for the careful monitoring of fluid balance to avoid the serious consequences of fluid overload
- Delivery should occur after stabilization; soon if more than 34 weeks; if <34 weeks, after senior decision and steroids. Vaginal delivery is preferable, but fetal condition, presentation, and cervical favourability will determine the mode
- After the acute phase, thromboprophylaxis, documentation, and close monitoring are very important. The woman should be reviewed before discharge, as late seizures may occur, and follow-up arranged
- Syntocinon should be used and ergometrine/syntometrine avoided for prevention of postpartum haemorrhage (PPH). For the treatment of massive haemorrhage, however, ergometrine/syntometrine can still be used, especially if the patient is shocked and other medications unavailable

Useful tips
- In collapse, the first priority is ABC rather than drugs or FHR monitoring
- Maternal condition always takes priority over fetal condition
- You should never deliver an unstable patient even if bradycardia does not resolve
- Fetal bradycardia is common but usually resolves with maternal treatment. Remember that the first line of treatment for any fetal distress is *in utero* resuscitation, not delivery
- Women with pre-eclampsia or eclampsia die from pulmonary oedema, not renal failure. The often neglected chest examination is far more important than urine output in the acute phase. The latter can be dealt with once the patient is stable

Further reading

www.rcog.org.uk The management of severe pre-eclampsia/eclampsia. Clinical greentop guideline No. 10(A). RCOG, 2006.

www.cemach.org.uk Why Mothers Die 2000–2002, 6th report. RCOG Press, London.

Magpie Trial Collaborative Group. Do women with pre-eclampsia, and their babies, benefit from magnesium sulphate? The Magpie Trial: a randomised placebo-controlled trial. *Lancet* 2002; **359**:1877–90.

⊘ Box 10.2 Differential diagnosis of eclampsia

1. *Pseudoseizures:* atypical, downgoing plantar reflexes
2. *Postdural puncture:* 4–7 days after puncture, preceded by headache, relieved by lying
3. *Idiopathic epilepsy:* may first present in pregnancy
4. *Secondary:* CNS masses, antiphospholipid syndrome
5. *Cerebral vein thrombosis:* usually postpartum, signs of increased intracranial pressure, transient focal signs, fever, leukocytosis, and neutrophilia
6. *Stroke*
7. *Thrombotic thrombocytopenic purpura:* immediate post-natal period, normotensive
8. *Withdrawal:* drugs, alcohol
9. *Metabolic:* hypoglycaemia, hypocalcaemia, hyponatraemia
10. *Amniotic fluid embolism:* atypical convulsions, respiratory arrest before collapse

→ Box 10.3 Magnesium sulphate

- Relieves cerebral vasospasm
- MAGPIE study demonstrated that, used prophylactically, $MgSO_4$ reduces the risk of seizures by 58% and of abruption regardless of the severity of pre-eclampsia
- The number needed to treat to prevent one seizure is 109 for non-severe cases (63 for severe).
- It is used in severe pre-eclampsia when delivery has been decided and for 24 h after the last seizure or delivery, whichever is latest. It may be used in other clinical situations after senior individual case assessment.

Administration

- IV bolus—4 g over 5 min or in 40 ml over 20 min
- Infusion—1–2 g/h (remember to subtract from 85 ml/h)

Monitoring of magnesum toxicity

Clinical: Flushing, double vision, slurred speech
            Patellar reflexes—should not be lost
            RR <16 per min
            SaO_2 <90%
Levels if: Clinical signs of toxicity
            Poor urine output (e.g. <100 ml/4 h)
            Recurrent fits
            Therapeutic level = 2–6 mEq/l

If toxic levels or signs

- Stop $MgSO_4$ infusion
- Consider 1 g Ca^{2+} gluconate IV over 3 min

Recurrence

- 5–20% risk
- Mg^{2+} 2 g bolus once only (4 g if >70 kg). Check levels
- Diazepam 10 mg IV, only after senior decision
- Thiopentone infusion 50 mg IV
- Intubation, intermittent postive-pressure ventilation (IPPV), muscle relaxation

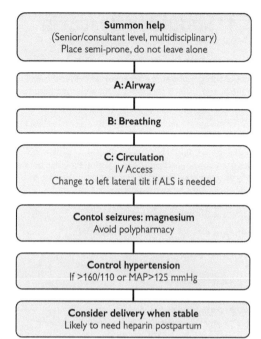

Fig. 10.1 Management algorithm in eclampsia.

10.4 Shoulder dystocia

Definition
The use of ancillary obstetric manoeuvres to deliver the fetal shoulders. Shoulder dystocia is associated with a prolonged head-to-body delivery time >60 s versus a mean of 25 s in births uncomplicated by shoulder dystocia.

Incidence
The incidence is 0.15–2% but may be affected by under-reporting. It results from bony impaction of the anterior shoulder behind the symphysis pubis (see Figure 10.2), or occasionally the posterior shoulder behind the sacral promontory, or both. The wide bisacromial diameter fails to rotate from the narrow AP diameter of the inlet to the wider transverse or oblique.

Significance
- Shoulder dystocia is associated with significant morbidity

Fetal
- Cerebral hypoxia and palsy
- Fractures of the clavicle or humerus (<10%)
- Brachial plexus injuries (~10%)
- Erb's ('waiter's tip' paralysis), C5–6 roots, 90% recovery
- Klumpke's ('claw hand'), C7–8+T1 roots, 40% recovery

Maternal
- Postpartum haemorrhage (PPH)
- Perineal tears, including fourth degree
- Uterine rupture
- Psychological injury
- Brachial plexus injuries are a significant cause of litigation

Risk factors
Mother
- Diabetes
- BMI>30
- Previous shoulder dystocia (10% recurrence risk)

Labour
- Prolonged first or second stage
- Induction, augmentation
- Assisted delivery

Fetus
- Macrosomia >4.5 kg or estimated fetal weight >97th centile
- Postmaturity

Prediction
- About half the cases occur in women without risk factors
- Conventional risk factors predict only 10–15% of cases
- US has a 10–15% error in estimating fetal weight and is not very reliable in detecting macrosomia
- The vast majority of macrosomic babies do not have shoulder dystocia (only 2–5% do)
- Most cases of shoulder dystocia do not result in injury
- About 2000 CSs would prevent one permanent injury
- Shoulder dystocia may still occur at CS. Cases of brachial plexus injury have been reported in CSs involving complex fetal manipulation (transverse lie, frozen pelvis)

Vigilance is therefore important in cases where known risk factors exist, e.g. availability of an experienced obstetrician.

Regular training of health professionals is equally important for the management of shoulder dystocia.

Signs
Signs of shoulder dystocia include:
- Difficulty delivering the head or chin
- The head remains tightly applied to the vulva or retracts ('turtle sign')
- There is no restitution
- The shoulders fail to descend and the anterior is still palpable abdominally

Prevention
- A 'prophylactic' McRobert's (before delivery) is frequently used in cases with risk factors to prevent shoulder dystocia at vaginal delivery. It is unclear whether the risk of shoulder dystocia is subsequently decreased. Further evidence is necessary before it is recommended
- Induction of labour (IOL) for suspected macrosomia has not been shown to alter maternal or neonatal morbidity, compared to expectant management. However, brachial plexus injury only occurred in cases managed expectantly
- IOL at term in women with insulin-requiring diabetes reduces macrosomia but not maternal or neonatal morbidity
- The only policy that is recommended is to consider an elective CS at term for mothers with diabetes and suspected fetal macrosomia (C)
- However, the trials addressing the above interventions were all underpowered. Large trials may be able to demonstrate differences in outcomes and some are under way

Management
- Help includes a midwife coordinator, additional midwives, an experienced obstetrician, and the neonatal team. An anaesthetist may be needed for third line procedures
- Aim to deliver within 5 min if possible, but always carefully. Between 30–60 s should be adequate for each manoeuvre, but time limits are arbitrary and evidence is inconclusive
- Routine traction should be applied after each manoeuvre. It should be similar to that applied in a normal delivery
- Lateral or downward traction or rocking should not be performed as they increase the risk of injury
- Fundal pressure should not be used, as it is associated with uterine rupture and may worsen the impaction. Maternal pushing has the same effect and should be discouraged until the shoulder is disimpacted by the use of manoeuvres
- McRobert's and suprapubic pressure (see Figure 10.3) combined (first line) will deliver the vast majority (80–90%) of cases when performed properly
- Flexing the thighs (at the hip and knee) twice may help to rotate the anterior shoulder and disimpact it
- Suprapubic pressure can be continuous or rocking. Both can be tried in succession
- Midwives may put the woman in the all fours position first
- Episiotomy is optional, not routine. It serves to facilitate the manoeuvres and will not disimpact the shoulder(s) per se
- The posterior arm is removed by inserting the whole hand in the presacral space. Episiotomy may help in nulliparas. The humerus is splinted with two fingers, the elbow flexed, and the hand grasped and swept across the face anteriorly (see Figure 10.4)
- The internal rotational manoeuvres consist of pressure on the shoulders in an effort to rotate them to the oblique or a full 180° before applying routine traction. Several manoeuvres exist. It is of paramount importance to apply pressure on the shoulders only (see Figure 10.5), with the hands inserted from the perineum (5 or 7 o'clock) upwards. Pressure on other areas may cause injury, as rotation of the body may occur with the shoulder(s) still impacted. It is also important either to continue suprapubic pressure if the two manoeuvres serve to rotate in the same direction, or to stop it if the direction is opposite
- Third line manoeuvres include fracture of the clavicle, symphysiotomy, and Zavanelli. The last consists of flexing the fetal head with tocolysis (e.g. terbutaline 0.25 mg SC), then replacing it in

the abdomen with a technique similar to manual rotations. A CS follows. The morbidity can be significant
- Documentation should include the time of delivery of the head, the direction it was facing initially, the manoeuvres performed, their sequence and timing, the time of delivery of the body, staff attendance and timing, the baby's condition, and the neonatal assessment

Further reading

www.rcog.org.uk Shoulder dystocia. Clinical greentop guideline No. 42. London: RCOG Press, 2005.

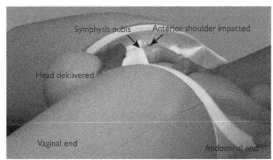

Fig. 10.2 Bony impaction of the anterior shoulder, demonstrating why pushing should be stopped until the shoulder has moved below the symphysis pubis with the use of obstetric manoeuvres.

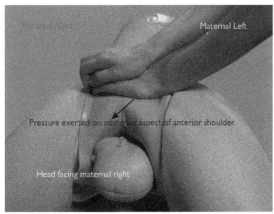

Fig. 10.3 Suprapubic pressure. The technique and force is similar to that for CPR.

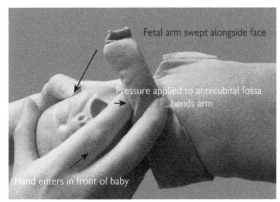

Fig. 10.4 Removing posterior arm. Easier to perform when the whole hand is inserted in the presacral space, then advanced in front of the baby. Pressure on the antecubital fossa bends the posterior arm, which is then grasped and swept in front of the face, like a cat licking its paws.

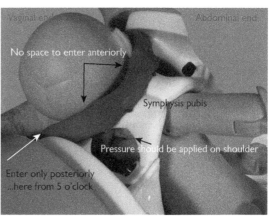

Fig. 10.5 Internal manoeuvres. Should not be performed unless the shoulder is reached otherwise they may result in brachial plexus injury.

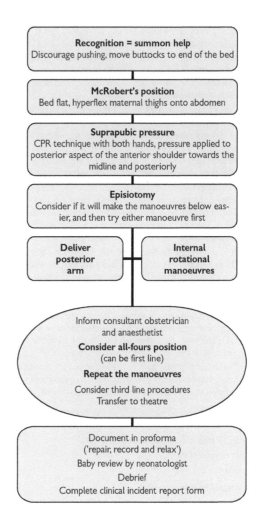

Fig. 10.6 Management algorithm for shoulder dystocia.

10.5 Cord prolapse

Definitions

Cord presentation—the presence of loop(s) of umbilical cord between the fetal presenting part and the cervical os.

Cord prolapse—the descent of the umbilical cord through the cervix alongside (occult prolapse) or past the presenting part (overt prolapse) in the context of ruptured membranes.

Incidence ranges from 0.1% to 0.5% of births.

Significance

Prolapse results in compression cutting off the blood supply to the fetus. Hypoxia may be followed by stillbirth, neonatal encephalopathy or cerebral palsy.

Cases of cord prolapse appear consistently in perinatal mortality inquiries. Prematurity and congenital anomalies account for the majority of adverse outcomes associated with cord prolapse, but death can occur in normal term pregnancies, if help is not readily available (e.g. home birth).

This is a mandatory labour ward Clinical Negligence Scheme for Trusts (CNST) standard.

Initial management

Summon appropriate help.

The following temporary measures can be undertaken (e.g. while preparing for delivery or expecting senior assessment):

- Knee–chest face-down position—this can be explained over the phone if at home, while waiting for transport. Alternatively, use a steep Trendelenburg (body laid flat on the back supine with the feet higher than the head)
- Wrap the cord in warm wet packs, if visible at the introitus, to prevent vasoconstriction
- Manual elevation of the presenting part vaginally until either the bladder is filled or prepared for delivery (e.g. a CS can be performed and ready for knife-to-skin). Once the presenting part is elevated above the pelvic inlet, suprapubic pressure with the other hand can keep it elevated
- Tocolysis—an injection of 0.25 mg terbutaline SC (0.5 ml of 0.5 mg/ml solution) can be given to relieve cord compression prior to delivery. Tocolysis may also enable regional (rather than general) anaesthesia
- Fill the bladder to lift the presenting part and inhibit contractions. Use a large (50–60 ml) syringe or a giving set with the end cut off to fit the Foley's catheter. The catheter must be clamped after instilling 500–700 ml. It is crucial to empty the bladder before any delivery attempt (vaginal or CS)
- Expectant management—in extreme prematurity (23–25 weeks), the temporary measures above have been used for hours to weeks. Delivery may be performed once optimum viability has been reached or there are signs of fetal distress
- Cord reduction manually back to the maternal abdomen has been used. Manipulating the cord can lead to vasoconstriction and be counterproductive so this is not recommended

Evaluation

History

- Risk factors for cord prolapse (see Box 10.4)
- Ruptured membranes
- Recent obstetric interventions

Observations and examination

A vaginal examination (VE) should be performed promptly after rupture of membranes (ROM) or with suspicious CTG abnormalities, to exclude cord prolapse.

Investigations

- CTG may show persistent variable decelerations or a profound bradycardia

- Abdominal USS (+ Doppler) to see cord presentation or occult prolapse only if time, i.e. there is no fetal distress

Delivery mode

Unless vaginal delivery is imminent, CS should be performed. Check viability (with Doppler or ultrasound) before the incision. Ventouse is appropriate in selected cases (engaged head and full dilatation are prerequisites, though senior obstetricians may attempt delivery of a parous woman at 9 cm dilatation).

Breech extraction may be performed under some circumstances, e.g. after internal podalic version for the second twin.

Tips

- The urgency is reduced if the CTG is normal and the presenting part is elevated manually or by a filled bladder
- A CS with a spinal rather than a general anaesthetic can be appropriate
- Do not forget to debrief the woman after delivery. Emergencies can be traumatic. A few sentences make all the difference

Further reading

Johansson R et al. *Managing Obstetric Emergencies and Trauma*. London: RCOG Press, 2004.

RCOG. Green top guideline No 50. Umbilical Cord Prolapse, April 2008 www.rcog.org.uk

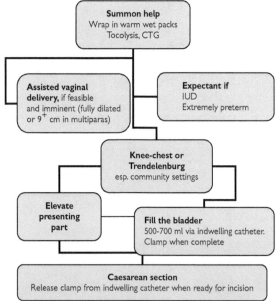

Fig. 10.7 Management algorithm for cord prolapse.

✚ Box 10.4 Risk factors for cord prolapse

- Transverse or unstable lie
- Breech presentation, particularly footling (up to 20% cord prolapse)
- Multiple pregnancy, particularly the second twin
- Prematurity, low birth weight
- Obstetric interventions (artificial rupture of membranes, external cephalic version, induction of labour)
- Unengaged head, parous, cephalopelvic disproportion
- Polyhydramnios
- Abnormal placentation (e.g. low)

Chapter 11

Postpartum care

Contents

Covered elsewhere

11.1 Postpartum haemorrhage

Although the maternal death rate in developed countries is relatively low, postpartum haemorrhage (PPH) remains a major cause of mortality. In Britain, the risk of death from obstetric haemorrhage is about one in 100 000 deliveries.

Major blood loss also causes severe morbidity, including:

- Hypovolaemic shock
- Disseminated intravascular coagulation (DIC)
- Renal failure
- Hepatic failure
- Adult respiratory distress
- Longer term anaemia and health consequences

Definitions

Primary postpartum haemorrhage
Loss of >500 ml of blood from the genital tract in the first 24 h after birth, or any loss <500 ml if associated with maternal haemodynamic changes.

Secondary postpartum haemorrhage
Abnormal or excessive bleeding which occurs between 24 h and 6 weeks postpartum.

Clinical evaluation

Estimation of blood loss
Blood loss in 'real time' is estimated by visual assessment and is likely to be imprecise and unreliable. The woman's general physical condition and vital signs should always be taken into account when assessing the importance of observed blood loss.

Signs and symptoms: emergency situation
- Visible, sudden, large volume of blood loss
- Maternal collapse

Signs and symptoms: raised concern
- Enlarged, soft uterus which lacks tone
- Rising pulse and restlessness
- Falling blood pressure
- Decreased urine output
- Pallor, dizziness, thirst

Causes and risk factors
The most important causes of primary PPH are:

- Uterine atony
- Retained placenta or placental fragments (see Section 11.2)
- Morbid placental adhesion
- Lower genital tract trauma

Rare causes include:

- Coagulopathy
- Uterine rupture
- Uterine inversion

Management of postpartum haemorrhage
The main objectives in management of a major PPH are to resuscitate the woman, stop bleeding, and stabilize her condition. Maternity care providers should draw up guidance for dealing with PPH as part of guidelines for emergency resuscitation. All healthcare staff offering postnatal care should be competent and confident to implement this effectively and efficiently.

Specific aspects of resuscitation relating to PPH
- Establish intravenous access to allow replacement and maintenance of circulating fluid volume and, where appropriate, administration of an oxytocic. A colloid infusion should be administered through one infusion line and a crystalloid through another until blood becomes available

- Obtain blood samples for:
  - Full blood count
  - Clotting screen
  - Urea and electrolytes
  - Crossmatching 6 units of blood
- Insert a urinary catheter with a urometer to empty the bladder and allow evaluation of output hourly
- Monitor heart rate, blood pressure, O_2 saturation (pulse oximetry), ECG
- Insert a central line
- A compression cuff and blood warmer should be used for transfusion of blood
- If a coagulopathy develops, it is vital to seek input from a haematologist and to obtain fresh frozen plasma, cryoprecipitate, and platelets

Communication
- A primary PPH is frightening. It is important for the whole team to communicate confidence and competence, not panic. As far as possible, the woman and her companions should be supported and cared for emotionally as well as physically whilst emergency treatment or urgent diagnostic tests and treatment are being carried out
- If a woman is able to give informed consent, treatment options should be discussed as fully as possible and consent obtained for intervention(s)
- When a woman has collapsed, she cannot give consent for interventions. It is important that she is given a clear explanation about the PPH, the reasons for the treatment she received as soon as she is able to participate in such a discussion
- As part of her postnatal care, the woman should be given opportunities to discuss the cause(s) for her PPH, including any implications for her future wellbeing and health

Uterine atony

Medical management
- Insert a urinary catheter to empty the bladder
- Stimulate contractions by massaging the uterus
- Administer an oxytocic

Drug therapy: uterotonics
- An IV bolus of 250 µg of ergometrine should be administered
- This is followed by an infusion of 40 iu syntocinon in 40 ml 0.9% saline given at a rate of 10 iu/h
- If bleeding persists, an IV bolus dose of 10 iu syntocinon should be given whilst performing bimanual compression of the uterus (one hand is placed over the fundus abdominally whilst the other is inserted vaginally in the posterior fornix, compressing the uterus concomitantly)
- If bleeding continues, administer 15-methylprostaglandin F2a (Haemobate®) 250 µg IM into the thigh or directly into the myometrium. This can be repeated every 15 min for a total of eight doses (i.e. 2.0 mg)
- If the bleeding is unresponsive to ergometrine and/or oxytocin, or if ergometrine is contraindicated, misoprostol 800 µg may be administered rectally (though unlicenced for this use, this is effective and accepted practice)

If bleeding persists in the absence of uterine atony, an examination under anaesthesia should be conducted to investigate the possibility of genital tract lacerations or retained placental fragments.

Uterine tamponade test

After coagulopathy and genital tract laceration have been excluded, the uterine tamponade test can detect whether a woman requires further surgical management.

In this procedure, a Sengstaken–Blakemore tube or Rusch balloon catheter is inserted into the uterine cavity and the balloon is filled with 500–700 ml of warm saline. The warm saline speeds up the action of the clotting cascade. If the observed bleeding is minimal, further surgery is not required.

Surgical management

If medical management is ineffective, there are a number of surgical strategies which can be considered.

Uterine compression sutures

The B-Lynch and modified B-Lynch suturing techniques involve inserting a brace suture that compresses and apposes the anterior and posterior walls of the uterus, thereby applying continuous compression.

This method is most effective when uterine bimanual compression induces marked reduction in blood loss.

Ligation of arteries

Bilateral ligation of the uterine arteries or internal iliac or hypogastric artery greatly reduces the blood flow to the uterus, improves clot formation and haemostasis.

This procedure has a success rate of 40–95%.

Arterial embolization

This is carried out by a specialized radiologist and involves passing a catheter under X-ray guidance through the femoral artery. Contrast dye is then injected to identify the site of bleeding. The feeder artery is embolized with absorbable gelatin sponge (usually reabsorbed in 10 days).

This procedure has several advantages, including shorter hospital stay, preservation of fertility, and it can be carried out under local anaesthesia.

However, there can be serious side effects for a minority of women which include ischaemia of the feet, bladder and rectal wall necrosis, sciatic nerve injury, and infertility.

Hysterectomy

Emergency hysterectomy should be reserved for women for whom all other available measures and surgical techniques which preserve fertility have been considered and/or have failed.

Such drastic intervention is only carried out when the woman is severely shocked, and in cases of coagulopathy where there is lack of replacement blood products.

If there is no active bleeding from the lower uterine segment or cervix, a subtotal hysterectomy may be performed. This is associated with less need for blood transfusion and reduced intraoperative and postoperative complications.

Although radical, an obstetrician should not hesitate to perform a hysterectomy if the woman's life is endangered.

Confidential Enquiries into maternal deaths in the UK repeatedly cite delay or failure to perform hysterectomy as an avoidable cause of death from PPH.

➕ Box 11.1 The main risk factors for PPH

Before onset of labour	During labour/delivery
Raised maternal age	Prolonged labour
Asian ethnicity	Pyrexia in labour
Obesity	Episiotomy
Previous PPH	Operative vaginal delivery
Nulliparity	CS
Placental abruption	Retained placenta
Placenta praevia	Full bladder
Multiple pregnancy	Physiological third stage
Pre-eclampsia	
Anaemia	

Useful tips

- Never be complacent with PPH. The gravid uterus has a blood supply of approximately 500 ml per minute, hence the potential for major bleeding in a very short time
- Have a low threshold for summoning help and transferring the woman to the theatre, where assessment of genital tract injury, especially cervical lacerations, can be achieved effectively
- As a rough guide, if bleeding caused by presumed uterine atony has not settled after two doses of Haemobate®, the woman should be transferred to theatre
- Another group of women that can collapse are those that 'trickle' unnoticed for hours after delivery

Further reading

Prendiville WJ, Elbourne D, McDonald S. Active versus expectant management in the third stage of labour. *Cochrane Database Syst Rev* 2000. A meta-analysis of randomized trials comparing active versus expectant management in the third stage of labour. www.mrw.interscience.wiley.com/cochrane

www.cemach.org.uk Saving Mothers' Lives Report, CEMACH 2003–2005. London, 2007.

11.2 Retained placenta and uterine inversion

Retained placenta

Definition
The placenta and membranes are undelivered 30 min (active management) or 60 min (physiological) after the vaginal delivery of the fetus.

This potentially life-threatening condition is often treated as a low priority compared with other obstetric emergencies, despite the associated risks of postpartum haemorrhage (PPH), infection, and procedural complications.

Incidence
- The incidence is ~0.6–2%

Causes
- Failed placental separation, e.g. morbid adherence (see Section 8.4)
- Succinturate lobe
- Cord detachment

Risk factors
- Previous retained placenta
- Preterm delivery
- Previous uterine surgery (e.g. curettage/CS)
- Young maternal age

Brandt–Andrews technique
Controlled cord traction (CCT) with countertraction above the level of the symphysis for delivery of the placenta results in a significantly lower incidence of PPH and retained placenta compared with a physiological third stage (see Figure 9.2, Section 9.1).

Clinical management
Principles of general care
- Keep the woman and her birthing partner informed
- Inform the anaesthetist, labour ward co-ordinator, and the senior obstetrician
- Record the time
- Establish IV access and start IV fluid replacement
- Send blood for FBC and G&S
- Insert an indwelling catheter
- Ensure adequate analgesia and reassess
- Inject a solution of 20 iu oxytocin in 20 ml saline into the umbilical vein; clamp the cord proximally; observe for 30 min
- The usual signs of placental separation may not be obvious, e.g. bleeding maybe concealed (see Box 11.2)
- If still undelivered, proceed to a manual removal (see Box 11.3)

Complications
Haemorrhage (primary and secondary)
In a study of secondary PPH, more than one-third had retained placental tissue (confirmed surgically). See Section 11.1.

Endometritis
There is no data to evaluate the efficacy of antibiotic prophylaxis against endometritis after manual removal of placenta (MROP) (Cochrane database).

Trauma
Increased risk of uterine perforation with instrumentation.

Recurrence
- Increased risk in subsequent deliveries

Useful tips
- If haemodynamically stable, wait for 30–60 min; otherwise resuscitate and proceed with MROP
- Although empirical, IV oxytocin infusions have been administered to assist the delivery of the placenta. The National Institute of Clinical Excellence (NICE) advise this should not be used

- Nitroglycerine tablets are not prescribed in UK practice owing to the associated drop in diastolic BP
- Acknowledge the mother's potential distress that the procedure is invasive (akin to veterinary medicine), especially if the woman is awake; keeping the baby with the mother is a welcome distraction
- The longer the third stage, the more difficult the MROP as the cervix may close. Hence the placenta may need to be removed piecemeal
- MROP at CS is associated with ↑ blood loss compared with CCT

Uterine inversion
This condition is very rare (1:2000 deliveries).

Risk factors
- Abnormalities of placentation, e.g. accreta
- Fundal placental insertion
- Any condition that predisposes to uterine atony and prolapse
- CCT without countertraction in an uncontracted uterus

Clinical management
- Attempt a manual replacement of the uterus (see Figure 11.2)
- Start maternal resuscitation
- Leave the placenta attached
- Arrange transfer to theatre for reduction under GA
- Try hydrostatic pressure in addition to manual pressure to reduce the uterus (using the gloved hand to seal off the vaginal entrance, pour saline into the vagina via two giving sets, or via a Silastic ventouse)
- If vital signs are stable and abnormal placentation is not suspected, uterine relaxants such as nitroglycerine, may be helpful during the manual replacement
- If all other methods fail, proceed with a transabdominal reduction
- Once the uterus is replaced, undertake a MROP
- Administer IV uterotonics

Complications
- Severe maternal shock
- Haemorrhage (primary and secondary)
- Sepsis
- Strangulation of the uterus

Further reading
Tandberg A, Alberchtsen S, Ivessen OE. Manual removal of the placenta. Incidence and clinical significance. *Acta Obstet Gynecol Scand* 1999; **78**:33–6.

Chongsomchai C, Lumbiganon P, Laopaidoon M. Prophylactic antibiotics for manual removal of retained placenta in vaginal birth. Cochrane Database of Systematic Reviews 2006, Issue 2 Art No. CD004904.

> **◎ Box 11.2 The four signs of placental separation**
>
> ***Cord lengthening:*** when the placenta separates, progressive uterine retraction forces the placenta into the lower uterine segment. A cord clamp near the perineum shows the lengthening. Traction on the cord without countertraction on the uterus above the symphysis may be mistaken for cord lengthening
>
> ***Uterus becomes globular and firmer:*** this change may be difficult to palpate
>
> ***Uterus rises in the abdomen:*** the descent of the placenta into the lower segment, and finally into the vagina, displaces the uterus upwards
>
> ***Gush of blood:*** retroplacental clot escapes as the placenta descends into the lower uterine segment. This is not a reliable indicator of complete separation

> **◎ Box 11.3 Manual removal of placenta (MROP)**
>
> (see Figure 11.1)
> - Counsel and consent (risks include infection, haemorrhage, and trauma to the womb and birth canal)
> - Inform the on-call consultant if not already done
> - Transfer to theatre
> - Regional anaesthesia is recommended. GA is less commonly used
> - Single dose of prophylactic IV antibiotics may be given intra-operatively
> - Prepare as for routine surgery but wear gauntlets (high-level gloves)
> - Lubricate your hand with an antiseptic cream, e.g. Hibitane®, before inserting into the vagina
> - Proceed to insert your hand into the uterine cavity
> - Place your other hand abdominally over the fundus to stabilize the uterus
> - Identify the plane between the placenta and uterus
> - With the hand, fingers together, proceed to separate the placenta in its entirety
> - Holding the placenta and membranes firmly, withdraw your hand. Simultaneously, position your other hand on the uterus to provide countertraction
> - Examine the uterine cavity for residual cotyledons or membranes
> - Commence IV oxytocin infusion to reduce the risks of atony and hence of PPH
> - Examine the placenta and membranes. If either appears incomplete, re-explore the uterine cavity
> - Continue close monitoring of the woman's vital signs, fundal height, and lochia
> - Measure blood loss and calculate running total
> - Repeat FBC and transfuse if clinically indicated

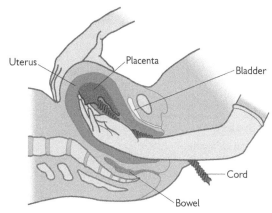

Fig. 11.1 Manual removal of placenta. One hand supports and guards the uterine fundus abdominally whilst the other (with the fingers held tightly together) advances along the line of cleavage of the placenta, separating it in its entirety. (Provided by Miss A Kumar.)

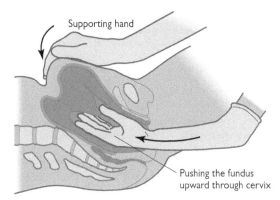

Fig. 11.2 Reduction of uterine inversion. The inverted uterus is replaced by applying firm pressure with a gloved hand. (Provided by Miss A Kumar.)

11.3 Perineal trauma

The perineum extends from the pubic arch to the coccyx, and can be divided into the anterior urogenital triangle and posterior anal triangle.

Incidence
- Up to 85% of women experience some perineal trauma during vaginal birth

Clinical relevance
In the first days postnatally, perineal trauma can be associated with considerable pain and discomfort, and interfere with breastfeeding and bonding. For a minority of women, it causes long-term physical and psychosocial morbidity.

Pathophysiology
Perineal damage occurs during birth in the following ways:
- Spontaneously when the presenting part tears the tissues
- From an episiotomy
- From instrumental or manipulation (e.g. MROP)

Clinical evaluation
- Systematic visual assessment should be carried out soon after birth to ascertain and classify the extent of any injury and therefore options for care
- Trauma is described as anterior or posterior to the vagina

Anterior perineal trauma
- Injury to labia, anterior vagina, urethra, and clitoris

Posterior perineal trauma
- Injury to the posterior vaginal wall, perineal muscles, anal sphincters, and anal epithelium
- Immediate visual assessment identifies around 2% of women as having damage involving the anal sphincter, whereas endoanal ultrasound identifies occult damage to the anal sphincter in up to 36% of women following vaginal delivery
- The clinical relevance of asymptomatic defects is unclear

Complications of trauma
The severity of trauma, timeliness, and effectiveness of treatment are important risk factors for developing complications.

Key factors which influence the outcome of repair are type of suturing material used, technique of repair, and skill of the operator.

Classification of trauma
A standard approach to describing classifying and recording trauma is recommended, as, for example, shown in Table 11.1.

Consent for perineal repair
Before initiating any assessment of trauma, the woman should be offered full information about why the procedure is recommended, the process involved, and her consent sought. The woman should be informed of the findings and given the opportunity to discuss options for treatment. Her consent to carry out treatment or care strategy (including non-repair of trauma) should be sought.

Operators should explain what they are doing during assessment and repair, and give the woman a written record of the trauma and treatment she has experienced and the plan for post-repair care.

Consent, assessment, repair, and treatment plan should be recorded in the woman's postnatal notes.

Methods and material for repair
The objectives of repair are to achieve haemostasis and approximate the disrupted tissue to assist natural healing. Good anatomical alignment is imperative.

Summary of the principles of perineal repair (Adapted from RCOG, 2004)
- Ensure that the woman has adequate analgesia and is as comfortable as possible throughout the initial assessment (systematic examination of the perineum, vagina, and rectum) and subsequent repair procedure
- Ask for more experienced opinion if any doubt about the extent of trauma or structures involved. The PR examination aims to detect any occult anal sphincter trauma
- Suture promptly after birth under aseptic conditions to reduce bleeding and risk of infection
- Check equipment and count swabs before starting the procedure; check and count again following completion of the repair
- Good lighting is essential to visualize and identify the structures involved
- Complex trauma should be repaired by an experienced operator in theatre under regional or general anaesthesia (good practice point). Following such repair, insert an indwelling catheter for 24 h to prevent urinary retention
- Perform a rectal examination after completing the repair to ensure that suture material has not been accidentally inserted through the rectal mucosa

Suture material
Rapid-absorption polyglactin 910 (Vicryl rapide) is less likely to cause pain and require suture removal compared to standard absorbable synthetic material. It is, therefore, the recommended suture material for non-complex perineal repair which does not involve the anal sphincter or rectum.

Method
Non-locking continuous suturing is recommended to re-approximate all layers. The procedure is outlined in Box 11.6.

Pain relief and care after repair
Unless contraindicated, administration of 100 mg diclofenac suppositories provides good, immediate pain relief.

In the first few days a woman should be advised to use:
- Topical cold therapy
- Oral paracetamol (unless contraindicated)
- Non-steroidal anti-inflammatories (NSAIDs), unless contraindicated

She should report any concerns about pain, discomfort or healing to the healthcare professional responsible for her care.

Although some women are apprehensive about showering or bathing after perineal repair, they should be reassured that bathing does provide relief from the discomfort they experience.

There is no evidence that additives such as salt or antiseptic solutions are beneficial to promote healing, reduce pain or, in the longer term, dyspareunia. Cleansing with water and, if required, mild soap, and gentle drying of the area should be advised.

Sexual health problems occurring after birth are common yet seldom identified by health professionals or indeed reported spontaneously by women. The risk factors include primiparity, mode of delivery, and perineal trauma.

A postnatal study of primiparous women post-delivery by Barrett et al. (2000) suggested that most women had resumed intercourse within 6 months. However, the majority of cases of first-onset dyspareunia occurred in the first 3 months following vaginal delivery. Between 2 and 6 weeks, it is therefore important to ask if a woman has resumed sexual intercourse and, if so, if she has experienced anxiety, pain or discomfort (NICE, 2006).

Management of postpartum dyspareunia ranges from pelvic floor exercises to the use of bath additives. A large survey of members of the National Childbirth Trust reported that some women rubbed oils or gels on their perineum or used vaginal lubrication to relieve soreness on penetration.

Repair of third or fourth degree tears

Repair of a third or fourth degree tear must be carried out by an operator with the appropriate levels of competence and experience. The procedure should take place in theatre to provide adequate lighting with the option of regional or general anaesthetic.

Method

Two methods are commonly used:

- **The overlap method**, which involves overlapping the torn ends of the anal sphincter and inserting interrupted sutures
- **The end-to-end method,** in which torn ends are re-approximated and repaired with interrupted mattress sutures

A monofilament suture material, such as polydioxanone (PDS), is recommended for sphincter repair as it has a longer half-life and carries a lower risk of infection.

A recent RCT suggests that the end-to-end method is better.

Care after repair

A course of prophylactic antibiotics and aperients (a stool softener and bulking agent) should be prescribed for 2 weeks after repair to reduce wound breakdown and to minimize straining during bowel movement (**C**).

Offering follow-up in a dedicated clinic for up to 1 year after birth so that the woman can review her experiences, healing and perineal function, and begin to discuss any issues about giving birth vaginally in future, has been shown to be of value to those who have experienced severe perineal trauma.

Further reading

Department of Health. National Maternity Statistics, England 89-90 to 94-95. London: HMSO, 1998.

Pendry E, Peacock J, Victor CR et al. 2000. Women's sexual health after childbirth BJOG 107;2:186–195.

Sultan AH, Kamm MA, Hudson CN, Bartram Cl. Third degree obstetric anal sphincter tears: risk factors and outcome of primary repair. BMJ 1994; **308:**887–91.

www.nice.org.uk Clinical guidelines and evidence review for postnatal care: routine postnatal care of recently delivered women and their babies. 2006 CG37 Postnatal care.

www.rcog.org.uk Methods and materials used in perineal repair. Guideline 23. RCOG, 2004.

Box 11.4 Risk factors for perineal trauma

Risk factors for perineal trauma

Primiparity	Ethnicity (Caucasian)
Fetal birth weight >4 kg	Raised maternal age
Prolonged second stage of labour	Tissue type
	Poor nutritional state
Instrumental delivery	Lack of antenatal perineal massage
Direct occipitoposterior position	
Precipitate birth	

Box 11.5 Complications of perineal trauma

Immediate	**Delayed**
Bleeding	Haematoma
Pain	Infection
Suturing through the rectum	Scarring
	Superficial dyspareunia
	Urinary incontinence
	Faecal incontinence
	Fistula formation

307

Table 11.1 Classification of perineal tears

Degree	Extent of trauma
First	Skin only
Second	Perineum involving the perineal muscles but not the anal sphincters
Third	Involvement of anal sphincter complex, (external anal sphincter (EAS) and internal anal sphincter (IAS)) divided into 3a <50% EAS thickness torn 3b >50% EAS thickness torn 3c (IAS)
Fourth	Involving anal sphincter complex and rectal mucosa

⊙ Box 11.6 Second degree perineal tear repair

Vaginal repair

- Locate the apex of the tear and assess if bilateral or unilateral (Figure 11.3)
- Secure any bleeding points by inserting suture above the apex (Figure 11.4)
- Apply a continuous non-locking stitch to the vaginal tissue (Figure 11.5)
- Deep tissue bites are recommended but should not be too tight
- Use the hymen remnants on either side as a landmark for correct vaginal mucosa reapproximation
- Once the fourchette has been reached, the needle should be inserted through the skin on one side and through deep tissue on the other to bury the knot. This is the first muscle stitch and it completes the vaginal repair (Figure 11.6)

Muscle repair

- Insert the non-suturing index finger to determine the depth of the defect and to push the rectum down and out of the way
- Begin a continuous stitch near the fourchette and emerge at the distal apex of the skin (Figure 11.7)
- Insert two layers of sutures, if necessary, to ensure no dead space remains (Figure 11.8)
- It may be necessary to place some single interrupted sutures to the muscle layer first if the tear is very deep

Skin repair

- Reverse the direction of the suture to close the subcuticular tissue
- Tie the loose stitch end to the starting end and bury the knot (Figure 11.9)
- It is unnecessary to insert sutures directly into the skin

Concluding procedure

- Examine the vagina to ensure that there is no bleeding
- Perform a rectal examination to ensure patency and check for misplaced sutures

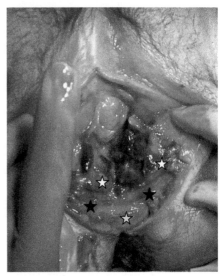

Fig. 11.3 Second degree tear. Torn mucosa edges (☆); torn perineal muscle (★); intact anal sphincter (☆).

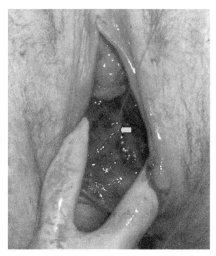

Fig. 11.4 First stitch secures the apex (⇦) of the mucosal tear.

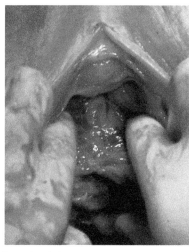

Fig. 11.5 Sutured vaginal mucosa.

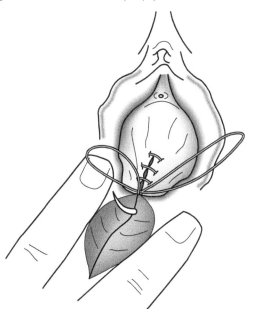

Fig. 11.6 Bury the knot after closing the vaginal mucosa.

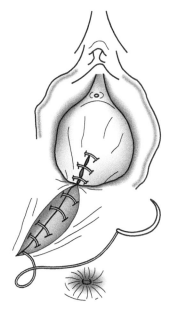

Fig. 11.7 Close the perineal muscles with a continuous stitch.

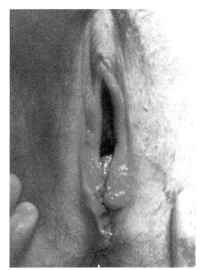

Fig. 11.8 Perineal muscles reapproximated.

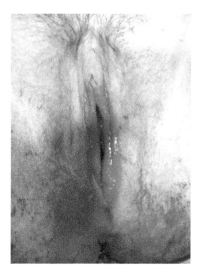

Fig. 11.9 Skin closed.

Maternal collapse

See also Sections 10.1, 10.2, and 10.3.

Postnatal maternal collapse may be sudden and unexpected, and may be a simple transient faint or a cardiac arrest. The underlying cause may be related to, or incidental and aggravated by, pregnancy.

The main causes of postnatal maternal collapse are:

- Postpartum haemorrhage (see Section 11.1)
- Cardiac arrest (see Section 10.2)
- Thromboembolic disease (see Sections 8.16 and 8.17)

Principles of management

Management aims at achieving resuscitation, stabilizing the woman's condition, diagnosis of cause, and prompt initiation of appropriate treatment. The outcome will largely depend on the success of management in the first few minutes.

Every maternity unit and trust providing maternity care should develop and implement guidelines for the management of obstetric emergencies such as maternal collapse.

All healthcare professionals offering postnatal care to women and babies should be sufficiently competent and skilled to implement these guidelines effectively and efficiently.

When a woman has collapsed, she cannot give consent for interventions and so it is important that she is given a clear explanation about the reasons for her collapse and recommended treatment as soon as she is able to participate in such a discussion. The principles of informed consent should be followed.

As far as possible, the woman and her partner or family should be supported and cared for emotionally as well as physically whilst emergency treatment or urgent diagnostic tests and treatment are being carried out.

Cardiac arrest

A woman experiencing cardiac arrest will have sudden, complete loss of consciousness with no vital signs.

The main objectives of management are to resuscitate the woman by beginning cardiopulmonary resuscitation within 3–4 min of onset, stabilize her condition, and diagnose and treat the underlying cause (for further information see ABCDE Boxes in Section 10.1).

All staff should regularly attend adult resuscitation 'skills and drills' courses so as to be prepard for this uncommon but increasing emergency.

Thromboembolic disease

Thromboembolic disease remains the principal cause of direct maternal death in the UK, with over half of deaths occurring in the puerperium.

Diagnosis and management of deep venous thrombosis (DVT) and pulmonary embolism (PE) are covered in Sections 8.16 and 8.17.

It is recommended that anticoagulant therapy is continued throughout pregnancy and for at least 6 weeks postnatally. Neither heparin nor warfarin is contraindicated in breastfeeding mothers. Women should be counselled about the choice of heparin or warfarin.

If warfarin is preferred, the need for regular blood test monitoring (INR level) should be discussed, especially in the first 7 days of treatment. It should also be noted that postpartum treatment with warfarin should not normally start until the second or third day after birth and later for women at increased risk of postpartum haemorrhage (PPH).

If the woman continues taking heparin postnatally, then the dosage should either be the same as used in pregnancy or the standard dose for a non-pregnant patient (e.g. enoxaparin 1.5 mg/kg once daily).

The haematologist will advise and arrange follow-up in an anticoagulation clinic.

Thromboprophylaxis

To avoid maternal death, it is vital that Trusts develop and implement clinical guidelines for thromboprophylaxis. Postnatal thromboprophylaxis can be planned at any stage, and written up in the notes at any time from booking until after delivery.

See Box 8.10 in Section 8.16 for risk factors for thromboembolic disease.

Puerperal pyrexia

Puerperal pyrexia is defined as a maternal temperature of ≥38°C or more recorded on two or more occasions within 2 weeks of birth. It is a cardinal sign of infection and other pathology, such as venous thrombosis or breast engorgement.

In 90% of cases, pyrexia is associated with genital or urinary tract infection. Uterine infection is associated with prolonged rupture of membranes and instrumental or CS delivery.

Differential diagnosis

- Endometritis
- Retained products of conception
- Wound infection (perineum, abdomen)
- Pelvic infection (haematoma, abscess)
- Urinary tract infection
- Mastitis or breast abcess
- Deep vein thrombosis
- Drug reaction
- Blood transfusion reaction
- Reactive pyrexia postoperative
- Retained swab
- Other infection

The most common sites for infection and causative organisms are listed in Table 11.2.

Investigation and diagnosis

It is most important to take a full history and perform a full physical examination of the woman, including vital signs, chest, heart, breasts, abdomen, perineum, and legs.

Relevant samples should be taken for microbiology before formulating a provisional diagnosis and prescribing any antibiotic.

A woman who has developed puerperal pyrexia may feel very unwell and anxious. As with any clinical evaluation or assessment, the healthcare professional should discuss the reasons for offering it, and seek consent before carrying out any procedure. As they are undertaking the examination they should describe what they are doing, why they are doing it, and give the woman opportunities to say how she is feeling and ask questions.

Management and antibiotic treatment

The results of any examination and tests should be fully discussed with the woman, along with options for care (including, for example, expected benefits and possible side effects, and duration of antibiotic treatment) before initiating treatment.

Management depends on diagnosing the specific organism causing the infection and the severity of the infection. Blind treatment of pyrexia is inappropriate practice, i.e. bacterial swabs and blood cultures must be taken and a working diagnosis made before initiating antibiotic treatment.

Where antibiotics are required, it is important to take into account medicines contraindicated when breastfeeding, e.g. tetracyclines.

For a woman suspected of having a pelvic infection, treatment should be initiated using a combination of amoxicillin (erythromycin in the case of penicillin allergy) and metronidazole or co-amoxiclav, before the results of a bacterial culture are available. As soon as the results are available, the treatment regimen should be reviewed to check that the antibiotics of choice are effective.

In cases of suspected skin infections, such as wound infections, flucloxacillin can be prescribed.

For urinary tract infection, trimethoprim is appropriate.

The choice of intravenous or oral antibiotic therapy will depend on the severity of the infection. For example, if the woman is vomiting, systemically unwell, or if pyelonephritis is suspected, intravenous therapy should be started.

Failure to respond to treatment may be as a result of prescribing an inappropriate antibiotic or undiagnosed pathology which requires further investigation and management.

A microbiology opinion should be sought. An ultrasound scan should be arranged urgently to rule out the possibility of a pelvic collection. If an abscess is detected, surgery may be required to drain it. The addition of gentamicin or a third generation cephalosporin to the antibiotic regime may be considered if results of cultures are not available at this point.

If β-haemolytic streptococcus, *Chlamydia* or *Neisseria gonorrhoea* are isolated, the paediatrician should be informed so that the baby can be tested and, if infected, offered treatment. If the mother and baby have been discharged home, the results should be communicated urgently to the GP so that the baby's condition can be checked.

In the 2003–2005 CEMACH report, 18 women died from sepsis; 78% of these were due to substandard care. If in doubt about any aspect of diagnosis or treatment, particularly in severe infections, contact a microbiologist and the senior obstetrician for advice and guidance.

Useful tips
- Vital signs are vital. Take tachycardia, tachypnoea, pyrexia, hypotension, and symptoms seriously
- In view of the lower staffing levels on postnatal wards where midwives care for both women and babies, it is very important to recognize sick postnatal women and transfer them in advance of collapse to a safer place (that might be the labour ward, high dependency or intensive care unit)
- Remember to consider thromboembolism prevention for all antenatal and postnatal patients

Further reading

www.library.nhs.uk Emergency ID=79009.

www.cemach.org.uk Saving mothers' lives. Report of Confidential Enquiry 2003–5, London 2007.

Table 11.2 Common sites of puerperal infection and causative organisms	
Site of infection	**Common causative organism**
Genital tract	*E. coli, Staphylococcus, Clostridium*
Urinary tract	*E. coli, Klebsiella, Proteus*
Lactation ducts (mastitis)	*Staphylococcus aureus*

11.6 Mental health in the puerperium

Mental illness in pregnancy is discussed in Section 7.1.

Although most new mothers experience a range of transient emotional states, women with pre-existing mental illness (such as bipolar disorder) are at higher risk of having an acute episode in the puerperium.

Mental health problems in general are as likely to be experienced by women after birth as other adults in the population. However, the care, treatment, and support offered for women in the perinatal period is influenced by the need to consider the baby's wellbeing and take into account the woman's wider family and social network.

It is important to remember that '…some changes in mental state and functioning are a normal part of the antenatal and postnatal experience and [clinicians] should, therefore, be cautious about basing any diagnosis largely on such features without careful consideration of the context. Such features include, for example, sleep disturbance, tiredness, loss of libido and anxious thoughts about the infant' (Antenatal and Postnatal Mental Health Guideline NICE, 2007).

Principles of care of women with mental health disorders (NICE, 2007)

After identifying a possible mental disorder in the postnatal period, further assessment should be considered, in consultation with colleagues if necessary.

- If the healthcare professional or the woman has significant concerns, the woman should normally be referred for further assessment to her GP
- If the woman has, or is suspected to have, a severe mental illness (for example, bipolar disorder or schizophrenia), she should be referred to a specialist mental health service, including, if appropriate and available, a specialist perinatal mental health service. This should be discussed with the woman and preferably with her GP

Postnatal blues ('baby blues')

This is a condition characterized by episodes of fatigue, tearfulness, anxiety, depression, confusion, headache, insomnia, and irritability. It usually peaks at day 4–5 postnatally. This cluster of symptoms is experienced by up to 85% of women. Usually self-limiting, medical treatment is inappropriate. Women should be offered reassurance and support.

Postpartum depression

The incidence of postnatal depression has been estimated to be 13%. The patterns of symptoms in women with postpartum depression are similar to those in women who have episodes unrelated to childbirth. An episode of depression is considered to have postpartum onset if it begins within 4 weeks after delivery. It has a recurrence rate of up to 70% in subsequent pregnancies.

Five or more of the following symptoms must be present daily for at least 2 consecutive weeks to make the diagnosis:

- Depressed mood
- Loss of interest or pleasure
- Significant increases or decreases in appetite
- Insomnia or hypersomnia
- Psychomotor agitation or retardation
- Fatigue or loss of energy
- Feelings of worthlessness or guilt
- Diminished concentration
- Recurrent thoughts of suicide

Postpartum depression usually resolves within 6 months and can be managed in the community by the woman's GP. Reassurance and support from her partner are important, and input from a social worker or group therapy may be of value.

Only a small number of women will need psychiatric management. In women diagnosed with major postpartum depression (typically lasting for more than 1 month), treatment with antidepressants and/or anxiolytics is appropriate.

Although all antidepressants are excreted in breast milk, when choosing an antidepressant for breastfeeding women, consider:

- Most tricyclic antidepressants have a higher fatal toxicity index than selective serotonin reuptake inhibitors (SSRIs)
- Imipramine, nortriptyline and sertraline are present in breast milk at relatively low levels
- Citalopram and fluoxetine are present in breast milk at relatively high levels
- The SSRI sertraline may be an appropriate first line treatment for breastfeeding mothers
- In extreme cases, electroconvulsive therapy (ECT) may be considered.

Puerperal psychosis

Puerperal psychosis is rare (incidence of 1–2:1000). Around 30% of prevalent cases are women with pre-existing mental illness (bipolar disorder, schizophrenia) who are at highest risk, with a recurrence risk in future pregnancies of up to 25%. It usually presents within the first month of birth. The woman may suffer bouts of restlessness, anxiety, and mania with paranoid thoughts or delusions.

Accurate and timely diagnosis is crucial to minimize danger to the mother and baby. For women who experience puerperal psychosis, the suicide rate is 5% and the infanticide rate is 4%. In the most acute phase the woman should be admitted to a specialist perinatal inpatient service which should:

- Provide facilities designed specifically for mothers and infants (typically with 6–12 beds)
- Be staffed by specialist perinatal mental health clinicians
- Be staffed to provide appropriate care for infants
- Have effective liaison with general medical and mental health services
- Have available the full range of therapeutic services
- Be closely integrated with community-based mental health services to ensure continuity of care and minimum length of stay

Post-traumatic stress disorder

This anxiety disorder may arise following a traumatic experience and for some women is the result of childbirth. Around 1.5% of women have been identified as having the symptoms of post-traumatic stress disorder (PTSD) at 6 weeks after birth.

Signs and symptoms
- Persistent experiencing of the traumatic event
- Persistent avoidance of stimuli associated with the event
- Numbing of general responsiveness
- Irritability
- Poor concentration
- Insomnia
- Increased arousal

Risk factors have been identified as including: perceived low levels of support from partners and staff, patterns of blame, and low self-control during labour and emergency CS delivery.

There is no convincing evidence to support drug treatment for PTSD. Psychological therapies should be considered.

Communication, information, and consent

At each postnatal contact, the healthcare professional should encourage the woman and her family to report concerns in relation to their physical, social, mental or emotional health, and discuss issues and ask questions.

Treatment and care should take into account the woman's individual needs and preferences. Women with mental disorders during pregnancy or postnatally should have the opportunity to make informed decisions about their care and treatment in partnership with their healthcare professionals.

If women do not have the capacity to make decisions, healthcare professionals should follow the Department of Health guidelines (Reference guide to consent for examination or treatment, 2001). As of April 2007, healthcare professionals need to follow a code of practice accompanying the Mental Capacity Act.

Good communication between healthcare professionals and women, and their partners, families and carers, is essential. It should be supported by evidence-based written information tailored to the woman's needs. The treatment and care, and information women are given about it, should be culturally appropriate. It should also be accessible to people with additional needs such as physical, sensory or learning disabilities, and to people who do not speak or read English.

Even though health professionals always need to ensure that there is a proper opportunity for confidential consultations (e.g. to enquire about prior pregnancies, domestic violence, etc.), carers and relatives should have the opportunity to be involved in decisions about the woman's care and treatment, unless the woman specifically excludes them.

Carers and relatives should also be given the information and support they need.

Further reading

American Psychiatric Association. Task Force on DSM-IV, 2000.

www.nice.org.uk Antenatal and postnatal mental health guideline. NICE, February 2007.

www.nice.org.uk Clinical guidelines and evidence review for postnatal care: routine postnatal care of recently delivered women and their babies. London: National Collaborating Centre for Primary Care and Royal College of General Practitioners, 2006. CG37, Postnatal care.

www.cemach.org.uk Confidential Enquiry into Maternal Deaths (CEMD). Why mothers die 2003–2005. London: RCOG, 2007.

www.sign.ac.uk/guidelines. Postnatal depression and puerperal psychosis. SIGN publication No. 60. June, 2002.

www.dca.gov.uk The Mental Capacity Act. Summary.

> **➕ Box 11.7 Risk factors for postpartum depression (Scotland Intercollegiate Guidelines Network, 2002)**
>
> **Absolute risk factors**
>
> Past history of postpartum depression
> Low social support
> Poor marital relationship
> Recent life events
> Postnatal blues
>
> **Possible risk factors**
>
> Parents' perceptions of their own upbringing
> Unplanned pregnancy
> Unemployment
> Not breastfeeding
> Antenatal parental stress
> Antenatal thyroid dysfunction
> Coping style
> Longer time to conception
> Depression in fathers
> Emotional lability
> Low quality social support
> Having two or more children

> **➕ Box 11.8 Risk factors for puerperal psychosis (Scotland Intercollegiate Guidelines Network, 2002)**
>
> Past history of puerperal psychosis
> Pre-existing psychotic illness
> Family history of affective psychosis in first or second degree relatives

11.7 Infant feeding

Breastfeeding is the healthiest way to feed a newborn, and provides benefits for both mother and baby. In 2005, only 77% of mothers breastfed at birth in the UK and very few continued for the recommended 6 months. It is important to offer a woman advice and support about breastfeeding before birth so as to make an informed decision about how she wants to feed her baby.

Physiology

The two main hormones involved in breastfeeding are prolactin and oxytocin. Prolactin is produced by the anterior pituitary and released into the circulation, and its levels are regulated by the dopaminergic system. It acts on the human breast to produce milk. Oxytocin is produced by the posterior pituitary and its release is stimulated by the action of suckling at the breast, resulting in milk ejection.

Benefits for baby
- Protection against infections, including gastrointestinal, urinary, respiratory, and middle ear
- Lower risk of atopic disease
- Lower risk of juvenile-onset diabetes

Benefits for mother
- ↑ likelihood of returning to pre-pregnancy weight
- ↓ risk of both oestrogen and progesterone receptor-positive and -negative breast cancers
- ↓ incidence of hip fractures
- ↑ bone density

Supporting a woman to decide about feeding

Obliging a woman to make the choice about how to feed her baby during pregnancy may lead her to opt for formula. Offering information about breastfeeding which helps her to make the right decision once her baby is born keeps all options open for her. This information should include details about local and national peer support groups for breastfeeding mothers.

Supporting breastfeeding initiation

Separation of a baby and mother should be avoided in the first hour after birth if at all possible. Bonding opportunities should take precedence over hospital or theatre routines. Early and prolonged skin-to-skin contact between mother and baby allows their relationship to develop and promotes hormonal changes needed to initiate and maintain breast milk production.

Hospital units should provide facilities for 24-h rooming-in, so they can remain together throughout their stay.

Culturally appropriate information about breastfeeding should be offered to women in the first 24 h after birth. This should describe colostrum, the high density low volume milk produced during early feeding. Normally, colostrum is replaced by 'full' breastmilk around day 3 when lactation is established and the women's milk 'comes in'.

From the earliest breastfeed, skilled support should be available to enable a woman to find a comfortable position and to help her ensure that her baby attaches correctly to her breasts. This will allow her to feed her baby effectively, prevent sore nipples and promote milk production.

Establishing breastfeeding may not be straightforward, and women need informed encouragement; conflicting advice from professionals can be very undermining. Women can be reassured that a healthy baby may safely lose up to 10% of its weight in the first week of life whilst establishing feeding.

Maintaining breastfeeding

Each baby has an individual feeding pattern and this will vary according to their physiological needs. Frequency of breastfeeding should not be restricted. A woman should be advised about indicators of good attachment and positioning of her baby.

These include:
- The baby's mouth is wide open before attachment
- Less areola is visible below the baby's chin than above the nipple
- The baby's chin should touch the breast, lower lip rolled down, nose free
- She should not feel pain

Indicators of effective feeding include:
- Audible and visible swallowing
- Sustained rhythmic sucking
- Baby's arms and hands relaxed
- Baby's mouth is moist
- Regular urine soaked nappies

Breastfed babies should not be offered any other fluids as they will reduce the need to suck at the breast to stimulate milk production.

Expressing breast milk

All breastfeeding women should be shown how to hand express their breast milk and advised how to store and freeze it correctly. Mechanical breast pumps should be available in maternity units, particularly for women who are separated from their babies because of need for care in a neonatal unit, so that they can continue to promote lactation and collect milk for their babies.

Formula feeding

Promotion of formula milk by health professionals and others undermines breastfeeding. Unless a woman chooses to offer formula or it is medically indicated, it should not be given to breastfed babies. Medical indications include:
- Very low birth weight, dysmature or sick babies or those in need of surgery in the care of a paediatrician
- Babies whose mothers have severe maternal illness
- Babies whose mothers have HIV (see Section 6.7)
- Babies with inborn errors of metabolism
- Mothers who are taking medication which is contraindicated when breastfeeding (very few)

If a woman chooses to formula feed, she should be offered tailored advice to ensure feeding is undertaken safely (e.g. how to make up and store feeds, cleanse bottles, and teats).

Weaning

Whether women breastfeed or formula feed they are advised to do so exclusively for 6 months before introducing any solids. Duration of breastfeeding is a personal decision and therefore varies from woman to woman.

Further reading

Amir LA, Garland SM, Lumley J. A case-control study of mastitis: nasal carriage of *Staphylococcus aureus*. *BMC Family Practice* 2006; **7:**57.

www.breastfeeding.nhs.uk NHS National Breastfeeding Awareness Week.

www.babyfriendly.org.uk/health.asp UNICEF UK Baby Friendly Initiative. Health benefits of breastfeeding. Promotion of breast-feeding initiation and duration: evidence into practice briefing, July 2006.

www.dh.gov.uk *Birth to five: feeding your child.* 04135770 DH 2006, Chapter 5.

www.dh.gov.uk 04136429, DH *The Pregnancy Book*, Chapter 8. The feeding question, 2006.

www.ic.nhs.uk/pubs/breastfeed2005 National Statistics 2005. Infant Feeding Survey 2005: Early Results.

www.nice.org.uk Clinical guidelines and evidence review for postna-tal care: routine postnatal care of recently delivered women and their babies. London: National Collaborating Centre for Primary Care and Royal College of General Practitioners, 2006. CG37 Postnatal care

www.patient.co.uk 27000668, Mastitis.

Table 11.3 Breastfeeding concerns and problems and outline actions

Nipple sensitivity/ pain	Transient at start of feeds in early postnatal period
	Caused by enhanced lactational hormones
	Check baby's attachment at breast
	Reassure woman that not uncommon
Engorgement	Advise women that breasts often feel tender, firm, and painful when milk comes in around 3 days after birth
	Advise a woman to wear a well-fitting bra that does not restrict her breasts
	Treat with frequent unlimited feeding, including from the affected breast
	Oral analgesia
	Tip: do not mistake the engorged axillary tail of the breast for an abnormal mass
Mastitis	Presentation ranges from local inflammation (tenderness, erythema, warmth, hardness) with few systemic symptoms, to abscess and septicaemia
	Continue breastfeeding; however, if too painful, express
	Oral analgesia
	Antibiotic therapy if no improvement
	If poorly managed, can lead to breast abscess
Breast abscess	Typically, maternal pyrexia, breast red with swollen area, infected discharge sometimes present
	Continue breastfeeding. However, if too painful, express
	Antibiotic therapy required
	Oral analgesia
	May require surgical drainage in severe cases

11.8 Neonatal assessment and resuscitation

Before birth, if resuscitation is unlikely to be needed, the mother should be asked whether she would like her baby to be born onto her abdomen for immediate skin-to-skin contact.

Almost immediately after birth, a baby should have a brief examination to ensure there are no gross physical abnormalities. This is normally carried out by a health professional birth attendant.

Later, a comprehensive physical examination should be performed, ideally within 24 h and certainly within 72 h. In a maternity unit, it is usually undertaken before discharge. The examination should be repeated at 6–8 weeks of age.

Assessment at birth

Most babies will breathe and some may cry at the moment of birth. If the baby does not needs immediate resuscitation (see below), there should be no delay in birthing the baby onto the mother's abdomen or handing the baby to the mother. Delaying cord clamping by 2 min after birth is associated with improved iron stores at 6 months, with no identified increase in morbidity such as jaundice. The baby should be covered in a warm towel to preserve heat while still maintaining skin-to-skin contact. Separation of mother and baby in the first hour for postnatal routines such as weighing or bathing should be avoided unless requested by the mother.

If the baby needs further evaluation or to support breathing then he or she should be transferred onto a firm flat surface, such as a resuscitaire, to allow full examination and other intervention.

Recording baby's condition

Baseline assessments of condition at 1 and 5 min after birth are made and recorded. In the UK, the Apgar score (see Table 11.4) is commonly used to indicate early neonatal condition. A systematic review suggested that the Apgar score is a moderate level predictor for neonatal death and the development of cerebral palsy. It generally serves to identify the need for resuscitation rather than predict hypoxic injury. It can be affected by maternal drugs (anaesthetic agents, opiates), and other causes.

If a baby is born with an Apgar score $\leq$5 at 1 min post-delivery, cord blood gas sampling is indicated.

With these observations, babies can be categorized:

1. Healthy (Apgar score 7–10)
Adequate respiration, heart rate >100 bpm, pink and crying.
The majority of babies fall into this category and do not require any support or resuscitation.

2. Primary apnoea (Apgar score 4–6)
Some respiratory effort, heart rate >100 bpm, cyanosed. Some tone and response to stimulation. Basic resuscitation involving gentle stimulation and ventilation with room air via an open mask is indicated. The baby usually begins to breathe spontaneously. Ventilate through a bag and mask using O_2 if there is no response after 1 min.

3. Terminal apnoea (Apgar score 1–3)
Apnoeic, heart rate <60 bpm, pale and floppy. Immediate bag and mask ventilation with O_2 is required. If the baby does not respond, intubation and cardiac compressions should be used.

4. Fresh stillbirth (Apgar score 0)
Apnoeic, no heart rate, pale and floppy. Immediate full cardiopulmonary resuscitation is required.

Meconium-stained liquor

Significant meconium staining is defined as the presence of liquor which is dark green or black and thick, or any liquor containing lumps of meconium. The passage of meconium before birth is associated with an increased incidence of perinatal morbidity and mortality. Aspiration of meconium can lead to meconium aspiration syndrome, which accounts for 2% of perinatal deaths. If meconium stained liquor is identified, a paediatrician should be present at delivery.

Resuscitation

Anticipation

Having highly trained paediatric staff present at every delivery is a waste of resource, yet only attending when problems arise puts babies at risk by potentially delaying effective resuscitation. Appropriately anticipating the need for resuscitation is key.

Risk factors which indicate that a paediatrician/health care professional with high level skills in neonatal resuscitation should be present at birth are shown in Box 11.9.

Having a baby who needs resuscitation causes considerable anxiety for parents, and clear sensitive communication is likely to reduce their distress.

Before the birth of a baby who may need resuscitation, it is important to inform the parents what is likely to happen, e.g. if there is meconium and the paediatrician is to check the baby immediately after birth, it is far better to explain to the parents why they may not hear their baby cry immediately, than to have them fear that their baby has died.

If it is not possible to discuss resuscitation before birth, then as soon as is feasible offer support to the parents by describing what is being done for their baby and why.

Preparation of equipment before birth
- Switch the resuscitaire light and heater on
- Ensure that warm dry towels are available
- Check all necessary equipment is available and functioning

The ABC of resuscitation
ABC stands for Airway, Breathing, and Circulation. Adequate temperature control is also needed. The baby should be kept dry and warm to reduce the risk of hypoglycaemia and acidosis.

Stimulation
Several methods of stimulation are used. Rubbing thoroughly dry with a warm towel achieves immediate stimulation as well as ensuring the baby will not get cold. Whether tactile stimulation is effective can easily be assessed by applying a single finger flick to the sole of the foot. If stimulation works this is likely to produce facial grimace or even a cry. It is important not to cause significant pain and under no circumstances should it cause bruising. Another method involves gentle rubbing of the back. Previous approaches such as back slapping and sternal pressure can cause injury and therefore should not be used.

Airway
The baby should be positioned supine with its head in the neutral position. As newborn babies have large occiputs, this causes them naturally to adopt a flexed position, so the use of a towel (or a hand) under the shoulders is helpful. Lift the chin slightly to prevent the tongue from obstructing the airway.

Most babies do not require airway clearance. However, if there is meconium in the airway, aspirate this using suction. Avoid blind deep pharyngeal suction as this may produce reflex apnoea, vagally induced bradycardia, and worsen existing hypoxia.

Breathing
Babies with shallow irregular respirations, heart rates <100 bpm or with apnoea should be ventilated with a bag and mask. The mask

should be large enough to cover the face from the bridge of the nose to below the mouth. The bag is connected to an oxygen supply and a rate of 30–40 per minute should be maintained until spontaneous, reliable respiration is achieved. It is also possible to use a T-piece for ventilation. This has the advantage of requiring only one hand to operate and a more flexible pressure control.

For babies with terminal apnoea or asystole, or with primary apnoea that does not respond to bag and mask ventilation, tracheal intubation will be required. A rate of 30–40 breaths/min with an inspiratory time of approximately 0.5 s should be maintained. It is crucial that, following intubation, the chest is inspected for bilateral chest movements, bilateral and equal breath sounds on auscultation, and absence of breath sounds over the stomach.

Circulation

Babies with a heart rate of <60 bpm despite effective ventilation require cardiac compression. There are two techniques:

1. Apply two fingers over the lower third of the sternum about one finger's breadth below the inter-nipple line. Care should be used to avoid compressions near the xiphoid process as these are likely to cause visceral damage (Figure 11.10)
2. Position both thumbs on the sternum one finger's breadth below the inter-nipple line and encircle the chest with both hands so that the fingers lie behind and support the baby (Figure 11.11)

The sternum should be depressed at a rate of 120 compressions/min at a depth of 1–2 cm. In practice, this is difficult to sustain and a rate of 90 compressions/min is acceptable. Three compressions are given for every ventilation.

Drugs used in resuscitation

Drugs are administered if ventilation with 100% O_2 and compressions fail to achieve a heart rate >60 bpm.

- Adrenaline (epinephrine) can be given IV (10 µg/kg) or via the endotracheal tube (20 µg/kg). Between 10 and 30 µg/kg can be given every 3–5 min
- Sodium bicarbonate 1 mmol/kg can be administered IV if the heart rate remains <60 bpm despite adrenaline
- Naloxone is reserved for specific cases where there is persistent apnoea and a maternal history of opiate analgesia. It should not be used if the heart rate is <60 bpm or if the mother is opiate-dependent

When should resuscitation stop?

It is standard practice to provide full cardiopulmonary resuscitation to any baby born with signs of life. However, if there is no improvement after 15 min, it is unlikely that it will be possible to revive the baby. Normally, the most senior paediatrician present should determine if and when to abandon resuscitation.

The parents of a baby who has not responded to resuscitation deserve particularly sensitive communication and support. Local trust guidelines should be developed and implemented to care for their needs.

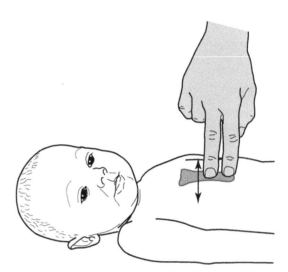
Box 11.9 Indicators of the need for neonatal resuscitation

Maternal factors	Fetal factors
Pre-eclampsia	Abnormal presentation
Heavy sedation	Multiple pregnancy
Diabetes mellitus	Preterm (<34 weeks)
Chronic illness	Post-term (>42 weeks)
Drug addiction	Growth restriction
Maternal haemorrhage	Fetal abnormality
Prolonged labour	Rhesus isoimmunization
Assisted delivery	Polyhydramnios
Emergency CS	Oligohydramnios
	Intrauterine infection
	Fetal distress
	Thick meconium-stained liquor

Fig. 11.10 Chest compression with two fingers (↔: inter-nipple line).

Table 11.4 Apgar score system			
Score	0	1	2
Heart rate	Absent	<100 bpm	>100 bpm
Respiratory effort	Absent	Irregular, slow	Regular, cry
Muscle tone	Limp	Some flexion in limbs	Well flexed limbs
Reflex irritability	Nil	Grimace	Cough/cry
Colour	Pale	Blue	Pink

Further reading

www.also.org Newborn

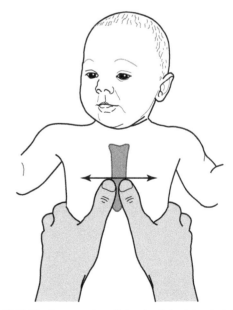
Fig. 11.11 Chest compression with two hands (↔: inter-nipple line).

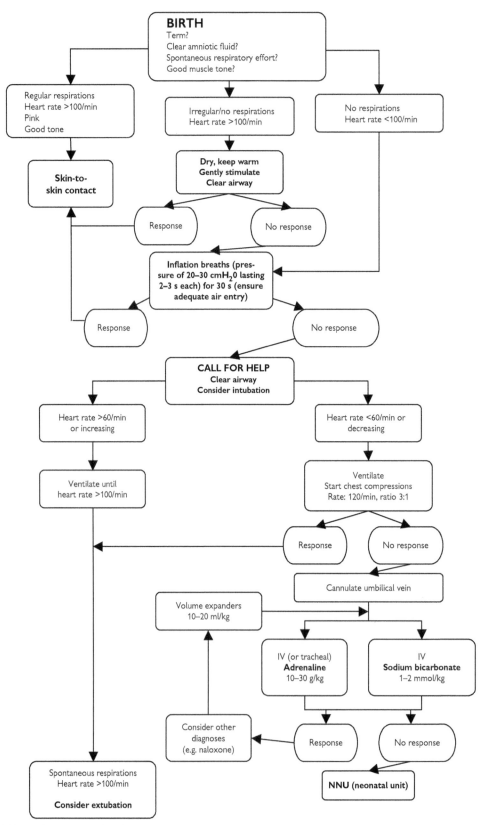

Fig. 11.12 Neonatal resuscitation algorithm.

Chapter 12

Menstrual disorders

Contents

Covered elsewhere

- Menstrual dysfunction in adolescence (see Section 2.8)
- Dysfunctional uterine bleeding and dysmenorrhoea in adolescence (see Section 2.9)
- Dysmenorrhoea (see Section 13.1)
- Hysterectomy (see Sections 13.6 and 13.7)

Physiology and embryology

Hypothalamic regulation of ovarian function

The ovary is regulated by pituitary hormones that are under the direct control of the hypothalamus.

Neurons in the hypothalamus secrete gonadotrophin-releasing hormone (GnRH), a peptide hormone made up of 10 amino acids, in a pulsatile fashion. This hormone passes along the portal vessels on either side of the pituitary stalk to reach the anterior pituitary. There it binds to the basophil gonadotroph cells to cause the synthesis and release of the gonadotrophin hormones LH and FSH that regulate ovarian hormone production and the growth and release of eggs (see Figure 12.1).

Clinical relevance—administration of GnRH in a pulsatile manner stimulates LH and FSH, but when given in a constant high dose, it desensitizes the GnRH receptor to reduce LH and FSH secretion and inhibit ovarian function.

Development of oocytes in the ovary

In the very early fetus, oocytes migrate to the gonadal ridge from extraembryonic tissue close to the yolk sac.

In the ovary they divide and increase in number until reaching a maximum in the late second trimester of pregnancy. The oocytes start the process of meiosis but are arrested at the first prophase until they are ovulated in later life. A thin layer of cells surround the oocytes to form the primordial follicle. Oocytes that have not formed follicles are lost from the ovary and the number of oocytes decreases markedly before birth.

At birth the ovary contains approximately just under 1 million oocytes. No new oocytes are formed. Every day throughout life a proportion of primordial follicles activate and start growing until the ovaries have run out of eggs.

Towards the time of menopause cycles become anovulatory.

Follicular activation

Understanding of what causes primordial follicles to activate and start to grow is incomplete. The oocyte begins to increase in size. The flattened surrounding pregranulosa cells become bigger. This is known as a primary follicle. The granulosa cells form into layers around the oocyte and begin to induce the formation of theca cells from the fibroblasts surrounding the follicle. Spaces appear within the granulosa cells and an antral cavity appears, containing follicular fluid. By this stage the follicle has developed an independent blood supply in the thecal layer and is a few millimetres in diameter. The process takes 3 months and occurs at a constant rate in the presence or absence of hormones.

The early follicular phase

At any time there are up to 20 antral follicles that have now developed the capacity to respond to LH and FSH. At the time of menstruation there is an increase in FSH and this stimulates the follicles to grow. Small follicles secrete inhibin B which feeds back to inhibit basal FSH secretion.

Follicular development

As the follicles grow they secrete increasing amounts of oestradiol. The synthesis of oestradiol requires both LH and FSH, as well as granulosa cells and theca cells. LH causes theca cells to produce androgen. This androgen is converted to oestrogen under the influence of FSH in the granulosa cells.

As follicles grow, the increasing oestradiol feeds back to the pituitary to lower FSH secretion. As smaller follicles need more FSH to survive than larger follicles, the largest follicle survives but the smaller follicles undergo atresia. The negative feedback on FSH is the main reason that only one follicle becomes dominant and ovulates each month.

Ovulation

During the 14-day follicular phase, the dominant follicle grows to ~20 mm in diameter. The granulosa cells develop receptors to LH during maturation to make up for the reduced FSH and prepare for ovulation. When the follicle is fully mature, the high concentrations of oestradiol cause a change at the hypothalamus and pituitary to cause a positive feedback effect. This causes a surge in LH.

Follicular rupture

The LH surge activates the oocyte and it enters metaphase of meiosis 1. The oocyte continues to develop until it fully completes the meiotic process around the time of fertilization. In addition, the LH surge activates a cascade of processes akin to an inflammatory response. This thins the follicle wall and 36 h later the oocyte is released. Several factors are involved in this process, but prostaglandins are key regulatory molecules.

The LH surge also luteinizes the granulosa cells, giving them the enzymatic machinery to synthesize progesterone in response to LH stimulation. This process is not dependent on prostaglandins.

The corpus luteum

The remaining granulosa and theca cells form the corpus luteum.

As the granulosa cells were avascular prior to ovulation and the corpus luteum is arguably the most vascular structure in the body, luteal formation is associated with massive angiogenesis. This is caused by local production of vascular endothelial growth factor (VEGF) from the steroidogenic cells.

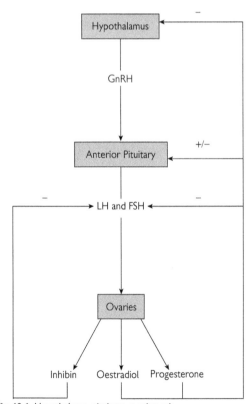

Fig. 12.1 Hypothalamo–pituitary–ovarian axis.

At its peak, the corpus luteum measures up to 20 mm in diameter and produces large amounts of progesterone to stabilize the endometrium in preparation for pregnancy.

Luteolysis

Luteal progesterone production is dependent on LH. As the corpus luteum matures, it becomes less sensitive to LH, progesterone secretion declines, and the corpus luteum begins to disappear from the ovary.

The luteal phase lasts 14 days and this is constant, unlike the follicular phase, which can be variable. The corpus luteum secretes inhibin A and oestradiol as well as progesterone. These feed back to inhibit FSH secretion during the luteal phase.

The corpus luteum has a central role in the regulation of menstruation and the progesterone it secretes is crucial for the establishment of pregnancy. The high levels of progesterone act on the endometrium to provide a suitable environment for blastocyst implantation. If this occurs, human chorionic gonadotrophin (HCG) rescues the corpus luteum and progesterone secretion is maintained to support early embryonic growth.

However, if conception does not occur, the corpus luteum regresses, progesterone levels fall, and menstruation is initiated. The withdrawal of progesterone causes menstruation and the increase in FSH required to stimulate the next cycle (see Figure 12.2).

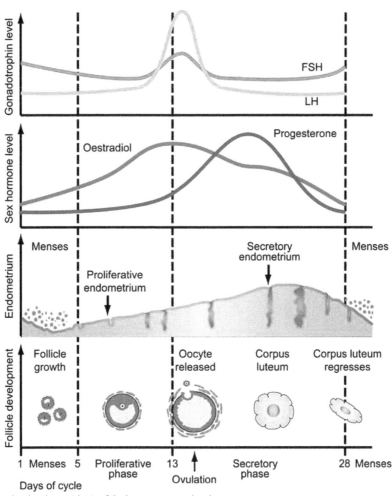

Fig. 12.2 The hormonal and endometrial axis of the human menstrual cycle.
After menstruation, rising levels of oestrogen exert a negative feedback, reducing FSH release. Towards midcycle, still higher levels of oestrogen then exert a positive feedback, causing a sudden peak release of LH, which induces ovulation. An increased level in FSH also occurs. The endometrium during this phase has a thin surface epithelium and the glands are straight, short, and narrow (proliferative/follicular). In the luteal phase, LH levels maintain the corpus luteum, the source of progesterone. The endometrial glands become more tortuous during this phase (secretory/ luteal) with secretion in the lumen and increasing fluid separating the stromal cells. If an embryo fails to implant, the corpus luteum deteriorates after about 7 days, with a resulting fall in progesterone and oestrogen concentrations.

12.2 Basic anatomy

External female genitalia and the perineum

See figures 12.5, 12.6, 12.7, and 12.8.

Uterus and cervix

The uterus is a muscular organ situated midline in the pelvis, with the bladder anteriorly and the rectum posteriorly.

It consists of a body and cervix, and joins the vagina inferiorly. Viewed anteriorly, it is an inverted triangle. Each of the superior corners, the cornu, is continuous with the Fallopian tubes, and the inferior corner forms the cervical os. The rounded superior end of the uterus is the fundus (see Figure 12.3).

Supports of the uterus

The uterus is supported by the pelvic floor and the surrounding viscera (e.g. the bladder and rectum). The main support is from the cervical ligaments. These consist of the uterosacral ligaments posteriorly, the pubocervical ligaments anteriorly, and the transverse cervical ligaments medially and laterally.

The round ligaments of the uterus also provide a degree of support. They run from the uterus, anterior and inferior to the Fallopian tubes, between the layers of the broad ligament to the lateral pelvic walls. Here they cross the pelvic brim to enter the inguinal canal, ending at the labia majora (see also Section 14.1).

Clinical relevance—in 80% of women, the cervical ligaments hold the uterus in an anteverted position, i.e. tilting up towards the abdominal wall. In the remaining 20% the uterus tilts back into the pelvis—retroversion.

The wall of the uterus consists of a thick wall of smooth muscle, the myometrium. This is lined internally by glandular epithelium, known as the endometrium. The outer coat is the serosa and is made up of peritoneum posteriorly.

Anteriorly, the peritoneum covers the uterus until it reaches the bladder, where it is reflected over the anterior surface of the bladder (the uterovesical fold). This peritoneum extends bilaterally to form the broad ligaments that connect the uterus and pelvic side wall. This broad ligament encloses the Fallopian tubes and round ligaments superiorly and the uterine arteries, ureters, and parametrium inferiorly.

Blood supply

The uterus is supplied by a rich anastomosis of the uterine and ovarian vessels. The uterine artery, derived from the anterior branch of the internal iliac artery, crosses over the ureter just lateral to the cervix (remembered by using the phrase 'water under the bridge'). At this point it gives off a vaginal branch, which runs downwards along the lateral vaginal wall.

The main artery follows a tortuous course along the lateral wall of the uterus, giving off numerous branches into the substance of the uterus. It finally diverges laterally into the broad ligament to anastomose with the ovarian artery (see Figure 12.4).

Clinical relevance—it is possible to ligate both internal iliac arteries to reduce bleeding from the uterus and still maintain viability of the pelvic organs due to collateral blood flow from the ovarian vessels.

Ovaries and Fallopian tubes

The ovaries, like the testes, develop in the abdominal cavity and descend into the pelvis before birth. Unlike the testes, the ovaries do not migrate through the inguinal canal but stop on the lateral pelvic wall just below the pelvic inlet.

Each ovary is attached to the broad ligament by the mesovarium. The infundibulopelvic ligament attaches each ovary to the pelvic side wall and contains the ovarian vessels, nerves, and lymphatics. The ovarian ligament connects the ovary to the uterus.

The ovary itself is comprised of an outer epithelial layer. This surrounds an inner medulla, containing connective tissue and blood vessels, and a follicle-containing cortex. Each month an ovum is released from the ovary into the peritoneal cavity, where it is directed by cilia into the Fallopian tube. It enters the trumpet-shaped end of the tube, the infundibulum.

Medial to the infundibulum, the tube expands to form the ampulla where fertilization usually takes place. The tube then narrows to form the isthmus, before joining with the uterus at the cornua.

Blood supply

The blood supply to the ovaries is from the ovarian artery. This is derived directly from the aorta (see Figure 12.4).

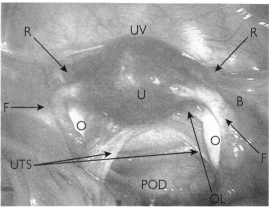

Fig. 12.3 Laparoscopic view of female pelvis demonstrating the uterovesical fold (UV); uterus (U); round ligaments (R); Fallopian tubes (F); ovaries (O); ovarian ligament (OL); broad ligament (B); uterosacral ligaments (UTS); and pouch of Douglas (POD).

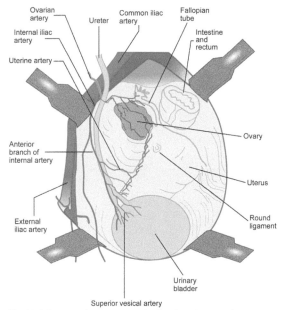

Fig. 12.4 Diagram demonstrating the female pelvic vasculature.

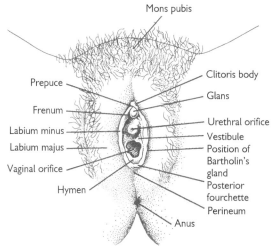

Fig. 12.5 Anatomy of the external genitalia. Reproduced with permission from Collier, Longmore and Brinsden. *Oxford Handbook of Clinical Specialties*, 7th edn. Oxford University Press, 2006.

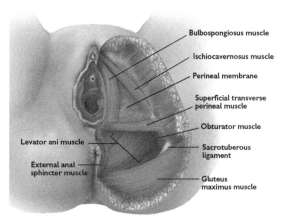

Fig. 12.6 Anatomy of the female perineum (Reproduced with permission from C.R. Bard, Inc.)

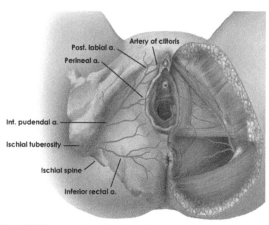

Fig. 12.7 Blood supply to female perineum. a: artery, post.: posterior, int: internal (Reproduced with permission from C.R. Bard, Inc.)

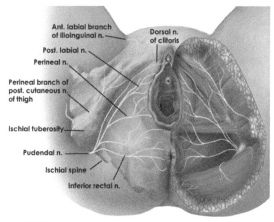

Fig. 12.8 Nerve supply to female perineum. n: nerve, ant: anterior, post: posterior (Reproduced with permission from C.R. Bard, Inc.)

CHAPTER 12 **Menstrual disorders**

323

12.3 Heavy menstrual bleeding—menorrhagia

Incidence
One in 20 women aged 30–49 years old present to medical services with heavy periods. Heavy menstrual bleeding (HMB) has a major effect on a woman's quality of life, raising physical, psychological, social, and financial issues for the patient and her gynaecologist to address.

Definition
HMB is both an objective and subjective diagnosis (see below).

Objectively, HMB is defined as a blood loss of >80 ml per menstruation. Studies have revealed that the average blood loss per cycle is 30–40 ml. Thus, women who objectively have HMB are at risk of symptoms of anaemia.

Subjective HMB is a complaint of excessive menstrual blood loss over several consecutive cycles. These women may not have a blood loss of >80 ml per cycle, but their symptoms have a considerable impact on their lives, making intervention necessary (Box 12.1 and Figure 12.9).

Differential diagnosis of heavy menstrual bleeding
Anatomical local
- Fibroids and polyps
- Pelvic infection (chlamydia)
- Endometrial (and cervical) carcinoma

Systemic
- Coagulopathy
- Thyroid disease

Iatrogenic
- Anticoagulation therapy
- Copper intrauterine contraceptive devices (IUCDs)

Unexplained (no systemic/pelvic pathology)
- Primary endometrial disorder

Pathophysiology
HMB may be caused by any of the anatomical or systemic pathologies listed. Irregular, heavy menstruation may be associated with anovulation.

HMB commonly occurs at the extremes of reproductive life. In the majority of cases, no organic cause for HMB can be found. It seems likely that the precise cause of HMB lies at the level of the endometrium itself.

Mechanisms contributing to causes of heavy bleeding remain undefined. A fibrinolytic system is known to be present in the human endometrium. This system appears to be more active in women who experience HMB, and its inhibition can lead to effective reduction in blood loss. Previous research has also demonstrated increased levels of total prostaglandins (PG) in the endometrium of women with HMB. There is a reduction in menstrual blood loss with inhibitors of PG-synthesizing enzymes (e.g. mefenamic acid).

Clinical evaluation
History
A good history is essential and should include a full gynaecological history. The following factors should be asked about specifically to determine the nature of the bleeding problem and any potentially serious pathology:
- The amount and timing of bleeding
- A menstrual diary is often helpful
- Flooding and clots may indicate significant loss

- Intermenstrual bleeding (IMB) and postcoital bleeding (PCB) suggest an anatomical cause
- Pelvic pain and its relation to the menstrual cycle
- Pressure symptoms, including bowel and urinary tract
- Abnormal vaginal discharge
- Smear history
- Sexual and contraceptive history (including desire for future pregnancy as this affects management)
- A history of a coagulation disorder, i.e. a history of excessive bleeding since menarche, a history of postpartum haemorrhage, surgery-related bleeding, bleeding associated with dental work, or a history of two or more of the following: bruising greater than 5 cm or epistaxis once a month, frequent bleeding or a family history of bleeding symptoms

Examination
- General—to exclude signs of anaemia
- Abdominal—for a pelvic mass
- A speculum—to assess the vulva, vagina, and cervix
- A bimanual—to elicit uterine and adnexal enlargement or tenderness

Investigations
If the history and examination strongly suggests heavy bleeding without the presence of pathology in a woman <45 years old, it is appropriate to implement first line medical treatment without further investigation.

In older women, and in younger women in whom medical treatment has failed, further investigation is warranted:
- Full blood count
- A coagulation screen is indicated if a focused history is suggestive of a coagulation disorder
- Thyroid function tests should only be taken from women with other symptoms of thyroid disease
- Cervical smear test
- Endocervical or high vaginal swabs
- Pelvic ultrasound is a useful first line diagnostic tool for structural pathology, such as fibroids or polyps
- Endometrial biopsy is indicated in symptomatic women >45 years old, in younger women when medical treatment has failed, and in all women prior to surgical intervention (see Box 12.2 and Figure 12.10)
- Hysteroscopy with biopsy may be helpful when women have IMB or PCB, irregular heavy menstrual loss, suspected structural pathology, or when medical management has failed (see Section 12.4)

The following studies raised concerns about conceptualization and assessment of menstrual complaint and the appropriateness of healthcare provision. They highlighted the importance of considering the diagnosis of heavy menstrual bleeding as a subjective, rather than a purely objective, diagnosis.

- Warner P, Critchley HO, Lumsden MA, Campbell-Brown M, Douglas A, Murray G. Referral for menstrual problems: cross sectional survey of symptoms, reasons for referral, and management. *British Medical Journal* 2001; **323**:24–8.

This study demonstrated that discordance exists between symptoms and both referral and diagnostic pathways, arising from a disproportionate focus on menstrual bleeding (Figure 12.9). It showed that, among women referred with heavy menstrual bleeding, volume of bleeding was not a key symptom.

- Warner PE, Critchley HO, Lumsden MA, Campbell-Brown M, Douglas A, Murray GD. Menorrhagia II: is the 80-mL blood loss criterion useful in management of complaint of menorrhagia? *American Journal of Obstetrics and Gynecology* 2004; **190(5)**:1224–9.

This study demonstrated that the 80 ml criterion for menorrhagia was of limited clinical usefulness because it is prognostic neither for pathology, nor iron status, and does not seem to guide management either.

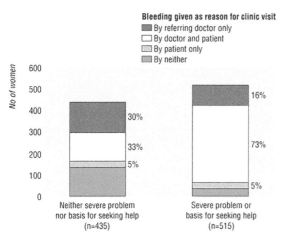

Fig. 12.9 Graphical representation of the frequency with which the doctor, the patient, or both gave 'excessive bleeding' as the reason for the clinic visit in a cross-sectional survey of women referred with menstrual problems. Reprinted with kind permission from Warner et al. *British Medical Journal* 2001; **323**:24–8.

Box 12.2 Technical skills: Outpatient endometrial biopsy

There are various of samplers available for endometrial biopsy. The most commonly used is the Pipelle de Cornier™ suction curette (see Figure 12.10). As it is only 3 mm in diameter, the procedure may be carried out in the outpatient setting and takes only a few minutes. The aim is to pass the curette through the cervical canal into the endometrium to obtain a sample for histological analysis. This is usually a simple procedure but may be more uncomfortable in nulliparous women.

- A chaperone should always be present throughout the procedure
- Verbal consent to perform the biopsy should be obtained
- The procedure should be explained and it should be made clear to the patient that she may experience some crampy pain as the sampler passes into the uterus
- The following equipment should be available: sterile gloves, a speculum with ratchet, lubricating jelly, a vulsellum, a Pipelle™ curette, a pathology specimen container, and a good light source
- The patient should be asked to position herself as for a vaginal examination, a speculum passed, and the cervix visualized
- The sampler should be gently passed through the cervical canal, and held between finger and thumb to avoid excessive pressure
- If the sampler does not pass easily, the vulsellum may be used to grasp the anterior lip of the cervix and straighten the canal to aid passage of the curette, or a uterine sound can be gently passed first
- The sampler should be advanced gently until it reaches the uterine fundus. Record the endometrial depth as the curette may have entered the cervical canal but not the uterine cavity
- At this point the inner lumen of the sampler should be revealed by withdrawal of the inner plunger. The exterior should be held at the fundus while the plunger is being pulled back by using traction on the posterior end of the sampler. This will create a negative pressure and a dead space into which the endometrial biopsy will enter
- To obtain the sample, the Pipelle™ should be moved back and forth in the cavity and rotated simultaneously to obtain tissue from 360° of the endometrial wall
- The Pipelle™ should then be removed and the plunger pushed in to release the sample into the pathology container
- The vulsellum, if used, should be removed before the speculum
- The patient should be warned that she may experience some vaginal spotting and mild cramping pains for a short time after the procedure

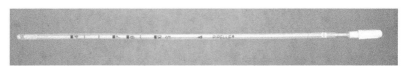

Fig. 12.10 Pipelle™ endometrial sampler.

12.4 Management of heavy menstrual bleeding

After exclusion of anatomical and systemic disorders, symptom management of heavy menstrual bleeding (HMB) becomes a priority. An improvement in the patient's quality of life should be used to gauge the success of any treatment.

Conservative

- Explanation and reassurance are most important
- Exclusion of pathology will allay fears and may avoid the need for further treatment

Medical

If a woman wishes to conceive, hormonal treatments and most surgical interventions are unacceptable.

Non-hormonal treatment

- Antifibrinolytics, such as tranexamic acid, reduce blood loss by up to 50% by inhibiting endometrial fibrinolysis
- Side effects are rare but include gastrointestinal symptoms. Inhibitors of fibrinolysis should not be used in women with a history of, or risk factors for, thromboembolism
- *Usual prescription:* tranexamic acid 1 g TDS or QDS PO when bleeding
- Prostaglandin (PG) synthetase inhibitors, such as non-steroidal anti-inflammatories (NSAIDs), inhibit endometrial PG production, leading to decreased menstrual blood loss.
- Mefenamic acid is the most frequently used agent and reduces blood loss by approximately 25%. The drug is taken during menstruation and has the advantage of containing analgesic properties. It is associated with gastrointestinal side effects.
- *Usual prescription:* mefenamic acid 500 mg TDS PO when bleeding

The use of NSAIDs or tranexamic acid should be stopped if there is no symptomatic improvement after 3 months. They may be continued indefinitely if they are found to be beneficial and can be used as adjuvant therapy alongside other agents.

Hormonal treatments

- The COCP usually produces an estimated reduction in blood loss of 50%. Risks of treatment are higher in older women, particularly smokers, and include thromboembolic disease and migraine
- The progestogen (levonorgestrel; LNG)-releasing intrauterine contraceptive system (IUS) or Mirena™ system (see Figure 12.11) can decrease menstrual loss by up to 96% after 1 year and is a real alternative to surgical management (**A**). In addition, it is an excellent contraceptive. It acts by releasing levonorgestrel, which prevents proliferation of the endometrium. As its action is local,

the progestogen-related side effects are much less than with oral agents. Women should be fully counselled that they are likely to experience daily vaginal spotting for the first 3–6 months. Perseverance for at least 6 months is required for benefits to be appreciated and side effects to subside. The Mirena™ IUS may be inserted as an outpatient (see Box 12.3) and should be changed every 5 years

- Oral progestogens, e.g. norethisterone 5 mg TDS prescribed from days 5–26 of the cycle, have a useful role in the regulation of irregular heavy bleeding. Side effects include weight gain, abdominal bloating, and headache
- Limited use of gonadotrophin-releasing hormone (GnRH) analogues may be considered when all other management options, including surgery, are contraindicated. They act by downregulating the hypothalamo–pituitary–ovarian axis and induce ovarian suppression, leading to amenorrhoea. Although effective in reducing blood loss, menopausal side effects limit their use beyond 6 months. If used >6 months, 'add-back' HRT therapy is recommended
- Danazol and gestrinone are no longer recommended for routine use in the treatment of HMB owing to their unacceptable side effects

Surgical

Surgical intervention should be considered when medical management has failed or as an initial treatment after full discussion of side effects and alternative treatment options. Typically, surgical management is only considered in women who have completed their family, with the exception of myomectomy, where fertility may be retained.

- Endometrial resection or ablation removes the first few millimetres of the endometrium and improves symptoms in up to 80% of women (see Section 12.8)
- Myomectomy is the surgical removal of fibroids (see Section 12.6)
- Hysterectomy is an established, effective treatment of HMB (**A**), but should only be considered when other surgical treatments have failed or are contraindicated. Potential complications and the resulting infertility should be discussed (see Sections 13.6 and 13.7)

Further reading

NICE. Heavy menstrual bleeding. CG44 2007. www.nice.org.uk

RCOG. The management of menorrhagia in secondary care. National evidence based clinical guideline, 2007.

⦿ Box 12.3 Insertion of Mirena™ intrauterine system

- Verbal consent should be obtained for insertion of the Mirena™ IUS after full discussion of its actions and side effects
- Ensure a chaperone is present
- Equipment—sterile gloves, speculum with ratchet, lubricating jelly, a vulsellum, sterile uterine sound, sterile Mirena™ IUS, and a good light source
- The IUS should be prepared on a sterile field by releasing the threads and pulling them until the IUS is in the insertion tube. The threads should be tightly fixed in the cleft at the end of the inserter
- The patient should be asked to position herself as for a vaginal examination and the cervix should be visualized with a speculum
- The cavity should be measured with a uterine sound and the flange on the Mirena™ insertion system set to the sound measurement
- The IUS should be held with the thumb on the slider and carefully inserted into the uterus until the flange is 2 cm from the cervix
- At this point the slider should be pulled back until it reaches the mark. This will open the arms of the IUS
- The inserter can now be gently pushed inwards until the flange touches the cervix. This will place the IUS in the fundal position
- The slider should be pulled down all the way prior to removal of the insertion system from the uterus. This will release the IUS from within the insertion tube
- The vaginal part of the threads should be trimmed, leaving 2 cm visible outside the cervix
- The woman is asked to feel for the threads of the IUS in 6 weeks so as to ensure that it has not been expelled
- The incidence of uterine perforation at the time of insertion is 1:1000

Useful tip

After insertion of the IUS, the strings are cut. Let the woman feel the end of the strings that are left so she knowns what she is feeling for at her 6-week position check.

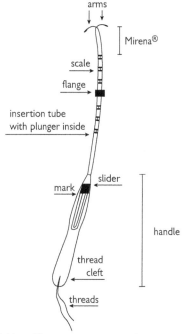

Fig. 12.11 Mirena™ intrauterine system and its inserter. (Reproduced with kind permission from Bayer Schering Pharma AG.)

Fibroids

Fibroids, or leiomyomata, are benign tumours of the myometrium and vary in size from a few millimetres to massive tumours filling the whole abdomen. They are formed from smooth muscle and fibrous elements.

Incidence and demographic factors
- They occur in almost one in three women >30
- More common as women approach the menopause
- Fibroids are more common in Afro-Caribbean women

Classification

Fibroids may be classified as subserosal, intramural or submucosal (see Figure 12.12). Each location is associated with particular signs and symptoms.

Clinical evaluation

History
- Asymptomatic—about 50% of fibroids cause no symptoms and are found incidentally
- Heavy menstrual bleeding (HMB) may occur, especially with submucosal or intramural fibroids
- Haematological disorders—anaemia may occur with HMB or polycythaemia owing to massive fibroids
- Dysmenorrhoea may be present, but pain is rare unless complications occur
- Pressure effects—the urinary system is most commonly affected, causing frequency, retention or hydronephrosis. Tenesmus may be troublesome if the rectum is affected
- Infertility—it has been suggested that distortion of the uterine cavity due to submucosal fibroids can lead to implantation failure
- Pregnancy—red degeneration of fibroids (see Section 8.5) is much more common. Other problems include premature labour, malpresentation, fetal obstruction, postpartum haemorrhage, and puerperal infection

Examination

Abdominal and pelvic examinations may reveal a pelvic mass, not separate from the uterus. This can be smooth and easily mistaken for a gravid uterus. An irregular, nodular mass may be palpated if there are multiple fibroids present

Investigations
- A full blood count is useful in women suffering from HMB
- Tumour markers, such as CA125 and carcinoembryonic antigen (CEA) may aid differential diagnosis e.g. from an ovarian mass
- Ultrasound—the characteristic ultrasonographic appearance is differential, variegated echogenicity in the substance of the myometrium. Confusion can occur with subserous fibroids, which may be difficult to delineate from ovarian pathology (see Figure 12.13)
- MRI is not usually a first line investigation
- Endometrial biopsy is indicated in older women with menstrual disturbance to exclude concurrent pathology
- Hysteroscopy assesses the endometrial cavity and may allow resection of submucosal fibroids (see Figures 5.1 and 12.14)
- Diagnostic laparoscopy or laparotomy may be the only way to distinguish fibroids from ovarian pathology

Differential diagnoses

Ovarian cancer or cyst, hydrosalpinx, bowel adherent to uterus, appendix abscess, bladder mass

Complications
- Degeneration (hyaline change, calcification, red)
- Torsion of pedunculated fibroid
- Infection with pyometra
- Malignancy (rare)—leiomyosarcoma

Degeneration of fibroids

Deposition of mucopolysaccharide around the muscle fibres leads to hyaline change and occurs in two-thirds of fibroids. Calcification is common after the menopause, when fibroids usually regress owing to lower hormone levels. Red degeneration occurs because of inadequate blood supply. Blood supply to fibroids is usually poor because of the local high pressure. If this delicate supply is compromised, further haemorrhage and infarction occur, causing necrosis, pain, and uterine tenderness.

Useful tip: it is very unwise to diagnose fibroids in a postmenopausal woman with an abdominal mass. Neoplasm must be excluded.

Leiomyosarcoma

(See also Section 15.10)
- Leiomyosarcoma is a pure sarcoma of the uterus, and the treatment of choice is TAH & BSO
- It arises from a fibroid or de novo from the myometrium
- Of 1000 women with fibroids 1–2 will have malignant change
- Fibroids most likely to be malignant include those with rapid growth, growth in the postmenopausal woman not on HRT, and those with a poor response to gonadotrophin-releasing hormone (GnRH) agonists.

Endometrial polyps
- Thought to result from focal stromal and glandular hyperplasia
- They can be an incidental finding or present with intermenstrual bleeding or HMB
- They vary in size and may be sessile or pedunculated
- Larger polyps may prolapse through the cervix
- Although mainly benign, they may rarely contain endometrial hyperplasia or carcinoma
- They are usually diagnosed by ultrasound (see Figure 12.15) or at hysteroscopy (see Figure 12.16), when they can be resected
- Small endocervical polyps can be avulsed in the outpatient setting by grasping with sponge-holding forceps and twisting, but never pulling, until the polyp is removed.

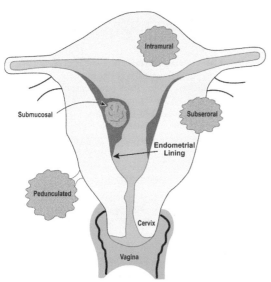

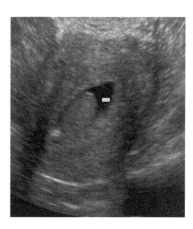

Fig. 12.15 Ultrasound image of an endometrial polyp with saline infusion (⇦). (Kindly provided by Dr Jane Walker.)

Fig. 12.12 Diagram demonstrating the potential locations of uterine fibroids: pedunculated, subserosal, intramural, and submucosal.

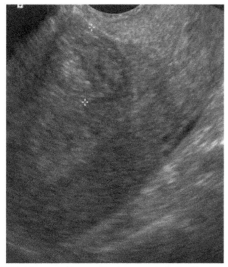

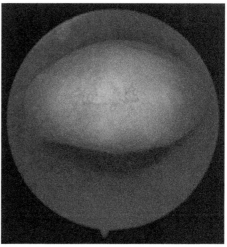

Fig. 12.16 Hysteroscopic view of an endometrial polyp (compare to Fig. 12.19).

Fig. 12.13 Ultrasound image of an intramural uterine fibroid (callipers). (Kindly provided by Dr Jane Walker.)

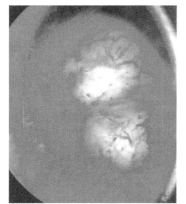

Fig. 12.14 Hysteroscopic view of a submucosal fibroid. (Kindly provided by Dr Sue Milne.)

12.6 Management of fibroids

Conservative

If women are asymptomatic with small or slow growing fibroids, no treatment is necessary. Women with larger fibroids who do not wish treatment may benefit from serial US to monitor growth.

Medical

- Tranexamic acid and non-steroidal anti-inflammatory drugs (NSAIDs) are often ineffective in heavy menstrual bleeding (HMB) secondary to fibroids
- As fibroids contain oestrogen and progesterone receptors, they respond to hormonal treatment. In particular, gonadotrophin-releasing hormone (GnRH) agonist therapy shrinks fibroids and decreases their vascularity. This is most useful prior to surgery. Owing to menopausal symptoms and risk of osteoporosis, this treatment is not usually given for >6 months
- The LNG-IUS (Mirena™) may be helpful in women suffering from HMB. Unfortunately, it may be difficult to insert when fibroids distort the uterine cavity and is more frequently expelled in these patients

Surgical

- Women with symptomatic fibroids often respond poorly to medical treatment, so surgery is often required.
- Hysterectomy is unacceptable for women who have not completed their families.
- The traditional surgical alternative is myomectomy and this can be carried out via a hysteroscopic, laparoscopic or abdominal route depending on their location and size.
- More recently, uterine artery embolization has also been utilized in the treatment of fibroids.

Myomectomy

This involves surgical removal of fibroids from the uterine wall with conservation of the uterus and is a treatment for women with HMB who wish to conserve their fertility. It may be carried out with the aim of improving fertility.

Gonadotrophin agonist therapy is often used for 3 months prior to surgical intervention in an attempt to reduce the vascularity of the fibroids. However, the fibroid capsule loses its clear demarcation at open surgery. Alternatively, the vasoconstrictor Pitressin can be injected directly into the fibroid at the time of surgery.

In women with multiple fibroids or a significantly enlarged uterus, the abdominal approach is most appropriate. If the fibroid protrudes into the uterine cavity, it may be removed hysteroscopically using diathermy or laser. Small subserosal fibroids can be treated laparoscopically, when a harmonic scalpel may be used to minimize blood loss.

Complications

- Immediate complications usually relate to blood loss
- Difficulty achieving haemostasis occurs more frequently than at hysterectomy
- A blood transfusion may be required intraoperatively or postoperatively
- Progression to hysterectomy to control blood loss is not uncommon and patients should be carefully counselled preoperatively about this risk
- There is also the risk of bowel or bladder damage at the time of surgery
- Intermediate risks include postoperative infection and bleeding

- The major late complication associated with myomectomy is recurrence. After an abdominal procedure, the recurrence rate is estimated at 5.7–11%. Up to 17% of women require further surgical intervention following myomectomy
- There is insufficient and conflicting evidence regarding the risk of uterine rupture in labour following a myomectomy. However, a vaginal delivery following an uncomplicated myomectomy appears to be safe

Uterine artery embolization

Uterine artery embolization (UAE) is a well established technique for the control of postpartum haemorrhage but has only recently been employed in the treatment of fibroids (see Figure 12.17). The procedure is carried out by an interventional radiologist, usually under local anaesthetic ± sedation.

The femoral artery is canalized on one or both sides and fed via the iliac into the uterine artery. Angiography is carried out to confirm the correct position before introduction of the embolic agent.

Blockage of both uterine arteries results in fibroids becoming avascular and shrinking. As the normal myometrium subsequently derives its blood supply from the vaginal and ovarian vasculature, it is thought to have no permanent effect on the rest of the uterus.

The procedure requires only a short hospital stay and may be done as a day case in selected women.

After UAE, a mean reduction of fibroid volume of 40–75% has been reported. Symptomatic improvement has been reported in 62–95% of women.

Complications

Immediate and intermediate

- Patients may experience ischaemic pain. This usually responds to simple analgesia
- Infection may be a problem post-UAE
- Subserosal fibroids may be adherent to the bowel and UAE can lead to bowel necrosis and peritonitis
- Uterine fibroids may prolapse through the cervix following UAE. The rapid change in uterine size can result in passage of the fibroid vaginally

Late

- There is a small risk of premature ovarian failure after UAE. The embolic agent could enter the ovarian artery due to its anastomosis with the uterine artery. The resulting decreased blood supply to the ovary may trigger ovarian failure, and amenorrhoea has been reported in 3% of women <40 years and 41% of those >40 years of age
- Because of these statistics and lack of studies assessing pregnancy rates post-UAE, the procedure is not currently recommended for women who wish to retain their fertility

Further reading

NICE. Uterine artery embolisation for fibroids. Interventional procedure guidance No. 94, 2004. www.nice.org.uk

Lumsden MA. Embolization versus myomectomy versus hysterectomy. Which is best, when? *Human Reproduction* 2002; **17**:253–9.

- Myomectomy
- Hysteroscopic
- Laparoscopic
- Laparotomy
- Uterine artery embolization
- Hysterectomy (see Section 13.6 and 13.7)

→ **Box 12.5 Landmark research**

- Edwards RD, Moss JG, Lumsden MA, Wu O, Murray LS, Twaddle S, Murray GD (CREST). Uterine-artery embolization versus surgery for symptomatic uterine fibroids. *New England Journal of Medicine* 2007; **356(4):**360–370.

A randomized controlled trial (RCT) that compared uterine artery embolization and surgery in women with symptomatic uterine fibroids found that there were no significant differences between groups in the primary outcome of quality of life at 1 year. The embolization group had a shorter median duration of hospitalization and a shorter time before return to work.

At 1 year, symptom scores were better in the surgical group. After the first year of follow-up, 14 women in the embolization group (13%) required hospitalization, three for major adverse events and 11 for reintervention for treatment failure.

The study concluded that, in women with symptomatic fibroids, the faster recovery after embolization must be weighed against the need for further treatment in a minority of patients.

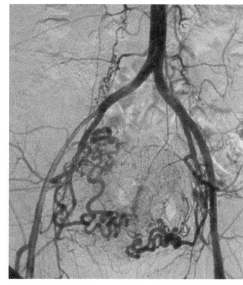

(a)

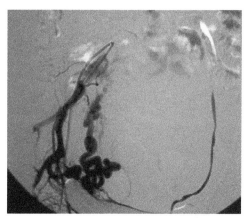

(b)

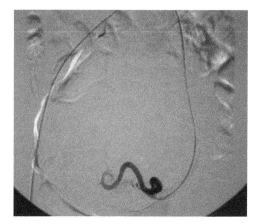

(c)

Fig. 12.17 Angiogram demonstrating fibroid embolization. The femoral artery is canalized and fed via the iliac into the uterine artery. Angiography is carried out to confirm the correct position before introduction of the embolic agent (**a** and **b**). Blockage of both uterine arteries (**c**) results in fibroids becoming avascular and shrinking. (Kindly provided by Dr Mustafa Fleet.)

12.7 Hysteroscopy

Diagnostic hysteroscopy can be carried out under general anaesthesia or in the outpatient setting ± local anaesthetic.

Indications
- Abnormal uterine bleeding
- Subfertility
- Retrieval of coil
- Polypectomy
- Hysteroscopic myomectomy
- Endometrial resection
- Division of synechiae
- Sterilization

Equipment
(see Figure 12.18)
- Endoscopes are flexible or rigid
- Rigid telescopes are available with different directions of view: 0°, 15° or 30°
- A 30° or flexible telescope is normally used for diagnosis
- Correct distension of the uterine cavity is vital. The most common distension media include carbon dioxide, electrolyte (e.g. saline), and hypertonic solutions (e.g. glycine or sorbitol). A diagnostic sheath slides over the telescope to allow flow of the medium
- A high-quality light source is required, e.g. xenon
- A camera at the end of the optic allows a clear view
- An operating sheath is used for procedural hysteroscopy. It contains an additional port, through which instruments can be passed, e.g. scissors, grasping or biopsy forceps, and diathermy
- When monopolar diathermy is used for endometrial resection, it is essential that a non-conducting hypertonic solution is used. Saline is used with bipolar diathermy

Technique
- The light source, camera, and appropriate distension media should be connected to the hysteroscope and sheath
- With the patient in the lithotomy position, a bimanual examination is performed to assess uterine size and position
- The cervix should be visualized
- Sometimes it is helpful to grasp the anterior lip gently with vulsellum forceps
- Cervical dilatation may occasionally be required in the nulliparous patient
- In most cases, the hysteroscope can be inserted into the cervical canal with the pressure from the distension media
- The vaginoscopic method may also be used, precluding the need for speculum or vulsellum (the vagina is filled with saline and the hysteroscope gently introduced into the cervix)
- Once the internal os has been passed, the distension medium should be allowed to fill the uterine cavity to give an adequate view of the endometrium
- Both ostia should be located, followed by a systematic visualization of 360° of the cavity (see Figure 12.19)
- A directed biopsy, excision of small polyps or fibroids, or division of adhesions can be performed by passing scissors and forceps through the diagnostic sheath (see Figure 12.20)
- After assessment of the cavity, the hysteroscope should be withdrawn slowly through the cervical canal, inspecting for pathology

Potential complications
- Perforation
- Damage to bladder, bowel, blood vessels
- Haemorrhage
- Infection
- Fluid overload

This last unusual complication is mainly restricted to resection procedures and is caused by absorption of distension medium. Hyponatraemia, cerebral oedema, and cardiac overload may ensue.

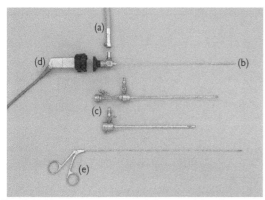

Fig. 12.18 Hysteroscopy equipment: light source (**a**); endoscope (**b**); components of operating sheath (**c**); camera (**d**); and biopsy forceps (**e**).

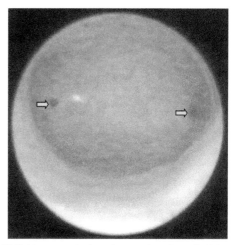

Fig. 12.19 Hysteroscopic view of a normal uterine cavity (⇨ ostia).

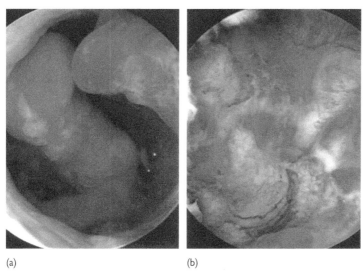

(a)   (b)

Fig. 12.20 Hysteroscopic view of endometrial polyps before (a) and after (b) resection. (Kindly provided by Dr Sue Milne.)

12.8 Endometrial ablation

This procedure aims to reduce menstrual bleeding by destroying the entire thickness of the endometrium and some of the underlying myometrium.

Techniques

First generation techniques include transcervical resection of the endometrium, using an electrical diathermy loop, and roller ball ablation (see Figure 12.21).

Simpler, quicker, second generation alternatives have subsequently been developed. These include fluid-filled thermal balloon endometrial ablation (see Figure 12.22), microwave ablation (see Figure 12.23), and impedance-controlled endometrial ablation (see Figure 12.24).

Indications

Ablation offers an alternative to hysterectomy in women with failed medical management of heavy menstrual bleeding (HMB).

The technique is suitable for women who have completed their family and in whom all organic and structural causes of HMB have been excluded (small fibroids are an exception).

Contraindications

- Desire for future fertility
- Classical CS
- Myomectomy
- Malignancy or premalignant disease of the endometrium

Method-specific contraindications are shown in Box 12.6.

Procedure

All can be performed as day case procedures, sometimes under local anaesthetic in the outpatient setting.

Endometrial thinning agents, such as gonadotrophin-releasing hormone (GnRH) analogues, are not usually indicated for the newer ablative techniques but can be employed at the operator's preference for endometrial resection.

It is recommended that pre-ablation histology of the endometrium is ascertained and that a hysteroscopy is performed before (following cervical dilatation) and after the procedure.

Postoperatively, patients suffer transiently from crampy abdominal pain and have a watery brown discharge for between 3 and 4 weeks.

Prophylactic antibiotic therapy is often used to decrease the risk of endometritis.

Outcomes

- Between 70–90% of women undergoing ablation have reported lighter bleeding levels at 12 months*
- Up to 40% of women are reported to have amenorrhoea 12 months after treatment*
- Longer term success rates are less good
- Up to 30% of women require further treatment of HMB (repeat ablation or hysterectomy) 12 months post-procedure

*The success rates of each technique vary.

Complications

- Device failures at time of procedure
- Bleeding
- Endometritis
- Haematometra
- Fluid overload owing to absorption of distension medium (resection only)
- Perforation with or without intra-abdominal injury
- Visceral burns

Further reading

NICE. Fluid filled thermal balloon and microwave endometrial ablation technology for heavy menstrual bleeding. NICE technology appraisal No. 78, 2004. www.nice.org.uk

> ### ✚ Box 12.6 Method-specific contraindications to endometrial ablation
>
> **Thermal ablation**
> - Large or irregular cavity (including fibroids). The balloon must have direct contact with the uterine wall
> - Uterine length over 10–12 cm
> - Latex allergy
>
> **Microwave ablation**
> - Myometrial thickness <10 mm on USS in three areas with attention to lower segment if previous CS
> - Previous ablation
> - Uterine cavity length greater than 14 cm
> - Any mechanical preparation of cavity, e.g. pre-treatment curettage
>
> **Impedance-controlled ablation**
> - Large or irregular cavity (including fibroids). The system must have direct contact with the uterine wall
> - Uterine length over 10 cm

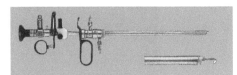

Fig. 12.21 The resectoscope for transcervical resection of the endometrium.

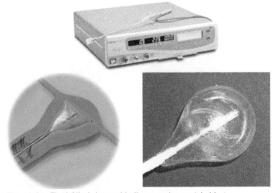

Fig. 12.22 Fluid-filled thermal balloon endometrial ablation (Thermachoice™). (Reproduced with kind permission from Gynecare and Ethicon Women's Health and Urology.)

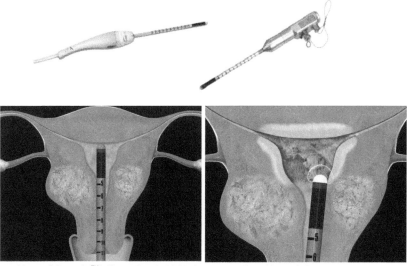

Fig. 12.23 Microwave ablation (Microsulis™). (Reproduced with kind permission from Microsulis.)

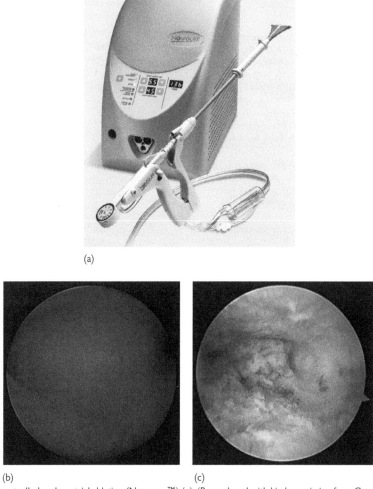

(a)

(b)   (c)

Fig. 12.24 Impedance-controlled endometrial ablation (Novasure™) (a). (Reproduced with kind permission from Cytec.) Endometrium before (b) and after (c) ablation. (Kindly provided by Mr J D S Goodman.)

Definition

Amenorrhoea is the absence of menstruation. It may occur as a physiological phenomenon, such as pre-puberty, during pregnancy or after the menopause. Alternatively, it can indicate a gynaecological disorder.

To menstruate normally, a woman requires a functional hypothalamic–pituitary–ovarian axis with a response endometrium and a patent genital outflow tract. In addition, she must have a normal chromosomal complement and no endocrine or systemic disease.

Primary amenorrhoea is the failure to establish menstruation by 16 years. During female puberty, secondary sexual characteristics usually develop by the age of 14 years. Menstruation should then occur within 2 years. Delay of either of these processes merits investigation.

Primary amenorrhoea may be because of congenital abnormalities of the chromosomes and/or genital tract and an aberration in the endocrine regulation of puberty (see Section 2.8).

Secondary amenorrhoea is defined as cessation of previously normal menstruation for a period of 6 months or more.

This section focuses on the diagnosis and management of secondary amenorrhoea.

Aetiology of secondary amenorrhoea
See Figure 12.22.

Hypothalamic causes

- Low body mass index (BMI)—fat appears to be essential for normal secretion of gonadotrophins. Weight loss of 10–15% of the expected normal usually results in reduced gonadotrophin-releasing hormone (GnRH) release, reduced follicle stimulating hormone (FSH) and luteinising hormone (LH) release, hence lower oestradiol levels, i.e. causes hypothalamic hypogonadism
- Excessive exercise—amenorrhoea is more common in athletes undergoing intensive training compared to the general population. This could be secondary to low BMI or may be an independent risk factor
- Hypothalamic lesions, such as craniopharyngiomas, gliomas, and dermoid cysts, can cause amenorrhoea. They disrupt hypothalamic function by either compressing the hypothalamic tissue or by blocking dopamine, a prolactin inhibitor, causing hyperprolactinaemia
- Systemic disorders can interfere with hypothalamic function, e.g. sarcoidosis, tuberculosis
- Head injury or cranial irradiation will also result in hypogonadotrophic hypogonadism

Pituitary causes

- Prolactin-secreting pituitary adenomas result in hyperprolactinaemia and a decrease in GnRH release. Tumours can be microadenomas (<1 cm) or macroadenomas (>1 cm) and are usually benign (see Figure 12.23)
- Sheehan's syndrome results from prolonged, severe hypotension following a major obstetric haemorrhage. During pregnancy the pituitary gland is enlarged and sensitive to hypoxic insult. FSH and LH secretion are reduced secondary to pituitary infarction.

Ovarian causes

- Polycystic ovarian syndrome (PCOS) is one of the most common causes of secondary amenorrhoea and is discussed in detail in Section 12.11
- Premature ovarian failure is defined as cessation of periods before 40 years old with elevated gonadotrophin levels. In most cases this phenomenon is unexplained. The commonest recognized cause is autoimmune disease and ovarian autoantibodies are commonly found in these patients. In addition, premature ovarian failure is associated with chromosomal disorders. Although Turner's syndrome is associated with primary amenorrhoea, Turner's mosaic (46XX/45XO) may be a cause of premature ovarian failure. Other causes include infection and previous chemotherapy or radiotherapy

Genital tract abnormalities

- Asherman's syndrome (see Figures 12.24 and 12.25) describes intrauterine adhesions, usually following curettage of the uterus or endometritis. There is failure of cyclical endometrial thickening and amenorrhoea ensues
- Cervical stenosis prevents passage of menstrual blood through the cervical os. It occurs rarely and there is usually a history of treatment to the cervix

Adrenal causes

- Virilizing adrenal tumours and late onset congenital adrenal hyperplasia are rare causes of secondary amenorrhoea

Drugs

- Previous or current use of progestogens or HRT can result in iatrogenic amenorrhoea
- Dopamine antagonists such as phenothiazines, domperidone, and metoclopramide can result in hyperprolactinaemia and secondary amenorrhoea

Systemic causes

- Any chronic disease has the potential to affect the hypothalamic–pituitary–ovarian axis. Renal failure, liver disease, thyroid disease
- Cushing's disease, and diabetes mellitus may all cause secondary amenorrhoea

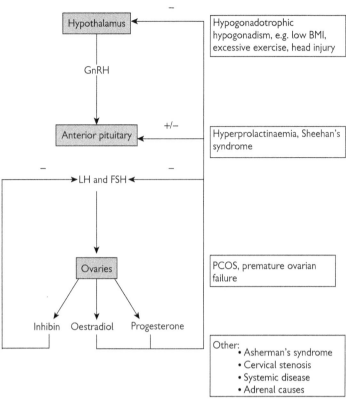

Fig. 12.25 Diagram illustrating hypothalamo–pituitary–ovarian axis and its pathologies.

12.10 Clinical evaluation and management of amenorrhea

Clinical evaluation

History

A comprehensive gynaecological history with a focus on:

- Age at menarche
- Details of previous menstrual cycle
- Any triggers of amenorrhoea, such as weight loss, emotional stress, excessive exercise
- Symptoms of the menopause, e.g. hot flushes, vaginal dryness
- Ask specifically about galactorrhoea as some women will not admit this symptom without direct questioning
- Obstetric history and any fertility problems
- Details of previous uterine surgery
- Drug history
- Family history of early menopause, infertility or autoimmune disease
- Detailed systemic enquiry to identify symptoms of systemic disease

Examination

- General—BMI, inspection of stature and body form. Document presence or absence of secondary sexual characteristics; hair growth, breast development. Signs of endocrine disease must not be missed. Hyperandrogenism may present with hirsutism, acne or balding. Cushing's disease classically gives findings of central obesity, abdominal striae, moon face, buffalo hump and increased bruising. Signs of hyperthyroid disease include goitre, weight loss, tachycardia, and exophthalmos. In contrast, hypothyroid patients have mental slowness, bradycardia, myotonia, and dry thin hair
- Breast examination is required to look for excess hair growth and to elicit galactorrhoea
  Useful tip: prolactin levels should be measured prior to breast examination as this can falsely elevate serum levels
- If a pituitary lesion is suspected, examination of the visual fields is necessary to exclude bitemporal hemianopia, a sign of pressure on the optic chiasm. If elicited, urgent treatment is required
- External genitalia and a vaginal examination

Investigations

- Pregnancy should be excluded
- A hormone profile includes the following: LH, FSH, oestradiol, prolactin, testosterone, sex hormone-binding globulin, and thyroid function tests
- ↑ gonadotrophin levels indicate failure of negative feedback from ovarian hormones, i.e. ovarian failure
- ↑ LH with normal FSH can be caused by the preovulatory LH surge or may indicate a diagnosis of PCOS (see Section 12.11)
- ↓ gonadotrophin levels suggest a pituitary or hypothalamic cause
- Many factors cause an ↑ in prolactin levels (see Box 12.7), which can make interpretation of results difficult
- However, as a general rule, a prolactin of >1000 miu/l on two occasions merits further investigation
- CT or MRI is used to exclude hypothalamic or pituitary tumours (see Figure 12.26)

Other investigations

- Karyotyping and an autoantibody screen may be indicated in women with premature ovarian failure
- Measurement of bone mineral density (BMD) is necessary in amenorrhoeic women with low oestrogen levels
- Hysteroscopy is indicated in amenorrhoeic women with a history of endometrial curettage and a normal hormone profile. In Asherman's syndrome, adhesions bridge the anterior and posterior walls of the uterine cavity (see Figure 12.27)
- US is useful for diagnosis of PCOS

Management

Hypothalamic causes

- In patients with low BMI, dietary advice and psychological support are the mainstays of treatment
- Treatment of infertility in very low weight women is controversial as pregnancy is associated with increased complications. These patients are at risk of osteoporosis and will benefit from oestrogen replacement therapy
- Hypothalamic lesions are usually treated surgically, with additional radiotherapy if required
- HRT is required in patients not wishing to conceive
- Pulsatile GnRH or FSH therapy may be used to induce ovulation

Pituitary causes

- Hyperprolactinaemia is usually treated with a dopamine agonist to increase the negative feedback on prolactin production
- Prolactin levels show a rapid response, decreasing significantly within a few days
- Most dopamine agonists result in decreased tumour bulk within 6 weeks
- Cabergoline is the most commonly used agent
- It is commenced at a low dose and gradually increased to limit the troublesome side effects of nausea, headache, postural hypotension, Raynaud's phenomenon, and aggression
- Failure of medical treatment is an indication for surgery
- This usually takes the form of a trans-sphenoidal adenectomy

Ovarian causes

- Premature ovarian failure results in all the complications associated with the menopause but at a much younger age
- The increased risk of osteoporosis may be limited by early diagnosis and treatment with HRT
- Limitation of cardiovascular risk factors, such as hyperlipidaemia and smoking, is essential
- If pregnancy is desired, oocyte donation as a part of *in vitro* fertilization is required

Genital tract abnormalities

- Asherman's syndrome is treated by adhesiolysis at hysteroscopy
- An intrauterine contraceptive device can be inserted postoperatively for a few months to prevent recurrence of adhesions
- Fertility is significantly reduced in severe cases, and pregnancy post-treatment is associated with an increased risk of placenta accreta
- Cervical stenosis is treated by careful cervical dilatation.

Systemic disorders

- Management of these patients is by careful treatment of the underlying systemic disorder.

> ### ⊙′ Box 12.7 Causes of hyperprolactinaemia
>
> *Mild elevation (<1000 miu/l)*
> Stress
> Recent breast examination
> Vaginal examination
> Venepuncture
> Hypothyroidism
> PCOS
>
> *Moderate elevation (>1000 miu/l, <5000 miu/l)*
> Hypothalamic tumour
> Non-functioning pituitary tumour compressing the hypothalamus
> Microprolactinoma
> PCOS
> Drugs, e.g. domperidone, phenothiazines
>
> *Extreme elevation (>5000 miu/l)*
> Macroprolactinoma

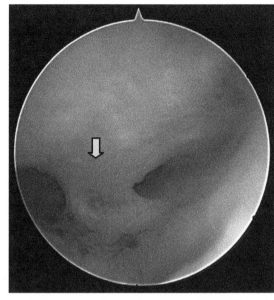

Fig. 12.27 Hysteroscopic view of intrauterine adhesions (⇩) (compare to Fig. 12.19). (Kindly provided by Mr J D S Goodman.)

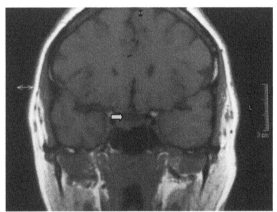

Fig. 12.26 Magnetic resonance imaging of a micro-prolactinoma (⇨). (Kindly provided by Professor Richard Anderson.)

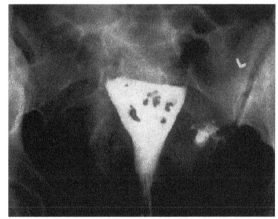

Fig. 12.28 A hysterosalpingogram demonstrating Asherman's syndrome. The cavity is filled with radio-opaque dye and the intrauterine adhesions cause filling defects. (Reproduced with kind permission from www.ivf.com.)

12.11 Polycystic ovary syndrome

Polycystic ovary syndrome (PCOS) is the most commonly diagnosed endocrine disorder in women of reproductive age. It has a wide clinical spectrum from asymptomatic to menstrual disturbance, signs of androgen excess, infertility, and obesity. Diagnosis requires two of the three following criteria:

- Oligomenorrhoea and/or anovulation
- Clinical and/or biochemical signs of hyperandrogenism
- Polycystic ovaries on ultrasound examination

Pathophysiology

Susceptibility to PCOS may be genetic. Its inheritance appears to be autosomal dominant, although a specific gene is yet to be identified. The fundamental endocrine abnormality in women with PCOS is raised levels of ovarian androgens. This high level of androgens results in multiple ovarian follicle formation and a polycystic appearance.

High ovarian androgen levels may occur via a number of mechanisms:

- Extraovarian production of androgens can lead to a polycystic ovary, e.g. congenital adrenal hyperplasia (CAH), Cushing's syndrome, androgen-secreting adrenal tumours, and steroid abuse
- ↑Luteinizing hormone (LH) levels. As described in Section 12.1, ovarian androgen production occurs in the theca cells under the control of LH. ↑LH levels will result in ↑ androgen production
- ↓Levels of sex hormone binding globulin (SHBG)—60% of patients with PCOS have normal LH levels. In these patients, ovarian androgen production may be normal but the level of active hormone in the circulation is increased. When bound to SHBG, androgens are inactive. Low levels of SHBG result in ↑ free androgen and clinical signs of androgen excess. SHBG levels are inversely proportional to BMI, and overweight women are therefore more likely to have severe PCOS.
- ↑ Insulin levels—it has been proposed that insulin acts to augment the activity of LH, resulting in increased ovarian androgen production. Patients with insulin resistance have hyperinsulinaemia and may develop hyperandrogenism. Obese women are more likely to have insulin resistance

One, or a combination of the above mechanisms, may be present in a woman with the PCOS phenotype.

Differential diagnosis

PCOS is a diagnosis of exclusion, and disorders that mimic the phenotype, such as late onset CAH, Cushing's syndrome, and androgen-secreting tumours should be ruled out.

Clinical evaluation

History

- Hyperandrogenism, e.g. hirsutism, acne, male pattern balding (see Figure 12.29)
- Infertility
- Obesity and metabolic dysfunction
- Menstrual disturbance, i.e. oligomenorrhoea (infrequent periods) or amenorrhoea
- Women may be entirely asymptomatic
- Family history of PCOS or infertility

Examination

- BMI and inspection of the distribution of fat, i.e. identification of truncal obesity
- Hirsutism should be assessed using a standardized system, e.g. the modified Ferriman–Gallwey system
- Full abdominal and gynaecological examination to exclude other causes of menstrual or endocrine disturbance

Investigations

- Pregnancy test to exclude physiological amenorrhoea
- Measurement of serum FSH and oestradiol levels will exclude hypogonadotrophic hypogonadism or premature ovarian failure
- Prolactin levels will help exclude hyperprolactinaemia but women with PCOS can have elevated prolactin levels
- Morning 17-hydroxyprogesterone level to exclude CAH
- Free testosterone, free androgen index, and SHBG levels should be measured in all women suspected to have PCOS
- Classically, high free testosterone and low SHBG are seen
- A ↑ LH:FSH ratio will support the diagnosis of PCOS but does not form part of the diagnostic criteria
- Definition of polycystic ovaries at ultrasound includes the presence of 12+ follicles in each ovary, measuring 2–9 mm in diameter, or an ovarian volume >10 ml (see Figure 12.30)
- PCOS is associated with a number of long-term metabolic complications (see Box 12.8). The main risk factor for these appears to be insulin resistance
- Therefore, women with PCOS may benefit from assessing fasting glucose, cholesterol, lipids, and triglycerides (**C**)
- Severe oligomenorrhoea and amenorrhoea can lead to endometrial hyperplasia, which is a risk factor for endometrial carcinoma
- Women with persistently thickened endometrium on ultrasound scan may benefit from an endometrial biopsy and/or hysteroscopy

Useful tip: a hormone profile should be checked within 1 week of LMP to avoid the physiological LH surge.

Management

Management should focus on individual problems and limitation of the long-term consequences of the syndrome (see Box 12.8).

Weight reduction

Weight reduction, through diet and exercise, leads to improved endocrine function, ovulation, safer pregnancy, and may reduce the incidence of long-term complications. This should be the first line treatment of PCOS in overweight women.

Menstrual disturbance

Women with PCOS have unopposed oestrogen owing to lack of cyclical progesterone. If regular menses do not occur, this unopposed oestrogen increases the risk of endometrial hyperplasia and cancer. Regulation of menstruation in women not wishing to conceive is with the COCP. An alternative is to use a progestogen for 12 days every 3 months to induce endometrial shedding (**B**). Metformin 850 mg BD PO is a non-hormonal alternative.

Infertility (see also Section 5.3)

Between 40 and 50% of women with PCOS are overweight.

Ovulation rates at 6 months are:

- 79%   BMI up to 25
- 12%   BMI>35

Cycles are anovulatory in women with PCOS. Clomiphene citrate, an anti-oestrogen, 50–100 mg on days 2–6 of the cycle is licensed for 6 months as an induction agent. Follicle tracking is useful to prevent multiple pregnancies (10% rate). The conception rate is 40%.

Metformin, an insulin-sensitizing agent, is unlicensed for this use but has an 8% conception rate.

If this treatment fails, gonadotrophin therapy may be used. Hormonal treatments are associated with an increased risk of multiple pregnancy and ovarian hyperstimulation syndrome.

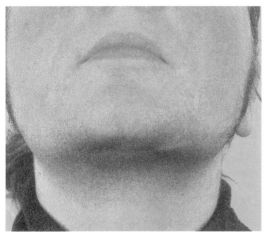

Fig. 12.29 Clinical manifestations of PCOS (hirsutism and acne). (Kindly provided by Professor Richard Anderson.)

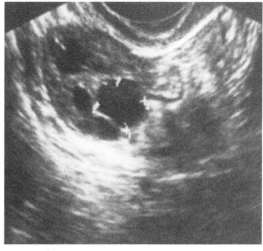

(a)

Surgical management in the form of laparoscopic ovarian diathermy or ovarian drilling (see Figure 5.2 in Section 5.3) is indicated in clomiphene-insensitive cases and is an alternative where follicle tracking is unavailable. This has replaced wedge resection of the ovaries (associated with premature ovarian failure). The mechanism of action is unknown but it ↓ LH and ↑ SHBG levels.

Hirsutism

Cyproterone acetate is an anti-androgen that can stop further progression and decrease the rate of hair growth. Oestrogens are used in combination with anti-androgens as they increase hepatic production of SHBG.

The two agents can be used cyclically or in combination in the Dianette® pill (monitor liver function if taking long term). This is also a useful treatment for acne. Alternatively, topical agents may be used. Eflornithine (Vaniqa®) is an antiprotozoal drug that reduces growth of unwanted facial hair.

These drug therapies may take 2–9 months to have an effect.

Cosmetic therapies, such as waxing, bleaching, electrolysis, and laser therapy can be used as an alternative or adjuvant to medical therapy.

Further reading

The Rotterdam ESHRE/ASRM-sponsored PCOS consensus workshop group. Revised 2003 consensus on diagnostic criteria and long-term health risks related to polycystic ovary syndrome (PCOS). Human Reproduction 2004; 19:41–7.

RCOG. Long-term consequences of polycystic ovary syndrome, RCOG guideline No. 33, 2003. www.rcog.org.uk

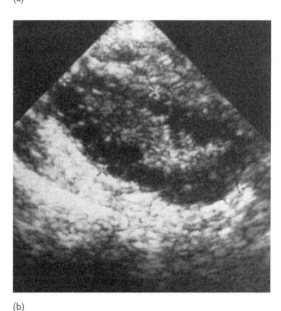

(b)

Fig. 12.30 Ultrasound scan of normal (a) and polycystic (b) ovary. (Kindly provided by Dr Colin Duncan.)

→ Box 12.8 Long-term consequences of PCOS

- Type II diabetes (11% prevalence)
- Gestational diabetes
- ↑Cardiovascular risk and ↑BP
- Endometrial hyperplasia and carcinoma

Definition and incidence

Premenstrual syndrome (PMS) is a cyclical disorder, occurring in the latter half of the menstrual cycle. Symptoms may be physical and psychological, and usually resolve following the onset of menstruation. Premenstrual symptoms occur in 95% of women of reproductive age, but only 5% have severe, debilitating symptoms. Premenstrual dysphoric disorder is the term used for the severe end of the spectrum with extreme mood symptoms.

Aetiology

The exact aetiology remains unknown. Women with PMS have normal hormone levels, but cyclical changes appear to trigger symptoms in sensitive women. This may be mediated through changes in neurotransmitters. PMS resolves after the menopause. There appears to be symptom correlation between women in the same family. Other theories are unsubstantiated.

Clinical assessment

Symptoms include:

- Mood swings and irritability
- Depressed mood, hopelessness, guilt
- Anxiety
- Poor concentration and clumsiness
- Fatigue, sleep disturbance
- Food craving or increased appetite
- Headache
- Generalized aches
- Fluid retention and bloatedness
- Breast pain

The key to making the diagnosis of PMS is the cyclicity and severity of symptoms. Ideally, women should be asked to keep daily symptom diaries over 2–3 months. The diaries should show a build-up of symptoms pre-menstrually which then resolve with the onset of menstruation. Coexisting menstrual problems are common. There are no abnormalities to find on examination, and it is usually not necessary to do any investigations if there is a clear history of severe, cyclical symptoms.

Management

Listening to and taking the complaint seriously are therapeutic in themselves. Trials of PMS therapies reveal a high placebo response, of at least 60%. The rationale of medical intervention is either to eliminate the cyclical hormone fluctuations or to modify the neurotransmitter response. These treatments have potential side effects but can be effective in severe PMS.

Psychological therapies

Cognitive behavioural therapy helps by developing the woman's coping mechanisms. The evidence base of effectiveness is limited and it can be difficult to access this clinical service.

Physical therapies

Complementary therapies such as bright light therapy, chiropractic manipulation, reflexology, and relaxation are popular with some women. Again, their evidence base is very limited beyond the placebo response but there are few side effects. Regular exercise, e.g. 20 min three times/week, improves mood and helps general fitness.

Dietary supplements

Some evidence exists that pyridoxine (vitamin B6) 50 mg BD PO is effective at relieving mild symptoms, but prolonged high doses can cause peripheral neuropathy. Evening primrose oil may relieve breast tenderness. Although specific diets are unsupported by clinical trials, a 'no sugar' diet may be helpful. There is limited evidence for either calcium or magnesium supplements, but a multivitamin preparation containing these agents is often recommended.

Drug therapies

- Selective serotonin reuptake inhibitors (SSRIs) relieve psychological and somatic symptoms when prescribed either continuously or intermittently in the second half of the cycle. This effect may arise from the cyclical nature of PMS and may reflect SSRI action at a different receptor site from that of affective disorders. Studies show an improvement in around 60–70% of women with severe PMS. However, the benefits have to be weighed against the side effects, such as nausea, fatigue, headache, and fear of addiction
- Hormone manipulation—oestrogen has antidopaminergic properties and progesterone modulates γ-aminobutyric acid, the neurotransmitter involved in emotional control. True PMS is caused by the fluctuation of hormones in the second half of the menstrual cycle, hence eliminating the cycle by various means may be effective. If there is no improvement, PMS is unlikely
- Contraceptives which abolish ovulation can be helpful in individual women, particularly if they require contraception. The COCP, Depo-Provera, and the progestogen-only pill Cerazette® can be tried. The COCP containing the progestogen drospirenone is the preparation of choice for women with moderate–severe PMS
- The levonorgestrel-releasing intrauterine device may be effective in some, although it may make some women worse
- Suppression of ovulation with high-dose oestrogen has been shown to be effective. Women can be prescribed oestrogen implants or 100–200 μg transdermal patches. The success of these regimens is limited by possible side effects and the need to add adjunctive progestogens which may cause a recurrence of PMS-like symptoms
- The role of progesterone is uncertain and a systematic review, which found only two trials suitable for inclusion, concluded that there is little evidence of any efficacy. Hence progesterone and progestogens are rarely used in clinical management
- In extreme, unresponsive cases, treatment may resort to an artificial menopause with gonadotrophin-releasing hormone (GnRH) agonists, with add-back oestrogen therapy. GnRH analogues are highly effective but menopausal symptoms, particularly loss of bone density, limit their long-term use. Use of a GnRH analogue on a trial basis to assess response prior to considering surgery can be helpful
- Bromocriptine and tamoxifen can be helpful in women with severe breast pain

Surgery

This option is reserved for women with very severe PMS or those who have significant coexisting gynaecological problems. Hysterectomy and bilateral salpingo-oophorectomy should not be undertaken without careful and considered discussion. Postoperative oestrogen replacement therapy should be considered to reduce the risks of induced premature ovarian failure.

Further reading

Kwan I, Onwude JL. Premenstrual syndrome. *Clinical Evidence* 2006; **15**:1–3.

Chapter 13

Benign gynaecology

Contents

Covered elsewhere

13.1 Pelvic pain

Definitions

Pelvic pain may be associated with menstruation (dysmenorrhoea), sexual intercourse (dyspareunia) or neither. Dysmenorrhoea is a common gynaecological complaint.

It is defined as primary when there is no specific underlying organic pathology found.

Secondary dysmenorrhoea and deep dyspareunia are generally associated with pelvic pathology. All may lead to chronic pelvic pain, but this term encompasses disease processes from numerous organ systems (Box 13.1).

Chronic pelvic pain is defined as pain not occurring exclusively with menstruation, intercourse or pregnancy, causing distress and/or disability that has lasted for >6 months.

It can be divided into four broad categories:

- Chronic organic pain—caused by a pathology causing continuing tissue damage, e.g. endometriosis
- Chronic psychological pain, which can occur without tissue damage
- Chronic cancer pain
- Chronic benign pain occuring despite tissue healing, e.g. postoperative adhesions

Pathophysiology

Primary dysmenorrhoea is thought to be caused by prostaglandin production in the myometrium during menstruation, triggering contractions and increasing uterine tone. This results in decreased blood flow and subsequent pain.

Secondary dysmenorrhoea and deep dyspareunia may be caused by endometriosis, adenomyosis, fibroids or adhesions.

The aetiology of endometriosis and adenomyosis is described in Section 13.2 and of fibroids in Section 12.5.

Adhesions may be the result of pelvic infection or previous surgery. The mechanism by which adhesions result in pelvic pain remains unresolved. Some patients with mild adhesions have severe pain and some with severe adhesions may be entirely asymptomatic.

Clinical evaluation

History

Age—primary dysmenorrhoea is commoner in women <30 years. Secondary dysmenorrhoea usually occurs in women between 30 and 45 years.

Assessment of pain—onset, duration, severity, location, radiation, character, aggravating and relieving factors, and triggers must be elicited.

- Pain occurring with onset of menstruation is indicative of primary dysmenorrhoea
- Pain preceding periods and relieved by menstruation is more likely to be caused by secondary dysmenorrhoea
- Non-cyclical pain is suggestive of a non-gynaecological pathology
- It is important to assess bowel habit and urinary symptoms thoroughly
- Associated heavy menstrual loss may indicate a gynaecological pathology such as fibroids
- Previous pelvic infection or surgery must be documented to assess risk of adhesion formation
- A past obstetric history is important. Endometriosis may be associated with subfertility
- Eliciting the patient's concerns and expectations is vital for appropriate management. It is often very informative to ask the woman what she thinks is causing her pain, and what causes it to fluctuate
- A psychosocial assessment of pain should be carried out, e.g. the impact of pain on her work/education, daily activities, emotional state, and relationships with partner, family friends and others

Examination

- Abdominal examination to exclude a pelvic mass and to elicit tenderness
- Pelvic examination is necessary to exclude fibroids
- Rectal examination should be performed if there is a positive history of altered bowel habit

Investigations

- Suitable samples should be taken to screen for infection, particularly chlamydia and gonorrhoea, if there is any suspicion of pelvic inflammatory disease (PID)
- Ultrasonography is useful in the diagnosis of fibroids and to screen for and assess adnexal masses
- MRI may be useful to diagnose adenomyosis
- Diagnostic laparoscopy may be required to diagnose endometriosis or pelvic adhesions. It may also have a role in management of a woman's beliefs about her pain

Management

- Primary dysmenorrhoea will usually respond to treatment with non-steroidal anti-inflammatory analgesics. These limit production of prostaglandins and reduce myometrial contractility. Alternatively, the COCP can be used to alleviate symptoms
- The management of identified causes of secondary dysmenorrhoea, deep dyspareunia, and chronic pelvic pain are addressed in the relevant pathology sections
- Women with a history and examination suggestive of non-gynaecological pathology will require referral to an appropriate specialist, e.g. gastroenterologist, psychologist

There is a proportion of women with chronic pelvic pain in whom no treatable pathology is identified. These women are best managed by a multidisciplinary team. Specialized pain clinics can combine pharmacology, physiotherapy, and psychology to allow women to manage their pain symptoms.

Pharmacological therapy

Simple, non-opioid analgesics are used as a first line, with opioid analgesia added in if necessary. Familiarity with the WHO analgesic ladder provides a framework for analgesia prescribing.

Physiotherapy

This is a vital treatment of referred musculoskeletal pain. In addition, abnormal posture can exacerbate pelvic pathology. Strengthening musculature can aid mobilization and restore function.

Psychological therapy

It is important that the woman is prepared for the therapy. This is particularly important if a referral to a psychologist is proposed, as patients may react negatively. This involves an explanation of why gynaecology is not able to help further and the expectation of what the new referral will bring to help the woman's problems.

The way the doctor suggests the referral will affect the woman's willingness to accept it.

For example, phrases such as 'we cannot find a cause, see a psychologist' might suggest it is unreal/not genuine/she's making it up, and are particularly unhelpful.

Conversely, saying something like 'It's good that we haven't found something serious like endometriosis or PID. There's no continuing internal damage or disease, but we still want to help you cope or deal with the pain you are suffering. There are treatments that colleagues such as psychologists are expert with that I think may help', is more likely to achieve cooperation.

- A clear and simple explanation of pain in lay terminology may reassure women that their symptoms are not caused by serious pathology
- If the pain is exacerbated by movement, many women will avoid movement. Careful explanation, supported by written material and diagrams, can help the woman to understand that pain does not equate to tissue damage
- A further common unhelpful belief is that, despite investigations, something has been missed. Patients will often respond to reassurance, though the effect can be short-lived
- When such beliefs do not change after careful and sensitive education, formal therapies such as cognitive behavioural therapy can be useful
- These methods aim to modify unhelpful beliefs about the ongoing health problem and reduce negative thoughts about pain. Such thoughts typically revolve around themes of uncertainty, helplessness, predictions of the condition worsening, and the condition's impact upon daily life becoming more extreme
- Breakdown of incorrect beliefs can lead to behavioural change and prevent avoidance of activities. Most effective cognitive behavioural strategies will involve exposure to the avoided stimuli
- Communication is vital in the treatment of chronic pain
- A woman's social support will have a huge impact on her perception and experience of pain
- The anxious concern of family and friends can lead them to encourage the woman with pelvic pain to continue to seek a cure, even when the clinical team have determined that further investigations will no longer be useful
- Occasionally, although the woman's pain is 'real' to her, she might be benefiting from some 'secondary gain' (e.g. in the form of avoidance of work or sex, attracted attention, etc.), which makes the lived experiences difficult to change
- Involving significant others in explanations and consultation, with the patient's consent, can help family members to adjust towards a self-management perspective
- This is a skilled task and needs appropriate experience to be undertaken well

Alternative therapies

- Acupuncture, transcutaneous electrical nerve stimulation (TENS), and homeopathy are very effective therapies in some patients.
- Although their evidence base is limited, adjunct management options should not be ignored in the treatment of chronic pain.

Further reading

RCOG. Greentop guideline No. 41. The initial management of chronic pelvic pain, 2005. www.rcog.org.uk

www.pelvicpain.org. The international pelvic pain society.

www.who.int/cancer/palliative/painladder/en/index.html World Health Organisation

Box 13.1 Differential diagnosis of chronic pelvic pain

Gynaecological	Primary dysmenorrhoea
	Adenomyosis
	Endometriosis
	Fibroids
	Infection
	Postoperative pelvic pain
Gastrointestinal	Irritable bowel syndrome
	Inflammatory bowel disease
	Diverticulitis
	Colon or rectal carcinoma
Urological	Chronic urethral syndrome
	Chronic bladder inflammation
Musculoskeletal	Referred pain from lower back
Psychological	Depression
	Sexual abuse
	Psychosomatic

Endometriosis

Definition and incidence
Endometriosis is the presence of tissue outside the uterine cavity that is similar to normal endometrium.

It can be found deposited throughout the pelvis, most commonly on the uterosacral ligaments and ovaries.

Ovarian endometriosis can lead to accumulated altered blood, causing an endometrioma or 'chocolate cyst'.

Occasionally, endometriosis affects the vagina, umbilicus, abdominal wound scars, bladder, rectum, and even the lungs.

Its prevalence is uncertain, as it varies depending on the population examined. Its incidence varies from 6 to 25% (in women undergoing sterilization or hysterectomy). It is most common in nulliparous women of higher socioeconomic class.

Pathophysiology
- Implantation theory—menstrual fluid can travel along the Fallopian tubes in a retrograde manner, introducing endometrial cells to the peritoneal cavity
- Coelomic metaplasia theory—embryologically, the coelomic epithelium gives rise to the epithelium of the Mullerian duct, the peritoneal and pleural cavities, and the ovaries. An unknown induction agent may stimulate endometrial differentiation of these tissues
- Embolization theory—endometrial cells may spread via the lymph or blood vessels to ectopic sites

Clinical evaluation
History
The presenting complaint may be one or a combination of:
- Pelvic pain and secondary dysmenorrhoea
- Pain is common and typically precedes menstruation and eases during bleeding
- Deep dyspareunia, particularly if there are deposits in the vagina or pouch of Douglas
- Subfertility
- Alteration in bowel habit, including rectal bleeding, particularly with bowel endometriosis
- Haematuria in urinary tract endometriosis

The predictive value of any one or set of symptoms remains uncertain. Women may be entirely asymptomatic.

Examination
Abdominal and pelvic examinations are usually unremarkable, with the exception of women with severe disease.
- Abdominal examination may reveal a mass. Ruptured cysts can present with an acute abdomen
- Speculum examination may show bluish discoloration of the cervix or vagina if the lower genital tract is involved
- Bimanual examination may elicit thick nodules or tenderness in the vagina, posterior fornix or uterus
- The uterus is characteristically immobile and retroverted with extensive disease
- Examination of the adnexa may reveal ovarian masses

Investigations
- Laparoscopy is the gold standard diagnostic test for endometriosis (see Figure 13.1). It is used to stage and treat the disease. The American Fertility Society's scoring system is the most widely used for classification of endometriosis. It grades women as having mild, moderate, severe, and extensive disease, depending of the extent of lesions and associated adhesions
- US is helpful in detection of endometriomas (see Figure 13.2)
- MRI may be useful to assess extraperitoneal lesions and to delineate the contents of pelvic masses

Management
The choice of treatment will depend on age, fertility plans, the severity of symptoms, and site of disease.

Conservative
Some women choose to use simple analgesia. This avoids hormonal preparations and is useful in women trying to conceive. Patient support groups can provide valuable advice and counselling for women with endometriosis.

Medical
The aim of hormonal medical treatment is to cause atrophy of ectopic endometrium. The COCP, progestogens or gonadotrophin-releasing hormone (GnRH) agonists may be used. All have been shown to be equally effective at reducing pain associated with endometriosis (A). Their use is limited by side effects. GnRH agonists are sometimes combined with 'add-back' HRT. Symptom recurrence is common with cessation of treatment as the primary biological mechanism is not addressed.

Surgical
- Laparoscopic ablation (with laser or bipolar diathermy; see Figure 13.3) and excision (with laser or harmonic scalpel) appear to be effective treatments for pain associated with endometriosis (A)
- Up to 70% of women with mild to moderate disease report symptomatic improvement. Benefits appear to be more longlasting than with medical treatments. Up to 90% of women continue to report symptomatic relief at 1 year. GnRH agonist use postoperatively significantly prolongs the pain-free interval. Laparoscopic ablation may also improve fertility rates (A)
- Endometriomas can be de-roofed and removed laparoscopically
- TAH & BSO are occasionally performed to alleviate symptoms. This operation is often technically difficult and should be a last resort, when all other treatment has failed and the woman has completed her family

Adenomyosis
- This is the presence of endometrial tissue within the myometrium.
- Risk factors for adenomyosis include high parity and vigorous curettage of the uterus. It occurs most often in multiparous women at the end of their reproductive life.
- Presenting complaints are usually of heavy menstrual bleeding, progressive dysmenorrhoea, and deep dyspareunia.
- Examination will reveal a symmetrically enlarged uterus that may be tender.
- MRI can sometimes be helpful, but the diagnosis is usually made histologically after removal of the uterus at hysterectomy (see Figure 13.4).
- Unfortunately, adenomyosis has a limited response to hormonal treatment and often requires hysterectomy to alleviate symptoms.

Further reading
RCOG. Greentop guideline No. 24. The investigation and management of endometriosis. www.rcog.org.uk

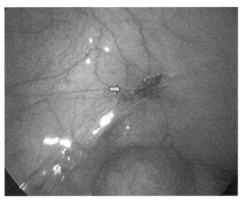

Fig. 13.1 Laparoscopic image demonstrating endometriosis (⇨) on the peritoneal surface of the anterior abdominal wall.

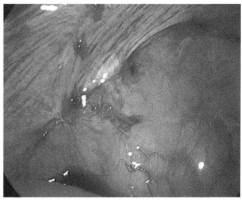

(a)

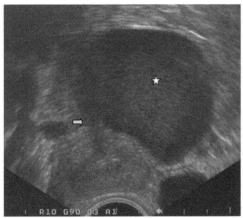

Fig. 13.2 Ultrasound of an endometrioma. The cyst is adherent to the posterolateral uterine wall (⇨). Notice the 'ground glass' appearance of the cyst (☆).

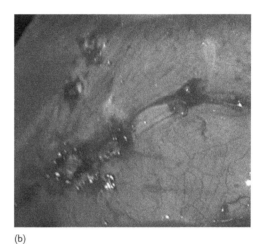

(b)

Fig. 13.3 Endometriosis in the Pouch of Douglas, before (a) and after (b) ablation.

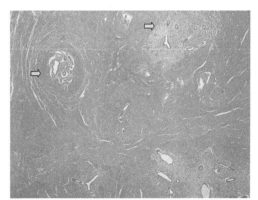

Fig. 13.4 Haematoxylin & eosin stained section of uterus with evidence of adenomyosis (⇨). (Kindly provided by Dr Alistair Williams.)

13.3 Benign ovarian cysts

Incidence

Complications of ovarian cysts are the fourth leading cause for gynaecological admissions, predominantly affecting women of the reproductive age group. The cysts are usually benign (for malignant cysts see Sections 15.6 and 15.7).

Pathophysiology

(see Box 13.2)

Physiological or functional cysts

These cysts arise from the normal physiological process of folliculogenesis (see normal physiology of the ovary, Section 12.1).

They may be subdivided into follicular and luteal cysts:

Follicular

- Commonest type of cyst
- Up to 10 cm in diameter
- Thin-walled, unilocular
- May secrete oestrogen, resulting in menstrual irregularities and endometrial hyperplasia

Multiple follicular cysts arise in:

- Hydatidiform moles
- Choriocarcinoma
- Ovarian hyperstimulation syndrome (OHSS)
- Preterm female babies

Luteal

- Less common
- Right > left
- >3 cm in diameter

Endometriomas ('chocolate' cysts)

These arise as a complication of endometriosis (see Section 13.2).

- The ovary is a common site for endometriotic deposits
- The chocolate describes the appearance of the accumulated menstrual blood in the cyst
- Size varies
- Usually multilocular
- Often found in women presenting with symptoms typical of endometriosis or dysmenorrhoea. They can present in women with subfertility (however, this might be an incidental finding) or with a cyst complication (see Section 13.4)

Polycystic ovaries

(see Section 12.11)

It is not unusual to receive referrals for women with polycystic ovary (PCO) as ovarian cysts. The follicles in PCO measure 2–9 mm in diameter (see Figure 12.30). These are tiny and do not cause the symptoms associated with ovarian cysts.

Abnormal development of ovarian tissue occurs in all the following benign tumour types:

Germ cell tumours

There are two main types: dermoids (mature cystic teratomas) and mature solid teratomas.

Dermoid cysts (mature cystic teratomas)

In most cases cells are derived from all three germ cell layers but may also arise from one (monodermal teratomas) or two of the layers.

These comprise 40% of all ovarian tumours, predominantly arising in children and young adults (usually <30 years). They can be cystic, solid or a combination of both.

Cyst characteristics include the following:

- May be bilateral (11%)
- Are unilocular
- Are usually <15 cm in diameter
- May contain structures of epidermal origin, e.g. hair (see Figure 13.5), teeth, and mesodermal origin, e.g. bone

Dermoids may rupture (up to 4%) or undergo torsion (up to 10%), with the risk of the former increasing during pregnancy. The risks are greater in large cysts (>5 cm). Up to 20% of dermoid cysts contain thyroid tissue; however, symptoms of hyperthyroidism are rare.

Mature solid teratomas

- Uncommon—usually in women <30 years and are cystic, solid or a combination of both.
- As they are predominantly solid, malignancy must be excluded.

Epithelial tumours

- Women are older, often >40 years.
- These are divided into cystadenomas (serous, mucinous, and endometrioid), Brenner, and clear cell tumours
- Serous cystadenomas are the commonest in this group of cysts.

Cystadenomas

- Serous cystadenomas are characteristically unilocular, with papillary projections on the inner surface. They are bilateral in 10%.
- Mucinous cystadenomas are larger than serous ones and in contrast are multilocular with a smooth surface (see Figure 13.6). They account for up to 25% of all cysts. These cysts can also be unilocular.
- Endometrioid cystadenomas are differentiated from endometriosis histologically and are often malignant.

Brenner tumours

- These tumours comprise approximately 2% of the caseload. They are small, solid cysts but are mostly benign. Fifteen per cent are bilateral.

Clear cell tumours

- Clear cell tumours are largely malignant.

Sex cord stromal tumours

Affecting all age groups, these tumours present with symptoms secondary to hormone secretion.

There are four types:

- Granulosa cell tumours (malignant, slow growing)
- Theca cell tumours
- Fibromas (uncommon, affect women >50 years); see Figure 13.7
- Sertoli–Leydig cell tumours (androblastomas)

Theca cell tumours affect women >60 years. The majority secrete oestrogen.

Sertoli–Leydig cell tumours are rare and benign. They affect a younger age group, i.e. 30-year-olds.

Clinical evaluation

History

- Usually asymptomatic and often a coincidental finding at clinical examination or a pelvic US.
- Commoner in women of reproductive age.

Symptoms:

- Pressure on adjacent organs
- Pain caused by
  - Torsion
  - Rupture
  - Haemorrhage
- Menstrual irregularities
- Bloating, weight loss in malignant change (see Section 15.6)
- Dyspareunia

- Hirsuitism or unusual hair growth on the face in cysts, with increased production of masculinizing hormones
- Acute urinary retention in large cysts

Examination
- Abdominally, a mass may arise from the pelvis
- There may be distension, ascites or an acute abdomen
- Fullness and/or tenderness may be found on bimanual examination

Investigations
Ultrasound
Preferably transvaginal or, in the case of larger cysts, a combination of transvaginal and transabdominal

Provides details of:
- Size
- Site
- Nature of the cyst (solid and cystic components)
- Presence and thickness of septae or papillae
- Free fluid in the pouch of Douglas and/or ascites
- Doppler flow to detect neovascularization
- Presence of 'daughter cysts'
- Omental thickening
- Mobility of the cyst/mass (i.e. fixed to surrounding tissues or not)

CT or MRI
- Discriminates between the tissue planes and provides additional information, i.e. lymphadenopathy.

Tumour markers
- Overall these have poor sensitivity. Serum maybe tested for elevated levels of:
  - CA125 (elevated in epithelial tumours and endometriosis; however, this can also be elevated in other benign gynecological pathologies such as fibroids)
  - HCG (elevated in germ cell tumours)
  - CA19-9
  - Carcinoembryonic antigen (CEA)
  - Alpha fetoprotein (elevated in yolk sac tumours)
  - Androgens (elevated in Sertoli–Leydig cell tumours)

Differential diagnosis
- Hydrosalpinx and pyosalpinx
- Fimbrial cysts
- Pseudocysts—encysted peritoneal fluid in adhesions or consequent to pelvic inflammatory disease (PID)

⊙ Box 13.2 Types of benign ovarian cyst

- Physiological or functional cysts
- Endometriotic 'chocolate' cysts
- Polycystic ovary (PCO)
- Benign germ cell tumours
- Benign epithelial tumours
- Benign sex cord stromal tumours

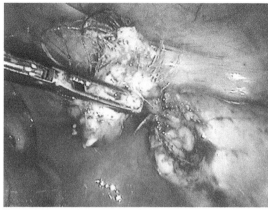

Fig. 13.5 Dermoid cyst containing hair.

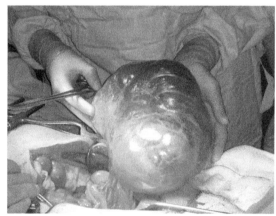

Fig. 13.6 Mucinous cystadenoma.

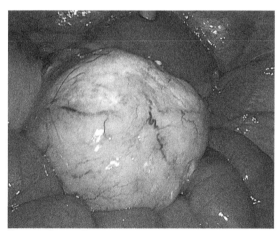

Fig. 13.7 Ovarian fibroma.

13.4 Complications and management of benign ovarian cysts

Complications

Pain

Acute pain arises with haemorrhage into the cyst (see Figure 13.8), torsion, infection, and rupture. Deep dyspareunia may occur with an ovarian cyst though more commonly with endometriosis.

Pressure effects

Large cysts may cause pressure effects, e.g. symptoms of urinary frequency and stress incontinence.

Torsion

The cyst (or the entire adnexal structures, including the Fallopian tube and ovary) twists itself, resulting in occlusion of its vasculature and ischaemia. Expeditious surgery and correction of the torsion reduces the chance of ovarian infarction (see Figures 13.9 and 13.10). Cystectomy ± oophorectomy (if non-viable ovarian tissue) should be performed. The risks are greater in larger cysts. Certain types of cyst are more likely to tort than others. Dermoids do so more frequently. Endometriomas tend to adhere to surrounding structures and hence are less likely to tort.

Rupture

All cysts are at risk of rupture (see Figure 13.11). However, the contents of endometriomas and cystadenomas are highly irritant and are more likely to cause peritonitis.

Malignancy (see Sections 15.6 and 15.7)

Malignant changes are more likely in postmenopausal women; see Figure 13.13.

Hormone secretion

Brenner tumours have been found to secrete oestrogen, thus often presenting with irregular vaginal bleeding.

General management principles

Management depends on the nature of the cyst and on any presenting symptoms, but aims to exclude malignancy. Two useful management algorithms are summarized in Figures 13.12 and 13.13. For RMI (Risk of Malignancy Index) calculation see Section 15.7.

An acute abdomen warrants urgent exploratory surgery; otherwise an elective diagnostic laparoscopy or laparotomy is indicated (depending on size).

If required, conservative surgery is preferred in younger and nulliparous women guided by the histological diagnosis.

Psychological support is important as the fear of cancer is common.

Always keep in mind that the majority of functional cysts resolve spontaneously.

In women with recurrent symptomatic functional cysts, it may be worth considering preventive measures such as the use of the COCP.

Further reading

www.rcog.org.uk RCOG greentop guideline No. 34. Ovarian cysts in postmenopausal women, 2003.

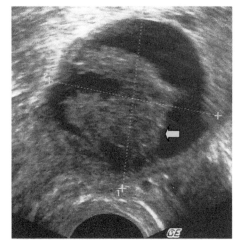

Fig. 13.8 USS image of a haemorrhagic cyst. Note the clot (⇦)within the fluid-filled cyst.

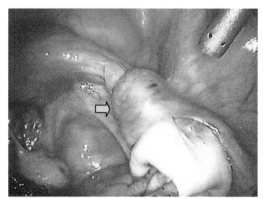

Fig. 13.9 Ovarian torsion. The cyst has been aspirated. Note how the ovary is twisted around its pedicle (⇨).

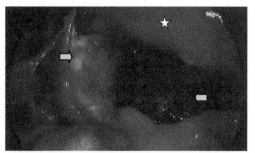

Fig. 13.10 Ovarian torsion. Note that the right ovary is black and gangrenous (⇦). The healthy left ovary is seen next to it for comparison (⇨). Uterus (☆).

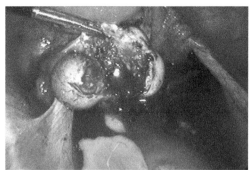

Fig. 13.11 Ruptured ovarian cyst. (Kindly provided by Mr F. Odejinmi.)

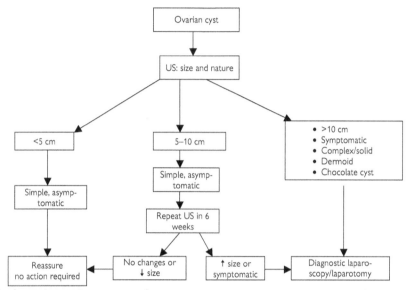

Fig. 13.12 Algorithm for ovarian cysts in premenopausal women.

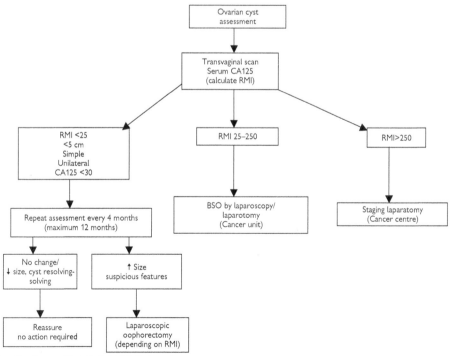

Fig. 13.13 Algorithm for ovarian cysts in postmenopausal women.

13.5 Laparoscopy

There is clear evidence that laparoscopic surgery provides significant benefits for patients compared with laparotomy. However, specific surgical training is required. The benefits include decreased mortality, reduced operative pain, less visible scarring, and quicker recovery times. Hospital stay is shorter, and inpatient and social costs are reduced.

Indications
- Diagnosis and investigation of chronic pelvic pain or infertility
- Treatments, such as:
  - Tubal sterilization
  - Salpingectomy/salpingotomy for ectopic pregnancy
  - Ovarian pathology, e.g. cyst aspiration, cystectomy, oophorectomy
  - Excision, diathermy or laser of endometriosis
  - Division of pelvic adhesions
  - Electrodiathermy of polycystic ovaries
  - Myomectomy
  - Hysterectomy
  - Urogynaecological surgery
  - Lymph node dissection

Contraindications
Patients must be clinically stable. Haemodynamic shock is an absolute contraindication. Mechanical and paralytic ileus, Crohn's disease, and morbid obesity are also contraindications owing to increased risk of bowel trauma.

Laparoscopy increases the anaesthetic risk of cardiac and respiratory diseases, and may be contraindicated in patients with severe disease.

Relative contraindications include previous multiple abdominal surgery, significant obesity, uterine size >12 weeks, and abdominal sepsis.

Equipment
(see Figure 13.14)
- A laparoscopic 'stack': a video screen (ideally with recording and printing system), a video camera which fits onto the end of the telescope, and a xenon light source
- An insufflator with the capacity to insufflate up to 15–30 l/min and to maintain a constant intra-abdominal pressure (safety limit of 12–16 mmHg)
- An electrosurgical unit (bipolar and unipolar)
- A suction irrigation system (important for maintaining a clear operative field)
- A telescope and light cable—the 0° angle of vision telescopes (either 5 or 10 mm) are generally preferred by gynaecologists
- A Veress needle to introduce a pneumoperitoneum. This consists of a sharp outer needle with a spring-loaded blunt gas channel. The needle only protrudes when passing through tissue and retracts in the abdominal cavity to allow free flow of gas
- Trochars/accessory ports (5–12 mm) to permit access to the intraperitoneal cavity
- A wide range of instruments is available to help the surgeon carry out procedures, e.g. grasping forceps, scissors, needle holders, clamps, and diathermy probes

Procedure
Position the woman in lithotomy with legs in comfortable supports. Port insertion is usually undertaken in the supine position.

The primary port is inserted at the umbilicus by either a 'closed' (favoured by gynaecologists) or 'open' (favoured by general surgeons) technique. In closed laparoscopy, a Veress needle is inserted through a vertical skin incision at the base of the umbilicus. Two 'clicks' can be felt/heard as the needle passes through the sheath and then peritoneum.

There is no current evidence that closed laparoscopy is more or less dangerous than the open technique. The open technique involves dissecting the skin, fascia, and peritoneum under direct vision, with insertion of a blunt-ended trocar.

The position of the needle can be tested by Palmer's test. A saline-filled syringe is connected to the Veress needle. Aspiration should not reveal blood or bowel content. Saline is injected into the abdomen and should occur without resistance. Re-aspiration should not elicit any fluid if the needle is positioned correctly.

A pneumoperitoneum is induced with CO_2. An initial flow of 1 l/min is recommended, increasing after confirmation of correct position of the Veress needle. Before increasing the flow rate, inform the anaesthetist. A pressure of 20–25 mmHg is recommended prior to trocar insertion. A good flow rate and low intra-abdominal pressure initially is a good way to confirm correct introduction of the Veress needle.

After removal of the Veress needle, a trocar and port are inserted vertically through the base of the umbilicus. As soon as the cavity is entered, the sharp trocar is withdrawn to leave an entry port.

The laparoscope should be immediately inserted to inspect for adherent or damaged bowel and bleeding. Tilting the patient head down will assist visualization of the pelvis (see Figure 12.3 in Section 12.2).

Accessory ports are inserted in the lower abdomen, avoiding the medial umbilical ligament (representing the obliterated umbilical artery) and inferior and superficial epigastric vessels. Both the medial umbilical ligament and the inferior epigastric vessels run below the rectus muscle and can be visualized with the laparoscope (see Figure 13.15). The midline or the point one-third of the way from the anterior superior iliac spine to the umbilicus are the safest insertion sites.

The rate of urinary tract injuries (bladder and ureters) will vary with the procedure. Preperitoneal emphysema secondary to incorrect Veress needle position is not uncommon but the incidence is unreported.

Complications of laparoscopy
- Mortality rate—0.08/1000
- Overall complication rate—3–5/1000
- Abdominal wall vessels injuries—3/1000
- Large retroperitoneal vessel injuries—0.9/1000
- Bowel injuries—1.3–1.8/1000
- Incisional hernias—1.7/1000

Further reading
RCOG. Consent advice 2. Diagnostic laparoscopy, 2004. www.rcog.org.uk
RCOG greentop guideline No.49 Preventing Entry-related Gynaecological Laparoscopic Injuries. May 2008 www.rcog.ork.uk

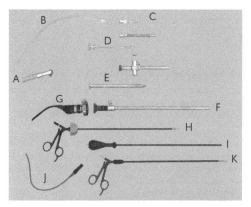

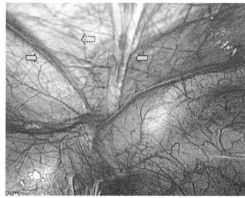

Fig. 13.15 Laparoscopic view of left medial umbilical ligament (⇦), inferior epigastric artery (⇨) and vein (⟨⋯⟩).

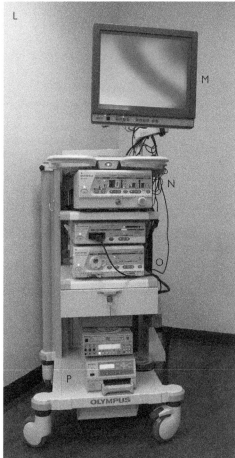

Fig. 13.14 Equipment for laparoscopy: light source (A), insufflator tubing (B), Veress needle (C), 5-mm (D) and 10-mm (E) trochar with port, laparoscope (F), camera (G), scissor (H), probe (I), diathermy leed (J), forceps (K), laparoscopic stack (L) with monitor (M), pressure leed controls (N), light source (O), and printer (P).

13.6 Hysterectomy—part 1

Hysterectomy is the most commonly performed major gynaecological operation in the world. Its most frequent indication is heavy menstrual bleeding (HMB), usually secondary to fibroids. Other indications are listed below. Hysterectomy should be considered as a treatment for HMB after a woman has completed her family and when medical and less invasive surgical options have failed or are inappropriate. Hysterectomy is an established, effective treatment for HMB (A) that induces amenorrhoea, but this must be balanced against its potential morbidity and mortality.

Possible indications for hysterectomy

- HMB— endometrial bleeding after failed medical management
- Fibroids
- Uterovaginal prolapse
- Malignant disease—endometrial, ovarian, and cervical
- Chronic pelvic inflammatory disease (PID)
- Endometriosis

The NICE guidelines for HMB (2007), supported by landmark research (Box 13.3) advised the hysterectomy route for HMB:

- First line: Vaginal
- Second line: Abdominal

354

Vaginal hysterectomy

The main indication is uterine prolapse but it is also appropriate for benign conditions with a small uterus. It may be the most appropriate approach in the woman with abdominal obesity. It is much less common to remove the ovaries at vaginal hysterectomy owing to their relative inaccessibility. Advantages of this route include absence of an abdominal wound and minimal disturbance of the intestines. This results in less postoperative pain, earlier mobilization, and earlier discharge.

Preoperatively

Informed consent is obtained for the operation after detailed discussion of the risks, benefits and recognized complications of the surgery. Blood should be sent for a FBC and 'group and save'.

Procedure for vaginal hysterectomy

Usually carried out under GA, but regional techniques can be used as an alternative or adjunct. The patient is positioned in lithotomy position and the skin prepared and draped. A bimanual examination is performed by the surgeon to assess size and descent of the uterus.

The cervix is grasped with two vulsella. Some surgeons infiltrate the subepithelial tissues with 10–15 ml of 1–2% lignocaine and 1:200 000 adrenaline to define tissue planes and reduce perioperative bleeding. A circumferential incision is made around the cervix with a knife or diathermy and the vaginal skin is reflected upwards (Figure 13.16). The cervicovesical ligament is divided anteriorly with scissors to allow reflection of the bladder off the cervix, taking particular care laterally to reflect the ureters upwards (Figure 13.17). In straightforward cases, the peritoneum overlying the uterus should become visible.

The cervix is lifted upwards to reveal the pouch of Douglas peritoneum, which is opened with blunt scissors (Figure 13.18). A marker suture is attached to the posterior edge.

Moving the cervix to the patient's right, the surgeon inserts a finger posteriorly, behind the cardinal and uterosacral ligaments. A tissue forceps (e.g. Zeppelin) is passed to surround the ligaments, which are cut medial to the forceps and ligated laterally (Figure 13.19). The suture is left long and attached to the drapes. The process is repeated on the right.

The uterovesical peritoneal pouch is then opened to allow clamping, dissection, and ligation of the uterine vessels bilaterally (Figure 13.20).

The round ligament, ovarian ligament, and Fallopian tube are clamped, divided, and ligated (Figure 13.21). Once completed on both sides, the uterus and cervix can be removed (Figure 13.22). The ovaries should be inspected at this stage.

The uterosacral ligaments may be reinforced with a further suture which then includes the posterior peritoneal edge and the lateral angles of the vaginal vault (Figure 13.23). Apposition of these secondary pedicles will provide vault support and may reduce enterocoele formation in the future.

The pedicles are checked for haemostasis and the vaginal vault is closed with continuous or interrupted sutures. At the end, it is recommended that an indwelling urinary catheter is left for 24 h. Some surgeons choose to insert a vaginal pack.

Suture material is polyglycolic acid (Vicryl) or polyglactin (Dexon).

Complications of hysterectomy

A prospective observational study of >10 000 hysterectomies in Finland revealed an overall complication rate of 23.3% for vaginal, 17.2% for abdominal, and 19% for laparoscopic hysterectomy. Mortality is a recognized complication. The risk of death for the abdominal approach is estimated as 1 in every 4000 procedures. This risk is not insignificant considering there were 38 000 abdominal hysterectomies in England 2000–2001, . Notwithstanding complications, patient satisfaction following hysterectomy for HMB is as high as 95%.

Serious risks include:

- Damage to the bladder and/or ureters—7/1000*
- Damage to the bowel—0.4/1000
- Major haemorrhage—15/1000*
- Return to theatre—6/1000
- Infection/pelvic abscess—2/1000
- Venous thromboembolism or pulmonary embolism—4/1000

*Risks highest with laparoscopic approach

Frequent risks include:

- Wound infection and bruising
- Frequency of micturition
- Delayed wound healing
- Keloid formation

> **Box 13.3 Landmark research**
>
> Johnson N, Barlow D, Lethaby A Tavender E, Curr L, Garry R. Methods of hysterectomy: systematic review and meta-analysis of randomised controlled trials. *British Medical Journal* 2005; 30(7506):1478.
>
> This study was performed to evaluate the most appropriate surgical method of hysterectomy (abdominal, vaginal or laparoscopic) for women with benign disease. The authors concluded that vaginal hysterectomy is preferable to abdominal where possible, owing to significantly speedier return to normal activities and other improved secondary outcomes; shorter duration of hospital stay and fewer unspecified infections or febrile episodes. However, they also stated that, where vaginal hysterectomy was not possible, laparoscopic hysterectomy is preferable to abdominal, although a higher chance of bladder or ureter injury.

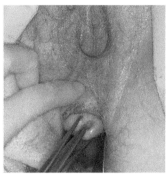

Fig. 13.16 An incision is made around the cervix and the vaginal skin is reflected upwards.

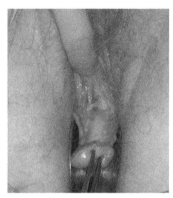

Fig. 13.17 The cervicovesical ligaments are divided and the bladder reflected.

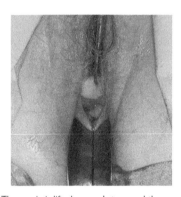

Fig. 13.18 The cervix is lifted upwards to reveal the pouch of Douglas peritoneum which is opened.

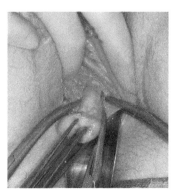

Fig. 13.19 The cardinal and uterosacral ligaments are clamped, divided, and ligated.

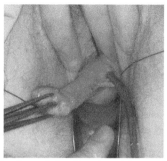

Fig. 13.20 The uterovesical peritoneal pouch is opened to allow clamping and ligation of both uterine vessels.

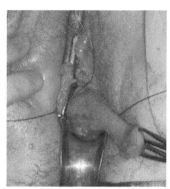

Fig. 13.21 The round ligament, ovarian ligament, and Fallopian tube are clamped, divided, and ligated.

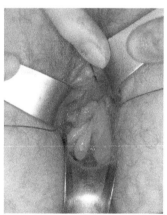

Fig. 13.22 The uterus and cervix can be removed.

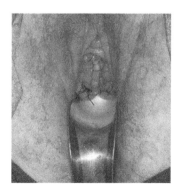

Fig. 13.23 The uterosacral ligaments may be reinforced with a further suture which then includes the posterior peritoneal edge and the lateral angles of the vaginal vault. The vaginal vault is closed.

Abdominal hysterectomy

An abdominal approach is necessary in women with:

- A uterine size more than 12 weeks pregnancy size
- Endometriosis or a history of pelvic inflammatory disease
- A history of previous CS
- Malignant disease for attempted clearance or cytoreduction and for staging of disease
- A long vagina and/or narrow pubic arch, making the vaginal approach technically difficult

It involves removal of the uterus with or without the cervix (total and subtotal, respectively) through an abdominal incision under GA. Subtotal hysterectomy may be performed for patient preference or technical difficulty, e.g. adhesions or endometriosis. If a subtotal hysterectomy is performed, patients must be advised to attend for cervical smears and that they may get cyclical spotting or bleeding. In young women with HMB, the ovaries are usually conserved but bilateral salpingo-oophorectomy may be carried out simultaneously after detailed discussion, with particular attention to family history and the need for HRT.

Preoperatively

The patient provides informed consent for the operation after detailed discussion of the risks, benefits, and recognized complications. Blood should be routinely sent for FBC and 'group and save'.

Procedure for abdominal hysterectomy

Under GA, the bladder is catheterized with an aseptic technique. A bimanual examination assesses size and mobility of the uterus. The skin is prepared with antiseptic wash and draped. The incision may be subumbilical midline or lower transverse, depending on uterine size.

The rectus sheath is incised in the same plane and extended with dissecting scissors. The rectus muscles are separated with the fingers. The peritoneum is entered carefully either bluntly or with scissors to avoid bowel injury. A retractor (e.g. Balfour self-retaining) may be used to assist visualization of the pelvis. Loops of bowel are moved out of the pelvis with the aid of a head-down table tilt and insertion of a moist pack.

The pelvic organs should now be clearly visualized. Medium-sized, straight tissue forceps (e.g. Kocher) are placed on either side of the uterus, over the Fallopian tubes and round ligament, to allow mobilization (Figure 13.24).

On elevation, the round ligaments can be seen extending anterolaterally. They are clamped with curved tissue forceps (e.g. Mayo) at the midpoint and cut, either with scissors or diathermy, medial to the forceps (Figure 13.25). The posterior fold of the broad ligament is then bluntly dissected with the surgeon's finger pressing from behind. To conserve the ovaries, a larger tissue forceps (e.g. Zeppelin or Maingot) is placed medial to the ovary, across the Fallopian tube and ovarian ligament, with division medial to the clamp (Figure 13.26). To remove the ovaries, a Zeppelin is placed lateral to the ovaries, across the infundibulo-pelvic ligament. The ureters are vulnerable to surgical damage at this point and should be identified as they enter the pelvis under the lateral origin of the infundibulopelvic fold.

Next, the bladder is reflected off the surface of the uterus by incision of the uterovesical peritoneum across the front of the uterus at the bladder–uterine junction with scissors or diathermy (Figure 13.27). Gentle downward pressure allows the bladder to separate from the cervix and upper vagina. Adequate bladder reflection minimizes the chance of bladder damage and moves the ureters away from the lateral cervix and upper vagina.

The uterine artery must be clamped and ligated safely. Again, the ureter is vulnerable to surgical damage as it passes under the uterine artery and it must be identified (by palpation or direct visualization). The artery runs along the lateral aspect of the uterus and a Zeppelin is placed at the midpoint of the uterus at right angles to its axis (Figures 13.28 and 13.29). It is cut medial to the forceps and ligated securely.

The paracervical tissue is clamped with a Zeppelin, to reach the vaginal angles (Figure 13.30). No vaginal epithelial tissue should be included in the clamp. Incision of the tissue medial to the forceps is with a knife, to improve accuracy. The uterosacral ligaments may be clamped and ligated separately in a similar fashion.

After adequate reflection of the bladder, a knife is passed into the anterior fornix of the vagina and dissected to the right and left. The posterior fornix is then incised under direct vision to remove the uterus and cervix (Figure 13.31). The paracervical and uterosacral pedicles are then ligated (to prevent vault prolapse).

The vaginal vault may be left open, but is more usually closed in continuous or interrupted sutures (Figure 13.32). If left open, the lateral angles must be securely sutured to prevent bleeding.

Suture material used is Vicryl or Dexon. After inspection for haemostasis of the pedicles and vault, the abdomen is closed. The peritoneum is left open, as closure has no postoperative benefits and results in prolonged operating time and anaesthetic exposure (A). The sheath is closed using a continuous suture (either Vicryl or PDS). Patients with adipose tissue deeper than 3 cm may benefit from sutures to appose the subcuticular fat. The skin is closed with staples, interrupted sutures or a subcuticular suture.

It is recommended that an indwelling urinary catheter is left for 24 h.

Laparoscopic hysterectomy

The proportion of hysterectomies performed laparoscopically has gradually increased and, although the procedure takes longer, proponents have emphasized several advantages. These include the opportunity to diagnose and treat other pelvic diseases (such as endometriosis), to carry out adnexal surgery, the ability to secure thorough intraperitoneal haemostasis at the end of the procedure, and a rapid recovery time.

Laparoscopic hysterectomy should be used as a general term, whereas operative laparoscopy before hysterectomy, laparoscopically-assisted vaginal hysterectomy (with or without laparoscopic uterine vessel ligation), laparoscopic total and subtotal hysterectomy should be used to describe the types of laparoscopic hysterectomy. In laparoscopically-assisted vaginal hysterectomy (LAVH), the procedure is performed partly laparoscopically and partly vaginally, but the laparoscopic component does not involve uterine vessel ligation. In uterine vessel ligation laparoscopic hysterectomy, although the uterine vessels are ligated laparoscopically, part of the operation is done vaginally. In total laparoscopic hysterectomy, the entire operation, including suturing of the vaginal vault, is done laparoscopically. These methods require more specific surgical training.

Further reading

RCOG. Consent advice 4. Abdominal hysterectomy for heavy periods, 2005. www.rcog.org.uk

RCOG. Peritoneal closure. Greentop guideline No. 15, 2002. www.rcog.org.uk

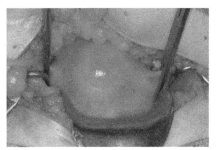

Fig. 13.24 The uterus is mobilized.

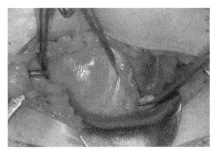

Fig. 13.25 The round ligaments are clamped, divided, and ligated.

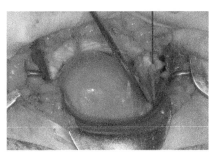

Fig. 13.26 The ureters are identified and the posterior fold of the broad ligament is dissected. To remove the ovaries, the infundibulo-pelvic ligament is clamped, divided, and ligated.

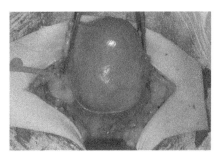

Fig. 13.27 The bladder is reflected off the uterus.

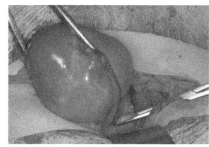

Fig. 13.28 The uterine artery is clamped.

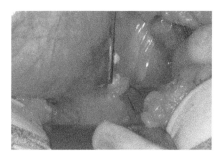

Fig. 13.29 The uterine artery is divided and ligated.

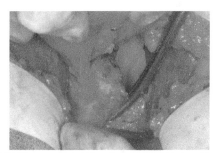

Fig. 13.30 The paracervical tissue is clamped, divided, and ligated.

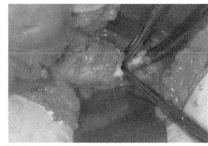

Fig. 13.31 The vaginal vault is opened.

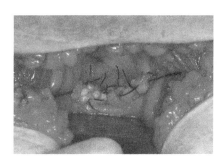

Fig. 13.32 The vaginal vault is closed.

13.8 Benign disease of the cervix

Anatomy

The uterine cervix is the inferior part of the uterus between the isthmus (internal os) and the vagina. The endocervical canal is lined with columnar epithelium. The vaginal part of the cervix (ectocervix) is lined with stratified squamous epithelium. The junction between them is the squamocolumnar junction (SCJ).

Pathophysiology

With increased levels of oestrogen (at puberty, in pregnancy or with the COCP), the cervix enlarges. This exposes the columnar epithelium on the ectocervix (eversion of the cervix). The single layer, less resistant columnar epithelium is then gradually replaced by a process of squamous metaplasia, giving rise to a new, more distal, SCJ. The area between the original and the new SCJ is known as the transformation zone (TZ).

The cervix can be affected by a variety of benign conditions, including inflammatory, infectious, and traumatic processes. Malignant and premalignant conditions (cervical intraepithelial neoplasia or CIN) are discussed in Sections 15.2 and 15.3.

Cervicitis

Cervicitis is infection of the cervical epithelium. It may be acute or chronic. Predisposing factors include multiple sexual partners, inconsistent use of condoms, cervical trauma (childbirth, retained tampons, pessaries), poor hygiene, and immunosuppression.

Common causative organisms are *Chlamydia trachomatis*, *Neisseria gonorrhoea*, *Candida albicans*, *Trichomonas vaginalis*, herpes simplex virus and bacterial vaginosis.

The condition usually presents with mucopurulent vaginal discharge, and vaginal irritation (itching or burning). It can be asymptomatic in a high proportion of patients (up to 50–70%, depending on the causative organism). It may be associated with postcoital bleeding and, more rarely, with intermenstrual bleeding, menorrhagia, dyspareunia, dysmenorrhoea or lower abdominal pain.

Polyps

These are benign tumours arising from the cervical epithelium, most commonly the endocervix. They are generally pedunculated but may have a wide base (see Figure 13.33).

- Polyps are frequently diagnosed incidentally in asymptomatic women. They can present with abnormal bleeding or vaginal discharge
- Differential diagnosis includes neoplasia and endometrial polyps or uterine fibroids prolapsing through the cervix
- Malignant transformation is uncommon (<1%)
- Recurrence after treatment is common

Ectropion

Ectropion is a red ring around the external os caused by the exposure of the more delicate columnar endocervical epithelium on the ectocervix (see Figure 13.35). It is a normal phenomenon, but occasionally can be associated with bleeding or infection.

Nabothian cysts

The replacement of columnar epithelium by stratified squamous epithelium on the ectocervix (squamous metaplasia) can block the opening of glands of columnar epithelium with consequent mucus retention. This is a normal phenomenon but rarely may be associated with discharge.

Trauma

There can be lacerations or ulcerations of the cervix, more commonly owing to repeated trauma (e.g. tampons or pessaries) or secondary to childbirth. Criminal assault or self-harm should also be considered.

Cervical stenosis

Cervical stenosis usually happens as a consequence of surgery (e.g. diathermy, cryotherapy, large loop excision of the transformation zone (LLETZ) or cone biopsy), but can also be congenital, inflammatory or neoplastic. If severe, it can present with haematometra (uterine enlargement with retention of altered menses), which requires drainage.

Benign cervical disease

Clinical evaluation

History

Presenting symptoms of benign cervical disease vary depending on the underlying pathology. Most commonly:

- Vaginal discharge
- Postcoital or intermenstrual bleeding
- Menorrhagia
- Dyspareunia
- Dysmenorrhoea
- Vaginal irritation
- Lower abdominal pain

Assessment of smear test history is essential.

Physical examination

Speculum examination is important to aid diagnosis (see Box 13.4)

Investigations

- High vaginal and endocervical swabs
- If gonorrhoea or chlamydia are suspected, a urethral swab is also indicated
- Smear test if clinically indicated, e.g. cytology not current, abnormal-looking cervix
- Colposcopy referral if suspected malignancy and/or abnormal smear

Management

Cervicitis

Treatment depends on the specific pathogen:

- Chlamydia—doxycycline 100 mg BD for 7 days or azithromycin 1 g orally single dose. Alternative regimens are: erythromycin 500 mg BD for 14 days or ofloxacin 200 mg BD or 400 mg OD for 7 days
- Gonorrhoea—ceftriaxone 250 mg IM or cefixime 400 mg orally or spectinomycin 2 g IM as a stat dose
- Trichomonas—metronidazole 400 mg BD for 7 days or 2 g as single dose
- Herpes—aciclovir 200 mg five times a day for 5 days. Although treatment does not affect the natural history, it may give symptom relief

Other pathogens are treated with appropriate antibiotic therapy.

Local measures such as vaginal acidification, avoiding irritants (vaginal deodorants, soaps, some underwear materials, etc.), and improving hygiene may be beneficial.

Severe chronic cervicitis may require local surgical treatment such as cryotherapy.

Polyps

Treatment is resection. Polyps can be avulsed in outpatient settings, sometimes requiring local anaesthetic (paracervical block). If wide-based, they may need excision in theatre with or without curettage or diathermy to the polyp bed (see Figure 13.34).

Ectropion and Nabothian cysts

These conditions rarely require treatment unless symptomatic. If necessary, treatment options include diathermy and cold coagulation after normal smear result is confirmed.

Lacerations and ulcerations

If symptomatic or associated with recurrent infection, these may be amenable to local treatment (diathermy, cold coagulation).

Cervical stenosis

Treatment involves dilatation of the cervix with local (paracervical block—see Box 13.5) or general anaesthetic.

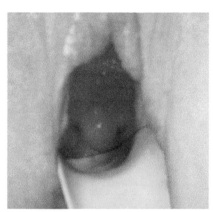

Fig. 13.33 Cervical polyp.

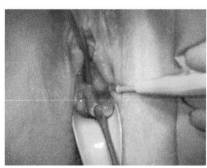

Fig. 13.34 Excision of cervical polyp.

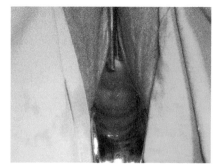

Fig. 13.35 Cervical ectropion.

◎ Box 13.4 Speculum examination

- Advise woman about procedure
- Ensure privacy, no risk of intrusion
- Obtain verbal consent and offer chaperone
- The woman should be comfortable and adductors relaxed
- Ensure good light
- Lubricate, and warm the speculum
- Explain what you are doing and make no sudden, unexpected movements
- If you cannot see the cervix completely, ask the patient to cough and/or put her fists or a cushion under the buttocks
- If she is very anxious or finds speculum insertion painful, offer the option of self-insertion

---

◎ Box 13.5 Paracervical block

- Ensure good visualization of, and access to, all four cervical quadrants
- Up to 20 ml of a solution of lidocaine 2% with adrenaline (1:80 000) is infiltrated using a dental syringe with a small gauge needle (27G), dividing the volume in the four quadrants (at 12, 3, 6 and 9 o'clock; alternatively, at 2, 4, 8 and 10 o'clock)
- To minimize discomfort, put the needle tip in contact with the cervix and ask the patient to cough (distracting her attention) while very gently inserting the needle
- Once in, aspirate before infiltrating to make sure the needle is not in a blood vessel. If blood is aspirated, the needle should be removed and reinserted. (IV injection of lidocaine can cause serious events, including convulsions and even death)

13.9 Benign disease of the vulva and the vagina

Many benign conditions can affect the vulva and vagina. This section looks at important or common conditions. Premalignant and malignant diseases are discussed in Sections 15.10 and 15.11).

Vulval symptoms are common, but only in recent decades has vulval disease been related to defined conditions with specific treatments. Controversy remains regarding terminology, clinical, and histopathological aspects of vulval disease.

Anatomy

The vulva comprises the labia majora, labia minora, mons pubis, clitoris, perineum, and vestibule(see Section 12.2). From puberty, the mons pubis and labia majora contain hair follicles, sebaceous and sweat glands. The labia minora contains sebaceous glands, and has a rich vascular and nerve supply. The clitoris contains erectile tissue attached to the crus to the puboischial ramus on each side. It has a rich blood supply from the pudendal artery. The vestibule is the area between the hymeneal ring and the labia minora. It contains the greater and lesser vestibular and periurethral glands, and is covered by non-keratinized squamous epithelium.

The vagina is surrounded by longitudinal and circular muscle layers and connective tissue. It is lined by non-keratinized squamous epithelium which forms transverse rugae on both the anterior and posterior walls. Before puberty and after the menopause, the vaginal epithelium is thin and atrophic; it is thicker in women of reproductive age.

Clinical evaluation

History

Vulval complaints such as pain, burning, itching, and soreness are often longstanding and distressing, with a significant effect on quality of life. Little is known of the prevalence. Women might have tried numerous topical treatments before being referred.

A multidisciplinary approach, including clinical psychologists, psychosexual counsellors, and pain specialists, may be necessary.

Symptoms are not specific to particular conditions and include:

- Pruritus
- Pain—this may be described as burning, irritation, stinging, rawness or soreness. Such chronic vulval discomfort is defined as vulvodynia
- Superficial dyspareunia
- Asymptomatic lesions

Physical examination

General examination should include all skin surfaces, looking for dermatological conditions, as well as the conjunctivae and the buccal and gingival mucosa. Evidence of systemic disease such as diabetes, renal, hepatic, and haematological disease should be sought.

Examination of the vulva should be performed on a tilting chair that allows a good view of the perineum and perianal area with adequate lighting. Examination of the vagina and the cervix may not be necessary or even possible in all patients (those with lichen sclerosus and pain may not tolerate speculum examination).

A speculum examination is mandatory in women with suspected neoplasia or in those with specific vaginal symptoms.

Examination of the vulva can be aided by vulvoscopy (colposcopy of the vulva). This is not necessary if there is an easily diagnosable lesion but might be useful in symptomatic patients with no obvious lesion, when there is difficulty defining the limits of visible lesions, or sometimes to select an appropriate site for biopsy. It is not clear whether vulvoscopy has similar predictive value to colposcopy.

Investigations

- Most vulval diagnoses are made on history and physical examination
- Infectious diseases require microbiological tests while other specific conditions can be confirmed by histopathology

- Vulval biopsies can be obtained in outpatient settings under local anaesthetic using a 4- or 6-mm Stiefel disposable sterile biopsy punch (see Box 13.6). Haemostasis is achieved by applying a silver nitrate stick or ferric subsulphate (Monsel's solution) to the biopsy area
- Clinical photography may be useful to assess treatment response

Classification

The vulval conditions discussed in this and the subsequent two sections can be grouped into:

- non-neoplastic epithelial disorders (lichen sclerosus, squamous cell hyperplasia, and other dermatoses);
- vulvodynia or vulval pain syndromes (vulval vestibulitis syndrome, essential or dysaesthetic vulvodynia, cyclical or episodical vulvitis, vestibular papillomatosis, and vulval dermatoses);
- vulval infections;
- benign tumours

For a more comprehensive classification of vulval pathology, refer to the International Society for the Study of Vulvovaginal Disease (ISSVD, www.issvd.org).

Lichen sclerosus

Lichen sclerosus is a common condition that affects up to a quarter of vulval clinic attenders. It affects women of all ages, including before puberty, but it is more common postmenopause. It is often related to squamous hyperplasia. The two conditions can occur separately or together at different stages of the disease.

The aetiology remains unknown. Hormonal, genetic, diet-related, and infectious theories have been proposed without conclusive supporting evidence. It has been suggested that lichen sclerosus may be caused by an autoimmune process, but no specific antibody has been found. Many affected women have features of autoimmune disorders such as hypothyroidism, vitiligo, and arthritis.

Lichen sclerosus may be associated with squamous vulval carcinoma in 2–5% of patients. The mechanism is unknown, and no factors have been identified that determine which women with lichen sclerosus are at increased risk.

The vulval skin appears thin and crinkly with pearly white appearance, but may be hyperkeratotic if there is concurrent squamous hyperplasia. Lesions are often bilateral and symmetrical (see Figure 13.36). Changes may be localized or in a 'figure of eight', encircling the vulva and the anus. They do not extend into the vagina or anal canal. There is often shrinkage of the introitus with loss or fusion of the labia minora (see Figure 13.37). In almost one-fifth of patients it may affect the limbs and trunk as well. The histopathology includes epidermal atrophy, hyalinization of the dermis, and underlying lymphocytic infiltrate.

Treatment is with topical steroids and bland emollients, e.g. simple aqueous cream. Topical steroids are graded by potency:

- Mild—e.g. hydrocortisone 1%
- Moderate—e.g. clobetasone butyrate 0.05%
- Potent—e.g. betamethasone 0.1%; triamcinolone acetonide 0.1%
- Very potent—e.g. clobetasol propionate 0.05%; diflucortolone valerate 0.3%

Most patients will require a potent or very potent preparation to gain relief. Once this is achieved, the steroid can be changed to a less potent preparation or the frequency of application reduced. A commonly used regime is clobetasone propionate nightly for up to 12 weeks, followed by application twice a week or only during flare-ups (depending on severity).

Past treatments such as topical oestrogens or testosterone do not offer any advantage and are not recommended. Surgery (cryotherapy, laser ablation, and vulvectomy) does not seem justi-fied. Occasionally, division of vulval adhesions may be required.

Because of the risk of vulval carcinoma, women with lichen sclerosus should have long-term follow-up in vulval clinics, usually every 6–12 months, depending on the severity.

Vaginal atrophy

This is a condition commonly found in clinical practice, mainly in postmenopausal women, but sometimes in prepubertal girls and during periods of prolonged lactation. The vaginal mucosa looks pale and dry with loss of rugal folds. Women can present with vaginal bleeding and are prone to infection.

Treatment is with topical oestrogens. There are many preparations (oestriol, oestradiol or conjugated oestrogens) at different concentrations. Treatment should be kept to the minimum effective dose for the shortest period of time to minimize adverse effects.

A typical regime is one application nightly for 2–3 weeks, reduced to twice a week. The need to continue treatment should be assessed at 3 months. However, it has been suggested that a low maintenance dose of 25 μg twice a week can be used indefinitely provided there is no bleeding.

Female genital mutilation (FGM)

Partial or whole removal of external female genitalia at any age (infancy to young adulthood).

A common social custom, with neither medical nor religious indications. It is practised in certain communities (especially African).

This is an illegal practice, contravening human rights.

Complications

Immediate—infection, haemorrhage

Long-term—keloid scarring, impaired sexual function, recurrent UTIs, anxiety, and depression

Obstetric—higher incidence of obstructed labour and CS, postpartum haemorrhage, episiotomy, prolonged inpatient admission, and perinatal death.

Further reading

www.lichensclerosus.org

www.who.int/reproductive-health

Rahman A, Toubia N. *Female genital mutilation: a guide to law and policies worldwide*, 2000.

> **Box 13.6 Punch biopsy**
> - Aseptic technique
> - Infiltrate the area with local anaesthetic
> - Hold the vulval skin firmly between finger and thumb
> - Place the Stiefel biopsy punch perpendicular to the skin surface and gently apply pressure against it while rotating the blade (like an apple corer)
> - Lift the loose piece of tissue, cut the stalk with a knife, and place it in a labelled pot
> - The hole can be left to heal by secondary intention if a small Stiefel has been used (3 mm), with application of silver nitrate or Monsel's solution for haemostasis. It can be sutured with absorbable material (e.g. rapid absorption polyglactin) or the edges approximated using Steri-strips

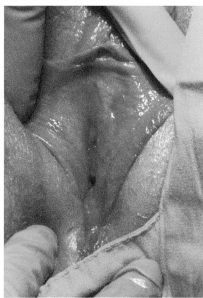

Fig. 13.36 Lichen sclerosus.

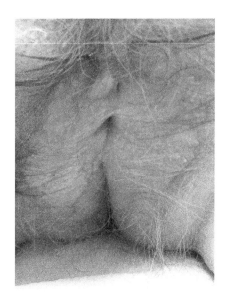

Fig. 13.37 Lichen sclerosus. The lesion is bilateral and symmetrical, with shrinkage of the introitus and fusion of the labia minora.

Vulval vestibulitis syndrome

Vulval vestibulitis syndrome (VVS) is a condition characterized by severe disproportionate pain (hyperalgesia) provoked by touching the vestibule or attempting vaginal entry, and erythema of the vestibule or gland openings. In 1987, Friedrich proposed three criteria for diagnosis: severe pain on vestibular or attempted vaginal entry; tenderness to pressure localized within the vestibule; and erythema confined to the vestibule. However, only the second criterion is specific to VVS.

The pain can be provoked using a Q-tip or cotton bud to apply pressure on the vestibule. Alternatively, it can be quantified using a vulval algesiometer to measure pressure, although these devices are not routinely available.

VVS affects mainly Caucasian women aged 20–40 years, with higher social class distribution and no history of psychosexual problems or abuse during childhood.

The aetiology of VVS remains unknown. A history of vulvo-vaginal candidiasis is the single most consistently reported feature, but many studies of this association rely on self-reporting without confirmatory microbiology. Animal studies have suggested a cross-reaction between *Candida albicans* antigens and certain tissue antigens in genetically susceptible individuals. However, candidiasis is no more common in women with VVS than controls.

Aetiology

Other postulated aetiological factors include iatrogenic causes (topical agents, previous laser or surgical therapies); genetic predisposition; diet (it has been suggested that direct contact of the vulva with oxalate crystals combined with calcium cause vulvovaginal burning); hormonal factors; and pelvic floor muscle tension (women with VVS have been shown to have levator ani instability, poor muscle recovery after contractions, and increased resting baseline tension on EMG).

VVS seems to have an analogy with interstitial cystitis. The bladder trigone, urethra, and vestibule all originate embryologically from the urogenital sinus. Increased nerve density (neural hyperplasia) has been found in vulval specimens of women with VVS and bladder biopsies from women with interstitial cystitis. The neurophysiological findings represent an interesting development, but there is no specific histopathology.

Treatment

- First line treatment includes avoidance of irritants and tight clothing, and the use of local anaesthetic gels and emollients
- Steroids have been used but their role remains unclear
- Some advocate a low oxalate diet and calcium citrate supplements
- Capsaicin, ketoconazole, and interferon have all been tried, but results are variable and proper controlled trials are lacking
- Pelvic floor muscle training with or without biofeedback (to aid pelvic floor relaxation) may also be helpful
- Surgery has been used, and the best results achieved with modified vestibulectomy, which involves resection of a horseshoe-shaped area of the vestibule and inner labia fold
- Up to 30% of women with VVS have resolution of symptoms without treatment.

Dysaesthetic vulvodynia

This is characterized by poorly localized constant vulval pain, often described as burning, and can also affect the perineal area. The pain can be provoked by touch or pressure, but, unlike VVS, it persists after cessation of the stimulus.

Women are typically peri- or post-menopausal. Vulval examination is normal, as the problem is neuropathic, not cutaneous. Psychological co-morbidity is significantly higher in this condition, as well as VVS, compared with asymptomatic women. However, the association is less clear when compared to patients with other vulval conditions.

Treatment is with tricyclic antidepressants, usually amitriptyline, starting at 10 mg at night and increasing to a maximum of 150 mg. Antidepressants improve neuralgic pain by inhibiting the reuptake of monoamines at neuronal junctions in peripheral nerves and modifying the sensitivity of adrenaline receptors. Newer antidepressants such as serotonin reuptake inhibitors may be tried if the former are not tolerated. It should be explained that these drugs have an effect on peripheral nerves so that women do not refuse treatment in the belief that they are merely being treated for depression. An alternative is gabapentin, incrementally increased to 3.6 g daily for up to 8 weeks.

Cyclical or episodic vulvitis

This is characterized by recurrent symptoms associated with menstruation and sexual intercourse, with no symptoms in between. It is associated with changes in vaginal pH owing to recurrent candidiasis or bacterial vaginosis.

Vestibular papillomatosis

The presence of multiple papillae covering the mucosal surface of the labia minora was thought to be due to human papilloma virus (HPV). However, papillae are commonly seen in asymptomatic women, and their clinical significance is unknown. They are thought to be the consequence rather than the cause of irritation and there is debate as to whether they need any treatment.

Dermatoses

A significant proportion of women with chronic vulval symptoms will have manifestations of dermatitis elsewhere. The commonest dermatoses affecting the vulva are:

- **Lichen simplex chronicus**—characterized by dry, scaly skin lesions, usually non-symmetrical, and sometimes with fissures due to scratching. Treatment is with emollients or low potency steroids, sometimes with addition of night sedation to stop nocturnal scratching
- **Lichen planus**—an autoimmune disorder affecting skin and/or mucosal surfaces. Classically it presents with itchy purple papules on the vulva, which may become white (see Figure 13.38). Wickham's striae, lacy white pattern on the vulva, flexor aspects of the wrists, gingival margins, and oral mucosa are often seen. It can extend into the vagina where it can cause adhesions and stenosis. It is a clinical diagnosis—biopsies often show non-specific inflammation (dermal lymphocytic infiltrate with liquefaction of the basal epidermal layer, acanthosis, and parakeratosis). Topical steroids are indicated. Systemic or intravaginal steroids may be necessary. It is associated rarely with vulval carcinoma.
- **Psoriasis**—this condition affects 2% of the population. There is usually a family history. Vulval lesions are different to psoriatic lesions elsewhere (see Figure 13.39): they are pink, rather than white or silvery, have irregular borders, and present satellite lesions. Treatment is with topical steroids

- **Eczema**—looks different from other areas of the skin owing to the moist area. There may be other areas affected and a history of atopy. A short trial of steroid cream may be useful
- **Contact dermatitis**—a wide range of allergens can cause allergic dermatitis: topical medications, perfumes, clothing, washing powder, barrier contraceptive materials, etc. Lesions are typically areas of diffuse erythema and oedema. Treatment is with mild steroids or moisturizing cream. Patch testing may identify the allergen to avoid

Further reading

www.vulvalpainsociety.org

www.bad.org.uk British Association of Dermatologists

www.womens-health-concern.org

Edwards S et al. National guideline on the management of vulval conditions. *International Journal of Sexually Transmitted Diseases and AIDS* 2002; **13:** 411–15.

Friedrich E.G., Jr (1987) Vulval vestibulitis syndrome. J Reprod. Med 32(2): 11 and 14.

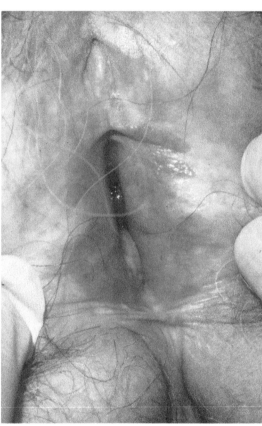

Fig. 13.38 Lichen planus.

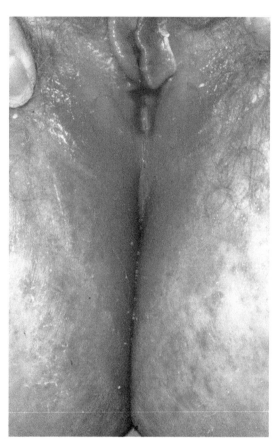

Fig. 13.39 Psoriasis affecting the vulval and perianal area.

Vulval and vaginal infections

A number of bacterial, viral, fungal, and parasitic infections may affect the vulva and vagina (see Chapter 3). Infection of the Bartholin gland's duct is the commonest bacterial vulval infection.

Bartholinitis

This is an infection of the Bartholin gland's duct. Acute blockage of the duct will cause an abscess (see Figure 13.40), but if infection is recurrent or low grade, a cyst may form instead. Although it usually affects women of reproductive age and some organisms may be sexually transmitted. Bartholinitis is not necessarily associated with sexual activity. It is usually unilateral and does not always compromise the gland. In postmenopausal women the edges of the cyst should be sent for histology to exclude Bartholin carcinoma.

The differential diagnosis includes sebaceous and inclusion cysts, congenital abnormalities, and malignant tumours either primary or metastatic.

Treatment is with appropriate antibiotics and analgesia. If a cyst or abscess is present, surgical drainage is required (see Figure 13.41). Marsupialization involves the creation of a permanent fistula by everting the cyst wall's edges and suturing them to the vulval skin with absorbable sutures (see Figure 13.42). This is recommended to avoid recurrence. Rarely, it may be necessary to excise the entire gland surgically. Swabs taken during surgery or after spontaneous rupture of a cyst or abscess will allow identification of any causal organism.

Benign tumours of the vulva

Multiple benign tumours can affect the vulva and vagina. They can be divided into cystic and solid lesions.

Cystic lesions

- *Epidermal cysts* are usually small, single, and asymptomatic lesions. They occur most commonly in the labia majora
- *Mucinous cysts* are common and mainly affect adult women. They are secondary to obstruction of vestibular glands. They are lined by mucinous epithelium which occasionally may show squamous metaplasia
- *Sebaceous and sweat gland cysts* almost invariably involve the labia majora. Blockage of sebaceous glands leads to formation of papules, nodules, and cysts, which are generally multiple and, if symptomatic, may require surgical excision (see Figure 13.43)
- *Hidradenitis suppurativa* is an inflammatory condition affecting the apocrine glands in the anogenital area, especially the groin, but also the axillae and breasts. The aetiology is uncertain. Although bacterial proliferation is frequently found in the glands, it is not thought to be causative. Hyperandrogenism has been implicated, but evidence is inconsistent.

  The disease is characterized by tender nodules which may lead to abscesses. In severe cases, there is widespread tissue destruction with formation of sinuses and scarring.

  First line treatment is usually a combination of long-term antibiotics and antiandrogens. Surgery may be necessary in severe cases.

Solid lesions

- *Fibroepitheliomas or 'skin tags'* are small polyps formed of epithelial elements. They are usually single, soft lesions, generally small and wrinkled
- *Squamous papillomas* are caused by an overgrowth of epidermis. They clinically resemble fibroepitheliomas and only differ from them by having a higher epithelial:stroma ratio

- *Lipomas and fibromas* are mesodermal tumours similar to those elsewhere in the body. They are the commonest non-epithelial benign tumours of the vulva

Vulval fibromas usually occur on the labia majora and can be pedunculated. Lipomas are generally soft, rounded masses, which usually arise from the fat tissue in the labia majora, although they can arise from other structures in the vulva

- *Pigmented naevi* should be viewed cautiously as they can give rise to malignant melanomas. Appropriate investigation and follow-up is required
- *Haemangioma* of the vulva is primarily a condition of infancy and childhood, which possibly indicates its hamartomatous nature. They are rarely clinically significant and usually too small for parents to seek medical help
- *Angiomyofibroblastomas and cellular angiofibromas* occur almost exclusively in the vulvovaginal area, nearly always in the labia majora, and can clinically be confused with Bartholin's cysts. They are generally asymptomatic, well circumscribed masses, which may reach several centimetres in size. Histologically, they show abundant capillary blood vessels, surrounded by spindled and oval stromal cells, which can be multinucleated. These tumours are always benign and are cured by local excision
- *Granular cell tumours* arise from peripheral nerves (Schwann cells) and present as painless subcutaneous nodules. They can happen exclusively in the vulva, but sometimes are a component of granular cell tumours elsewhere. They affect mainly the labia and can affect women of all ages. The vast majority of granular cell tumours are benign, with only very few reports in the literature of recurrence and local metastasis after excision
- *Neurofibromas* can happen in the vulva as part of von Recklinghausen disease (neurofibromatosis). Solitary lesions can be treated by local excision. The nature of the condition is usually that of multiple lesions which, together with high recurrence rates, make surgical treatment unsatisfactory

Most benign tumours of the vulva do not require treatment unless they are symptomatic or a malignancy is suspected, in which case excision biopsy is usually sufficient.

Benign tumours of the vagina

Benign vaginal tumours are uncommon.

- *Condyloma acuminata (warts)* due to HPV infection are by far the commonest vaginal tumours (see Section 3.7)
- *Mesonephric (Gartner's) or paramesonephric cysts* are rarer masses which can happen in the vagina and the vulva. In the vagina, they usually appear in the upper third. They are thin-walled and contain clear fluid. They rarely require treatment unless symptoms develop
- *Endometriosis* of the vagina and the vulva is uncommon. It can occur in an episiotomy scar and appears as a painful, blue or purple nodule, which may enlarge during menstruation

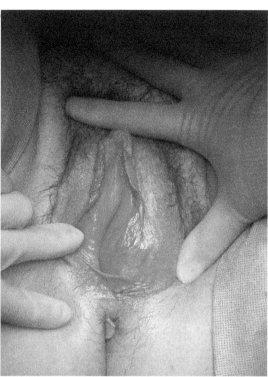

Fig. 13.40 Left Bartholin gland abscess.

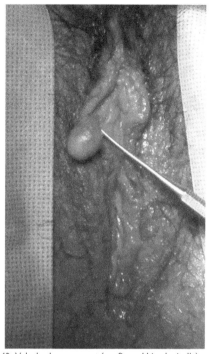

Fig. 13.43 Vulval sebaceous cyst (confirmed histologically).

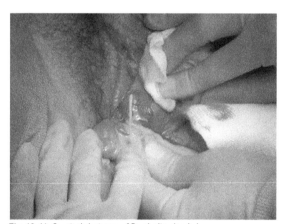

Fig. 13.41 Surgical drainage of Bartholin gland abscess.

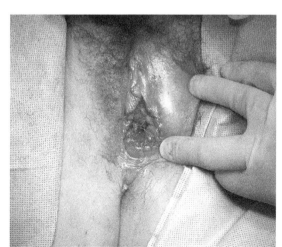

Fig. 13.42 Appearance of Bartholin gland following marsupialization.

13.12 Urinary tract infection

Definitions

A urinary tract infection (UTI) refers to bacterial or fungal infection of the kidneys, pelvis, ureters or bladder. Viruses may infect the urinary tract but this is usually as part of a systemic viral infection, e.g. Hantaan viral infection. Pyelonephritis refers to an infection involving the kidneys and collecting systems. Cystitis refers to infections localized to the urinary bladder.

Recurrence is defined by repeated episodes of infection, whether this is by the same or a different organism. A relapsing or persistent infection is caused by the continued presence of the same organism which has either been suppressed or not by antibiotic treatment. These infections are more likely to reflect abnormal host defences, i.e. either abnormal anatomy or function. These infections may result in irreversible renal damage unless the underlying cause is treated. An uncomplicated UTI occurs in an anatomically and functionally normal urinary tract.

Demographics

- UTIs are very common in women
- Three per cent of girls will develop a UTI
- Fifty per cent of women have a history of at least one episode of UTI
- Each year around 60 women per 1000 population visit their GP for a UTI
- Asymptomatic bacteriuria is found in 20% of elderly women

Aetiology

The commonest causative organisms are bacteria, most often Gram-negative gut bacteria, and most commonly *Escherichia coli*. *Proteus* is another important causative organism, as is *Staphylococcus saprophyticus* in sexually active young women.

Fungal infections are rare in the non-immunocompromised but most commonly are due to *Candida*. This infection may be present in those with a long-term catheter, ureteric stent, previous wide spectrum antibiotic therapy, diabetes or on immunosuppressive drugs.

Schistosomiasis is an infection of the venules of the urinary bladder and may cause irritative symptoms and terminal haematuria starting about 2–3 months after infection. Although rare in the UK, it is worth considering in those returning from travelling or recent immigrants.

Genitourinary tuberculosis is uncommon and a late manifestation of tuberculosis which is often clinically silent and seeds by haematogenous spread.

Pathophysiology

Most infections are due to organisms ascending the urethra. Most of these reach the urinary tract via the perineum and urethra. Very few infections are caused by haematogenous spread, e.g. TB or vesicoenteric fistulas.

The uroepithelium is impermeable to toxins and water. This is because of tight junctions between the surface cells. Experimental models have shown that infection causes these tight junctions to dysfunction, allowing urine to permeate the epithelium. In doing this they stimulate pain fibres and a local inflammatory reaction involving cytokine release. Successful bacteria colonize the gut and perineum and are able to adhere to the uroepithelium glycoproteins with adhesins expressed on its surface. Some bacteria are effective at colonizing foreign surfaces, e.g. *Proteus* with massive flagella to move against the flow of urine, and are therefore found to be the causative organism in infections of patients with catheters.

To cause an infection, the number of organisms present in the urine needs to reach a certain concentration. Thus, increased oral intake, larger volume of urine produced, and increased frequency of voiding all reduce the likely establishment of infection. Some women who suffer with recurrent UTIs report self-treating by increasing oral intake significantly. Incomplete voiding increases the risk of infection.

During normal micturition there is no retrograde flow of urine into the ureters because the vesicoureteric junctions close as the bladder contracts. However, abnormal insertion of the ureters into the bladder or an abnormally high intravesical pressure causes retrograde flow which increases the risk of infection in the bladder as there is incomplete voiding. It also increases the risk of pyelonephritis as the infected urine ascends up the ureters.

Foreign bodies such as catheters and stones provide a protected site where organisms can adhere and multiply. It can be impossible to treat an infection effectively as prolonged use of antibiotics merely encourages resistance to develop. The only effective treatment is antibiotics combined with foreign body removal.

Many women experience cystitis soon after becoming sexually active. UTIs are associated with vaginal intercourse and are exacerbated with condom use. They are more likely to occur with a new partner. This is explained by the mechanical effect of intercourse encouraging spread of perineal organisms to the urethral opening. Spermicides used either with diaphragms or condoms increases the risk of UTI. This is probably due to nonoxinol-9, the active ingredient, which is bactericidal to lactobacilli. This encourages colonization of the perineum by gut commensals.

A normal acidic pH of the vagina also suppresses the growth of some uropathogens so suppression of this, e.g. in bacterial vaginosis increases the risk of ascending infection. Atrophic vaginitis caused by oestrogen deficiency is also associated with the absence of lactobacilli that protect the vulva and periurethral area against colonization with uropathogens.

Clinical assessment

History

In lower urinary tract infection

- Dysuria, commonly worse at the end of micturition
- Frequency
- Urgency
- Urge incontinence
- Strangury—the feeling of needing to pass urine even if just micturated
- Offensive smelling urine, often described as fishy
- Macroscopic haematuria
- Lower abdominal pain, constant
- Non-specific malaise, e.g. aching, nausea, tiredness

These symptoms are not specific to UTIs and only some may be present. Differential includes vaginitis and drug-induced cystitis.

Asymptomatic bacteruria

- An incidental finding in patients whose urine is cultured in the absence of symptoms
- Only significant in pregnancy because of the risk of pyelonephritis and consequent increased risk of premature delivery and fetal growth retardation (20–30%). Thus, antibiotic treatment is needed
- Elderly women with asymptomatic bacteriuria are at increased risk of death. However, antibacterial treatment has not been shown to improve survival

In pyelonephritis

- Flank pain, usually unilateral
- Fever

- Rigors
- Increased inflammatory markers, e.g. C-reactive protein
- Neutrophilia
- Positive midstream urine culture

Studies have shown that correlation between the classical symptoms of pyelonephritis and the actual site of infection is poor. Some patients with cystitis may also have systemic symptoms, an acute phase response and flank pain. This makes the distinction between cystitis and pyelonephritis difficult.

Examination
Clinical findings may include all, any or none of:
- Pyrexia >38°C
- Lower abdominal tenderness
- Flank tenderness, usually unilateral

There should be no signs of peritonism, i.e. rebound, guarding, or percussion tenderness.

Investigations
- Urine inspection—classically it is cloudy and offensive smelling
- Urine dipstick—this is a commonly used investigation and classically it will be positive for blood, protein, leukocyte esterase, and nitrite
- Urine—microscopy, culture, and sensitivity. Microscopy allows quantification of the number of white cells in the urine, i.e. degree of pyuria. Some patients with significant pyuria and negative culture may have vaginal discharge contaminating the specimen, but they may have a chlamydia urethral infection, or a low count bacteruria owing to a slow-growing organism. Significant growth will be reported if there is pure growth of one organism, it is a recognized pathogen, it is above the laboratory's quantitative result and/or there is significant pyuria. Mixed growth can be seen in some infections and all the true urinary pathogens may not be recognized. Low count of bacteria may be present in infection, especially if the patient's fluid intake is very high and the urine is dilute
- Blood tests may show a neutrophilia in bacterial infection, or eosinophilia in schistosomiasis

Further investigations are not required in uncomplicated UTI. Investigations may be required if symptoms are recurrent, or they present abnormally and may include plain abdominal imaging (with ultrasound or intravenous urography), cystoscopy, and bladder voiding studies

Differential diagnosis
- Chlamydial urethritis
- Renal stones
- Appendicitis
- Pelvic inflammatory disease
- Atrophic vaginitis
- Bacterial vaginitis
- Urethral syndrome
- Interstitial cystitis
- Drug-induced cystitis, e.g. NSAIDs, acrolein, ifosfamide, danazol

 Box 13.7 Urine sample collection and dipstick interpretation

A midstream urine sample should be obtained to reduce the contamination from vaginal discharge. Ideally, a sample would be obtained by suprapubic aspiration or by catheterizing the bladder. However, these are not practical and have a risk of infection of 1–2%.

The woman should be asked to part the labia with one hand, pass some urine, stop, start to micturate again, collect a sample, stop, and then finish voiding into the toilet.

Washing the vulva with water or antibacterial solutions has not been shown to reduce the contamination rate.

Urine dipsticks are commonplace and must always be interpreted in light of the clinical story with the exception of pregnancy, when asymptomatic bacteruria should be treated.

- Cloudy urine can be caused by bacteruria and pyuria. However, in normal urine, as it cools, amorphous phosphate crystals form, causing it to be cloudy
- Macroscopic haematuria can occur in severe cystitis. It may also be caused by glomerular bleeding or urothelial tumours or stones
- Microscopic haematuria is not sensitive or specific for UTI
- Proteinuria can occur in UTIs as protein is released from white cells involved in the immune response, but it is not sensitive or specific
- Leukocyte esterase is an enzyme released from white cells. The transport medium boric acid causes a false negative result as it inhibits the enzyme, so always dipstick urine before putting in the transport container if it contains transport medium
- Nitrite is produced by most uropathogens which reduce urinary nitrate to nitrite. Exceptions are Gram-positive organisms, e.g. Staphylococcus saprophyticus. A positive test is highly suggestive of a UTI. False negatives occur in patients with low dietary nitrate (so therefore low nitrate levels in the urine) and those taking high dose ascorbic acid

The sensitivity of the urine dipstick is 83% and specificity is 71%. A negative dipstick for both nitrite and leukocyte esterase makes the diagnosis of UTI highly unlikely.

13.13 Management of urinary tract infection

Management

- Analgesia
- Increase oral intake to 'flush out' the bacteria
- Alkalinizing agents, e.g. potassium citrate, work by reducing bladder irritability
- Fructose in many fruit juices inhibits the binding of E. coli fimbriae to the urothelium. Cranberry juice contains proanthocyanidin which also inhibits the binding of the fimbriae to the urothelium
- Empirical treatment should be started prior to the culture result
- Consult local guidelines as antibiotic resistance varies
- Trimethoprim is often first line, e.g. 200 mg BD PO for 3 days (longer increases the risk of side effects) or use β lactams, or penicillins
- Consider admission if the patient is pregnant, the symptoms are severe, she cannot tolerate oral therapy, or is not responding to previous oral treatment
- For pyelonephritis with septicaemia, patients should receive a quinolone, or aminoglycoside with ampicillin, or cephalosporin. Treatment should be for at least 7 days in mild disease, but 14 days for severe disease. IV antibiotics can be changed to oral once afebrile for 24 h and there is clinical improvement
- In pregnancy, asymptomatic bacteriuria should be treated empirically without waiting for the culture
- Recurrent UTI may be treated with each episode or by using low-dose long-term antibiotics. Prophylaxis can be considered in women with two symptomatic UTIs/year. Regimens include trimethoprim 100 mg PO nocte, nitrofurantoin 100 mg PO nocte (but monitor lung and liver function), rotating antibiotics every 3 months to minimize resistance

To prevent recurrent UTIs, advice should be given regarding wiping from front to back after micturition or defaecation, and micturating prior to, and immediately after, sex (although there is no good evidence base for the latter).

Complications

- Lower UTI ascending to cause pyelonephritis requiring hospital admission and intravenous antibiotics
- Renal scarring is thought to be unlikely due to pyelonephritis alone, but may be caused by undiagnosed reflux nephropathy or other complicating factors such as stones, obstructive uropathy, diabetes or chronic alcoholism

Prognosis

Patients respond well to correct antibiotic therapy, either oral or intravenous.

If not, then investigations should be carried out to exclude the causes of complicated UTIs.

It is important to exclude an obstructed ureter in pyelonephritis which is not responding to antibiotic treatment by ultrasound or intravenous urography.

Management in pregnancy

See Section 8.6.

Further reading

www.womens-health.co.uk (useful to give patients for their information).

Smaill F. Antibiotics for asymptomatic bacteriuria in pregnancy. The Cochrane Library, Issue 1, Updated Software, Oxford, 2002.

Vazquez JC, Villar J. Treatment for symptomatic urinary tract infections during pregnancy. *The Cochrane Database of Systematic Reviews* 2003; **4:** CD002256.

Chapter 14

The pelvic floor and continence

Contents

Covered elsewhere

- Vaginal hysterectomy (see Section 13.6)

14.1 Pelvic organ prolapse—background information

Definition
Pelvic organ prolapse (POP) is the herniation of pelvic or abdominal organs through the vaginal canal.

Prevalence
- There are few epidemiological studies
- In the UK, the prevalence of prolapse has been calculated at 204 per 1000 woman years
- A fifth of patients on gynaecological waiting lists are scheduled for prolapse surgery
- In the USA, the lifetime risk of requiring an operation for prolapse or incontinence by the age of 80 years is 11%
- A 29% reoperation rate
- Estimates suggest an increase of 45% in the demand for prolapse surgery over the next three decades

Aetiology
The aetiology of POP is complex. Risk factors include:
- *Age*
- *Parity and vaginal delivery* are the most significant risk factors, with a 4-fold increase in the risk of developing a prolapse after vaginal delivery of the first child, and 11-fold increase after four or more vaginal deliveries. Direct neuromuscular or connective tissue damage from childbirth leads to weakening of the supportive ligaments and connective tissue, with progressive descent of pelvic organs through the urogenital hiatus

  However, avoidance of vaginal deliveries is not completely protective. Pregnancy itself is associated with connective tissue changes, albeit reversible. Qualitative and quantitative collagen changes have been observed in nulliparous women, with both prolapse and incontinence presenting in these patients. Furthermore, it has been estimated that three elective CS may have a similar effect in pelvic floor dysfunction as one vaginal delivery
- *Postmenopausal oestrogen deficiency* affects vaginal and periurethral collagen metabolism
- *Obesity and chronic increase in intra-abdominal pressure*, e.g. chronic cough, heavy lifting, constipation, etc.
- *Neurological conditions* such as spina bifida and muscular dystrophy
- *Genetic connective tissue disorders*, e.g. Marfan's and Ehlers–Danlos syndrome
- *Hysterectomy* is traditionally associated with pelvic floor dysfunction. However, a recent review suggests that hysterectomy for benign conditions other than prolapse does not seem to be a risk factor for POP

Pathophysiology
Mechanical support of the vagina relies on three mechanisms:
- Vertical suspension at the apex from the uterosacral and cardinal ligaments
- Closure at the introitus by pelvic floor muscles which form a muscular plate upon which pelvic organs can rest
- Valve effect created by the horizontal position of the vagina in the pelvic floor

Muscular support is given mainly by the levator ani muscles. These contain two fibres: type 1, or slow-twitch, which provide resting tone; type 2, or fast-twitch, which respond to stress or intra-abdominal pressure to maintain urethral and anal closure.

Ligamentous support is given by the endopelvic fascia, a layer of fibromuscular tissue that surrounds each pelvic organ and forms condensations or ligaments.

There are three anatomical levels of vaginal support (see Figure 14.1).
- Level I—vertical suspension of the uterus, cervix, and vagina provided by the uterosacral and cardinal ligaments, at the apex or upper third of the vagina
- Level II—lateral attachment of the vagina in its middle third, provided by connective tissue known as paracolpium or paravaginal (part of the endopelvic fascia, which surrounds the vagina and pelvic organs). It connects the vagina to the 'white line' or arcus tendineus fascia pelvis (ATFP), which in turn is part of the origin of the levator ani muscles
- Level III—the lower third of the vagina is supported by the fusion of the vaginal endopelvic fascia to the perineal body posteriorly, the levator ani muscles laterally and the urethra anteriorly

Somatic nerve supply to the pelvic floor is provided by the pudendal nerve, arising from the anterior rami of sacral roots S2–S4. The inferior hypogastric plexus, which carries both sympathetic and parasympathetic fibres, gives autonomic supply to the pelvic organs.

Neuromuscular or connective tissue damage at any of those three levels may lead to POP or incontinence, e.g. level I, uterine or vault prolapse; level II, cystocele; and level III, rectocele, urethral mobility, and stress urinary incontinence (SUI).

Classification of POP
In 1996 the International Continence Society (ICS) introduced a system of standard terminology for the evaluation of POP called the Pelvic Organ Prolapse Quantification system or POP-Q (see Box 14.1). It has been adopted by the Society of Gynaecologic Surgeons and the American Urogynecology Society, and has become the most commonly used grading system in the literature.

The concepts of *anterior vaginal wall prolapse* and *posterior vaginal wall prolapse* replace the previous terms cystocele, urethrocele, rectocele, and enterocele. The latter imply certainty as to the organs protruding through the vaginal canal, which could only be confirmed by ancillary tests that are not routinely used.

The POP-Q system uses the hymen as the fixed anatomical landmark of reference and defines six points, two in each vaginal compartment (anterior, superior, and posterior), which are located in relation to this.

The hymen is defined as zero and the distance to the six defined points is measured in centimetres above the hymen (negative number) or below the hymen (positive number).

Box 14.1 The POP-Q system

From Bump RC et al. The standardisation of terminology of female pelvic organ prolapse and pelvic floor dysfunction. *American Journal of Obstetrics and Gynecology* 1996; **175**:10–17 (see Figure 14.2).

Reference point:
- Hymenal ring, defined as zero

Two points are located on the anterior vaginal wall:
- Point Aa, located in the midline, 3 cm proximal (–3 in the absence of prolapse) to the external urethral meatus. It corresponds approximately to the urethrovesical crease. By definition, the range of movement will be between –3 and +3 cm in relation to the hymen
- Point Ba is the most distal (dependent) position of any part of the upper anterior vaginal wall between point Aa and the anterior vaginal fornix (or vaginal vault after hysterectomy)

Two points are located in the superior vagina:
- Point C represents the most distal (dependent) edge of the cervix or the leading edge of the vaginal vault after hysterectomy
- Point D is the posterior fornix or pouch of Douglas in a woman who still has a cervix. It represents the attachment of the uterosacral ligaments to the cervix. Its measurement allows differentiating suspensory failure of the uterosacral ligaments from cervical elongation. If point D is significantly more negative (i.e. greater than 4 cm) than point C, the cervix is elongated. Point D is omitted in the absence of cervix

Two points are located on the posterior vaginal wall:
- Point Ap is located in the midline 3 cm proximal to the hymen (–3 in the absence of prolapse). Its range of movement will be from –3 to +3
- Point Bp represents the most distal (dependent) position of any part of the upper posterior vaginal wall between point D (or vaginal vault after hysterectomy) and point Ap

The POP-Q system incorporates three other landmarks and measurements:
- The genital hiatus (gh), measured from the middle of the external urethral meatus to the posterior midline hymen. If the location of the hymen is distorted (usually by scars from surgery or episiotomy repair), the firm tissue of the perineal body is the posterior margin for this measurement
- The perineal body (pb) is measured from the posterior margin of the gh to the midanal opening
- The total vaginal length (tvl) is the greatest depth of the vagina when point C or D is reduced to its normal position

There are five ordinal stages for POP:
- Stage 0—no prolapse is demonstrated
- Stage I—the leading edge of the prolapse is not lower than 1 cm above the level of the hymen
- Stage II—the leading surface of the prolapse is between –1 and +1 cm in relation to the hymen (see Figure 14.3)
- Stage III—the most distal portion of the prolapse is from 1 cm beyond the hymen but without complete eversion
- Stage IV—complete vaginal eversion

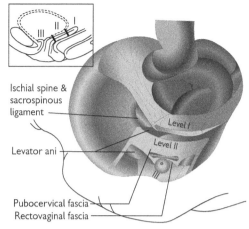

Fig. 14.1 Anatomical levels of vaginal support. The uterus is absent. The pubocervical and rectovaginal fascia are part of the endopelvic fascia. The inset shows a lateral view of the three levels of support. (Reproduced from DeLancey JO Anatomic aspects of vaginal eversion after hysterectomy. *American Journal of Obstetrics and Gynecology* 1992; 166:1717–28, with permission from Elsevier.)

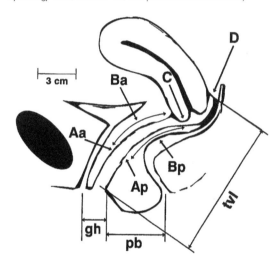

Fig. 14.2 The POP-Q system, showing points Aa and Ba in the anterior vaginal wall; Ap and Bp in the posterior wall; and point C and D superiorly. Gh, pb, and tvl measurements are also demonstrated. (Reproduced from Bump RC et al. The standardisation of terminology of female pelvic organ prolapse and pelvic floor dysfunction. *American Journal of Obstetrics and Gynecology* 1996; 175:10–17, with permission from Elsevier.)

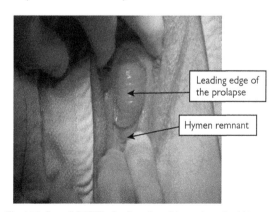

Fig. 14.3 Stage II POP. The leading edge of the prolapse is within +/−1 cm of the hymen.

History

Symptoms of prolapse are variable and not specific to different compartments. Many are not well characterized, especially functional deficits.

Symptoms

- Pressure or heaviness in the vagina, dragging sensation, awareness of vaginal protrusion or bulge
- Urinary symptoms: urgency, frequency, urge (UUI) or stress incontinence (SUI), feeling of incomplete emptying, hesitancy, manual reduction of prolapse or positional changes to accomplish voiding
- Defaecatory symptoms: faecal incontinence, urgency, incomplete rectal emptying, excessive straining, need for perineal or vaginal pressure or digitation to accomplish defaecation
- Sexual dysfunction: difficulty with intercourse, lack of sensation, dyspareunia, anorgasmia
- Low back pain has been traditionally related to prolapse, although recent studies have failed to confirm this
- Pain is not a symptom of POP. If present it may suggest pudendal neuralgia, which could be worsened by vaginal surgery
- The vaginal symptoms questionnaire from the International Consultation on Incontinence (ICIQ-VS) is a useful validated tool to assess POP symptoms

Physical examination

The conditions of the examination are very important and should be specified. The aim is to reproduce the maximum protrusion noted by the patient in her daily activities.

She should be examined in the left lateral or occasionally in lithotomy, using an appropriate vaginal speculum, most commonly Sims.

Anterior vaginal wall prolapse is demonstrated by retracting the posterior vaginal wall with the speculum blade. Similarly, retraction of the anterior wall allows demonstration of posterior wall prolapse.

Maximum uterine descent is achieved by applying gentle traction to the cervix using a single tooth vulsellum.

Straining (e.g. Valsalva manoeuvre, cough) and/or examining the patient in the standing position might help to demonstrate the maximum prolapse.

Other techniques that may need to be used for a comprehensive assessment of the prolapse and preoperative planning include: digital rectovaginal examination; measurements of perineal descent and transverse diameter of the gh; examination techniques for differentiating between various types of defects (e.g. central versus paravaginal defects of the anterior vaginal wall); inspection and palpation of the pelvic floor muscles (pelvic floor contraction causes inward movement of the perineum, while straining or a Valsalva manoeuvre causes the opposite); and prolapse reduction test for SUI ('occult' SUI, i.e. *de novo* occurrence of SUI after POP surgery).

Investigations

POP is a clinical diagnosis. Ancillary tests are not routinely recommended, but they may help in selected patients and research.

- Endoscopy—cystoscopy and sigmoidoscopy may occasionally have a role in POP, e.g. bowel peristalsis under the bladder base observed at cystoscopy might identify an anterior enterocele
- Imaging techniques—might be more accurate than physical examination in determining the organs involved in POP. However, they lack standardization and validation. Ultrasonography allows for observation of dynamic events in real-time. Contrast radiography may illustrate static or dynamic events of micturition and defaecation. CT and MRI are promising and currently good research tools but they are not available for routine use (see Figure 14.4)
- Pelvic floor muscle testing—its clinical use in POP assessment is still unclear and remains experimental. It includes electromyography and measurements of urethral, vaginal, and anal pressures
- Urodynamics—may be useful if there is a positive POP reduction test for occult SUI and in the presence of symptoms of UUI as the results potentially influence the choice of therapy offered
- Anorectal manometry and endoanal ultrasonography assess the degree of anal incontinence, demonstrating the involvement of sphincters and nerve damage

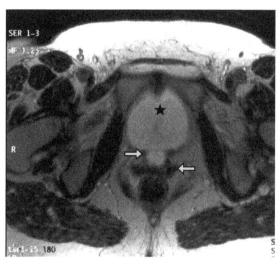

Fig. 14.4 MRI showing a cystocele (central defect). The circular light grey area in the middle is the bladder (★). Note the herniation of its neck (⇨) into the vagina (⇦). (Courtesy of O. Adekanmi and R. Freeman.)

Uterine and anterior vaginal wall prolapse

Definition

Failure of the apical support of the vagina and/or the anterior vaginal wall support leads to uterine prolapse (see Figure 14.5), and anterior vaginal wall prolapse (see Figure 14.6), respectively.

Prevalence

Up to 20% of asymptomatic postmenopausal women may have uterine or vault prolapse, and 51% may have anterior vaginal wall prolapse. A significant proportion of women may have a combined prolapse of these two compartments.

Anatomy

The main support to the uterus is given by the uterosacral ligaments, which extend from the back of the cervix to the sacrum; and the transverse cervical or cardinal ligaments, which extend laterally from the cervix to the pelvic side wall. Failure of this supporting mechanism leads to uterine or vault prolapse, characterized in the POP-Q system by lower points C and D in women with uterus or low point C in women with vault prolapse.

Support to the anterior compartment is mainly from the pubocervical fascia (part of the endopelvic fascia). It extends from the anterior part of the cervix to the posterior aspect of the pubic bone and laterally to the ATFP (arcus tendineus fascia pelvis). The posterior pubourethral ligament, which extends from the posterior and inferior aspect of the symphysis pubis to the middle third of the urethra and bladder, maintains bladder neck elevation and probably has a role in maintaining continence.

Anterior vaginal wall prolapse can result from:

- Defects in the midline (central defects)
- Lateral detachment of the pubocervical fascia from the ATFP (lateral or paravaginal defects)
- Loss of bladder neck support
- Superior transverse defects near the attachment of the pubocervical fascia to the cervix (high central prolapse)

History

Symptoms of prolapse of the anterior and middle compartments also include lower urinary tract symptoms and voiding difficulty.

Assessment

Examination

Clinical evaluation using the POP-Q system will show points Aa or Ba as the leading edge of the anterior compartment prolapse, and point C as the leading edge of uterine or vault prolapse. Several examination techniques allow differentiation between central and lateral defects of the anterior compartment, but none has been validated.

Posterior vaginal wall prolapse

Prevalence

Posterior compartment prolapse is common, with reported rectocele prevalence ranging between 20–80% of the general population. Assessment of the symptoms is paramount, as small rectoceles can be found in up to 70% of asymptomatic women. Spontaneous regression of stage I rectocele is not uncommon. As with prolapse of other compartments, the size of posterior vaginal wall prolapse correlates poorly with the severity of symptoms.

Anatomy

The rectovaginal septum, or Denonvilliers' fascia, is the posterior equivalent to the pubocervical fascia in the anterior wall. It is a fibromuscular layer that extends from the vaginal apex (cervix) to the perineal body (see Figure 14.1). Between the rectovaginal septum and the rectum is the pararectal fascia, which extends medially from the pelvic side walls dividing into anterior and posterior sheaths, encompassing the rectum and providing additional support to the anterior rectal wall. It extends down from the posterior aspect of the uterosacral ligaments to the upper margin of the perineal body and laterally to the levator ani fascia.

Posterior vaginal wall prolapse includes: rectocele which arises from defects in the rectovaginal fascia or septum with herniation of the rectum into the vaginal lumen (see figure 14.7), cul-de-sac (pouch of Douglas) hernias, enterocele, and sigmoidocele. The latter is a peritoneal herniation through the upper posterior vaginal wall, between the vagina and the rectum. The contents can include sigmoid colon, omentum, and small bowel.

History

Risk factors for posterior wall prolapse are the same as POP, although obstetric injury (vaginal and perineal tears, poor episiotomy repair, etc.) is a major predisposing factor. Posterior compartment prolapse is quite common after colposuspension, owing to the change in the vaginal axis.

Symptoms of posterior compartment prolapse often include disorders of defaecation, e.g. incomplete rectal evacuation.

Assessment

Examination

Points Ap and Bp are the leading edge of the prolapse.

Vaginal vault prolapse

Definition

Prolapse of the vaginal vault or cuff (point C on the POP-Q system) following hysterectomy.

Pathology

Although the aetiology is multifactorial, including genetic predisposition, surgery is by far the most significant factor. Vault prolapse is more likely when the hysterectomy has been performed for prolapse (11.6% versus 1.8% for other indications).

During hysterectomy, the uterosacral and cardinal ligaments are detached from the vaginal apex, leading to vault prolapse. This can be prevented by reattaching those ligaments to the vaginal cuff at the time of hysterectomy (see Section 13.6).

History

Symptoms of vault prolapse are similar to those of POP in general.

Assessment

Examination

Physical examination will typically reveal a transverse band of scar tissue at the vaginal apex with a dimple at either end of the band, representing previous attachment sites of uterosacral and cardinal ligaments. These are a useful landmark for identification of the vault.

There is a high incidence, up to 50%, of 'occult' SUI in these patients. Therefore, a good assessment of bladder function with the prolapse reduced before surgery might be necessary to plan concomitant or delayed procedures for SUI.

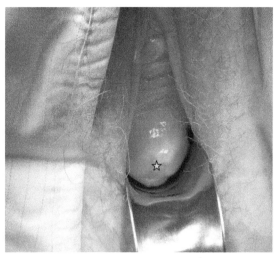

Fig. 14.5 Uterine prolapse. The cervix, point C, (☆) prolapses down to the introitus while the speculum's blade is retracting the posterior vaginal wall. This represents a stage II prolapse on the POP-Q system.

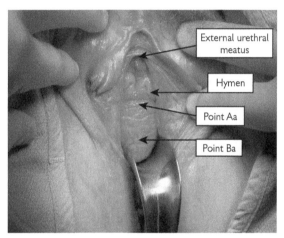

Fig. 14.6 Anterior vaginal wall prolapse. Note that point Aa maintains its relation to the urethra (3 cm away) but has descended to the level of the hymen (0 cm on POP-Q). Ba is at +1 cm, representing a stage II prolapse.

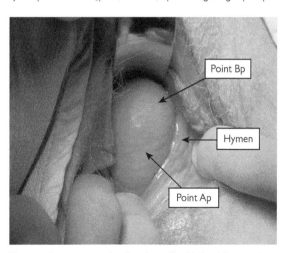

Fig. 14.7 Posterior vaginal wall prolapse. The blade of the speculum is retracting the anterior vaginal wall. Point Ap is at the level of the hymen (0 cm), while point Bp is descending further (+1 cm).

14.4 Management of the anterior compartment and uterine prolapse

Management of pelvic organ prolapse (POP) depends on multiple factors, including:

- Specific compartment affected or combinations of them:
- Co-morbidities (especially urinary or faecal incontinence)
- Coital activity and patient expectations

Treatment modalities include:

- Conservative management
- Mechanical devices (pessaries)
- Surgery

In general, conservative treatment and mechanical devices are considered for women with mild to moderate prolapse, those who want more children, frail patients, and those wishing to avoid or delay surgery. They can be used in any type of prolapse, unlike surgery which is specific for different compartments.

Conservative management

Conservative management includes lifestyle advice and pelvic floor muscle training. It is of doubtful benefit in POP.

A recent Cochrane review found no relevant randomized controlled trials and therefore concluded that there is no rigorous evidence for the use of conservative interventions in managing POP.

Mechanical devices

Pessaries have been used to treat POP for many years. In recent times there has been a resurgence in their use owing to the increase in the elderly population requiring non-surgical treatment. Historically, they have been made from a wide variety of materials, but currently most are made of silicone or inert plastic.

Although physical examination, including measurement of vaginal length, may give an estimate of pessary size, it is usually assessed by 'trial and error' (see Box 14.2). The right size pessary should stay in place during daily activities without causing pain or discomfort.

There are multiple shapes and sizes of pessaries available. They can be divided in two types: those that give support, e.g. Ring, Gehrung, and Hodge; and those that function as 'space-occupying' devices, e.g. for stages III and IV POP, including Shelf, Gelhorn, Donut, Cube, and Inflatoball devices.

Complications of long term pessary use include;

- Vaginal discharge
- Vaginal ulcerations (which might lead to vesicovaginal or rectovaginal fistulae)
- Formation of fibrous bands attaching the pessary to the vagina

To avoid some of these, pessaries should be changed regularly, usually every 6 months. The vagina should be inspected at every visit to exclude ulcerations or take biopsies if there is any suspicious lesion.

In addition, women should be encouraged to use topical oestrogen, which helps make the vaginal mucosa more resistant to trauma and treats minor symptoms such as vaginal irritation and discomfort. A typical regimen is one applicator dose or vaginal tablet or pessary (dose varies depending on the type of oestrogen) two nights per week, which has not been shown to result in significant endometrial hyperplasia.

Women who are able to remove and reinsert the pessary may be advised to remove it nightly, or at least two nights per week, which may lengthen the interval between gynaecological examinations and ring changes.

Despite their common use, a recent Cochrane review on mechanical devices for POP found no evidence from randomized controlled trials on their effectiveness. The authors also concluded that there was no consensus on the use of different types of devices, the indications, and the frequency of replacement or follow-up care.

Surgery

Surgery is the mainstay of POP management and aims to restore pelvic anatomy and function.

Surgical repair can be performed via a vaginal, abdominal or a laparoscopic approach. The appropriate choice depends on several factors, including the type of defect(s), the presence of co-morbidities (urinary or faecal incontinence), history of previous pelvic surgery, particularly failed prolapse surgery, the surgeon's training and skills, as well as patient factors such as age, obesity, and fitness for anaesthesia.

Uterine prolapse

Vaginal hysterectomy corrects uterine prolapse in women who do not want to preserve fertility. It can be combined with surgery to repair anterior and/or posterior compartment defects. It involves careful dissection and displacement of the bladder anteriorly and the rectum posteriorly, and ligation of three main pedicles on each side: uterosacral, uterine artery, and ovarian pedicles. The uterosacral ligament pedicles are attached to the posterior fornix to restore vaginal cuff support, and the vault is closed (see Section 13.6).

Abdominal sacrohysteropexy can be performed by open surgery or laparoscopically in women who want to conserve their uterus. Sutures or mesh can be attached inferiorly to the junction of the cervix and uterus (and uterosacral ligaments) and superiorly to the anterior longitudinal sacral ligament over the first or second sacral vertebra.

Sacrospinous fixation is an alternative where the cervix is attached to the sacrospinous ligament (see Section 14.5).

The latter two are not common procedures, but small case series have shown no significant intraoperative or postoperative complications (III).

Total vaginal mesh also allows for conservation of the uterus (see Section 14.5). However, long-term data on efficacy and complications are lacking.

Anterior compartment

This is the compartment most likely to have recurrent prolapse after surgery, with reported anatomical recurrence rates as high as 40%. However, symptomatic recurrences can be less.

Anterior colporrhaphy—this is the commonest technique for transvaginal correction of anterior vaginal wall prolapse. It involves a midline incision in the anterior vaginal mucosa with lateral dissection of mucosal flaps to separate the vaginal epithelium from the endopelvic fascia, exposing the bladder and proximal urethra. The endopelvic fascia is then plicated in the midline with absorbable mattress sutures, thereby elevating the anterior vagina (see Figure 14.8). Further plication of the periurethral tissue under the bladder neck (Kelly plication) may give additional support to this structure. The surplus vaginal skin is then excised and sutured in the midline with absorbable suture.

Outcomes of anterior colporrhaphy are largely limited to case series and retrospective studies, with wide variations in rates and definitions of cure and/or recurrence

Paravaginal repair—this procedure aims to correct lateral defects by reattaching the lateral vaginal sulcus to the ATFP/white line. This can be accomplished either abdominally or vaginally.

Once the retropubic space has been accessed, the bladder is dissected medially to expose the paravaginal space and four to six interrupted permanent sutures are placed to reattach the lateral vagina to the ATFP. Cystoscopy with intravenous indigocarmin (5 ml of 0.8% in 100 ml 50% dextrose) is recommended to detect any ureteric trauma.

The success rate of paravaginal repair ranges from 92–97% for the abdominal route, and 76–100% for the vaginal approach, with reported recurrence rates of up to 33%. Some studies have reported a longer time to recurrence for abdominal compared to vaginal repair

Abdominoperineal or four corner repair—this procedure, suggested by Raz in 1989, involves placing four sutures: two paraurethral and two more proximally through the entire vaginal wall, which are then transferred to the abdomen using a double-pronged needle through a suprapubic incision. The elevation of the bladder neck is adjusted via cystoscopy and the sutures are tied abdominally over the rectus sheath. Initial success rates of up to 90% have been quoted but recurrences are as high as 33%. Therefore this procedure does not seem to have significant advantages over anterior colporrhaphy

Mesh repairs—one recently developed technique involves an incision and repair similar to an anterior colporrhaphy, but incorporating the use of a biological or synthetic mesh to support the repair. The graft has four arms, two on each side, which are externalized using helical needles through the obturator foramen with two small incisions on each side (one for each arm of the mesh); see Figure 14.9. This new technique requires further evaluation

Other organic and synthetic grafts have been used for the management of anterior wall prolapse. Data on the use of these prostheses are limited.

A Cochrane review on the surgical management of POP found that standard anterior repair was associated with higher recurrence rates than when supplemented by Vicryl mesh (RR 1.39, 95% CI 1.02–1.90, evidence level **Ia**). However, data on morbidity and long-term outcome were too few for comparison or not available. The same review found no randomized controlled trials comparing anterior colporrhaphy and abdominal paravaginal repair.

Complications
Complications specific to anterior vaginal wall surgery include:

- Injury to adjacent structures—bladder, ureters, urethra, genitofemoral or ilioinguinal nerves (rates range from 0.5%–2%)
- Urinary complications—retention, recurrent UTI, *de novo* stress or urge incontinence or enterocele
- Erosion—of mesh or suture material through adjacent tissues
- Dyspareunia (more common with posterior repairs)

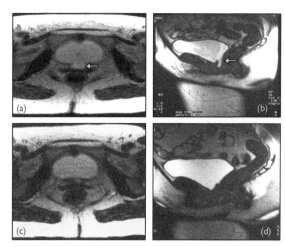

Fig. 14.8 MRI of cystocele repair. Transverse and sagittal views of a cystocele (⇐) before (a and b) and after (c and d) repair. (Courtesy of O. Adekanmi and R. Freeman.)

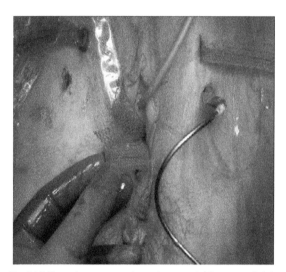

Fig. 14.9 Transobturator anterior prolapse repair. The surgeon's left hand holds the synthetic mesh. The mesh's two upper arms are exteriorized whilst the helical needle is externalizing one lower arm (on patient's left). (Reproduced from Perigee™ with permission from American Medical Systems, Minnetonka, Minnesota.)

⊙ Box 14.2 Fitting a ring pessary

- More comfortable if patient has emptied her bladder and bowel
- Woman in supine position
- Soften the pessary in hot water and cool before insertion
- Squeeze the pessary and gently insert through the introitus (an introducer is available to minimize patient discomfort during insertion of the ring pessary)
- Check that ring encircles the cervix and its supported anteriorly by the pubic bone
- Ask the woman to squat and bear down and also walk around to assess retention of the pessary and comfort
- The patient should not feel uncomfortable with the pessary

14.5 Management of the posterior compartment and vault prolapse

Posterior compartment

Surgical management of the posterior vaginal wall has been generally successful at restoring anatomy, but the results regarding functional outcome are conflicting, especially with regard to postoperative bowel dysfunction and dyspareunia.

Several procedures are available to the pelvic floor surgeon, with posterior colporrhaphy being the commonest amongst gynaecologists.

For obstructed defaecation associated with rectocele, a proctogram is recommended to exclude intussusception.

Posterior colporrhaphy—two clamps are placed bilaterally in the hymen to make the base of an inverted triangular skin incision whose apex is lower on the perineal body skin. Sharp dissection is then performed to separate the rectovaginal fascia from the posterior vaginal mucosa with a midline incision in the vaginal mucosa. This is enlarged as the dissection progresses until the upper edge of the rectocele is reached. The dissection is furthered laterally to the vaginal sulcus and the rectovaginal fascia is plicated in the midline with interrupted sutures to depress the anterior rectal wall. Redundant vaginal epithelium is then trimmed and the incision closed with absorbable suture. The procedure is commonly accompanied by plication of the transverse perinei muscles (perineorrhaphy) to reinforce the perineal body and give further support. However, care should be taken to avoid narrowing of the introitus.

As with anterior colporrhaphy, outcomes for posterior repair are mostly from retrospective studies, with wide variation in definitions of cure and other outcomes.

A common postoperative problem is new onset or worsening dyspareunia, which some attribute to levator ani plication, causing this practice to be abandoned by many surgeons

Site-specific fascial defect repair—involves dissecting the rectovaginal fascia in a similar way to a posterior repair, allowing the identification of all fascial tears. These are then repaired separately, as opposed to midline repair, with interrupted permanent or preferably delayed absorbable sutures.

A few studies have shown improvement in bowel and sexual function with this technique, but its major advantage seems to be reduction in complications rather than long-term improvement. Results are generally poorer than with traditional fascial repair. Some suggest that these defects might be created by the dissection during this procedure

Transanal repair—this procedure is usually performed by colorectal surgeons but is not primarily aimed at rectocele repair. Its main indication is disordered defaecation. An anterior rectal mucosa incision is performed about 1 cm above the dentate line, and the rectum is dissected to about 10 cm above the anal margin. The rectovaginal septum and rectal muscle are then plicated with interrupted absorbable sutures, and the redundant mucosa is trimmed.

This technique appears to improve bowel function, but data regarding prolapse and sexual function are lacking.

Stapled transanal rectal resection (STARR)—a new procedure performed by colorectal surgeons to treat rectal outlet obstruction caused by rectal intussusception. It involves placing three semicircular sutures in the ventral rectal side 2 cm apart, with the lowest 4 cm above the dentate line, followed by resection of mucosal flaps using a circular stapler. The procedure is then repeated on the posterior side. The posterior vaginal wall and the rectal wall are protected throughout. It aims to remove the rectocele and the redundant mucosa.

There are very early data on this procedure and further research is required.

Vaginal enterocele repair—the enterocele sac is reached and dissected from the vagina and rectum in a similar fashion to a posterior colporrhaphy. The sac is entered sharply, aided by traction with two clamps, followed by closure with absorbable purse-string, circumferential sutures, with or without involvement of the uterosacral ligaments.

This procedure can also be accomplished by open abdominal surgery or laparoscopy

A Cochrane review on surgical management of posterior wall prolapse found only two small studies comparing vaginal and transanal approaches, and concluded that the vaginal route had a lower rate of recurrence (RR 0.24, 95% CI 0.09–0.64), but it had a higher blood loss and postoperative narcotic use (evidence level **Ia**). There were no studies comparing the vaginal versus the abdominal approach. Data on the use of meshes or the effect of surgery on bowel function were insufficient.

Complications

Complications specific to posterior wall surgery include:

- Dyspareunia
- Worsening of bowel symptoms
- Rectal injury
- Vaginal shortening
- Pudendal neuralgia

Vaginal vault repair

Surgical repair of vaginal vault prolapse can be approached vaginally or abdominally, the latter via either laparotomy or laparoscopy. Several operations have been described, including high posterior repair, colpocleisis, culdoplasties (McCall, Halban, and Moschowitz), uterosacral vault suspension, sacrospinous fixation, posterior intravaginal slingoplasty, sacrocolpopexy, and mesh procedures (such as the total vaginal mesh). Laparoscopic approaches include ventrosuspension, cervicopexy, high McCall culdoplasty, hysteropexy, sacrospinous fixation, and sacrocolpopexy. The most commonly performed and generally widely accepted alternatives are described.

Abdominal sacrocolpopexy—this is considered the gold standard for vaginal vault repair. It involves the use of a mesh to suspend the vault to the sacral promontory. An abdominal incision is performed and the sacral promontory is exposed by dissecting the peritoneum and clearing the periosteum of connective tissue. Two or three nonabsorbable sutures are placed through the periosteum. The vaginal vault is identified and the bladder dissected off the anterior wall. Three rows of sutures are placed as far down the posterior vaginal wall as possible to correct posterior compartment prolapse, and two rows along the front wall of the vagina to correct concomitant anterior wall prolapse. Finally, all sutures are secured to a mesh and this is suspended to the sacral promontory with minimal tension.

The laparoscopic approach is similar to the open procedure. Recovery might be reduced but there are no comparative studies to assess this.

Success rate of this procedure ranges between 90 and 98%. Complications include bleeding, rectal trauma, ileus, mesh erosion, 'occult' stress urinary incontinence (SUI), and sacral osteomyelitis

Sacrospinous fixation (SSF)—this involves the attachment and subsequent elevation of the vaginal apex to the sacrospinous ligament using a delayed absorbable suture. It can be performed unilaterally (usually the right side) or bilaterally. Via a posterior wall dissection, the pararectal space is entered, and the ischial spine and sacrospinous ligament are identified and the suture inserted through the ligament using an appropriate suture carrier, e.g. Miya hook.

The success rate of this procedure has been consistently over 90% in different series. The reported complications, though few, are potentially serious, e.g. pudendal neurovascular damage, risk of cystocele formation (20–30%) owing to the exaggerated horizontal axis of the vagina resulting from this procedure, buttock pain, and sexual dysfunction

Posterior intravaginal slingoplasty (IVS)—recreates the suspensory ligament to the vaginal apex. A tape is secured to the vaginal apex through bilateral pararectal incisions 3 cm lateral and posterior to the anus. The tape is introduced using a metal tunneller onto the endopelvic fascia and immediately anterior to the ischial spines and sacrospinous ligament.

It gives a more physiological vaginal axis and is therefore suitable for women who have a short vagina.

There are no long-term follow-up data and more research is required for further evaluation.

Complications include rectal trauma and sepsis

Mesh repairs—biological or synthetic grafts have also been employed in repairs of the vault and the posterior compartment to enhance their longevity (see Figure 14.10). Polypropylene (type 1) has been the material most commonly used owing to its relatively low erosion rate and its large pore size which allows the passage of phagocytes. However, high rates of dyspareunia have been reported and so alternative mesh should be considered.

Total vaginal mesh—a recently developed technique which allows mesh augmentation of all the compartments: anterior, vault, and posterior, with a single piece of graft, for women with advanced POP. Risks of mesh augmentation include erosion and infection, and the long-term effect on bladder, bowel, and sexual function should be determined before their generalized use can be recommended

Colpocleisis—this is a vaginal closure which is indicated for elderly patients with POP who no longer want to have sexual intercourse. It involves removal of the vaginal mucosa and inversion of the vagina using purse-string sutures. It is highly effective but the rate of reoperation is unknown

A Cochrane review on surgical management of vault prolapse concluded that abdominal sacrocolpopexy had a lower recurrence rate, less dyspareunia, and a trend towards lower reoperation rate than sacrospinous fixation (Ia). However, the latter was quicker and cheaper. Data comparing intravaginal slingoplasty and sacrospinous fixation were too few and there were no trials comparing laparoscopic versus open surgery.

Further reading

Cochrane database of systematic reviews. www.mrw.interscience. wiley.com/cochrane for a) Surgical management of POP in women b) Conservative management of POP in women, and c) Mechanical devices for POP in women

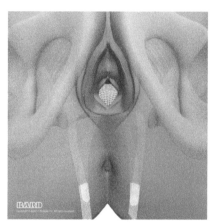

Fig. 14.10 Posterior prolapse repair with mesh. (Reproduced with permission from CR Bard, Inc.)

14.6 Urinary incontinence

Definition

Urinary incontinence (UI) is defined as the complaint of any involuntary urinary leakage. It is a common symptom that can affect women of all ages. It is rarely life-threatening, but can seriously affect physical, psychological, and social wellbeing. UI can result from functional abnormalities of the lower urinary tract, which will be discussed in this section. Other conditions (neurological, metabolic, psychiatric or surgical, e.g. fistulas) are outside the scope of this chapter.

Prevalence

There is wide variation in the epidemiology of UI, mostly owing to differences in study populations, definitions and measurements of UI, and survey methods.

For less severe or transient UI ('ever', 'any', or 'at least once in the last 12 months'), the prevalence ranges from 5–69% in women >15 years old, with most studies in the range of 25–45%.

The prevalence of more severe UI is more consistent, with estimates for daily UI in the general population of 4–7% in women <65 years and between 4–17% in those >65 years. In a large study carried out in Norway in 2001 (the EPINCONT study), with over 27 000 women, the reported incidence of UI was 25%. The prevalence among nulliparous women ranged from 8–32%. In the UK, the Leicestershire MRC Incontinence Study found that 34% of women over 40 years reported UI, but only 3.5% of these had daily incontinence.

The prevalence of UI tends to increase up to the age of 50, then plateaus or falls between 50 and 70 years, and steadily increases thereafter. This pattern seems to be related to variations in the types of UI—overall, stress urinary incontinence (SUI) is the commonest form (approximately 50% of cases); followed by mixed stress and urge urinary incontinence (MUI); with the smallest proportion being urge urinary incontinence (UUI); SUI appears to decrease after the age of 50, with UUI and MUI increasing over the age of 60 years.

Data suggests that UI is commoner among Caucasians, but there is paucity of data for other racial groups. Although the natural history of UI is not fully known, remission can occur but little is known about its predictors. Between 5 and 10% of women with overactive bladder syndrome (OAB) can remit.

Aetiology

The aetiology of UI is multifactorial. Well controlled, longitudinal studies to identify risk factors are scarce, and most have been identified from cross-sectional studies. These only identify association and not causation. Among the possible risk factors, age, parity, and obesity have been the most rigorously studied.

The established and suggested risk factors for UI are:

- **Age**—this is the most consistent risk factor reported in the literature (see prevalence above)
- **Parity**—the effects of pelvic floor damage during childbirth, discussed earlier for POP (see Section 14.1), apply similarly to UI. However, some studies have shown that the association between parity and UI seems to decrease and even disappear with age, which supports the idea that age is a stronger risk factor than parity. It is less clear whether age at delivery or time since delivery may influence the effect of parity
- **Obesity**—there is strong evidence that supports the causal role of obesity in UI. There are intervention studies showing that drastic weight reduction results in subjective and objective resolution of UI in the short term
- **Pregnancy**—UI during pregnancy is a self-limiting condition for many women. Incontinence in pregnancy has been shown to be a predictor of incontinence postpartum and at 5 years' post-delivery. However, it is debatable whether pregnancy per se

contributes to UI or whether the association is related to vaginal delivery

- **Obstetric and fetal factors**—forceps and vacuum delivery, episiotomy and vaginal or perineal tears, induction of labour, duration of second stage, and birth weight have all been associated with UI, but reports in the literature show an inconsistent relationship. UI may arise following bladder overdistension injury, e.g. after premature catheter removal or poor bladder management when using regional anaesthesia
- **Menopause and oestrogen deficiency**—oestrogen receptors are abundant in the urethra, bladder, and trigone. Oestrogens help maintain normal urinary function and its deficiency predisposes to urinary tract infections (UTI), frequency, urgency, dysuria, vaginal dryness, and dyspareunia. However, there is inconsistency in the literature with regard to the role of oestrogen deficiency in UI
- **Hysterectomy**—can predispose to UI by two different mechanisms: either via neuromuscular or connective tissue damage to the bladder and pelvic side wall during the procedure or via a hormonal mechanism if a bilateral oophorectomy is performed simultaneously. In a recent systematic review by Brown et al., the risk of developing UI after hysterectomy was increased by 60% in women who were >60 years (OR 1.6, 95% CI 1.4–1.8) but not in younger women
- **Lower urinary tract infection**—there is an association between UTI and UI
- **Cognitive (dementia) and functional impairment (reduced mobility)** can cause failure of inhibition of the sacral reflex controlling voiding, leading to detrusor overactivity and urge urinary incontinence
- **Smoking**
- **Family history** (possible connective tissue weakness)

Pathophysiology

Neuromuscular or connective tissue damage at any of the three levels of pelvic organ support might lead to POP or UI as described (see Section 14.1). Here, the mechanisms of micturition and how these can be affected in UI are explained.

Urinary continence is a complex dynamic process involving a low pressure reservoir (bladder) with a high pressure sphincter (urethra).

Low intravesical pressure is maintained by:

- The hydrostatic pressure in the bladder—this works against the mechanisms of urethral closure but is insignificant if there is adequate urethral resistance. It rarely amounts to >10 cmH$_2$O
- Transmission of intra-abdominal pressure—pressures are usually transmitted to bladder, bladder neck, and proximal urethra. After an increase in intra-abdominal pressure (e.g. coughing), the pressure rises in the urethra before it rises in the bladder, which helps to maintain continence
- Tension in the bladder wall—this is partially a passive phenomenon owing to the distensibility of the bladder wall, which allows it to store large volumes with little rise in pressure (compliance), and partially an active phenomenon owing to the neurological control of the detrusor muscle

Urethral function is maintained by:

- The watertight seal—the hermetic seal of the urethra is maintained by a rich venous supply to the submucosa which engorges the tissues, and by urethral secretions. This may fail in postmenopausal women
- Intrinsic and extrinsic muscles—in the mid-urethra at rest, closure is mainly maintained by constant pressure of the intrinsic striated muscle of the rhabdosphincter, and to a lesser degree by intrinsic smooth muscle contraction. During stress (increased intra-abdominal

pressure), the extrinsic striated muscles of the pelvic floor also contract to maintain urethral closure. Urethral pressure studies have shown that resting urethral pressure is caused by striated muscle effect, smooth muscle effect, and to vascular supply. The pudendal nerve innervates the urethral sphincter. Failure of the striated or smooth muscle sphincter function, mucosa seal function or pudendal innervation may result in SUI, i.e. intrinsic sphincter deficiency (ISD)

- Urethral support—it is postulated that urethral support is maintained by a 'hammock'. The urethra is supported posteriorly and inferiorly by the anterior vaginal wall. The pubocervical fascia that lies between them attaches laterally to the ATFP (arcus tendineus fascia pelvis), which in turn attaches to the pubococcygeus muscles. Their contraction can produce urethral elevation. During rises in intra-abdominal pressure, the urethra is supported by its lateral attachments and is therefore compressed by the downward force of intra-abdominal pressure against the resistance offered by the anterior vaginal wall. Failure of this mechanism can cause stress incontinence as a result of urethral hypermobility (see Figure 14.11)

- Two condensations of the endopelvic fascia connecting the urethra to the pubic bone, known as the anterior and posterior pubourethral ligaments, provide further urethral support. Some investigators have postulated that elongation of these ligaments may contribute to stress incontinence

Voiding is normally under voluntary control mediated by the pontine reticular formation centre located in the cerebellum. Neurological control of detrusor contractility is dependent on a sacral spinal reflex controlled by several higher centres. Urethral function is controlled by pudendal innervation. The micturition cycle involves three phases: storage, initiation, and voiding.

During the early stages of bladder filling, sensory receptors in the bladder wall pass impulses via the pelvic splanchnic nerves to the sacral roots S2–S4, which then ascend to higher centres via the lateral spinothalamic tracts. The descending impulses inhibit detrusor contraction. This inhibition is mediated by the sympathetic nervous system through α- and β-receptors. The former are located along the bladder neck and urethra, and the latter are spread throughout the detrusor muscle. Stimulation of α-adrenergic receptors increases outlet urethral resistance. Stimulation of β-adrenergic receptors causes detrusor smooth muscle relaxation which accommodates bladder filling. At approximately half of bladder capacity, a first sensation to void is appreciated. The impulses continue as the volume increases and reinforce conscious inhibition of micturition until an acceptable place to void is found. This suppression of detrusor contraction may be accompanied by voluntary pelvic floor contraction to aid urethral closure.

The initiation phase begins with relaxation of the pelvic floor with simultaneous relaxation of extrinsic and intrinsic striated muscle, followed by suppression of descending inhibitory impulses leading to detrusor contraction. The parasympathetic system mediates inhibition of the resting tone of the urethral smooth muscle, resulting in relaxation. In addition, stimulated parasympathetic fibres from S2 to S4, via the hypogastric nerve, release acetylcholine which binds to M2 and M3 muscarinic receptors in the bladder, resulting in detrusor muscle contraction.

The voiding phase commences when rising intravesical and falling urethral pressures equate, leading to urine flow and bladder emptying. As the intravesical pressure falls towards the end of micturition, the pelvic floor and urethral muscles contract, causing urethral closure and interruption of flow, finalizing the cycle.

Detrusor overactivity and urge urinary incontinence may result from disruption at many levels of these complex mechanisms.

Further reading

Brown JS, Sawaya G, Thom DH, Grady D. Hysterectomy and urinary incontinence: a systematic review. Lancet 2000;**356**:535–9.

> **Box 14.3 Terminology of urinary incontinence**
>
> The International Continence Society has defined the types of incontinence and other common terminology in UI.
>
> - Urgency—the complaint of a sudden compelling desire to pass urine which is difficult to defer
> - Urge urinary incontinence (UUI)—involuntary leakage of urine accompanied by, or immediately preceded by, urgency
> - Stress urinary incontinence (SUI)—involuntary leakage of urine on effort or exertion, or on sneezing or coughing
> - Mixed urinary incontinence (MUI)—involuntary leakage associated with urgency and also with exertion, effort, sneezing or coughing
> - Overactive bladder (OAB) syndrome—urgency, with or without UUI, usually with frequency and nocturia. OAB wet is where UUI is present, and OAB dry is where incontinence is absent
> - Detrusor overactivity (DO)—an urodynamic observation characterized by involuntary detrusor contractions during the filling phase of cystometry that may be spontaneous or provoked
> - Urodynamic stress urinary incontinence (USI)—the demonstration of leakage of urine during increased abdominal pressure in the absence of detrusor contraction during filling cystometry

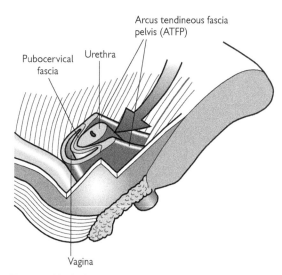

Fig. 14.11 Urethral support (Hammock theory). The downward force of increased intra-abdominal pressure (large arrow) compresses the urethra against the resistance offered by the pubocervical fascia. (Reproduced from DeLancey JO. Structural support of the urethra as it relates to stress urinary incontinence: the hammock hypothesis. *American Journal of Obstetrics and Gynecology* 1994; **170**:1713–23, with permission from Elsevier.)

History

The bladder has been said to be an 'unreliable witness', but this may be overcome with adequate history-taking. The aim of the initial clinical assessment is to categorize the woman's UI as stress UI (SUI), mixed UI (MUI) or urge UI/OAB (UUI) (see Box 14.3). Expert opinion from the NICE guideline on UI (2006) recommends that history-taking is sufficiently reliable to inform initial, non-invasive treatment decisions. If the initial diagnosis is MUI, treatment should be directed towards the predominant symptom.

Urinary symptoms can be divided into:

- **Storage symptoms**—frequency (daytime), nocturia (>1), urgency, UUI and SUI, or constant leakage (e.g. due to a fistula)
- **Voiding symptoms**—hesitancy, straining to void and poor or intermittent urinary flow
- **Postmicturition symptoms**—incontinence, sensation of incomplete emptying

It is important to differentiate urgency from urge to void: urgency is the compelling desire to pass urine which allows no delay, while urge to void is a strong sensation which can be delayed. Urgency is the main symptom of overactive bladder (OAB), and identification is important in the clinical history.

Other areas that require assessment include:

- **Bowel symptoms**—constipation might predispose to UI and affect surgical outcome; straining might contribute to weakening of the pelvic floor muscles
- **POP symptoms**
- **Obstetric and gynaecological history**—parity, number and mode of deliveries; menopausal status
- **Sexual history**—dyspareunia, vaginal dryness, coital incontinence
- **Medical history**—conditions that may coexist or exacerbate UI include diabetes, neurological disorders, e.g. multiple sclerosis, Parkinson's disease, cerebrovascular accident, spinal cord injury, cardiorespiratory and renal disease
- **Surgical history**—previous spinal or pelvic surgery, especially for UI or POP
- **Drug history**—e.g. diuretics
- **Occupation and social circumstances**
- **Lifestyle information**, including alcohol, smoking, and fluid intake
- **Psychological problems**
- **Family history**

There are several tools to supplement the clinical history. These include questionnaires and bladder diaries, and can provide valuable information that could otherwise be missed during the initial consultation. They may also give an indication of the impact of UI on quality of life (QoL), and can be used to assess outcomes of treatment.

There are many incontinence-specific symptoms and QoL questionnaires. NICE recommends eight which have shown the highest validity and reliability: International Consultation on Incontinence Questionnaire (ICIQ); Bristol Female Lower Urinary Tract Symptoms (BFLUTS); Incontinence Quality of Life (I-QOL); Stress and Urge Incontinence and Quality of Life Questionnaire (SUIQQ); Urinary Incontinence Severity Score (UISS); SEAPI-QMM; Incontinence Severity Index (ISI); and King's Health Questionnaire (KHQ). The ICIQ has a short form (ICIQ-SF), which has only four questions and is a good screening tool.

Bladder diaries, also known as frequency/volume charts, are a method of quantification of urinary frequency (diurnal and nocturnal), voided volume, urgency, incontinence episodes, pad changes, and total urine output. They can be 1-, 3- or 7-day diaries. NICE recommends these be used at the initial consultation over a minimum of 3 days, covering the woman's variations in her usual activities, i.e. work and leisure.

Clinical assessment

Physical examination

Examination should be performed to assist the diagnosis and management of UI, and to exclude other modifiable or related conditions:

- Body mass index (BMI)
- Abdominal and pelvic (bimanual and speculum) examination to assess for masses and POP, including cough stress test for SUI
- Vaginal examination can identify atrophic change. The strength of pelvic floor muscles can be assessed using the modified Oxford score system. This involves placing one or two fingers in the vagina and asking the woman to squeeze. The strength of pelvic muscles is graded on a 6-point scale from 0 (no contraction), 1 (flicker), 2 (weak), 3 (moderate), 4 (good, with lift), to 5 (strong contraction). The duration of the contraction should also be noted
- Neurological examination, with emphasis on sacral roots S2–S4: deep tendon reflexes at the knee and ankle; abduction and dorsiflexion of toes (S3); sensory innervation at the sole and lateral aspect of the foot (S1), posterior aspect of the thigh (S2), perineum (S3), and perianal area (S4)
- Assessment of cognitive impairment in women >75 years with complex co-morbidities. Also in younger women if indicated

Women should be examined with a comfortably full bladder to assess stress incontinence by cough stress test. If POP is present it should be reduced to determine 'occult' SUI. The examination should be performed both in supine and upright positions. The woman should be asked to bear down and cough to try to reproduce SUI. The examination should be repeated with the bladder empty. Attention should be given to patient dignity (e.g. offer a pad to avoid leakage, especially onto the floor if standing).

Investigations

Several tests may help in the assessment of UI.

Urinalysis

Urinalysis is used to detect blood (suggestive of infection, stone or cancer); protein (infection, renal impairment); glucose (diabetes mellitus); leukocytes and nitrites (infection). If consistently positive for blood, cystoscopy and renal ultrasound are indicated.

Urine dipstick test for leukocytes and nitrites has low sensitivity but high specificity for the diagnosis of UTI.

Women with symptoms of UTI, with either positive or negative urine dipsticks for leukocytes or nitrites, should have midstream urine (MSU) specimen sent for culture. The former should be prescribed antibiotics pending culture results. Women without symptoms but positive urinalysis for leukocytes/nitrites should also have a MSU, but treatment should not be commenced until the result is known.

Post-void residual volume

Post-void residual (PVR) is the volume of urine remaining in the bladder following a void. Large residuals may indicate outlet obstruction, detrusor failure or neurological disease. However, there is no accepted definition of 'normal' or 'high' residual volumes. Furthermore, they may vary between voids, making repeat measurements sometimes necessary. It seems that the percentage of the voided volume remaining in the bladder is important.

The PVR can be measured either by catheterization or, more commonly, by ultrasound using a portable bladder scanner. A NICE review found that the diagnostic accuracy of ultrasound in comparison with catheterization was within clinically acceptable limits, with the advantage of better acceptability and lower incidence of adverse events.

Pad test

The aim is to quantify urine loss by weighing a perineal pad before and after 'leakage provocation'. It can be performed as a short outpatient test (1 h) or at home over 24 h. It begins with a full bladder or a fixed known volume of saline instilled into the bladder and weighing of the pad before starting a series of standardized exercises or activities. A weight gain of >1 g during 1 h or >4 g in 24 h is considered positive.

There is no strong evidence to support the use of the pad test in the assessment of UI. NICE does not recommend its routine use. It may be useful for evaluating therapies.

A specific indication for pad testing is to differentiate urine loss from vaginal discharge or sweating. When urine cannot be demonstrated by other tests, the woman is given a short course of phenazopyridine hydrochloride (Pyridium®) 200 mg TDS orally for 48 h. This stains urine orange and UI can be confirmed.

Tests for urethral mobility

These tests assess urethral competence. Bladder neck mobility may also be assessed by radiology (bead chain cystourethrography or videocystourethrography) or more usually by ultrasound. The Q-tip test is used mainly for research but rarely in clinical practice and it is questionable whether it affects management. It involves placing a sterile, lubricated cotton swab in the urethra. With the woman at rest, a standard protractor is used to determine the angle of the Q-tip from the horizontal (resting angle). The woman is asked to bear down or strain and the angle of the Q-tip is measured again (straining angle). If the Q-tip moves more than 30° the test is considered positive.

Ultrasound

The commonest use of ultrasound in UI is to determine PVR. The PVR is measured using a portable bladder scan machine, which calculates the urine volume using preconfigured settings. It is useful in women with voiding difficulties and sometimes after postoperative catheter removal.

Ultrasound can also assess mobility and support of the bladder neck, with the advantage of avoiding irradiation. There are several

approaches: abdominal, vaginal, rectal, and perineal. The transabdominal route has the disadvantage of not having a fixed reference point and is more difficult in obese women. The reference point for the other approaches is the lower edge of the pubis symphysis. The perineal route is less likely to cause pelvic distortion, is better accepted by women, and is more reliable in obese women.

Another proposed use of ultrasound is to measure bladder wall thickness for the diagnosis of overactive bladder (OAB). There are reports suggesting that women with OAB have a thicker bladder wall than women with SUI or women without UI demonstrated on urodynamics. However, there is not enough evidence to support its routine use.

NICE does not recommend the routine use of ultrasound in UI other than for measurement of PVR.

Cystoscopy

Cystoscopy is the direct visualization of the bladder and urethra using a flexible or rigid cystoscope. It is not indicated in the routine assessment of UI but may be useful in cases of suspected urethrovaginal or vesicovaginal fistula, women with reduced bladder capacity at cystometry, and in women with pain or recurrent UTI. It is mandatory in women with haematuria, including persistent microscopic haematuria. Bladder mucosal biopsies may be taken during the procedure.

Electromyography (EMG)

EMG is the study of electrical potentials generated by neuromuscular units and can be used to assess pelvic floor denervation in women with UI or POP. It can be performed using surface or needle electrodes, and may provide useful information of urethral sphincter function and overall pelvic floor neuromuscular damage. It is not used routinely in the investigation of UI.

Urodynamics

Urodynamics are discussed in Section 14.8.

Further reading

www.nice.org.uk NICE guideline on urinary incontinence, October 2006.

14.8 Urodynamics

Definition

Urodynamic investigation is the functional assessment of bladder and urethral function. It aims to demonstrate an abnormality of storage or voiding. However, inconsistency between symptoms and urodynamic findings is quite common. Urodynamics comprise a number of tests which may provide useful information in determining the underlying pathology and in selecting the most appropriate intervention.

- **Uroflowmetry** is a measurement of the flow rate over time. It helps to diagnose or exclude voiding difficulties. The woman voids in a commode that funnels urine onto a device that measures the flow rate.

  The uroflowmetric parameters include maximum and average flow rate, flow time, and total volume voided. The total voided volume should be >150 ml for these parameters to be meaningful. A flow rate below 15 ml/s on more than one occasion is considered abnormal. Flow rates above 40 ml/s may indicate decreased outlet resistance and are commonly seen in women with SUI. The pattern of the flow curve is also observed. A normal flow pattern is a bell-shaped curve. Obstructed flow is characterized by low flow rate and prolonged voiding time with an intermittent or plateau-shaped curve. However, the diagnosis is confirmed by pressure–flow studies, i.e. voiding cystometry

- **Cystometry** is the measure of the pressure–volume relationship of the bladder during filling and voiding. It is usually carried out through concurrent measurement of intravesical and abdominal pressures using catheters inserted into the bladder and the rectum or vagina (multichannel cystometry). The pressure-recording catheters may be water-infused attached to external pressure transducers or microtip (solid state transducers). The former can have two lumens, one for filling and one for pressure monitoring, or three lumens to measure urethral pressure simultaneously. Measurements are made in centimetres of water (cmH_2O), with the zero reference being the upper edge of the pubic symphysis. The filling fluid may be saline, water or contrast media. The filling rate depends on the woman's bladder capacity, seen on the frequency volume chart/bladder diary. It can be from as slow as <10 ml/min to up to >100 ml/min.

  The parameters measured are the intravesical pressure (P_{ves}) and the intra-abdominal pressure (P_{abd}). Detrusor pressure (P_{det}) is calculated as $P_{ves} - P_{abd}$ The flow rate and filling and voided volumes are also recorded.

Many women find urodynamics embarrassing. It is important to maintain their dignity and ensure privacy throughout the procedure, keeping the number of observers to a minimum. Information leaflets given in advance are useful.

Uroflowmetry is performed before cystometry. The recording and filling catheters are then inserted and residual volume is noted. The woman is instructed to inhibit micturition. Bladder filling then begins and the volumes at which the woman indicates her first and maximal desire to void are noted. Provocative tests for stress urinary incontinence (SUI) (coughing) and detrusor overactivity (DO) (hand washing, listening to running water) are performed, and leakage and any detrusor contractions are noted. At the end of the procedure, the woman voids with the pressure lines still in place to measure pressure and flow.

DO is diagnosed during the filling phase if there are spontaneous or provoked detrusor contractions with the woman voluntarily trying to inhibit micturition (see Figure 14.12). The diagnosis of urodynamic stress incontinence (USI) is made if leakage occurs on coughing in the absence of detrusor contraction (see Figure 14.13).

Normal values

Although there is disagreement on some cystometric parameters, usually accepted 'normal' values include: residual volume of <50 ml; first desire to void between 150 and 200 ml; bladder capacity >400 ml (measured at maximal desire to void); no detrusor pressure rise during filling and a rise of <50 cmH_2O during voiding for a peak flow rate of >15 ml/s.

- **Ambulatory monitoring** can be performed in those women in whom laboratory urodynamics, i.e. static cystometry, give unexpected negative results. It involves using a small digital recording system with microtip pressure transducers and an electronic leakage (pad) detection system worn usually for 6 h. This technique is expensive but avoids the problems of an artificial environment and non-physiological bladder filling rate attributed to traditional cystometry. It helps diagnose DO, but not SUI, and is time-consuming

- **Urethral pressure profile** is a measure of urethral resistance along its lumen. There are several techniques, including the perfusion method and microtransducer system. The clinical value is debatable since there are few validity or reproducibility data, but it may be useful in women following failed surgery and for assessing urethral strictures and diverticula

- **Urethral retro-resistance pressure (URP)** is the pressure required to maintain the urethral sphincter open at rest. Data on the usefulness of this test are limited and its role in routine practice is still unclear. The URP is considered an indirect assessment of urethral function and is not a substitute for urodynamics

- **Leak point pressure** is the bladder pressure at which leakage occurs. An increased bladder pressure may be caused by detrusor contraction or a rise in abdominal pressure. Therefore, there are two leak point pressures: the bladder or detrusor leak point pressure, which is the detrusor pressure at which leakage occurs in the absence of raised intra-abdominal pressure; and the abdominal leak point pressure, which is the bladder pressure at which leakage occurs with increased abdominal pressure (cough or Valsalva manoeuvre) in the absence of detrusor contraction. It is a measure of urethral closure resistance but the technique is not standardized and is poorly reproducible. A low abdominal leak pressure point can be associated with intrinsic sphincter deficiency but the clinical value is unclear

- **Videocystourethrography (VCU)**—this technique involves combining routine cystometry (with contrast media as filling fluid) with radiological assessment of the bladder and urethra. Anatomical features and functional events are displayed and recorded simultaneously. VCU is used in patients with complicated lower urinary tract dysfunction, especially those with neurological conditions. It is not indicated as a first line in the routine assessment of UI, but is regarded as the 'gold standard' lower urinary tract investigation as it can reveal bladder neck opening, reflux, etc.

The NICE guideline on UI found no evidence to support the use of urodynamic testing prior to conservative treatment, nor to support its preoperative use in the small number of women with 'pure' SUI. They recommend multichannel cystometry before surgery in women in whom DO is suspected (i.e. symptoms of frequency or urgency), when there has been previous surgery for SUI or anterior wall prolapse, or when there are symptoms suggestive of voiding dysfunction (**D**).

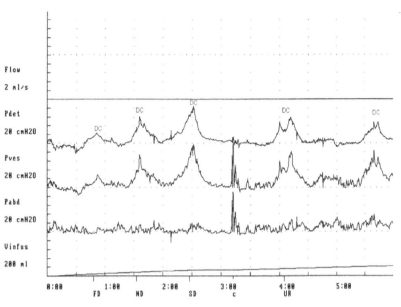

Fig. 14.12 Detrusor overactivity. There are unprovoked detrusor contractions (DC) on the detrusor pressure (Pdet) line, with consequent increases in bladder pressure (Pves), without increases in abdominal pressure (Pabd) during filling phase. Vinfus, volume of fluid infused in the bladder.

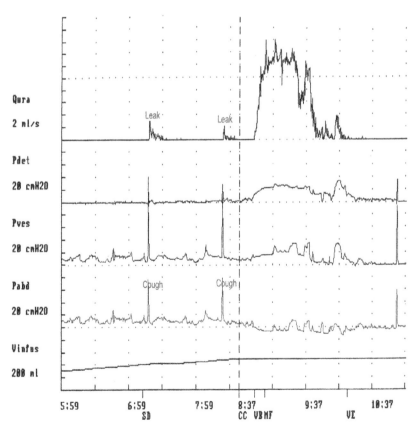

Fig. 14.13 Urodynamic stress incontinence. Note that increases in abdominal pressure (Pabd) during coughing are followed or accompanied by leakage. Qura, urine flow; Pdet, detrusor pressure; Pves, bladder pressure; Pabd, abdominal pressure; Vinfus, volume of fluid infused in the bladder.

14.9 Conservative management of urinary incontinence

The commonest types of urinary incontinence (UI) are stress (SUI), urge (UUI), and mixed urinary incontinence (MUI). Management depends on the underlying diagnosis. Treatments include conservative management (lifestyle interventions, physical and behavioural therapies), and pharmacological and surgical treatments.

Conservative interventions such as lifestyle changes, pelvic floor muscle training (PFMT), biofeedback, and electrical stimulation are indicated for all types of UI.

UUI and overactive bladder (OAB) syndrome treatments aim to improve central control of micturition (behavioural therapy) or to modify detrusor contractility (drugs or surgery).

SUI treatments aim to improve pelvic floor muscle function and/or increase urethral support.

For MUI, NICE recommends that treatment should be directed to the predominant symptoms.

Lifestyle interventions
Advice on lifestyle interventions can be beneficial for patients with any form of UI, and a trial should be recommended.
- Reducing daily fluid intake to 1–1.5 l/day
- Avoiding tea, coffee, and alcohol
- Dietary advice to improve constipation if present
- Weight loss
- Smoking cessation advice

The use of drugs such as diuretics and other medications affecting bladder function should also be reviewed.

Behavioural therapy
Behavioural modifications for UI include:
- **Bladder drill (re-training) for OAB**—the main component is timed voiding, which aims to increase the intervals between voids and the bladder capacity, as well as reduce the number of urge incontinence episodes. The woman is asked to void every hour for the first week, even if there is no desire to void, but not to void if there is urgency. Voiding intervals are then increased progressively by 15–30 min every week until a desired interval of 3–4 h is achieved.
  There is good evidence that bladder retraining is effective for UUI and MUI, with fewer adverse effects than pharmacological treatment. It should be offered as a first line treatment (NICE, **A**) but requires patient motivation and compliance. Relapse rates are high
- **Biofeedback** aims to teach voluntary inhibition of detrusor contractions in detrusor overactivity (DO) and improve pelvic floor muscle contraction in SUI. The patient gets information about this normally unconscious physiological process by auditory, visual or tactile signals. Vaginal or rectal pressure sensors or EMG electrodes are used and the patient is able to visualize, hear or feel the increase in pressures or the EMG activity. DO/UUI cystometric biofeedback involves conscious inhibition of DO while watching the overactive contractions on cystometry. Most data on biofeedback relates to its simultaneous use with PFMT in patients with SUI rather than as an isolated intervention for either UUI or SUI. Some studies have shown significant improvement in patients with UUI, but long-term results are poor
- **Hypnotherapy**—OAB has been thought to be exacerbated by underlying psychological factors. Some studies show that women correlate the onset of symptoms to untoward events. Hypnotherapy aims to improve symptoms by suggestion alone or by helping patients disclose 'repressed' emotions or memories. This was

first described in the early 1980s with short-lasting improvement. It is not currently widely employed in the management of UUI
- **Acupuncture** is thought to increase endorphin and encephalin levels in cerebrospinal fluid. The latter are known to inhibit detrusor contractions in vitro. Some studies have shown symptomatic improvement in women with OAB treated with acupuncture. It is an alternative for UUI/OAB only, but long-term studies are required

Physical therapies
- **Pelvic floor muscle training (PFMT)** is well established. NICE recommends it as a first line treatment for SUI or MUI (**A**). It can also be utilized as a preventive measure during and after pregnancy, as it has been shown to reduce the risk of developing UI postnatally.
  Women can be taught PFMT during pelvic examination at the initial consultation or can be referred for physiotherapy. The aim is to contract the pelvic floor muscles at least eight times on three occasions in a day. The examiner assesses pelvic floor muscle contraction by placing one or two fingers into the vagina as the woman squeezes. Thereafter she can monitor her own progress in the same way.
  Women who have difficulty in performing PFMT may benefit from biofeedback, electrical stimulation or vaginal cones.
  There is good evidence that daily PFMT is safe and effective for the management of SUI and MUI, and a trial of at least 3 months should be offered. PFMT is best done under supervision. It requires motivation. Compliance rates are poor and long-term results inconsistent
- **Vaginal cones** may help women train their pelvic floor muscles. They are available in sets of incremental weight. The woman inserts the lightest cone in the vagina and tries to retain it while walking. This causes the pelvic floor muscles to contract to keep the cone in the vagina. When successful, the next heavier cone is used. Vaginal cones represent a form of biofeedback, as the sensation of 'losing' the cone may prompt pelvic floor muscles contraction to retain it.
  There is wide variation in the weight of cones and the frequency of treatment. Studies comparing vaginal cones in combination with PFMT or versus electrical stimulation have generally shown vaginal cones to be as effective, but vaginal cones are no better than PFMT alone. However, withdrawal rates seem to be higher in vaginal cones users
- **Functional electrical stimulation** involves delivering short pulses of current through a probe placed in the mid-vagina. In DO this inhibits detrusor contractions through inhibitory pelvic floor reflexes, while in SUI it directly stimulates pelvic floor muscles. There is wide variation in the type and intensity of current used for both SUI and OAB, and the duration and frequency of the sessions. In general, stimulation parameters are tailored to the woman's tolerance.
  Other forms of electrical stimulation include transcutaneous electrical nerve stimulation (TENS) applied daily to S2–S4 dermatomes and the Stoller afferent nerve stimulator (a fine gauge needle in the posterior tibial nerve above the ankle, which carries electrical stimulation to the sacral spine).
  A NICE review found that study results were inconsistent, and electrical stimulation is not recommended for routine use in women with OAB, nor in combination with PFMT (**A**).

14.10 Pharmacological management of urinary incontinence

Pharmacological management of urge urinary incontinence /overactive bladder syndrome

Drug therapy plus behavioural modification are the mainstays of management of urge urinary incontinence (UUI) and overactive bladder syndrome (OAB).

- **Antimuscarinic drugs**—detrusor contraction is modulated by acetylcholine binding to muscarinic receptors, mostly M2 and M3, in the bladder (see Section 14.6). The agents used for OAB usually have antimuscarinic effects and this group is currently the mainstay of treatment. However, drugs differ in their selectivity for muscarinic receptors. All of them interact with muscarinic receptors in other organs to a greater or lesser degree, causing significant side effects, mainly dry mouth, blurred vision, tachycardia, drowsiness, and constipation. Central nervous system adverse effects include disorientation, hallucinations, convulsions, and cognitive impairment. Side effects often limit compliance.

  Oxybutynin has, in addition, direct muscle relaxant and local anaesthetic effects. Its efficacy and adverse effects are well documented. At the recommended dose of 5 mg TDS, many women find the side effects, especially dry mouth, more intolerable than the OAB symptoms. Compliance may be improved by reducing the dose (2.5 or 3 mg TDS), by a slow release preparation or by other routes of administration, i.e. rectal suppositories, transdermal or intravesical preparations for self-catheterizing patients.

  Tolterodine is an antimuscarinic drug that has no specificity for any particular receptor subtype but has high selectivity for bladder muscarinic receptors versus salivary glands, therefore causing fewer side effects. The recommended dose is 2 mg BD or 4 mg OD of the slow release preparation (shown to reduce the incidence of side effects compared with immediate release without affecting efficacy).

  Trospium chloride is a non-selective muscarinic receptor blocker which increases bladder volume at first unstable contraction and bladder capacity. It appears to be as effective as oxybutynin with fewer side effects. It does not cross the blood–brain barrier, thus reducing the risk of cognitive impairment and other central nervous system side effects.

  Propiverine is a smooth muscle relaxant which has anticholinergic and calcium channel blocking actions. It has relative selectivity for bladder and ileum. It is associated with an improvement in frequency and can be used for this in women with OAB, but is not recommended for the treatment of UI.

  Darifenacin is a highly selective antimuscarinic drug which has five times more affinity for bladder (M3) than salivary gland (M1) receptors. It has been shown to be effective and tolerated in placebo-controlled randomized controlled trials (RCTs).

  Solifenacin is a recently introduced drug that has been shown to be as effective as other antimuscarinics. RCTs comparing solifenacin with placebo or tolterodine 2 mg BD or 4 mg slow release have shown that solifenacin is not inferior to tolterodine and has comparable tolerability.

  NICE assessment of antimuscarinic drugs concluded that treatment with oxybutynin, tolterodine, trospium, darifenacin, and solifenacin improves frequency, incontinence, and quality of life in women with OAB. There is no evidence of a clinically important difference in efficacy. Based on cost analysis, NICE recommends non-proprietary oral immediate release oxybutynin (**A**). Women should be counselled about the adverse effects, especially dry mouth. Propiverine should be considered for the treatment of frequency in OAB, but is not recommended for UI (**A**)

- **Desmopressin** or DDAVP (1-desamino-8-D-arginine vasopressin) is a synthetic analogue of vasopressin which inhibits diuresis but avoids vasopressive effects. Used at night, especially in patients with nocturnal polyuria, it reduces nocturnal urine production by up to 50%. It can be used to treat nocturia and nocturnal enuresis

- **Oestrogens** have been used for many years in the management of UI, although their precise role remains unclear. They are important in helping to maintain healthy lower urinary tract tissues and normal urinary function. There is some RCT evidence that intravaginal oestrogens may improve symptoms of OAB in women with vaginal atrophy. There is no evidence to support their use in SUI. Systemic oestrogens confer no benefit to women with UI, and their use is not recommended for this indication (**A**)

- **Tricyclic antidepressants**—at therapeutic doses, tricyclic antidepressants can cause orthostatic hypotension, ventricular arrhythmias, hepatic dysfunction, tremor, and fatigue. Imipramine and other tricyclic antidepressants have been used to treat UI. There are no placebo-controlled RCTs evaluating this and no evidence to support their use in UI

Pharmacological management of stress urinary incontinence

Duloxetine is a serotonin and noradrenaline reuptake inhibitor introduced for the management of moderate to severe SUI. It is the only medication currently used for this indication. It acts in the sacral spinal cord where it is thought to increase pudendal nerve activity, thus increasing urethral sphincter closure.

Nausea is the most significant side effect (13–46%), accounting for a high proportion of withdrawals. Others include vomiting, constipation, dry mouth, insomnia, somnolence, and dizziness. The incidence of side effects can be reduced by escalating the dose from 20 mg BD for 2 weeks to 40 mg BD thereafter.

Short-term placebo-controlled studies have shown that duloxetine is associated with reductions in incontinence episodes and improvement in quality of life in women with SUI and MUI, but clinical differences are small. The combination of duloxetine with PFMT is better than no treatment or placebo. It remains unclear whether the combination is better than either treatment alone.

NICE does not recommend duloxetine either as a first line treatment for SUI or as a routine second line treatment unless the woman prefers to avoid, or is unsuitable for, surgery (**A**).

Physical interventions

These include intravaginal and intraurethral devices, bladder catheterization, absorbent products, and toileting aids.

A number of urethral and vaginal devices have been developed and marketed for the management of UI, especially SUI. The urethral devices occlude the urethra externally (at the external meatus) or are intraurethral. They require high patient motivation and manual dexterity. Their disadvantages include the possibility of migration, infection, and the woman's adherence to treatment. Vaginal devices aim to support the bladder neck during activities likely to cause SUI, e.g. sports. They include pessaries and bladder neck support prostheses. They can cause irritation or vaginal erosion.

Bladder catheterization, intermittent or indwelling (urethral or suprapubic), can be considered for women with intractable incontinence who are not fit for other treatments. It is not helpful in women with UUI as bypassing is likely.

Physical interventions should not be considered active treatment but rather part of a containment strategy, since there is no evidence that they improve UI.

14.11 Surgical management of stress urinary incontinence

Surgical procedures for stress urinary incontinence

Over 100 surgical procedures to treat stress urinary incontinence (SUI) have been described. Only those currently used in clinical practice are discussed.

Surgical interventions can be divided into those that might augment urethral closure (e.g. intramural urethral bulking agents and artificial urinary sphincters) and those that support the bladder neck and urethra (e.g. colposuspension, biological or synthetic sling procedures, anterior vaginal and paravaginal repairs, and needle suspension procedures).

Anterior colporrhaphy and paravaginal repairs have been described as anti-incontinence procedures for decades. Long-term results are disappointing. They are no longer a primary procedure for SUI but still have a role in pelvic organ prolapse (POP; see Section 14.4).

Needle suspension procedures (such as Pereyra, Raz, and Stamey) were popular and involve suspending paraurethral tissue, usually to the rectus sheath. They have low success rates and have been largely superseded by other techniques.

Burch colposuspension

This was developed in the 1960s as a modification of the Marshall–Marchetti–Krantz (MMK) procedure. It was the gold standard surgical treatment for SUI, but has been superseded by mid-urethral sling operations (e.g. the tension free vaginal tape, TVT). However, it remains the procedure against which other techniques are compared.

Open colposuspension is performed through a Pfannenstiel incision. The retropubic space is accessed by blunt dissection. The surgeon's non-dominant hand is placed in the vagina to identify the bladder neck and elevate the anterior vagina while the other hand, in the retropubic space, is used to sweep the periurethral fatty tissue and expose the paravaginal fascia. Two non-absorbable sutures are then placed through the full thickness of the paravaginal fascia on each side at the level of the bladder neck. Each suture is attached to the iliopectineal ligament about 3 or 4 cm from the midline of the pubic bone.

There are no significant clinical differences between open and laparoscopic colposuspension, but the laparoscopic approach consumes more time, the learning curve is longer and long-term data are lacking. NICE does not recommend the routine use of laparoscopic colposuspension in the treatment of SUI.

The success rate of open colposuspension is between 85 and 90% at 1 year, which falls to 70% at 5 years and thereafter.

Complications include:
- Voiding difficulties (median 6%)
- *De novo* detrusor overactivity (DO) (22%)
- POP, mainly posterior vaginal wall (up to 30%)
- Dyspareunia (3%)
- Recurrent UTI (5%)

The MMK procedure is no longer routinely used owing to the additional complication of osteitis pubis, and the fact that it does not offer significant advantages over Burch colposuspension.

Mid-urethral tapes

Tension-free vaginal tape

This involves placing a macroporous type I suburethral sling (Prolene) through a small vertical anterior vaginal wall incision at the level of the mid-urethra. The tape is passed to either side of the mid-urethra using specially designed needles, which are passed through the retropubic space and exteriorized through two small suprapubic incisions about 3–4 cm on each side of the midline ('bottom-up' approach). With the needles still in the retropubic space (see Figure 14.14), cystoscopy is performed. If bladder perforation has occurred (see Figure 14.16), the needle is withdrawn and reinserted; if not, the needles are pulled up through the suprapubic incisions, and the plastic sheath covering the tape is removed while ensuring the tape is under no tension (hence its name); see Figure 14.15. A cough test can be performed to adjust tension but there is no evidence this prevents voiding difficulty. Vaginal and suprapubic incisions are then closed with absorbable sutures.

The originators of the tension-free vaginal tape (TVT) claim it is an ambulatory procedure. In clinical practice it is done under local, regional or general anaesthetic, but the optimum anaesthetic has not been determined.

Randomized controlled trials (RCTs) comparing TVT to open colposuspension have shown similar effectiveness, with cure rates between 85 and 90% at 1 year, with similar longevity for both procedures at 3 years. Seven-year follow-up studies of TVT have shown 80% efficacy with 1% erosion rate. Bladder perforation is more common with TVT, but more women undergoing colposuspension require further surgery for POP. TVT has the added benefits of being a minimal access technique, using local or regional anaesthetic, and requiring a shorter hospital stay.

Complications of TVT include:
- Bladder perforation (median 4%)
- Urethral perforation (0.5%)
- Haematoma (1.5%)
- Nerve injury (0.7%)
- Voiding problems (11%)
- Need for long-term intermittant self-catheterization (ISC) (1.8%)
- *De novo* DO (6%)
- UTI (7%)
- Tape erosion (1.1%)
- Need for trimming or removal of the tape (1.2%)

Transobturator tape

The transobturator tape (TOT) is a relatively new technique, which involves placing a suburethral sling in a similar fashion to a TVT, but the tape is brought out through the obturator foramen instead of suprapubically. The tape can be inserted from the suburethral incision towards the obturator foramen (inside out technique) or vice versa (outside in). Since the retropubic space is not entered, it is claimed to reduce the risk of bladder, bowel and vascular injury, and eliminates the need for routine cystoscopy.

Comparative studies of TOT and TVT with mean follow-up ranging from 7 weeks to 17 months have shown similar effectiveness. However, long-term outcome data for TOT are lacking.

Bladder perforation is significantly lower with TOT (mean 0.5% versus 4% for TVT), but urethral damage is significantly higher (mean 1% versus 0.5% for TVT). Other complications of TOT include voiding dysfunction (2%); *de novo* urgency (4%); vaginal erosion (2.5%); and vaginal perforation (0.7%). There are also anecdotal reports of groin pain after TOT.

Other sling procedures

Traditional pubovaginal suburethral sling procedures are recommended alternatives for the treatment of SUI. They involve a small horizontal incision 2 cm above the symphysis pubis and a small vaginal suburethral incision. The vaginal wall is dissected off the bladder and urethra; the rectus sheath is dissected and visualized abdominally. A curved instrument (Kelly clamp or Stamey needle) is then passed through the retropubic space from the abdominal incision ('top-down' technique), emerging through the vaginal incision. Cystoscopy is performed to exclude bladder injury. Then each end of the sling is pulled up through the retropubic space using the previously passed instruments. The two ends of the sling can be sewn to the rectus sheath or together in the midline, ensuring minimal tension of the sling.

Materials used can be autologous (rectus sheath, fascia lata, vaginal wall), allografts (cadaveric fascia lata or dura mater), xenografts (porcine dermis or small bowel mucosa), or synthetic. Autologous fascial slings are the most established biological option with longer data on efficacy and safety. There are no significant differences between short and full length slings.

The commonest reported complications with pubovaginal slings are voiding dysfunction, urgency, and urge urinary incontinence (UUI). Other complications include vaginal erosion, pain, infection, and haematoma.

Intramural urethral bulking agents

Periurethral or transurethral injection of bulking material into the urethral submucosa at the bladder neck is thought to improve SUI by increasing the resting tone and pressure of the sphincter, and possibly improving its support. The injection may be given transurethrally using an operative cystoscope or blindly using a non-endoscopic implantation device. Alternatively, a periurethral injection may be given passing a needle through the skin parallel to the urethra while simultaneously visualizing the bladder neck by cystoscopy. The injections are usually given under local anaesthesia.

A variety of biological and synthetic injectables are available, including collagen, autologous fat, porcine dermis, silicone, hyaluronic acid/dextran copolymer, polytetrafluoroethylene and carbon-coated zirconium beads. There is no evidence of one injectable being better than others (other than autologous fat—no better than placebo and less effective than collagen). Controlled trials on bulking agents are few, but the evidence suggests that injectables are less effective than open surgery for SUI. Their benefits reduce with time, making repeat injections necessary. However, they have fewer postoperative complications such as transient adverse events of infection, dysuria, haematuria, and UTI and de novo DO and UUI.

Their main use is in the elderly or unfit.

Artificial urinary sphincters

Artificial urinary sphincters (AUS) are complex devices comprising an occlusive periurethral cuff that remains inflated to exert constant urethral pressure. It is deflated by the woman using a small pump located in the labia when she wishes to void. They are generally used when other continence surgical procedures have failed.

Most studies evaluating AUS include different populations (men and patients with neurogenic bladder), and therefore data on women with idiopathic SUI are scanty. They seem to be highly effective, with success rates around 90%. They are expensive, and complications and associated morbidity are common, including injury to the vagina, bladder and urethra, infection, erosion, device malfunction, and surgical device revision or removal.

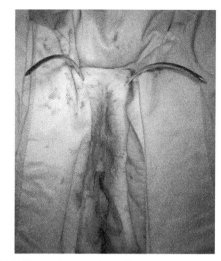

Fig. 14.14 Tension-free vaginal tape. The needles are still in the retropubic space.

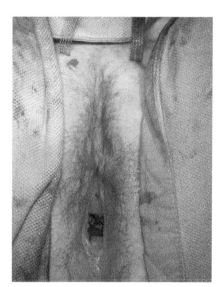

Fig. 14.15 Tension-free vaginal tape. The needles have been pulled up, the plastic sheath removed, and the tape is sitting tension-free under the mid-urethra.

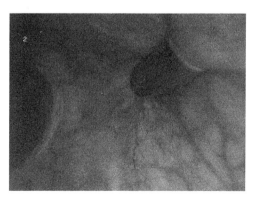

Fig. 14.16 Bladder perforation. The TVT needle has been inserted through the bladder.

Women with urge urinary incontinence (UUI) and detrusor overactivity (DO) who have not improved with conservative and pharmacological treatment can be considered for surgery.

Only a small proportion of studies in the literature concerning surgery for UI are randomized controlled trials (RCTs), making comparison of different interventions difficult. Most data come from case series with their inherent limitations. Furthermore, there is wide variation in the outcome measures used, even for the same intervention in different studies. All these caveats apply to surgery for both UUI and stress urinary incontinence (SUI).

Surgical procedures for DO aim to increase bladder capacity, modify the innervation and contractility of the detrusor muscle, or bypass the lower urinary tract. Women undergoing these procedures should be willing and able to self-catheterize, since voiding difficulty is common after surgery.

- **Sacral nerve root stimulation** relies on inhibition of the sacral bladder reflex by chronic electrical stimulation of the S3 roots. Women initially undergo a 'test' of percutaneous nerve stimulation using a needle inserted through the sacral foramina. Responders may proceed to a permanent implant.

  Cure or improvement rates vary between 39 and 77%, median 63%. The efficacy is sustained for 3–5 years.

  Side effects include pain at the site of implantation, infection, and device failure.

  Reoperation rate can be as high as 30%, and about 7% of patients may need permanent removal of the device

- **Botulinum toxin** blocks the release of acetylcholine and, when injected into the bladder wall using a flexible cystoscope, can relax the overactive detrusor muscle. There are two strains available for clinical use, A and B.

  Botulinum toxin B is only effective for up to 6 weeks and is not recommended for women with idiopathic overactive bladder syndrome (OAB).

  Botulinum toxin A is used in doses of 100–300 units injected in 10–40 sites in the detrusor muscle. Efficacy varies between 50 and 75%, with duration of benefit of 3–12 months. Its benefit in neurogenic DO has been established but not in 'idiopathic' DO.

  Adverse effects include urinary retention, dysuria, UTI, haematuria, and the need for repeat injections. Data on the use of botulinum toxin A are limited and long-term evaluation is lacking

- **Augmentation cystoplasty**, also known as clam cystoplasty or enterocystoplasty, aims to increase bladder capacity and reduce the effect of detrusor contractions. The bladder wall is bisected almost completely and a segment of bowel, usually ileum but sometimes also sigmoid or ileocaecum, is sewn in place to act as a reservoir. This prevents incontinence as urine enters the reservoir rather than the urethra.

  Case series have shown improvement in between 50–90% of patients.

  However, common side effects that patients must be counselled about include electrolyte disturbances, mucus retention, recurrent UTI, urinary retention, and the need for self-catheterization.

  Malignant transformation of the bowel segment has been reported. Lifelong follow-up, including cystoscopy, is recommended

- **Detrusor myectomy** involves excision of the whole thickness of the detrusor muscle at the fundus, while leaving the mucosa intact, and is an alternative to clam cystoplasty. The defect is usually covered with a segment of mobilized omentum. This procedure increases functional bladder capacity by creating a diverticulum with no intrinsic contractility. In theory, detrusor myectomy avoids the complications of bowel interposition.

  Case series involving patients with both neurogenic bladder dysfunction and idiopathic DO give conflicting results. The role in the management of UUI/OAB remains unclear

- **Urinary diversion** is used as a last resort in women who have not responded or are not suitable for other surgical procedures. It involves diverting the ureters to a segment of ileum with creation of a permanent abdominal stoma (ileal conduit), which can be incontinent or continent (catheterizable stoma).

  This has been mainly used in children and patients with neurogenic bladder dysfunction.

  Data on the outcomes of urinary diversion in women with UUI/OAB are scanty

Further reading

www.nice.org.uk/guidance NICE guideline on urinary incontinence, October 2006.

Chapter 15

Malignancy

Contents

Covered elsewhere

- Benign ovarian cysts (see Section 13.3 and Section 13.4)

15.1 Background

Incidence and trends in cancer

The incidence of gynaecological malignancies is increasing in the UK. This is thought to be caused by increasing obesity, as well as an ageing population. Both endometrial and ovarian carcinomas are in the top 10 cancers which affect women.

Risk factors

With any cancer it is worth considering:

- Which women are particularly at risk of cancer?
- Why are they at risk?

There may be:

- Inherited predispositions
- Environmental factors
- Sexually transmitted agents
- Hormonal milieu (which could be related to reproduction or obesity)
- Lifestyle issues such as declining to be screened

Diagnostic challenges

Some tumours are relatively rare (e.g. ovarian cancer). On average, a GP can expect to see one case every 4 years. The diagnosis presents such a challenge to GPs because the onset is often insidious, with vague symptoms of abdominal pain, change in bowel habit, and bloating. These women are often referred to gastroenterologists, or GI surgeons with suspected bowel pathologies.

This can be contrasted, for example, with endometrial cancer, which presents early and obviously (i.e. postmenopausal bleeding).

Screening principles

For a screening programme to be effective, the disease must have the following characteristics:

- Be serious
- Have a precancerous, or early, stage in which treatment is beneficial
- Have a high prevalence in population
- Have a known natural history

The screening programme must be:

- Inexpensive
- Easy to administer
- Acceptable to patients
- Valid, reliable, and reproducible

Cervical cancer fits this model well. It is the second most common cancer in women under 35 years. It is life-threatening if not treated, and, if detected at an early or premalignant stage is curable. Cervical cancer has a premalignant stage—cervical intraepithelial neoplasia (CIN). The natural history is that if this is untreated a proportion of women will progress to cervical cancer over a period of years. The cervical screening programme has been very successful, saving 4500 lives in England per year.

Ovarian cancer, however, is not so amenable to screening. It has no recognized premalignant phase; benign ovarian cysts do not develop into ovarian cancers if untreated. The natural history is known, but the majority of women present with symptoms once the cancer has spread. It is serious, but the majority of women present with advanced disease, which carries a poorer prognosis.

Future improvements

Improvements in care and outcomes may come from:

- HPV vaccine
- Genetic testing
- Improved screening
- Gradual improvements from randomized controlled trials (RCTs)

- Organization of care
- Raised standards

Quality of care

The simple, traditional gynaecology skills of diagnosis and surgery are inadequate alone in the modern-day treatment of gynaecological cancer.

A complex multidisciplinary team (MDT) and a number of organizational issues and non-core skills aid the delivery of high-quality care to cancer patients.

Organizational issues

The Calman–Hine report and Improving Outcomes Guidelines (1999) were government recommendations for the treatment of gynaecological cancers that led to important organizational changes in the delivery of care.

The key recommendations were:

- Dedicated diagnostic and assessment services in cancer units to which all women with possible or suspected gynaecological cancers are referred, including those with symptoms and through the cervical screening programme
- Specialist multiprofessional gynaecological oncology teams based in cancer centres responsible for the management of all women with ovarian cancer and the majority of women with other gynaecological cancers
- Clear local policies for the management of advanced or progressive disease designed to ensure the coordination of high-quality care between cancer centres, units, palliative care, primary care, and community services
- Rapid and efficient communication systems for liaison and cross-referral between all levels of service. Audit should take place across the entire service delivery network

There should be one gynaecological cancer centre per 1.5 million population. The other hospitals in the region, or network, are designated as cancer units. Women with the following cancers should be referred to a specialist gynaecological cancer centre:

- All stages of ovarian cancer
- All stages of vulval and vaginal cancers
- Endometrial cancer stage Ic or grade 3 and above
- Cervical cancer stage Ib and above

Early endometrial and cervical cancers may be treated at individual units.

Resources are concentrated at the cancer centre so that a specialized MDT can be created. It meets weekly at a formal MDT meeting and in clinical settings. The MDT is the focus of the treatment decisions for a woman so that all her complex needs can be assessed. The team includes surgeons, radiotherapists, chemotherapists, pathologists, and radiologists, along with clinical nurse specialists and palliative care specialists.

Palliative care

Palliative care is commenced when the patient cannot be cured. The aim is the alleviation of symptoms and is organized as close to home as possible.

Each cancer unit should have a palliative care team. This is usually based in the community, with a palliative care doctor and clinical nurse specialist in the hospital. Palliative care is organized at home with the GP, district nurse, and Macmillan nurse. A hospice should be available when needed and is organized by the Macmillan team.

Different patients use the services to different extents, and provision in different parts of the UK can be patchy. Palliation does not mean that nothing can be done—indeed, it is the beginning of an important, and highly meaningful, phase.

There are many taboos about dying. Euthanasia (deliberate killing) is not legal in the UK, although it is available in some European countries for terminal illness.

Many patients understand that they have to die at some stage, but they fear pain and loss of dignity. Reassure the patient that symptoms such as pain can be dealt with and that her dignity will be kept uppermost at all times.

Breaking bad news
- Make a special meeting and invite the relatives if the woman wishes to have them present
- Take a nurse with you, preferably the clinical nurse specialist or the palliative care nurse
- Start at the beginning
- Reiterate how you got to this point
- Get to the stage where you say, 'So we sent off the biopsy to the lab. This has come back showing a cancer of the [uterus/ovary/cervix]'
- Consider saying 'I understand this is a shock'
- Be honest, but kind
- Tell the truth, but pause to show empathy and check on the reaction
- Empathy means that you understand the pain of the situation that the patient is in
- Sympathy, indicating that you are sorry, is not so helpful
- Have a plan—either for treatment or palliation
- If you are honest, kind, show empathy, and are able to make a patient understand what is going to happen, she will thank you for delivering the news
- Uncertainty can bring more fear than the truth
- Remember that most patients fear they have cancer already—it is rarely a complete shock
- Do not try to do everything at once
- Sometimes it is better to have a series of shorter, specific communications at a pace set by the patient, than overwhelming her with information all at once
- Being the bearer of bad news is upsetting for staff
- Allow yourself some space to reflect on your feelings
- Ask witnesses (e.g. the nurse, students, your trainers, and even patients if appropriate occasions arise) what you do well and what you could do better
- Get feedback so that you can improve over time
- Take advice!

Useful tips on communication
See also Section 1.1.
- Remember what you were taught
- The techniques may seem irrelevant or impractical but they work
- Listening is more important than talking
- Use lay language not jargon
- Do not lecture. You are not trying to impress
- You are trying to make her understand
- Keep it simple
- Keep eye contact appropriately
- Look at the patient but do not stare her down
- Open with 'What do you think is going on?' or 'What are your worries?'
- Use pauses, allow or invite the patient to respond
- Follow verbal clues: if she says 'no', stop and take heed
- Follow non-verbal clues: if she is shaking her head and screwing her eyes up, she probably does not understand or does not agree
- Patients only remember about 10% of what is said
- Do not abandon the patient
- Make sure the forward plan is understood
- Ask her
- Offer further support or to return

Further reading
www.dh.gov.uk/ 4009609 Publications policy and guidance for NHS plan, 063067 Publications policy and guidance cancer waiting targets, and 4083846 Improving outcomes in gynaecological cancer.

http://www.nice.org.uk/ CG27 Referral for suspected cancer.

http://www.statistics.gov.uk/ Theme health 5099 for cancer trends in England & Wales.

15.2 Cervical screening and cervical intraepithelial neoplasia

NHS cervical screening programme

This began in 1988 and offers a cervical smear test to all eligible women by computerized invitation. Previously, screening was opportunistic. Since 1988, the incidence of cervical cancer in the UK has fallen by 7% every year (from 16 to 9/100 000 between 1985 and 2003, a total reduction of 42%).

- Screening is 3-yearly from 25–50 years and 5-yearly from 50–65 years of age
- Of eligible women, 84% have been screened

Annually;

- Smears performed–3 000 000
- Smear abnormalities detected–200 000
- Referred for colposcopy–40 000
- The programme costs £157 million
- The mortality rate is falling by about 7%
- Cases of cancer prevented–3900
- Lives saved in England–4500

Liquid-based cytology

Modern smear technology uses a plastic 'broom' swept over the transformation zone, aiming to remove a thin layer of cells. This is placed in liquid transport medium to be examined microscopically for any cells with dyskaryotic features.

This is preferred to conventional smear because:

- Clearer slides are provided
- Reduced inadequate smears (from 9% to 1–2%)
- It is more sensitive
- Quicker reporting time (reducing anxiety)
- HPV and chlamydia can be tested for simultaneously

Dyskaryosis is a cytopathological diagnosis. Assessment of dyskaryosis is based on nuclear enlargement, variation in size and shape of the nuclei, hyperchromasia, and reduction in the amount of cytoplasm altering the nuclear:cytoplasmic ratio. The nucleus enlarges and the amount of cytoplasm decreases as the severity of the dyskaryosis increases. In severe dyskaryosis, nuclear pleomorphism and occasional mitoses are also present.

Cervical intraepithelial neoplasia

Aetiology

HPV, especially oncogenic subtypes 16, 18, 31, 33, 35, 39, 45, 51, 52, 56, and 58.

Associated factors

- Smoking (affects local cervical immunity)
- HIV or immunosuppression
- Sexual activity

Facts about HPV

- All sexually active women are exposed to HPV
- Eighty per cent of women will clear the virus in 1–2 years
- Only a small percentage are unable to clear the virus
- Persistent, high levels of oncogenic HPV lead to cervical intraepithelial neoplasia (CIN)

Pathophysiology

At puberty, rising oestrogen levels cause the cervix to evert. The columnar tissue lining the cervical canal is everted onto the surface of the cervix. This area of columnar tissue in the centre of the cervix is known as an ectopy or ectropion (see Figure 13.35). Squamous metaplasia is a normal physiological process, caused by the acid conditions in the vagina, which causes columnar cells to transform into squamous cells. The area where this occurs is called the transformation zone. Squamous metaplasia is an ongoing process, occurring over many years. If oncogenic HPV affects the transformation zone, CIN may form instead of normal squamous tissue.

CIN is a *histological* diagnosis only made on biopsy.

CIN (dysplasia) is characterized by lack of differentiation and disordered cellular maturation involving the squamous epithelium but not the basement membrane. It is graded 1–3.

- Lower one-third of epithelium = CIN-1
- Lower two-thirds of epithelium = CIN-2
- Full thickness of epithelium   = CIN-3

Nuclear:cytoplasmic abnormalities increase from CIN-1 to -3.

CIN-3 shows almost no differentiation, with large, hyperchromatic nuclei, and increased mitotic figures.

Natural history

CIN is precancerous. Lesions may develop directly to CIN-3 rather than progressing stepwise.

- Between 60 and 90% of CIN-1 revert to normal within 10–23 months
- Thirty per cent of CIN-3 progress to cancer, typically over 10 years

Clinical evaluation

History

- Asymptomatic

Examination

- Very little to see on routine speculum examination

Colposcopy

Colposcopy entails examination of the cervix with bright light and magnification to identify any abnormal areas (see Figure 15.1).

- The whole transformation zone should be visualized
- Acetic acid (5%) is applied to the cervix
- CIN contains immature cells which contain higher levels of protein, and so appear white with acetic acid
- Other typical appearances include abnormal capillary patterns, such as punctation and mosaicism
- Iodine (Schiller's test) can confirm an abnormality as it is less well taken up by immature cells owing to lower intracellular glycogen
- Biopsies of abnormal areas should be taken

Management

CIN-1

- May be observed as many will regress spontaneously
- If the abnormal area is large, or the patient is anxious, treatment may be performed
- Destructive techniques may be used: cryotherapy or laser or cold coagulation

CIN-2 or -3

- Should treat with excision to a depth of 8 mm
- In the UK, 85% of treatments are by LLETZ (large loop excision of the transformation zone)
- Mostly performed in clinic under local anaesthesia

A single treatment is not thought to affect fertility. However, as more cervical tissue is removed, e.g. with repeat treatments, an increased risk of preterm deliveries (<37 weeks' gestation) occurs owing to a weakened cervix. Cervical stenosis may occur secondary to scar tissue formation.

Follow-up (NHSCSP guidelines)

- CIN-1—smear at 6 months, repeat at 6 months and 1 year. If normal, back to routine recall interval of 3 years
- CIN-2 or -3—smear at 6 months, repeat at 6 months. If normal, annual smears for 10 years

Survival and prognosis

- Of women having treatment for CIN, 95% have no further smear abnormalities
- Five per cent of women will have further abnormal smears and may require further LLETZ or a cone biopsy
- CIN is a premalignant condition and survival is 100%
- Women with a history of CIN have an increased incidence of cervical cancer compared to women whose smears have all been normal

Cervical glandular intraepithelial neoplasia

Cervical glandular intraepithelial neoplasia (CGIN) is:

- Rare—0.15% smears
- Tends to arise within the cervical canal

Smears detect glandular lesions less well than squamous lesions. This is caused by the position of the abnormality on the cervix and the appearance of the abnormal cells which are difficult to detect on the smear slide.

- Difficult to assess colposcopically
- Rarely visible with acetic acid
- Skip lesions occur
- Abnormal areas may exist further up the cervical canal

Treatment

- Knife cone biopsy (i.e. surgical excision under GA) to 25 mm depth to avoid missing skip lesions
- Hysterectomy should be considered if fertility is no longer required or the margins are not clear, owing to the inaccuracy of follow-up by either smears or colposcopy

HPV vaccines pros and cons

Since CIN is caused by HPV, vaccination against HPV should offer a degree of protection from CIN and cervical cancer.

A prophylactic vaccine against HPV 6, 11, 16, and 18 has been developed. Phase 2 clinical trials have demonstrated 100% vaccine efficacy in preventing HPV 6, 11, 16, or 18 related CIN grades 2 or 3, and adenocarcinoma *in situ* (AIS) in subjects naïve to the relevant HPV type (95% CI 55–100%).

- Licensed for 9–25-year-olds
- Should prevent 90% of warts and 60–70% of CIN
- Highly effective in preventing HPV-type related genital warts, vulval intraepithelial neoplasia (VIN)-1–3 and vaginal intraepithelial neoplasia (VAIN)-1–3
- Phase 3 trials are under way
- Long-term effects and duration of immunity are unknown
- Currently too expensive for use in developing countries
- UK immunization programme started in Autumn 2008 for all 12- and 13-year-old girls but with bivalent vaccine against HPV 16 and 18 only

- Recommended for USA school girls before the onset of sexual activity
- Controversial for some parents
- Does not replace the need for cervical screening

Smear results and actions

The possible results of a smear are shown in Table 15.1.

- Mild dyskaryosis suggests underlying CIN-1
- Moderate dyskaryosis suggests underlying CIN-2
- Severe dyskaryosis suggests underlying CIN-3

Table 15.1 Smear results and actions

Smear result	Action
Normal (90%)	Routine screening unless another reason
Borderline (4%)	Repeat in 6 months Three borderline smears ⇒ refer for colposcopy
Mild dyskaryosis (2%)	Refer for colposcopy
Moderate dyskaryosis (1%)	Refer for colposcopy
Severe dyskaryosis (0.7%)	Refer for colposcopy
?Invasive changes (0.02%)	Urgent colposcopy referral
Glandular abnormality (0.15%)	Urgent colposcopy referral
Inadequate (1–3% with liquid-based cytology)	Repeat in 6 months Three inadequate or inflammatory smears ⇒ refer for colposcopy

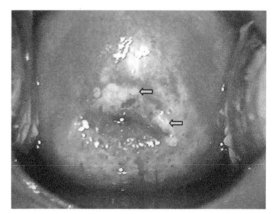

Fig. 15.1 Colposcopic view of CIN-3. The area of white on the anterior lip is an example of high-density aceto white as a result of staining of immature cells with acetic acid (⇐).

Further reading

www.bsccp.org.uk

www.rcog.org.uk

www.cancerscreening.nhs.uk/cervical/publications for NHSCSP guidelines

15.3 Cervical carcinoma

Incidence

- There were 2700 cases of cervical cancer in England and Wales in 2004
- This comprises 2.5% of all cancer cases in women
- Third commonest gynaecological malignancy in the UK
- Peak incidence for invasive carcinoma is 45–50 years
- Highest number of deaths occur in the 75–79-year age group

Aetiology

In 99.7% of cases, HPV (human papillomavirus) causes the precancerous changes that develop into cancer.

Oncogenic subtypes of HPV are 16, 18, 31, 33, 35, 39, 45, 51, 52, 56, and 58.

Non-oncogenic subtypes, e.g. 6 and 11, cause low-grade cervical lesions and genital warts.

Additional factors:

- Smoking
- HIV infection
- COCP

Pathophysiology

- Squamous cell carcinomas—70–80%
- Adenocarcinomas—20%
- Rare forms include malignant melanomas, sarcomas, lymphomas, and small cell carcinomas

Squamous cell carcinomas and adenocarcinomas develop from precancerous lesions, cervical intraepithelial neoplasia (CIN), and cervical intraepithelial glandular neoplasia (CGIN), respectively.

CIN develops in the transformation zone (see Section 15.2), usually on the ectocervix.

CGIN develops from columnar epithelium, and is found in the cervical canal or endocervix.

Spread

- Direct or local: down to vagina, anteriorly to bladder, laterally to parametrium, and posteriorly to bowel
- Lymphatic spread: via the parametrial nodes to internal, external and common iliac nodes and the obturator nodes. Presacral and para-aortic lymph nodes may be involved at a later stage
- Bloodborne spread occurs late to the lungs and liver

Staging

If radiation is used as a primary treatment, surgical pathological staging is not possible as lymph node status remains unknown. Thus lymph node spread is not included in the FIGO staging for cervical cancer (Box 15.1).

Clinical evaluation

History

- Postcoital bleeding
- Intermenstrual bleeding
- Postmenopausal bleeding
- Persistent, offensive, bloodstained discharge
- Pain (late disease)—lateral direct spread may obstruct the ureter, causing loin pain due to hydronephrosis. It may affect the sciatic nerve, causing pain in the buttock and back of the leg.
- Thrombosis in the pelvic veins may cause a swollen leg

Examination

- Speculum examination obligatory. Squamous carcinomas present as exophytic, friable lesions (see Figure 15.2)
- Hard, barrel-shaped cervix (more common with adenocarcinomas)
- Cervix may be fixed in advanced disease
- PR—hard, irregular mass palpable anteriorly

Investigations

- Colposcopy to examine cervix
- Cervical biopsy
- FBC (pretreatment assessment)
- U&Es (to assess likely ureteric involvement)
- LFTs
- MRI pelvis, although not part of FIGO staging, is used to assess tumour volume, size, local invasion, and pelvic lymph node spread to help plan treatment (Figure 15.3)
- CT of abdomen and chest (or CXR), in addition to pelvic MRI, is designed to look for metastatic disease

Staging

Staging is clinical and requires an examination under anaesthetic with cystoscopy and sigmoidoscopy.

🎯 Box 15.1 FIGO staging and 5-year survival of patients with cervical carcinoma

Stage	Definition	Pelvic lymph node involvement (%)	5-year survival (%)
I	**Carcinoma strictly confined to cervix**		
Ia	Microscopic invasive carcinoma		
Ia1	Stromal invasion ≤3 mm diameter ≤7 mm	0.6	98–99
Ia2	Stromal invasion > 3mm and ≤5 mm diameter ≤7 mm	4.8	95–98
Ib	Lesion >7 mm wide or >5 mm deep or visible	15.9	
Ib1	Clinical lesion ≤4 cm		60–95
Ib2	Clinical lesion >4 cm		60–80
II	**Carcinoma that extends beyond the cervix, but not to pelvic side wall or lower third of vagina**		60–80
IIa	No obvious parametrial involvement, involvement of up to upper two-thirds of vagina	24.5	
IIb	Obvious parametrial involvement, but not extending to pelvic side wall	31.4	
III	**Carcinoma has extended to pelvic side wall or lower third of vagina. All cases with hydronephrosis /non-functioning kidney**	44.8	40
IIIa	No extension onto pelvic side wall, but involvement of lower one-third of vagina		
IIIb	Extension onto pelvic side wall and/or hydronephrosis or non-functioning kidney		
IV	**Carcinoma has extended beyond the true pelvis, or involvement of bladder and/or rectal mucosa**		15–20
IVa	Spread to adjacent pelvic organs	55	
IVb	Distant metastasis		

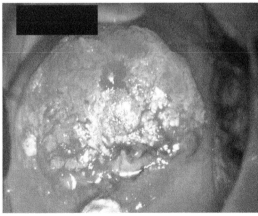

Fig. 15.2 Exophytic cervical carcinoma.

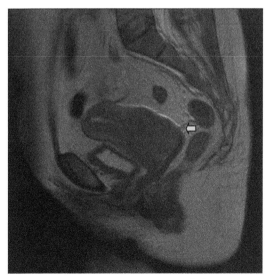

Fig. 15.3 2 MRI demonstrating cervical tumour (⟸)

Management

Women should be referred to regional cancer centres and treatment discussed at multidisciplinary meetings. Treatment is the same for squamous and adenocarcinomas, though it depends on stage, desire for future fertility, age, and concurrent medical conditions.

Stage Ia1—cone biopsy

- Lymphatic spread occurs in 0.6%
- Where excision margins are clear, no further treatment is necessary
- If excision margins are not clear, either a further cone biopsy should be performed or, if fertility is not an issue, a simple hysterectomy is recommended—particularly for adenocarcinoma, as follow-up may be difficult

Stage Ia2—modified radical or simple hysterectomy + pelvic node dissection

Lymphatic spread occurs in 4.8%, thus pelvic node removal is mandatory.

However, in a tumour <10 mm, spread to the parametrium occurs in 0.6% so simple hysterectomy is feasible.

Women desiring future fertility—repeat cone biopsy with laparoscopic pelvic node dissection is sufficient treatment.

Stage Ib1—radical (Wertheim's) hysterectomy and pelvic lymphadenectomy, or chemoradiation

- Cure rates are equal for both surgery and chemoradiation
- The side effects of radiation include vaginal stenosis and ovarian inactivation
- Hence, surgery is favoured in younger women where the ovaries can be conserved
- Although the vagina is shortened, sexual intercourse is relatively normal
- The disadvantage of surgery is that it does not fully treat the pelvic lymph nodes
- If metastatic disease is found on final histopathology, postoperative radiotherapy is indicated
- Using both surgery and radiation multiplies x 5 the chance of side effects such as leg lymphoedema, chronic bladder frequency or diarrhoea

Small stage Ib1 in women requiring fertility—radical trachelectomy (Figure 15.4) + laparoscopic pelvic node dissection

Low risk tumours <2 cm (i.e. not grade 3 and negative lymphovascular space invasion) may be treated with this fertility-preserving operation. Radical trachelectomy is a vaginal procedure to remove the cervix, parametrium, and a cuff of vagina. A permanent nylon suture is placed at the base of the uterus to replace the cervical function. Future birth is via a CS.

Stages Ib2–IVa—chemoradiation

Radiotherapy has an advantage over surgery in that it treats the central tumour and any metastases to the pelvic lymph nodes. The treatment consists of:

- Radical external beam radiotherapy for 30 min/day Monday to Friday for 5 weeks
- Weekly cisplatin chemotherapy is added as it increases the effectiveness of pelvic radiation by 30%

- Two internal radiation treatments (brachytherapy) are applied to the cervix under a 30-min general anaesthetic at the end of the external treatment. The internal treatments provide an intense boost of radiation to the cervix that represents 30% of the total radiation dose to the tumour itself. This final part of the treatment makes it as effective as surgery to remove the central tumour

Stage IVb

Treatment is palliative, aiming to control symptoms. Radiotherapy may be used to control vaginal bleeding if this is problematic.

Recurrent disease

If recurrences occur, these tend to be early; 50% are within the first year, and 90% within 5 years. Management depends on the primary treatment. Recurrence after surgery may be treated with chemotherapy. Central recurrence following radiotherapy may be amenable to exenteration—removal of tumour, bladder, and rectum.

Follow-up

There is a lack of evidence on follow-up after treatment for gynaecological malignancies and no national guidelines. Regional protocols exist and some units offer patient-initiated follow-up.

Typically, appointments in a multidisciplinary clinic are offered:

- 6 weeks' post-treatment
- Every 3–4 months for 1–2 years
- Annually for a total of 5 years

Involves direct questioning for symptoms such as weight loss, abdominal pain, and vaginal bleeding.

An abdominal and vaginal examination are performed at each visit

Vault smears may be performed but are difficult to read after radiotherapy.

Prognosis and survival

Prognosis is most importantly linked to stage. The size of the central tumour and the type affect the risk of metastatic disease, i.e. increase the stage.

Survival by stage is not very helpful as FIGO staging does not include lymph node spread. For instance, FIGO stage Ib1 may have clear lymph nodes or metastatic spread to nodes. If the nodes are clear, the 5-year survival is 90–95%. If the pelvic nodes have metastatic cells, the survival immediately drops to 60%. The more nodes involved, the worse the survival. If para-aortic nodes are involved, the survival will drop to 30–50% (see Box 15.1).

Cervical cancer in pregnancy

Incidence is 1.2 per 10 000 pregnancies.

- Biopsies should be taken under anaesthesia as the cervix is highly vascular in pregnancy and major haemorrhage may occur
- Staging is problematic. MRI can be safely used, but pregnancy hormone-induced changes of the cervix make parametral spread difficult to assess accurately
- Management decisions should be made at a multidisciplinary level, and involve the woman. These may prove ethically difficult as options include termination of the pregnancy, or delaying treatment to allow the fetus to achieve viability, which may adversely affect maternal prognosis.

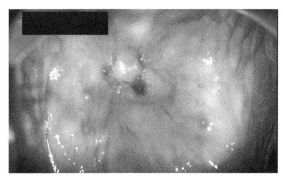
Fig. 15.4 Vagina after radical trachelectomy.

15.5 Endometrial carcinoma

Incidence
- There were just over 6000 cases of cancer of the body of the uterus in England and Wales in 2004
- These comprised 4% of all cancer cases in women
- Most common postmenopause, peak age 61 years
- 75% of women present with symptoms at stage I
- Prognosis is better than other malignancies
- Second commonest gynaecological malignancy
- Third commonest cause of death after ovary and cervix

Pathophysiology
Cancer of the endometrial lining of the uterus is caused by stimulation of the endometrium by oestrogen without the protective effect of progesterone. Progesterone is produced by the corpus luteum after ovulation, so anovulation is a risk. Anovulatory periods occur at the extremes of reproductive age and increase the amount of unopposed oestrogen exposure. Subcutaneous fat produces oestrogen postmenopausally owing to aromatization of adrenal steroids.

A small number are caused by an inherited gene mutation (e.g. hereditary non-polyposis colorectal cancers, HNPCC).

Risk factors
- Obesity
- Menstrual factors:
  - Early menarche
  - Late menopause
  - Low parity
- Anovulatory amenorrhoea, e.g. polycystic ovary syndrome
- Unopposed oestrogen HRT
- Oestrogen-secreting ovarian tumours
- Tamoxifen
- Family history of colorectal cancer, endometrial cancer, breast cancer (HNPCC)

Associations
- Diabetes mellitus
- Hypertension

This is due to their association with obesity.

Endometrial hyperplasia

Pathophysiology
Long periods of unopposed oestrogen lead to hyperplasia (endometrial thickening) which predisposes to cytological atypia. Atypical hyperplasia is precancerous and develops into invasive cancer in 10–50% cumulatively over 20 years. Clinical identification is not possible.

The three subdubdivisions are:
- Simple (cystic)
- Complex (adenomatous)
- Atypical

Simple hyperplasia
- Commonest of the three forms
- Often present at the either end of the reproductive lifecycle
- Glands are enlarged and may be pleiomorphic (simple atypical hyperplasia); mitoses are present but there is no cytological atypia

Complex hyperplasia
Atypical glandular picture with proliferation, irregular outlines, and obvious structural complexity

Atypical hyperplasia
- Glands have atypical nuclei, e.g. enlarged rounded nuclei, hyperchromatism, enlarged nucleoli, and abnormal mitotic figures
- Severe cases are indistinguishable from cancer
- Persistent untreated atypical hyperplasia has the highest rate of progression to malignancy

Treatment of endometrial hyperplasia
Management depends on symptomatology, surgical risks, and fertility wishes.

Simple and complex hyperplasia
- Conservative management
- Progestogens, e.g. Mirena™ intrauterine system, or cyclical Provera®, followed by repeat biopsy

Atypical hyperplasia
- High risk of coexistent carcinoma, so TAH + BSO recommended
- If surgery is medically contraindicated or declined, hysteroscopy and endometrial biopsy should be repeated after 3 months, or sooner if symptoms recur
- Regular surveillance is indicated
- Treatment with high-dose progestogens has been reported to result in regression, but studies are neither conclusive nor comparable
- The optimal dose and duration of therapy are unknown

Endometrial carcinoma
- Adenocarcinoma is the commonest carcinoma (95%)
- Majority are of endometrioid type
- Squamous metaplasia is often seen alongside
- Adenosquamous carcinoma (mixed adenocarcinoma and squamous cell carcinoma) is not uncommon
- Primary squamous cell carcinoma is very rare
- Less common types are papillary serous and clear cell
- Sarcomatous elements may be present alongside the glandular adenocarcinoma—a mixed Mullerian tumour

Papillary serous carcinoma, clear cell, and mixed Mullerian tumours are highly aggressive and carry the worst prognosis.

Spread
- The myometrium may act as a barrier and thus explain the tumour's early presentation and high cure rate
- Direct spread: through the myometrium, and down to the cervical stroma, or to the Fallopian tubes and ovaries. If the tumour reaches the serosal surface of the uterus, it can spread across the peritoneal cavity to involve omentum and the surface of other organs such as the bowel and liver
- Lymphatic spread: typically follows the uterine blood vessels to the pelvic lymph nodes. The para-aortic and rarely the inguinal nodes may be involved
- Spread via the bloodstream is to the liver and lungs

Staging
Staging is surgicopathological (i.e. determined by the results of histology following surgery) and follows the FIGO guidelines (see Box 15.2).

Clinical evaluation
History
- Postmenopausal vaginal bleeding (PMB)
- Defined as bleeding 1 year after the cessation of periods
- 10% of women with PMB will have a malignancy

- Premenopausal women may present with irregular, heavy or intermenstrual bleeding
- Menstrual irregularities in women >40 years require investigation

Examination

- Speculum examination to exclude other causes such as a cervical or vaginal lesion
- Fixed or bulky uterus occurs with advanced disease

Investigations

- Transvaginal ultrasound: may show endometrial thickness >5 mm (suspicious postmenopause), fluid within the cavity or a polyp

- Biopsy: Pipelle™ in clinic may obtain a fast diagnosis
- Hysteroscopy and biopsy: if Pipelle™ not possible, or if patient on tamoxifen. Endometrial carcinoma typically has an irregular, vascular appearance (see Figure 15.5) in Section 15.6
- MRI: to assess depth of myometrial invasion, cervical involvement, and lymphadenopathy
- CT abdomen and chest: if high-risk cancer, e.g. sarcoma

Stage	Definition	Pelvic lymph node involvement (%)	5-year survival (%)
I	**Carcinoma confined to the uterine corpus**	<20	80
Ia	Tumour limited to the endometrium		
Ib	Invasion confined to <50% of myometrium		
Ic	Invasion >50% of myometrium		
II	**Carcinoma confined to the uterine corpus and cervix, but not beyond the uterus**	20	65
IIa	Endocervical glandular involvement only		
IIb	Cervical stromal invasion		
III	**Carcinoma extends outside the uterus, but confined to the true pelvis**	35	30
IIIa	Tumour invades uterine serosa, and/or adnexa, and/or positive peritoneal cytology		
IIIb	Vaginal metastases		
IIIc	Metastases to pelvic and/or para-aortic lymph nodes		
IV	**Carcinoma involves bladder or bowel mucosa, or has metastasized to distant sites**	50	10
IVa	Tumour invasion of bladder and/or bowel mucosa		
IVb	Distant metastases, including intra-abdominal and/or inguinal lymph nodes		

Box 15.2 FIGO staging and 5-year survival of endometrial carcinoma

- Surgery is the mainstay of treatment
- Additional, or adjuvant, treatment depends on the stage of the disease and the physical health of the woman

Surgery

- Total hysterectomy, bilateral salpingo-oophorectomy, and peritoneal washings
- Hysterectomy may be laparoscopic, vaginal or open
- Laparoscopic surgery is helpful in obese women as this reduces the incidence of wound complications
- Pelvic lymphadenectomy is controversial
- Removing pelvic lymph nodes adds staging information but no survival benefit was seen in a large randomized controlled trial (RCT) (ASTEC study)

Adjuvant radiotherapy and chemotherapy

Stage I a&b, grade 1–2 disease—no adjuvant treatment
Prognosis is already excellent

Stage Ic or grade 3 disease—radiotherapy
External beam pelvic radiation + followed by vault brachytherapy (see Section 15.4) is offered as there is an increased risk of recurrence in these women

Stage II disease—radiotherapy
Pelvic radiation as above. Frail patients may be offered vaginal vault brachytherapy alone following surgery

Stage III disease—carboplatin + pacitaxel chemotherapy + pelvic radiation

The tumour has potentially spread intra-abdominally or into para-aortic nodes and is beyond the field of pelvic radiotherapy. Thus, carboplatin pacitaxel chemotherapy is administered initially, followed by pelvic radiation

Stage IV disease—a palliative approach is taken
Symptom control may be achieved by low-dose radiotherapy to the pelvis to stop vaginal bleeding, chemotherapy to prevent pain or other symptoms from distant spread.

Progesterone treatment (Provera® 100–200 mg BD) gives an improvement in symptoms in 30% of patients and occasionally gives longer term control of lung metastases.

Conservative medical treatment
Women desiring fertility with grade 1 disease on biopsy and stage la on MRI have been treated with progesterone alone. This is not standard, and published case series do not give full details concerning treatment failure.

Recurrent disease
- 95% of relapses occur within 2 years of initial treatment
- The vagina is the most common site of recurrence in women who have not received pelvic radiation. They can be treated with pelvic radiotherapy
- Pelvic recurrence is less usual where pelvic radiation has been administered. Para-aortic lymph nodes, lungs, and the abdominal cavity are more common
- Pelvic radiotherapy cannot be repeated, and treatment is palliative in intent—see stage IV disease above

Follow-up
- No national guidelines for follow-up exist
- Normally determined at a regional level

Typically women will be reviewed in a multidisciplinary clinic:
- 6 weeks' postoperatively
- Every 3–4 months for 2 years
- Annually to 5 years

At each appointment, symptoms such as vaginal bleeding, abdominal pain, weight loss, and poor appetite need to be sought.

Vaginal and abdominal examination are performed.

Prognosis and survival
This is determined by grade, type and stage, as well as patient age and treatment (See Box 15.2 section 15.5).

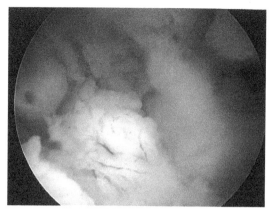

Fig. 15.5 Hysteroscopic view of endometrial carcinoma. The uterine cavity is filled with friable, irregular tissue.

15.7 Ovarian carcinoma

Incidence

- The commonest gynaecological malignancy
- There were 6600 new registrations in England and Wales in 2004, making it the fourth most common site in women (after breast, colorectal, and lung)
- The majority present with advanced disease, and so prognosis and survival remains poor
- The lifetime incidence of ovarian cancer is 1:80, affecting predominantly postmenopausal women

Aetiology

Unknown but two hypotheses:

- Incessant ovulation: each ovulation causes minor trauma to the surface epithelium. The more trauma, the higher the chance of malignant transformation
- Familial: 5–10% are familial and associated with the oncogenes BRCA1 and 2, and hereditary non-polyposis colorectal cancer (HNPCC)

Protective factors

- Parity and breastfeeding. 50% reduced risk with 3 children
- COCP—50% reduction in risk after 5 years, with some reduction after 6 months. The protective effect may last for 20 years after stopping
- Hysterectomy or tubal occlusion—raising the possibility of an environmental factor

Risk factors

- Fertility drugs stimulating ovulation, e.g. clomiphene citrate or gonadotrophins used in IVF

Pathophysiology

Epithelial tumours (cystadenocarcinoma)

Account for 90% of ovarian cancers:

- Serous—secrete CA125
- Mucinous—secrete CA19-9

These tumours have a borderline category.

Borderline tumours have cells which have malignant appearance but are not invasive. They have a better prognosis. Commonly, they are found in younger women and can be treated by removal of the affected ovary only.

- Endometrioid—secrete CA125
- Clear cell—rarer and associated with worse prognosis

Germ cell tumours

Account for 10% of ovarian cancers. These are commoner in younger women.

- Dysgerminomas—secrete lactate dehydrogenase (LDH)
- Yolk sac tumours—secrete alpha fetoprotein (αFP)
- Malignant teratomas
- Choriocarcinomas—secrete HCG

Sex cord stromal tumours

The smallest group, and occur at any age.

- Granulosa thecal cell tumours—secrete oestrogen
- Sertoli–Leydig tumours—secrete testosterone

Metastic tumours

Between 5 and 10% of ovarian tumours are metastatic from:

- Breast—most common primary site
- Colorectum
- Stomach
- Endometrium

If a tumour shows 'signet ring' cells on histopathology (cells containing mucin which pushes the nucleus to the periphery of the cell), it is called a Krukenberg tumour. These tumours most commonly originate from the stomach.

Spread

- Transperitoneal or transcoelomic: when ovarian cancers breach the capsule of the ovary, they are able to spread across the peritoneal cavity, typically to peritoneal surfaces, such as the diaphragm, bowel, and to the omentum
- Lymphatic spread: to para-aortic and pelvic lymph nodes
- Haematogenous spread: occurs late to lungs and liver

Staging

- Staging is surgical (see Figures 15.6 and 15.7) and follows FIGO guidelines (see Box 15.3)
- Early cancers of the ovary rarely produce symptoms unless an ovarian accident (torsion, haemorrhage, rupture)
- Most women present with the symptoms caused by disease that has spread across the peritoneum
- Thus, 75% of women present with stage III or IV disease

Clinical evaluation

History

- Abdominal pain and swelling
- Loss of appetite
- Bladder or bowel symptoms

Examination

- Adnexal or pelvic mass may be fixed disease in the pouch of Douglas
- Shifting dullness (ascites)
- Irregular abdominal mass (omental cake)

Investigations

- Ultrasound scan of ovaries (see Figures 15.8 and 15.9)
- CA125
- CA19-9 (raised in mucinous tumours, including pancreas)
- Carcinoembryonic antigen (CEA) (high levels indicate possible colorectal primary)
- αFP, HCG, and LDH in younger women
- Chest X-ray
- FBC, U&E, and LFTs
- CT abdomen and pelvis to assess metastatic spread
- Paracentesis of ascites or pleural tap for cytology

Ovarian carcinoma is very difficult to diagnose at an early stage as it is often asymptomatic until it has spread.

The symptoms are often non-specific, and many women are eventually diagnosed following investigations by gastroenterologists, or colorectal surgeons for non-specific abdominal symptoms.

→ Box 15.3 **FIGO staging of ovarian cancer and 5-year survival by stage**

Stage	Definition	5-year survival (%)
I	**Confined to one, or both ovaries**	80–90
Ia	Disease confined to one ovary, capsule intact, no ascites	
Ib	Limited to both ovaries, capsules intact, no ascites	
Ic	Ruptured capsule or surface disease on one or both ovaries, malignant ascites, or positive peritoneal washings	
II	**Spread to pelvic structures**	67–70
IIa	Spread to uterus or Fallopian tubes	
IIb	Spread to other pelvic tissues	
IIc	IIa or b with ruptured capsule or surface disease, malignant ascites, or positive peritoneal washings	
III	**Stage I or II plus peritoneal implants outside the pelvis or positive retroperitoneal lymph nodes**	29–59
IIIa	Microscopic peritoneal surface metastases	
IIIb	Peritoneal surface deposits of <2 cm, negative retroperitoneal lymph nodes	
IIIc	Peritoneal surface deposits of >2 cm, or positive retroperitoneal lymph nodes	
IV	**Distant metastases—liver, lung, or positive pleural effusions**	17

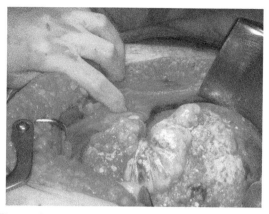

Fig. 15.6 Surgical staging of ovarian cancer.

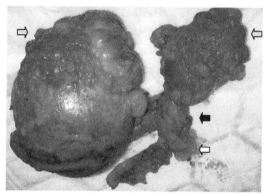

Fig. 15.7 Surgical specimen following staging laparotomy for ovarian cancer. Ovaries (⇨); uterus (◄■); cervix (⇦).

15.8 Management of ovarian carcinoma

Risk of malignancy index

One of the key problems in managing ovarian masses is to differentiate benign from malignant cysts, particularly if found incidentally on imaging.

The RMI (Risk of Malignancy Index) is a helpful calculation to assess whether a cyst is likely to be malignant.

RMI = CA125 x menopausal status x ultrasound features

- CA125 is measured in u/ml
- Premenopausal women score 1, postmenopausal 3
- US features: multilocularity, solid areas, papillary proliferations, bilaterality, ascites, intra-abdominal metastases (see Figures 15.8 and 15.9)
- If any US feature is present, a score of 1 is given
- If >1 features is present, a score of 3 is given

RMI of >200 confers an increased risk of malignancy

Elevated CA125

- Is found with endometriosis, other intra-abdominal malignancies and intra-abdominal TB
- Small rises can occur with cardiac, renal, and liver failure
- Of stage I ovarian cancers, 50% do not have elevated CA125

Tumour markers

- If ascites or intra-abdominal carcinomatosis are seen on CT scan, then test for tumour markers (CA125, carcinoembryonic antigen (CEA), and CA19-9)
- Tap the ascites to look for adenocarcinoma cells
- Perform CT- or US-guided biopsy for cytokeratins (CK). This distinguishes ovarian (CK 7 positive, CK 20 negative) and colorectal cancers (CK 7 negative, CK 20 positive)

Useful tip: primary peritoneal cancers appear identical to ovarian cancer but do not have a pelvic mass.

Treatment

There is a debate regarding the effectiveness of cyto-reductive surgery versus chemotherapy in women with advanced malignancy. The CHORUS trial aims to shed light on this.

Epithelial ovarian malignancies

The majority present in postmenopausal women.

Early cancer—isolated ovarian mass

- Extended midline laparotomy, full intra-abdominal examination of all peritoneal surfaces, such as the diaphragm, liver, bowel serosa, appendix, and para-aortic nodes
- Peritoneal washings for cytology
- TAH & BSO
- Omentectomy
- Para-aortic node dissection

This process is known as a 'staging' laparotomy. If the cancer is confined to the ovary with no spread, adjuvant treatment may not be required. If occult metastatic spread is identified, then adjuvant chemotherapy is required with carboplatin ± pacitaxel.

Late cancer—metastatic spread across the abdomen

- TAH & BSO
- Total omentectomy
- Debulking of all visible cancer to leave as little residual tumour mass as possible
- Chemotherapy—carboplatin and pacitaxel

The standard management involves primary 'cytoreductive' surgery with extended midline laparotomy. The aim of surgery is to remove as much tumour as possible. Optimal debulked if there are no single tumour deposits of ≥1 cm left. Maximum surgical removal of disease is associated with a longer disease-free interval.

Ovarian malignancies are chemosensitive. Platinum-based drugs have revolutionized survival rates. Ninety per cent of cases respond to carboplatin, with 60% achieving complete remission. The majority of women will have a recurrence. Although 5-year survival figures have increased to 40% for stage III disease, the median survival is 3 years. Response to treatment is monitored by CA125 levels and CT imaging.

Young women—where disease appears to be confined to one ovary. Where fertility is to be preserved, the principles are:

- Removal of the affected ovary
- Biopsy of the contralateral ovary
- Staging with peritoneal washings, omentectomy, para-aortic node dissection
- If tumour is endometrioid cystadenocarcinoma (see pathophysiology), an endometrial biopsy is required owing to the risk of synchronous endometrioid endometrial cancer

Minimally invasive surgical techniques may be considered. However, intraoperative rupture of the cyst will result in a higher stage which is associated with a worse prognosis. Laparoscopic TAH & BSO, omentectomy, and para-aortic and pelvic lymph node sampling may be performed. This is complex surgery and should be undertaken in specialist centres in carefully selected patients. Laparoscopy is also associated with port-site metastases.

Neoadjuvant chemotherapy

- Some women may not be suitable for primary surgery—e.g. elderly patients with advanced disease
- Chemotherapy may be used as a first line
- Cytoreductive surgery is performed after 3–4 cycles if a response has occurred

This is not standard therapy and studies are in progress to study the effectiveness.

Borderline tumours

These usually present at an early stage and are associated with a very good prognosis as they do not tend to be invasive. These should be managed with minimally invasive surgical techniques.

CA125 is often not raised in borderline lesions, and as a result the RMI may suggest a benign lesion.

Fertility-preserving surgery is possible if these are accurately diagnosed preoperatively. Adjuvant chemotherapy is not usually required.

These women should be followed-up postoperatively, but reassured that 5-year survival rate is >97%.

Germ cell tumours

As these usually occur in women of reproductive age, the aim should be for surgery to be as conservative as possible. Formal staging with laparotomy and washings should be performed. It is often possible to remove only the affected ovary. Tumours are very chemosensitive, and carry a good prognosis.

Germ cell tumours are managed with bleomycin, etoposide, and cisplatinum, achieving good response rates, whilst preserving ovarian function.

Follow-up can be by tracking tumour markers as these are usually elevated.

Sex cord stromal tumours

These tumours are associated with endometrial carcinomas as most are oestrogen-secreting. They should be managed as per epithelial tumours, except in young women.

Other surgery

Other surgery may be required, e.g. if there is bowel involvement, resulting in resection or stoma. Women must be warned of this and appropriate liaison made with surgical teams.

Radiotherapy

As ovarian malignancies tend to disseminate throughout the peritoneal cavity, radiotherapy is not usually possible owing to the adverse effect on the bowel and other structures. However, it can be used to treat small volume residual disease.

Follow-up

There are no nationally agreed follow-up protocols for ovarian carcinoma. Typically, women will be seen in a multidisciplinary clinic 6 weeks' postoperatively, and then every 3–4 months for 1–2 years, then annually to 5 years.

Direct questioning for symptoms of abdominal pain, bloating, and swelling, as well as appetite and weight loss, is usually followed by an abdominal and vaginal examination.

If CA125 or CA19-9 levels were elevated at initial presentation these may be used to monitor relapse. An increase in CA125 more than twice the upper limit of normal accurately predicts relapse with a sensitivity of 86%, and a positive predictive value of 95%, typically with a lead time of 2–4 months before symptoms occur.

Recurrent disease

If there has been a reasonable disease-free interval it may be possible to re-challenge women with platinum-based chemotherapy agents. Secondary surgery is rarely indicated.

Bowel obstruction is a common problem with recurrent disease and can be distressing. Palliative procedures may be considered to bypass a single obstruction. However, the bowel is extensively involved more often than not.

Ascites can cause abdominal distension, loss of appetite, and breathing difficulties (breathlessness). These symptoms can easily be relieved by ultrasound-guided paracentesis. Pleural effusions can also be drained to provide symptomatic relief.

The aim is to palliate the symptoms, and it is important to adopt a multidisciplinary team approach, involving cancer nurse specialists, oncologists, and palliative care specialists.

Prognosis and survival

Both depend on the stage and the general wellbeing of the patient (see Box 15.3, Section 15.5).

Research

Most cases of ovarian cancer are sporadic. In the absence of a reliable tumour marker it is difficult to screen the ovaries. Two large studies are currently under way involving the use of CA125 and transvaginal scan (TVS) ultrasound to assess the benefit of screening the general population (UKCTOCS) and women with a strong family history of ovarian cancer (UKFOCS).

Further reading

info.cancerresearchuk.org/cancerandresearch/cancers/ovarian/

www.ovacome.org.uk/Home

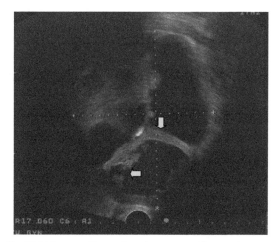

Fig. 15.8 Ultrasound image of ovarian serous papillary carcinoma. Multilocular cyst with thick, irregular septae (⇩) and papillary proliferations (⇦).

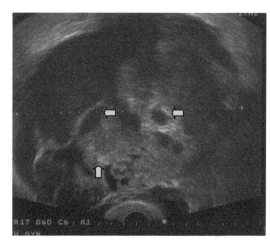

Fig. 15.9 Ultrasound image of ovarian mixed endometrioid serous carcinoma. Multilocular solid (⇧)/cystic (⇦) tumour.

15.9 Fallopian tube carcinoma

Incidence

Primary cancer of the Fallopian tube is rare.

- Typically unilateral (75%)
- Difficult to diagnose, but 50% present at stage I or II
- More common in postmenopausal women (60%)

Aetiology

Unclear—a small number of cases may be due to an inherited gene mutation e.g. BRCA1 and BRCA2.

Pathophysiology

- Of primary tumours, 90% are papillary serous adenocarcinomas. Rarer types include endometrioid, transitional cell, clear cell, undifferentiated, mixed, and sarcomas
- Behave similarly to epithelial ovarian carcinomas
- It may be difficult to identify the primary
- Metastatic tumours are commoner—mainly ovary, endometrium, breast, colorectal or stomach

Diagnostic criteria for a true Fallopian tube primary:

- Tumour arises from endosalpinx
- Histology reproduces epithelium of tubal mucosa
- Transition from benign to malignant epithelium seen
- Ovaries and endometrium are either normal, or contain tumours smaller than Fallopian tube

Spread

As with ovarian cancer this is largely transcoelomic.

- Direct spread through the tube and to other tube, ovaries, uterus, and adjacent pelvic structures
- Transperitoneal spread occurs early to involve the surface of the bowel, omentum, and liver
- Lymphatic spread is to the para-aortic and, rarely, to inguinal lymph nodes
- Haematological spread rarely to the liver and lungs

Staging

Staging is surgicopathological and follows the FIGO guidelines (see Box 15.4). This determines adjuvant treatment and prognosis.

Clinical evaluation

History

- Vaginal bleeding (34%)
- Pain (23%)
- Vaginal discharge (20%)—often watery and profuse
- Abdominal distension (9%)
- Abnormal glandular cervical smear with normal cervix and endometrium on investigation
- Cervical smear and endometrial biopsy may reveal cells suggesting adenocarcinoma in 25 and 50% of cases, respectively

Examination

- Speculum to exclude other causes of bleeding or discharge
- Adnexal mass may be palpable on bimanual examination
- Ascites is often present in advanced disease

Investigations

- Transvaginal scan may reveal a tubal cystic mass adjacent to the ovary, containing solid papillary proliferations and increased vascularity, or ascites in advanced disease
- CT or MRI may establish diagnosis and assess spread
- CA125 is elevated in 70% of cases

Management

This tumour is difficult to diagnose accurately preoperatively and often the diagnosis is made at laparotomy.

Surgery

- Midline laparotomy, TAH & BSO
- If no obvious metastatic disease—peritoneal washings, omentectomy, para-aortic node dissection

These will stage the tumour.

- If metastatic disease is apparent, optimal debulking should be performed with maximal removal of any visible disease along with omentectomy

Chemotherapy

Stage I grade 1 tumours:

- Evidence base for the effectiveness of adjuvant chemotherapy is lacking
- Some centres give single agent carboplatin (as the tumour had access to the peritoneal cavity through the fimbrial end). Other centres will observe

Stage I/II disease—adjuvant chemotherapy:

- Carboplatin only if no visible disease at end of surgery
- Clinical remission rates of 85% may be achieved

Stage III/IV disease—adjuvant chemotherapy:

- Optimal chemotherapy is carboplatin + pacitaxel
- Reserved for advanced disease as more side effects, including hair loss and joint pain, than carboplatin alone

Radiotherapy

Radiotherapy cannot be given effectively to the whole abdomen owing to the sensitivity of the small bowel. Fallopian tube cancer may spread across the whole peritoneal cavity. Thus chemotherapy is a better adjuvant treatment.

Recurrent disease

Local and distant recurrence can occur. If CA125 was elevated at initial diagnosis this can be used in follow-up to detect presymptomatic recurrence.

Rechallenging with chemotherapy is the normal management. If the disease recurs within 6 months it is thought to be resistant to platinum chemotherapy and the prognosis is very poor.

Repeat surgery may be used if there is one localized mass.

Prognosis and survival

See Box 15.4.

- Determined by FIGO stage
- Similar to epithelial ovarian malignancies
- Overall prognosis is better as more present early
- At presentation 35% of women will have spread to the para-aortic lymph nodes

Box 15.4 FIGO staging of Fallopian tube carcinomas and 5-year survival rates

Stage	Definition	5-year survival (%)
0	Carcinoma *in situ*	
I	**Tumour confined to Fallopian tube**	84
Ia	Tumour limited to one tube, without penetrating serosal surface, no ascites	
Ib	Tumour limited to both tubes, without penetrating serosal surface, no ascites	
Ic	Tumour limited to one or both tubes, with extension onto or through the tubal serosa, or with positive malignant cells in ascites or peritoneal washings	
II	**Tumour involves one or both Fallopian tubes with pelvic extension**	50
IIa	Extension and/or metastasis to uterus and/or ovaries	
IIb	Extension to other pelvic organs	
IIc	IIa or b with positive malignant cells in ascites or peritoneal washings	
III	**Tumour involves one or both Fallopian tubes with peritoneal implants outside the pelvis, and/or positive regional lymph nodes**	36
IIIa	Microscopic peritoneal metastasis outside the pelvis	
IIIb	Macroscopic peritoneal metastasis outside the pelvis ≤ 2cm in greatest diameter	
IIIc	Peritoneal metastasis >2 cm in greatest diameter and/or positive regional lymph nodes	
IV	**Distant metastasis beyond the peritoneal cavity**	20

15.10 Uterine sarcomas

Incidence
- Rare, <1% of all gynaecological malignancies
- Arise from the stroma (usually of myometrial muscle)
- Most commonly occur postmenopausally

Aetiology
- Unknown

Risk factors
- Between 10 and 25% occur in women who have undergone pelvic radiotherapy 5–25 years earlier
- Race: Black 2x > incidence than Caucasian or Asian women
- As for endometrial carcinoma (see Section 15.5), particularly tamoxifen

Pathophysiology
- Leiomyosarcomas—arise from myometrium, rarely from pre-existing fibroids. Histologically, they are characterized by >10 mitotic figures per high-power field, coagulative necrosis, and pleomorphic nuclei
- Endometrial stromal sarcomas—low- and high-grade forms, defined by number of mitoses per 10 high-power fields
- Mixed Mullerian tumours—areas of both sarcoma and carcinoma from glands are seen on histology
- Adenosarcoma—sarcoma and areas of benign glands

Spread
- Direct spread through myometrium and cervix
- Haematogenous spread to the lungs is common
- Lymphatic spread is less common

Staging
Staging is surgicopathological and follows the FIGO guidelines for endometrial carcinomas (see Box 15.2, Section 15.5).

Clinical evaluation
History
- Postmenopausal bleeding (PMB) or intermenstrual spotting occur in 85%
- Vaginal discharge without blood
- Pelvic pain and/or mass occur in 10%

The vast majority of sarcomas are leiomyosarcomas and are only diagnosed on histology examination of myomectomy or hysterectomy specimens. As such, they have not usually been suspected preoperatively as imaging is not usually able to distinguish between leiomyoma and leiomyosarcoma.

Possible diagnostic clues include:
- Rapidly growing fibroids
- Weight loss
- Pyrexia of unknown origin

Examination
- Speculum to exclude other causes of bleeding
- Enlarged uterus, often a palpable pelvic mass

Investigations
- Transvaginal US may show a vascular myometrial mass
- Endometrial biopsy, or hysteroscopy and biopsy, will often not detect the abnormality
- MRI to assess size, myometrial invasion, cervical, and lymphovascular spread
- CT chest to assess for lung metastases

Management
Surgery is the mainstay of treatment for all forms of sarcoma. Treatment should be planned with both the gynae-oncology and sarcoma multidisciplinary teams.

Stage I and II disease
- **Surgery**—total hysterectomy and bilateral salpingo-oophorectomy aiming to debulk maximally
- **BSO** is important as some tumours, e.g. low-grade endometrial stromal, have oestrogen receptors
- **Lymph node dissection** is not required if the lymph nodes are normal size, as these tumours rarely metastasize to nodes
- **Debulking** if the nodes are enlarged. Nodal debulking should be performed. Any other intra-abdominal deposits should be excised where technically possible
- **Adjuvant treatment** after full resection of early stage disease (see below). If the disease is stage I and low risk, then no adjuvant treatment is required. If it is high risk stage I or stage II then adjuvant treatment is required (see Box 15.5 to calculate risk of tumours)

Stage III and IV
- Individualized regimen of any or a combination of chemotherapy, radiotherapy. and surgery

Stage IV
- Tumours may be shrunk with chemotherapy to cause symptomatic relief
- Progesterone-like drugs or oestrogen-blocking drugs may provide symptom control in advanced endometrial stromal sarcomas
- Surgery to remove pelvic disease may be performed if distant metastatic disease is stable

Adjuvant therapy
Leiomyosarcoma
Adjuvant radiotherapy has been shown to reduce the risk of local recurrence, but does not improve survival rates.

Adjuvant chemotherapy comprises doxorubicin and ifosfamide. The concept of using adjuvant chemotherapy is attractive, given that > 80% of relapses are outside the pelvis.

There are no large randomized controlled trials (RCTs) as these tumours are rare. Thus, there is no evidence that survival will be improved with adjuvant chemotherapy. However, these drugs show significant activity in gynaecological leiomyosarcomas and their use should be discussed with the individual patient.

Endometrial stromal sarcoma—low grade
These tumours are often sensitive to oestrogen. Thus hormone manipulation is used as adjuvant treatment. Initial strategies are to perform a BSO at surgery and avoid HRT.

Oestrogen and progesterone receptor status should be routinely assessed on pathology specimens. Further treatments can be used if receptor status is positive.

First line adjuvant hormonal manipulation—aromatase inhibitors, e.g. letrozole or anastrozole prevent conversion of steroids to oestrogen in subcutaneous fat.

Second line—progestogens, e.g. medroxyprogesterone or megestrol acetate.

Adjuvant radiotherapy—consider for unresectable residual disease in the pelvis.

Endometrial stromal sarcoma—high grade

Adjuvant radiotherapy considered in all patients with stage I/II disease.

Adjuvant chemotherapy is not indicated.

Mixed Mullerian tumours

Treat as per high-grade endometrial carcinomas.
Adjuvant radiotherapy for stage 1b and above.

Adenosarcomas

Treat as per leiomyosarcomas.

Prognosis and survival

Staging is an important prognostic factor. However, the type of sarcoma is also relevant.

- Leiomyosarcoma
- Endometrial stromal sarcoma—high grade
- Mixed mullerian tumour
- Adenosarcoma

These are all aggressive and have a poor prognosis unless early stage and no high risk factors. Five-year survival by stage is:

- Stages I–II 50%
- Stage III 20%
- Stage IV <10%
- Endometrial stromal sarcoma
  - Low grade: has an indolent course
  - Often recur but after many years
  - Five-year survival is 70%.

→ **Box 15.5 Risk assessment index for predicting survival in leiomyosarcoma**

Variables	Score
• Age <51 years	1
• Tumour >5 cm	1
• FIGO stage 2–4	1
• Grade 3	2

Total score	Risk
0–1	Low
2–3	Intermediate
4–5	High

15.11 Vulval intraepithelial neoplasia and vulval cancer

Vulval intraepithelial neoplasia

Vulval intraepithelial neoplasia (VIN) is a squamous premalignant lesion classified as I, II, and III. It is not common, but may occur in young women.

Aetiology
- Oncogenic HPV

Associated risk factors
- Smoking
- Immunosuppression, e.g. HIV infection, medications

Pathophysiology
The histological appearances are the same as cervical intraepithelial neoplasia (CIN): lack of differentiation, disordered cellular maturation, and nuclear abnormalities. However, VIN occurs in original squamous epithelium rather than metaplastic tissue since there is no transformation zone on the vulva. Progression to invasive disease is lower than for CIN—approximately 6%.

Clinical evaluation
History
- Pruritis
- Pain
- Often asymptomatic

Examination
- Visible vulval lesion, but variable appearance
- White due to hyperkeratosis, red due to thin skin or brown due to increased melanin (Figure 15.10)
- Raised, papular and rough, or macular with indistinct border

Investigations
- Vulvoscopy—apply 5% acetic acid to reveal lesions
- Biopsy—multiple sites using punch biopsy (see Technical skills Box 13.6, in Section 13.9)

Management
- Local excision, but associated with high recurrence rate. Thus excision is reserved for florid or symptomatic lesions
- Topical imiquimod (immunomodulator cream) is widely used, but not yet licensed
- Long term follow-up. Be alert for signs of progression to cancer: ulceration, bleeding, swelling, soreness or irritation. Most VIN-related cancers occur within first decade following diagnosis and treatment

Vulval carcinoma

Predominantly affects older women, with 80% >65 years. It is a rare condition which should be managed at gynaecological cancer centres by multidisciplinary teams (MDTs) (RCOG guideline 2006).

Aetiology—premalignant lesions
Vulval cancers develop from a range of skin abnormalities which have malignant potential.
- Lichen sclerosis (see Section 13.9). Sixty-six per cent of vulval cancers occur in women with lichen sclerosis. However, only 2–5% of women with lichen sclerosis will go on to develop vulval cancer.
- VIN caused by oncogenic HPV
- Paget's disease—intraepithelial abnormal glandular cells (preinvasive lesion for adenocarcinoma of the vulva). Between 4 and 8% are associated with primary adenocarcinoma elsewhere

- Lichen planus—although rarely associated with development of vulval cancer, it is a recognized risk factor

Pathophysiology
- 85% are squamous cell
- 5% are malignant melanomas
- Basal cell carcinoma
- Adenocarcinomas arising from Bartholin's glands.
- Verrucous carcinoma is a rare variant of squamous cell carcinomas with slower growth and improved prognosis

Spread
- Local involving:
  - Vagina
  - Urethra and clitoris anteriorly
  - Rectum posteriorly
- Via lymphatics—groin (inguinofemoral) lymph nodes. Depth of invasion of tumour is predictive of lymph node involvement
- Haematogenous spread is rare

Staging
- Staging follows the FIGO guidelines (Box 15.6)

Clinical evaluation
History
- Pruritis vulvae
- Ulcer or mass
- Bleeding

Examination
- Ulcer
- Mass (see Figure 15.11)
- The labia majora is the most common location, followed by the labia minora, clitoris, posterior fourchette, perineum, and Bartholin's gland
- The cervix must be examined to exclude coexisting CIN or cervical carcinoma

Investigations
- Biopsy to confirm diagnosis and depth of invasion
- MRI for inguinal lymph node involvement

Management
Surgery is mainstay of treatment.

Stage Ia—wide local excision, aiming for adequate resection margins of 1 cm
In this early stage of vulval cancer, where invasion is <1 mm below the basement membrane, the risk of nodal metastases is <1%.

Thus local excision only is needed.

Stage Ib–IVa—Radical vulvectomy and bilateral groin node dissection
Separate incisions are performed for groin node dissection, as tumour metastases rarely occur in the skin between the vulva and groin. This has replaced the 'butterfly' excision in which the vulva and groin dissection is en bloc, leaving a huge skin defect to repair. The modern technique using three separate incisions for the vulva and groins reduces morbidity.

Despite this change in practice, 10% morbidity occurs owing to wound breakdown, infection, lymphocyst formation, and lymphoedema of the lower limbs. Suction drainage of the groins for 5–7 days postoperatively is used to reduce this.

Future development

Sentinel lymph node mapping—the sentinel node is the first node in the lymphatic chain to which the malignancy is likely to have spread.

A dye or radioactive isotope is injected into, or around, the cancer, which is then tracked. The first node that the dye or isotope reaches is the sentinel node. This can be surgically removed and sent for perioperative frozen section. If this is negative for malignancy, it is likely that the rest of the chain will also be, allowing the woman to be spared a formal groin node dissection.

This technique is still at the clinical trial phase, but has proved useful in breast malignancies and melanomas.

Other surgical procedures

The surgical procedure may be modified in certain situations:

Lateral tumours
- Modified radical vulvectomy of affected side

Ipsilateral groin nodes (guided by MRI)
- If ipsilateral lymph nodes are clear, the contralateral nodes will be clear
- If positive, the contralateral nodes require dissection

Stage III owing to local invasion of urethra or anus
- Radical excision, including the distal part of the urethra, or removal of the anus with colostomy formation and groin node dissection
- Adjuvant radiation is indicated if nodes involved
- Chemoradiation may be used to preserve sphincter function and avoid stomas
- Morbidity owing to intense skin desquamation and pain
- Cure rate uncertain as reports limited to small numbers

Stage III owing to unilateral positive nodal involvement on pathology
- Adjuvant radiation to groins and pelvis after surgery

Stage IVa owing to local extension to pelvic structures
- Consider initial groin node dissection
- Then radical exenterative surgery if nodes clear

Stage IVa owing to bilateral groin node involvement and stage IVb
- Prognosis is very poor, with 5-year survival rates of 10–15%
- Thus, treatment is individualized
- The focus is disease control, maybe combining surgery or radiation depending on the disease spread
- Associated with considerable psychosexual morbidity

Recurrent disease
- Further excision
- Lymph node recurrences may be treated with radiotherapy, if not used previously. This is mostly palliative

Prognosis and survival
Determined by stage, patient age, and treatment (see Box 15.6).

Further reading

www.rcog.org.uk/resources/Public/pdf/vulval_cancer.pdf

Box 15.6 FIGO staging and 5-year survival of vulval carcinoma

Stage	Definition	5-year survival (%)
Ia	Lesion confined to vulva and <1 mm of stromal invasion. No nodal metastases	98
Ib	Lesion confined to vulva, <2 cm in dimension, but with >1 mm of stromal invasion. No nodal metastases	
II	All lesions confined to vulva >2 cm dimension, with no nodal metastases	85
III	Adjacent spread to the lower urethra and/or vagina and/or anus, or unilateral lymph node metastases	74
IVa	Lesion involving upper urethra, bladder mucosa, rectal mucosa, pelvic bone or lesions with bilateral groin node metastases	10–15
IVb	Any distant metastases, including pelvic nodes	
	Node-negative disease	90
	Node-positive disease	60 or less

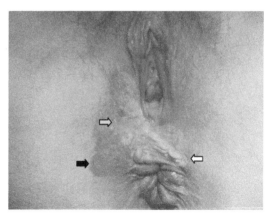

Fig. 15.10 VIN showing white lesions due to hyperkeratosis (⇦), brown lesions due to increased melanin (⇨), and red lesions due to thin skin (➡).

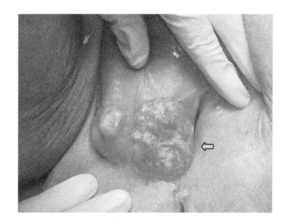

Fig. 15.11 Vulval cancer (⇦).

Vaginal intraepithelial neoplasia

Vaginal intraepithelial neoplasia (VAIN) is a squamous premalignant lesion, classified as VAIN-I–III, often seen in association with CIN.

Aetiology

- Oncogenic HPV

VAIN may be caused by extension of CIN onto vaginal fornices and is often found after hysterectomy for incompletely excised CIN. It may be found within the surgical margin at the vault.

Pathophysiology

- VAIN-I–III—as for CIN (Section 15.2), but no transformation zone
- Risk of invasive disease with VAIN-III is about 5–10%
- Uncertain percentage of women progress to carcinoma but should be less than CIN as no susceptible transformation zone

Clinical evaluation

History

- Asymptomatic—detected on colposcopy

Examination

- Colposcopy of vagina—acetic acid will show white changes

Investigations

- Biopsy, which must be full thickness to ensure invasion is not missed

Treatment

Localized areas of disease

- Laser vaporization for VAIN-I–II
- Excision

RCOG consensus suggests that excision is preferable for VAIN-III, especially if previous hysterectomy.

Widespread changes throughout the vagina

- Vaginectomy
- Imiquimod cream
- 5-fluorouracil cream
- Radiotherapy

Surgical excision by vaginectomy for recurrent widespread disease, especially if there is a possibility of early invasion on biopsies. In younger women, strategies to preserve the vagina are attempted. The treatments cause significant morbidity, and have varying success.

Vaginal carcinoma

Incidence

Rare, and less than 1% of gynaecological malignancies. The majority are secondary from cervical and endometrial primaries.

Aetiology

- HPV causes VAIN, a premalignant condition
- Associated with CIN, either because of lateral spread, or incompletely excised at hysterectomy
- More common in immunosuppressed

Pathophysiology

- Majority (92%) are squamous
- Malignant melanomas are rare and carry a poor prognosis, with early haematogenous spread
- Sarcomas—as for melanomas

- Clear cell adenocarcinoma—linked to in utero diethylstilbestrol (DES) exposure. DES was used 1945–1970 to prevent miscarriage. One in 1000 women whose mother took DES develop a clear cell vaginal malignancy, typically between 15–22 years.

Spread

Squamous tumours:

- Local to bladder or bowel
- Lymphatic to the pelvic nodes in proximal two-thirds of the vagina, and inguinal nodes if the distal one-third is involved
- Haematogenous spread is rare

Staging

Staging follows FIGO guidelines (Box 15.7)

Clinical evaluation

History

- Vaginal bleeding, vaginal discharge, pelvic pain

Examination

- Colposcopic examination with 5% acetic acid detects pre-existing VAIN, and reveals extent of the lesion
- Cervix must also be assessed to exclude coexisting lesion

Investigations

- Biopsy must be full thickness for formal histopathological staging. Depth of invasion into mucosa and muscle is significant in staging
- MRI pelvis assesses local invasion and lymph node involvement
- CT scans of the abdomen and chest for melanomas and sarcomas

Management

Stage I–III—chemoradiation including brachytherapy

The vaginal epithelium is thin, and bladder and rectum are nearby. Thus, surgical margins of 1 cm can be achieved only by removing the bladder for anterior lesions and rectum for posterior. Chemoradiation as primary treatment is organ-preserving.

Regimens are similar to cervical cancer, but the radiation fields are altered to concentrate radiation to the exact tumour site.

Stage IV—palliative intent

Treatment is individualized according to tumour site and symptoms. Combinations of radiotherapy and chemotherapy are used.

Radiotherapy is associated with significant morbidity and mortality, vaginal stenosis in 25–32% of cases, ulceration of the vaginal mucosa, and fistulae in 10%. Both bowel and bladder are sensitive to radiotherapy. Radiation cystitis is common, with burning sensation on urination, frequency, and incomplete voiding. Stress incontinence and urgency may also occur. Diarrhoea affects 50% of patients receiving radiotherapy, and may be permanent, occasionally causing faecal incontinence.

Recurrent disease

Exenterative surgery if localized.

Prognosis and survival

Determined by stage and general fitness of patient (Box 15.7).

Box 15.7 FIGO staging of vaginal carcinoma and 5-year survival rates

Stage	Definition	5-year Survival (%)
I	Tumour confined to vagina	80
II	Tumour invades paravaginal tissues, but not to pelvic sidewall	40
III	Tumour extends to pelvic sidewall	30
IVa	Tumour invades mucosa of bladder or rectum and/or extends beyond the true pelvis	10
IVb	All cases with distant metastases	

Chapter 16

Case-based discussions

Contents

16.1 Case-based discussion questions

1. Abdominal pain, bleeding, and rape

An 18-year-old attends the emergency department with abdominal pain and vaginal bleeding. Her last period was 1 week prior and she has not had intercourse since then. When taking the history she reports an alleged vaginal rape by a stranger 5 h prior to presenting. You are the first person she has told and she becomes very distressed

Discuss

1. How will you approach the history and examination?
2. Will you contact the police?

Case continued: she decides she does want police involvement. She is not using any regular contraception. She says the assailant ejaculated inside her vagina without a condom. He was a white male aged about 30 years. She has not been bitten and has noticed no other injuries.

3. What are the issues regarding pregnancy?
4. What are the issues regarding infection?

2. Unprotected sex

A 22-year-old attends her local family planning clinic requesting the 'morning after' pill. She had unprotected sex 5 days before. The first day of her last period was 22 days ago. She has had three episodes of unprotected sex since her period and has not taken emergency contraception in this cycle. Her cycle is regular and 32 days long.

She reports using condoms for protection but not all the time. She had 10 partners in the last 6 months and has no current symptoms of infection.

Discuss

1. Is the 'morning after' pill appropriate?
2. Are there other options to prevent a pregnancy?
3. What are her options regarding avoiding infection?
4. What follow-up should be provided?

3. Abnormal smear

A 25-year-old woman is found to have a mildly dyskaryotic smear. She is referred to your colposcopy clinic.

Discuss

1. What is meant by mild dyskaryosis?
2. What is the likely cause of this abnormality?
3. Her cervical biopsy is reported as CIN-1 with HPV. How would you proceed?
4. She asks about the new vaccine she has read about. Would this have prevented this smear result?

4. Labour and vulval pain

A 30-year-old primigravida 38/40 attends the labour ward contracting without ruptured membranes. She gives a 2-day history of increasing vulval irritation and 'sores'.

Discuss

1. What is the differential diagnosis?
2. What are the important features to elicit in the history and on examination?

Case continued: the 'sores' started 2 days ago and are painful. She has never had anything similar previously. She has dysuria and no discharge. She was screened negatively for STIs aged 25 and has been

in a monogamous relationship since. Her partner has no genital or labial symptoms. She is not sure if he has had STIs previously. She has no other medical conditions of note.

On examination, she has multiple painful ulcers around the vulval area and inguinal lymphadenopathy. The cervix is 4 cm dilated and membranes are intact and bulging.

3. What will you tell her and are tests warranted?
4. What is your management plan?

5. Collapse in labour

You are sitting in the coffee room waiting for hand-over. The emergency bell goes off and you rush to a delivery room. You find a heavily pregnant woman breathless and not communicating.

A short history from the attending midwife reveals that the woman had induction of labour (IOL) with a prostaglandin pessary for suspected pre-eclampsia. Spontaneous rupture of membranes (clear liquor) and onset of labour ensued and she was transferred to labour ward for further care an hour earlier. She is 38 years old, in her first pregnancy, and has no significant medical or obstetric history. Just before you attended, she suddenly lost consciousness and some involuntary spasms were noted, mainly of the upper limbs.

She is cyanosed, pulse and respiration are irregular, BP is 210/140, and fetal heart rate (FHR) auscultation reveals bradycardia. Temperature is 36.6°C.

Within 3 minutes, breathing stops, the pulse is not palpable and she shows no signs of life.

Discuss

1. What is your first action?
2. Which possible diagnoses should you have in mind?
3. What is the appropriate initial treatment prior to the maternal arrest?
4. Which treatment is the most important?
5. Is delivery indicated, when, and how?
6. What should happen after the event?

6. Incontinence treatment

A 65-year-old woman presents with a 2-year history of leaking urine. It happens mainly when coughing or sneezing, but sometimes without warning. She also complains of urgency of micturition, frequency, and nocturia. She does not have bowel problems and is not sexually active.

She does not have any significant medical problem. She has two children, one of them delivered by emergency CS. She had a hysterectomy in her late 40s for menorrhagia. She smokes 10 cigarettes a day.

She has a raised BMI of 34, but examination is otherwise unremarkable. You cannot reproduce urinary incontinence with Valsalva manoeuvre during examination.

Discuss

1. What is your clinical diagnosis?
2. What would be your initial management?
3. Would you consider urodynamics? If so, when?
4. Discuss subsequent management options.

7. Bloated abdomen

A 63-year-old woman presents to the emergency department with shortness of breath and abdominal pain, and a gynaecological opinion has been requested. She gives a history of abdominal distension and bloating for 4 months. She is also complaining of altered bowel habit and urinary frequency.

She is nulliparous, and underwent the menopause at 50. Her last cervical smear 4 years ago was normal. She has been previously diagnosed with diverticular disease, but has no other medical history of note.

She has been to see her GP on three occasions, and has been referred to the colorectal surgeons for investigation of her change in bowel habit.

On examination she has reduced air entry in the right lung base, and is dull to percussion on chest examination. She is obese, but her abdomen is grossly distended, and you are able to demonstrate shifting dullness.

Discuss

1. What is your clinical diagnosis?
2. What would be your initial management?
3. What investigations would you organize?
4. What is the likely stage of her disease?
5. What are the subsequent management options?

8. Prolapse with co-morbidity

A 68-year-old woman presents with a 1-year history of feeling 'something coming down below', which is worsening. It tends to be more noticeable towards the end of the day. She also complains of frequency of micturition and nocturia 3–4 times/night, but there is no incontinence. There are no bowel symptoms.

She has three children delivered vaginally: one by forceps and two normal deliveries. She has been menopausal for about 10 years but has never used HRT.

She is diabetic type 2, well controlled on glibenclamide 5 mg BD and takes bendroflumethiazide 2.5 mg OD for mild hypertension.

On examination she has a BMI of 31. She has a pelvic organ prolapse, with the uterine cervix as the leading edge at about 1 cm above the hymen; but there is also a degree of anterior vaginal wall prolapse (point Aa at –1 cm and point Ba at –2 cm). The posterior vaginal wall seems well supported.

Discuss

1. What other relevant information is needed from the history?
2. What are her risk factors for POP?

3. Which investigations, if any, may be necessary?
4. What are treatment alternatives?

9. Postmenopausal vaginal bleeding

A 70-year-old woman is referred urgently by her GP under a '2-week rule' with one episode of vaginal bleeding. This lasted for 1 day, and she experienced a 'period'-like pain before and after the bleed.

She has two children delivered vaginally. She underwent the menopause aged 56, and took HRT for 8 years. Her last cervical smear was at age 65, and was normal. She had a hysteroscopy approximately 20 years ago for benign polyps.

On examination she is slim and abdominal examination is unremarkable.

Discuss

1. What other examination would you perform in the clinic?
2. What are her risk factors for endometrial carcinoma?
3. Which investigations would you organize?
4. A transvaginal ultrasound scan reports an endometrial thickness of 8.5 mm. How would you proceed?

10. Itchy vulva

A 71-year-old woman has come for a follow-up appointment to the gynaecology outpatient department. She was seen 4 months previously by a colleague who made a diagnosis of lichen sclerosus and prescribed Dermovate® cream, which she has been using as prescribed. She still complains of itching and burning sensation, and doesn't think that her problem has improved.

On examination you notice that she has vulvovaginal atrophy, with pallor of the vulva, which is more pronounced on her right side, while on the left there seems to be a slightly darker area.

Discuss

1. What is the differential diagnosis?
2. What is your management?

16.2 Case-based discussion answers

1. Abdominal pain, bleeding, and rape

1. Don't panic and be sympathetic. Take a brief history—where, who, when, what happened in brief (document, making sure all is legible). Assess the vaginal bleeding from the history and examining the underwear or pad (which is minimal in this case).

2. Explain her options: 1) to report to the police; 2) to have evidence gathered to buy time whilst thinking about reporting to the police; 3) simply to have medical care (with the loss of high quality evidence if future legal proceedings).

   If she agrees, call the local police station for advice. Advise her not to wash and to 'drip-dry' if she goes to the toilet. Collect any sanitary wear in sample/histology pots and label with time, date, patient's name, and your name.

   As the police will organize a forensic examination, there is no need for vaginal examination or to document injuries.

3. Discuss emergency contraception. As her LMP was a week ago, and she had not had intercourse since, offer Levonelle® 1500, with advice that if she vomits within 2 h she needs another dose.

4. Offer hepatitis B vaccination and discuss post-exposure prophylaxis. The risk of HIV transmission with one episode is low, but the source risk is unknown. A starter pack should be available in the emergency department.

   She has not been bitten or noticed any other injuries so she does not need tetanus or antibiotic prophylaxis.

   Explain the risk of STI. She can have a full sexual health screen, ideally 10 days to 2 weeks afterwards, to allow for incubation period.

   Arrange follow-up with local GUM services; to rediscuss all the above issues and for repeat tests.

2. Unprotected sex

1. The hormonal contraceptive pill is unlikely to be effective 5 days after unprotected sex and there is already a risk of pregnancy from the previous episodes.

2. Her cycle is regular and 32 days long. She is likely to ovulate on day 18 (32 minus 14). A coil can therefore be safely fitted in this case until day 23 (18+5). As it is day 22, a coil can be fitted to protect her against pregnancy. This method is 99% effective.

3. Take triple swabs for STIs at the time of coil insertion and arrange how she will receive these results. The risk of pelvic inflammatory disease is higher in the 3 weeks after insertion.

   It may be worth giving prophylactic azithromycin to treat any asymptomatic chlamydia infection at the time of insertion. Warn her to observe for abdominal pain, offensive discharge, and dyspareunia, and to seek medical advice if these occur.

4. Briefly outline contraceptive choices and offer leaflets.

   Give her free condoms. Reiterate that only condoms will protect her against STIs (and even then not all of them). Go through the process of how to use the condoms.

   See again in 2–3 weeks for a pregnancy test. At this visit go through her choices for contraception.

3. Abnormal smear

1. Mild dyskaryosis is a cytological diagnosis suggestive of underlying CIN-1. This is related to the degree of cellular abnormality and nuclear atypia present in the cells.

2. The likely cause of the abnormality is HPV, especially serotypes 16 and 18.

3. Between 60 and 90% of cases of CIN-1 will revert to normal within 10–23 months. As her smear also comments on the presence of HPV, it is likely that she has been exposed to this virus recently, and will clear this.

   Management options should be discussed. It would be reasonable to adopt a conservative approach, with a repeat smear and colposcopy in 6 months. If the patient is particularly anxious and requesting treatment, a locally destructive technique such as laser or cold coagulation could be performed as an outpatient procedure.

4. Prophylactic vaccination against HPV 6, 11, 16, and 18 should prevent 60–70% of CIN, but does not replace the need for cervical smears.

4. Labour and vulval pain

1. The differential list is long (see Section 3.4)

2. History-taking includes: full history of symptoms, including previous episodes, change in discharge, sexual history and symptoms in partner, and other medical conditions or skin disease.

3. In this case the diagnosis is most likely to be herpes simplex. It is often difficult to establish whether it is a primary or secondary infection. If in doubt, err on the side of caution and treat as a primary infection. With this history and lymphadenopathy, it is likely to be a primary attack rather than recurrence.

   This is a challenging situation: the woman is in labour, in pain, and has to take on a distressing likely diagnosis. Be frank and explain the ulcers are likely to be herpes.

   Investigations are warranted: swabs should be taken from the ulcers, warning her that this will be painful, and syphilis serology (and repeat serology at follow-up).

4. Explain the risks. In a primary attack the risk of neonatal infection with vaginal delivery is 40%. Complications, if infected, affect the brain, eyes, and skin.

   There are only two options: to continue labour or CS. Recommend CS (as membranes intact and lymphadenopathy).

   Start aciclovir 200 mg five times a day for 5 days and monitor her urine output as she may go into retention.

   Inform the paediatric team.

   Other issues: partner notification and referral to the GUM clinic are appropriate after delivery. It may be useful to see the couple together, as the diagnosis may or may not mean one partner has been unfaithful. Explain the likelihood of recurrences and how to deal with these.

5. Collapse in labour

1. The first action should be to call for help. Summon the appropriate staff: midwife in charge, junior and consultant obstetrician, anaesthetist, paediatrician, extra midwives and porter.

   When arrest is confirmed, the arrest team should be summoned.

   The haematologist and biochemist will have to be informed for blood processing and any transfusion requirements.

2. The list is long, but the main ones are stroke, eclampsia, cardiac arrest, arrhythmia, pulmonary embolism, amniotic fluid embolism, epilepsy, concealed abruption (with Couvelaire uterus). Sepsis is less likely but should be considered.

3. The patient initially should be treated as eclamptic and management instigated as described in Section 10.3.

4. The ABCs of resuscitation should be assessed and once arrest is confirmed, advanced life support (ALS) with left lateral tilt.

5. Without maternal arrest, such a sick mother must be assessed and stabilized first before delivery of the baby even in the face of abnormal CTG.

After an arrest, a perimortem CS 'splash-and-slash' should be performed simultaneously with ALS in the delivery room, ideally within 5 min, but as soon as possible, primarily to assist the resuscitation but also to give some chance of saving the baby.

6. Documentation, debriefing, breaking bad news to relatives if necessary.

6. Incontinence treatment

1. The clinical diagnosis is mixed urinary incontinence, since there are symptoms of both stress urinary incontinence (SUI) and urge urinary incontinence (UUI).

2. Initial management depends on the chief complaint. If SUI, pelvic floor muscle training and lifestyle advice (weight reduction and smoking cessation) should be given. If the main problem is UUI, bladder training and lifestyle advice are the first line of treatment. Other measures to consider are caffeine reduction, drug therapy for overactive bladder syndrome (OAB), and tampon use to prevent SUI during exercise.

3. Urodynamics might be considered if there is no response to conservative management.

4. If her main complaint is SUI and she hasn't responded to pelvic floor muscle training, her options are surgery or duloxetine, if she wants to avoid an operation. Surgical alternatives include sling procedures—either TVT or TOT, Burch colposuspension (probably slightly riskier given her previous surgery and obesity), or intramural bulking agents (counselling her on the shorter duration and need for repeat procedures).

7. Bloated abdomen

1. The likely diagnosis is that of an advanced ovarian or primary peritoneal carcinoma.

2. Initial management is to make the patient comfortable, and would include analgesia and consideration of paracentesis to relieve her abdominal distension.

3. She needs to have bloods taken for FBC, U&E, LFTs, and tumour markers, including CA125. She should also have a chest X-ray in casualty. Once admitted, an abdominal ultrasound and CT chest abdomen and pelvis should be arranged. To obtain a diagnosis, an ascitic tap should be obtained for cytology, and a pleural tap to stage her disease accurately if a pleural effusion is present. She should be referred to the gynaeoncology team, and her case discussed at the multidisciplinary team meeting.

4. If her disease is confined to the ovaries, it is likely to be FIGO stage Ic; if it has spread outside the pelvis to involve the omentum it is stage III; if the pleural tap is positive for malignant cells the stage is IV.

5. The management is dependent on the stage. Stage I disease is managed surgically, with postoperative chemotherapy.

The CHORUS study is aiming to answer whether women with more advanced ovarian or primary peritoneal malignancies should be treated first with surgery followed by chemotherapy, or by neoadjuvant chemotherapy, with interval debulking surgery.

8. Prolapse with co-morbidity

1. Other helpful information to elicit includes: sexual activity (as this may affect treatment options—pessaries may not be suitable or acceptable for sexually active patients, although some women remove the ring themselves and reinsert after coitus); sexual dysfunction; voiding difficulty; difficulty with defaecation (digitation); smoking status; at what time she takes her diuretic (is usually prescribed to take in the morning, but if taken at night, might contribute to her nocturia).

2. Age, parity, obesity, and oestrogen deficiency.

3. A urine dipstick ± MSU should be performed to exclude UTI. A pelvic organ prolapse (POP) reduction test may help to elicit associated urinary incontinence. If positive, urodynamics might be indicated.

4. The alternatives are conservative management (ring pessary), or surgical treatment in the form of a vaginal hysterectomy and anterior colporrhaphy, bearing in mind her associated risks of obesity and co-morbidities. If she wishes to conserve the uterus, a sacrohysteropexy, sacrospinous fixation or total vaginal mesh can be considered (see Section 14.4).

9. Postmenopausal vaginal bleeding

1. A speculum examination must be performed to exclude a cervical malignancy, or polyp, as well as a bimanual vaginal examination to assess uterine size and any adnexal masses.

2. She had a late menopause and took HRT. It is important to establish whether she took a combined HRT or was exposed to unopposed oestrogens.

3. A transvaginal ultrasound examination must be arranged urgently.

4. This endometrial thickness is abnormal for a postmenopausal woman. An endometrial biopsy is needed, either as a Pipelle® biopsy in the outpatient clinic, at outpatient hysteroscopy, or as a day case procedure to exclude an endometrial malignancy. Ten per cent of women with postmenopausal bleeding (PMB) will be found to have a malignancy (see Section 2.12).

10. Itchy vulva

1. Given the lack of response to treatment and findings on clinical examination, the initial diagnosis should be questioned. Other differential diagnoses, including vaginal atropy and malignancy should be considered.

2. A punch biopsy of the darker area on the left vulva should be performed to exclude malignancy.

Index

Page numbers in *italics* refer to figures or tables.

423